Pediatric Infectious Diseases

MEDICAL OUTLINE SERIES

Edited by

CHENG T. CHO, M.D., Ph.D.
Professor of Pediatrics and Microbiology
Chief, Section of Pediatric Infectious Diseases
Department of Pediatrics
University of Kansas Medical Center
Kansas City, Kansas

and

BURTON A. DUDDING, M.D.
Professor and Chairman
Department of Pediatrics
University of Nevada School of Medical Sciences
Reno, Nevada

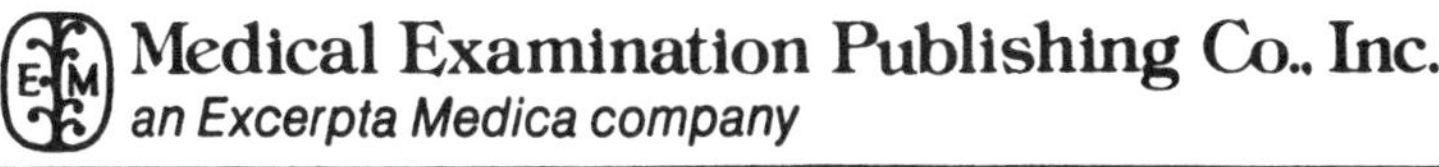

Medical Examination Publishing Co., Inc.
an Excerpta Medica company

969 Stewart Avenue   •   Garden City, New York 11530

NOTICE

The editors and the publisher of this book have made every effort to ensure that the drug dosage recommendations are in agreement with the standards accepted at the time of publication. Readers are advised, however, that the recommended dosage schedules are not absolute and they are only intended as a guide. The dosage schedules may change as additional clinical and laboratory studies accumulate. It is urged, therefore, that package insert information should be consulted for such details as dosage, administration, side effects, precautions, etc.

SIMULTANEOUSLY PUBLISHED IN:

Europe : HANS HUBER PUBLISHERS
Bern, Switzerland

United Kingdom : HENRY KIMPTON PUBLISHERS
London, England

South and East Asia : TOPPAN COMPANY (S) Pte. Ltd.
Singapore

Brazil : GUANABARA KOOGAN
Rio de Janeiro, Brazil

PREFACE

This book is written for students of Pediatric Infectious Diseases, by students of Pediatric Infectious Diseases. Most of the chapters have been written by faculty members in the Departments of Medicine, Community Health, Microbiology, and Pathology, at the University of Kansas School of Medicine. In addition, significant contributions were made by our pediatric colleagues at the Children's Mercy Hospital in Kansas City, Missouri. Several of the contributing authors are senior residents or fellows in the Department of Pediatrics, at the University of Kansas College of Health Sciences and Hospital.

Students of Pediatric Infectious Diseases may find this text useful for rapid review of selected topics. The authors in no way intend that their individual chapters stand as complete treatments of the topics. The first section of the book, which approaches infections from an organ system point of view, has been organized to include pertinent and current information concerning: 1) Introduction (including epidemiology); 2) Etiology and Pathogenesis; 3) Clinical Manifestations; 4) Diagnosis; and 5) Management of commonly occurring infections involving each organ system. In the second section, the authors have attempted to review selected diagnostic or management problems which are particularly germaine to pediatric patients with infectious diseases. A review of the subject of immunizations is also included. Finally, at the end of the text, the reader is provided with reference tables for anti-microbial therapy and for diseases acquired from animals and pets.

Emphasis was placed on preparing thorough, concise and well-referenced reviews of each subject, utilizing tables and illustrations to further abbreviate the material presented whenever possible. The reader is encouraged to utilize the references for more detailed and complete information regarding the topics reviewed in each chapter.

The editors wish to acknowledge the many patient and helpful secretaries who typed the copy for this text. Finally, the editors wish to express their deep appreciation to all of the authors who contributed to this book with special thanks for their enthusiasm, cooperation and interest in the project.

Cheng T. Cho, M.D., Ph.D.
Burton A. Dudding, M.D.

CONTRIBUTORS

LARRY H. BAKER, M.D., *Assistant Professor,* Department of Community Health, University of Kansas Medical Center (KUMC), Kansas City, Kansas.

JOHN R. CARLILE, M.D., *Resident,* Department of Pediatrics, KUMC.

TOM D. Y. CHIN, M.D., *Professor and Chairman,* Department of Community Health, *Professor of Medicine,* KUMC.

CHENG T. CHO, M.D., Ph.D., *Professor of Pediatrics and Microbiology, Chief,* Section of Pediatrics Infectious Diseases, Department of Pediatrics, KUMC.

ANTONI M. DIEHL, M.D., *Professor of Pediatrics, Chief,* Section of Pediatric Cardiology, Department of Pediatrics, KUMC.

BURTON A. DUDDING, M.D., *Professor and Chairman,* Department of Pediatrics, University of Nevada School of Medical Sciences, Reno, Nevada. (Former Professor and Chairman, Department of Pediatrics, KUMC.)

DOLORES FURTADO, Ph.D., *Associate Professor of Microbiology,* Department of Microbiology, KUMC.

NATHAN GOLDSTEIN, III, M.D., *Assistant Professor of Pediatrics,* Department of Pediatrics, KUMC.

DANIEL R. HINTHORN, M.D., *Associate Professor,* Division of Infectious Diseases, Department of Medicine, KUMC.

MARC S. JACOBSON, M.D., *Resident in Pediatrics,* Department of Pediatrics, KUMC.

RHONDA L. JEFFRIES, M.D., *Resident in Pediatrics,* Department of Pediatrics, KUMC.

STEVEN M. KALAVSKY, M.D., *Assistant Professor of Pediatrics,* Section of Pediatric Neurology, Department of Pediatrics, KUMC.

MARY ANN LAUVER, M.D., *Chief Resident of Pediatrics,* Department of Pediatrics, KUMC.

HUNTER C. LEAKE, III, M.D., *Associate Professor of Pediatrics, Chief,* Section of Ambulatory Pediatrics, Department of Pediatrics, KUMC.

NORMA J. LINDSEY, Ph.D., *Assistant Professor,* Clinical Laboratories, Department of Pathology and Oncology, KUMC.

CAROL B. LINDSLEY, M.D., *Assistant Professor of Pediatrics,* Department of Pediatrics, KUMC.

CHIEN LIU, M.D., *Professor of Medicine and Pediatrics, Chief,* Division of Infectious Diseases, Department of Medicine, KUMC.

THOMAS L. LUZIER, M.D., Fitzsimmon's Army Medical Center, Denver, Colorado.

VINCENT P. McCARTHY, M.D., *Fellow in Pediatric Infectious Diseases,* Department of Pediatrics, KUMC.

HERBERT C. MILLER, M.D., *Professor of Pediatrics,* Department of Pediatrics, KUMC.

LEONE F. MATTIOLI, M.D., *Professor of Pediatrics,* Section of Pediatric Cardiology, Department of Pediatrics, KUMC.

LLOYD C. OLSON, M.D., *Professor of Pediatrics,* The Children's Mercy Hospital and the University of Missouri-Kansas City School of Medicine, Kansas City, Missouri.

MYUNG K. PARK, M.D., *Assistant Professor of Pediatrics,* Section of Pediatric Cardiology, Department of Pediatrics, KUMC.

EDNA PEREZ, M.D., *Fellow in Infectious Diseases,* The Children's Mercy Hospital and the University of Missouri-Kansas City School of Medicine, Kansas City, Missouri.

F. BRUDER STAPLETON, M.D., *Fellow in Pediatrics Nephrology,* Department of Pediatrics, KUMC.

MIKE TORRENCE, M.D., *Resident in Pediatrics,* Department of Pediatrics, KUMC.

HERBERT A. WENNER, M.D., *Professor of Pediatrics,* The Children's Mercy Hospital and the University of Missouri-Kansas City School of Medicine, Kansas City, Missouri.

PEDIATRIC INFECTIOUS DISEASES

Medical Outline Series

CONTENTS

SECTION 1. GENERAL CONSIDERATIONS

SECTION 2. DIAGNOSTIC AND MANAGEMENT PROBLEMS

DEDICATION

The editors wish to dedicate this book to their former mentors: Dr. Herbert A. Wenner, Professor of Pediatrics, The Children's Mercy Hospital and the University of Missouri-Kansas City School of Medicine, Kansas City, Missouri; Dr. Chien Liu, Professor of Pediatrics and Medicine, University of Kansas School of Medicine, Kansas City, Kansas; and Dr. Lewis W. Wannamaker, Professor of Pediatrics, University of Minnesota School of Medicine, Minneapolis, Minnesota.

SECTION I. GENERAL CONSIDERATIONS

CHAPTER 1. RESPIRATORY INFECTIONS

1.1: COLDS, PHARYNGITIS, TONSILLITIS

INTRODUCTION: Although it may be possible to subdivide upper
respiratory infections into several clinical syndromes (rhinitis,
"common cold," nasopharyngitis, tonsillopharyngitis, etc.) it is
doubtful that such a classification has much utility in the clinical
setting wherein the busy practitioner is confronted by countless numbers of infants and children with upper respiratory infections. Thus,
for purposes of this discussion, an upper respiratory infection
(URI) will be used as an all inclusive term referring to any acute
illness manifested by signs and/or symptoms associated with infection limited to the upper respiratory tract.

EPIDEMIOLOGY: Of all infections known to occur in the pediatric
age group, infections of the upper respiratory tract are the most
common. The saying that a child will have 100 URI's in the first
10 years of life is nearly supported by data obtained from at least
three prospective studies of respiratory infections carried out during the past 25 years. (Dingle, et al, 1964; Lebowitz, et al, 1972;
Loda, et al, 1972.) In each study, children experienced an average
of 7-8 URI's per year in the first four years of life. Thereafter the
number gradually declined to an average of 3-4 per year in adolescence and adulthood.

The number of URI's experienced by any one child is highly variable
as illustrated in the data reported by Dingle (1964) in the Cleveland
Family Study. Some fortunate children rarely experienced clinically
manifest upper respiratory infections whereas others such as one
5-year-old who had 18 URI's recorded in a single year, were constantly afflicted.

A number of host and environmental factors have been shown to affect the incidence of URI's. Clearly age is an important factor as
previously noted. Irrespective of other factors, younger children
have more URI's than older children. Schools and homes contribute
to the high incidence of colds in children, providing environments
that facilitate transmission of the agents that cause URI's. Children
who attend kindergarten and first grade have more URI's than children of similar ages who stay at home. The incidence of URI's is
higher in preschool children who are siblings of school children than
in preschool children who do not have siblings attending school. Members of larger families have more URI's than members of smaller

11

families. If a child 1-4 years old introduces a URI into the household, subsequent spread to other household members is more likely than if a URI is introduced by an older child or adult. For the same reasons that homes and schools contribute to the high incidence of URI's in children by providing milieus favorable for exposure to and transmission of URI-producing agents to susceptible hosts, overcrowding and poorer hygiene may likewise contribute to the high incidence of URI's in children.

It is well known that climate, seasonal changes and geography affect the incidence of URI's in many different ways. Upper respiratory infections are a seasonable phenomena, especially in northern temperate climates. Certain climatic characteristics favor the survival and/or transmissability of certain bacteria and viruses. For example, the influenza virus seems to exert its greatest effect during cold, dry periods of winter. On the other hand, the Group A streptococcus seems to enjoy a greater pathogenic potential at high altitudes in cold weather. For many years it has been known that in states such as Colorado and Wyoming streptococcal upper respiratory disease is a significant problem in winter months whereas in non-mountainous neighboring states the incidence of streptococcal infections and their complications, is much lower.

There are a number of physical environmental factors which have not been shown to affect the incidence of colds under experimental conditions. These include having cold, wet feet; sitting in front of a draft; sudden exposure to a cold, chilling, etc., all conditions which laymen and many physicians claim are contributing factors to the cause of upper respiratory infections.

It is extraordinarily difficult to understand how all of these environmental factors are inter-related. In addition to the physical-environmental factors already noted, it is well known that the quality of the air we breathe may also exert an influence on the incidence of colds. Casell et al. (1971) have suggested that in order to determine the effect of air pollutants on the incidence of the common cold, one must use an empirically derived index incorporating the various air pollutants, wind velocity, temperature, relative humidity, etc. Use of this index makes it theoretically possible to correlate these factors with lower and higher incidences of common colds in various populations provided the various components are weighted properly.

1. ETIOLOGY

URI's are caused primarily by viruses but also by two bacterial species and one species of Mycoplasma. The major causes of URI's are listed in Table 1-1. Although all of the infectious agents or groups of agents shown in Table 1-1 have been associated with URI's in a variety of studies as cited in Cherry's excellent review article (1973) many of these agents are more commonly associated with other infections. For example, respiratory syncytial virus is a common

TABLE 1-1: ETIOLOGIC AGENTS IN URI'S

VIRUSES:

Picornaviruses: Rhinoviruses
Coxsackieviruses
ECHOviruses

Adenoviruses: Types 1,2,3,4,5,6,7,14 and 21

Myxoviruses: Influenza A, B and C
Parainfluenza viruses Types 1,2,3,4
Respiratory Syncytial virus
Mumps virus

Other: Coronoviruses
Epstein-Barr Virus

MYCOPLASA:

Mycoplasma pneumoniae

BACTERIA:

Streptococcus pyogenes, Groups A,B,C,G
Neisseria gonorrhea

cause of bronchiolitis in younger children, parainfluenza viruses
are commonly associated with laryngotracheobronchitis, and mumps
virus with parotitis. However, these same agents are also commonly associated with URI's as shown recently by Cooney, Fox and
Hall in the Seattle Virus Watch Program (1975).

Because of the multitude of etiologic agents that can cause URI's and
the virtually impossible task of distinguishing a URI caused by a
rhinovirus from a URI caused by a parainfluenza virus based on clinical
evidence alone, the most important question to be asked with respect
to the etiology of URI's is simply, in what situations should the clinician attempt to identify the etiologic agent responsible for a URI?
Since the vast majority of URI's are short-lived, uncomplicated illnesses which can neither be prevented nor treated, the clinician's
efforts to define the etiology of an URI must focus primarily on those
URI's associated with sequelae and complications which may be
ameliorated or prevented by specific treatment. This effort is directed primarily toward identifying URI's caused by Group A beta-
hemolytic streptococci. Although this topic will be discussed in the
sections entitled 3. Diagnosis and 4. Management, the reader is
referred to Dillon and Dudding's Chapter on streptococcal infections
in Brennemann's Practice of Pediatrics (1970) for a more extensive
review of this subject.

2. PATHOGENESIS AND CLINICAL MANIFESTATIONS

In the acute stages of URI's, mucous membranes are hyperemic and edematous. Serous and mucinous exudation tend to occur in viral URI's whereas in streptococcal URI's, the exudate is more prurulent, tending to contain more cellular debris and greater numbers of inflammatory cells (mostly polymorphonuclear cells). However, the latter finding is not useful in discriminating viral from streptococcal URI's. Mucous membranes throughout the upper respiratory tract may become congested and thickened or signs of infection may be limited to one or two anatomical areas within the upper airway passages. In the nose, ciliary activity may be affected, accompanied by depressed nasal mucociliary flow rates. Epithelial surfaces may become denuded.

URI's regardless of their etiology are manifested by a limited number of symptoms and signs of infection, in part because there are a limited number of ways that the mucous membranes lining the upper respiratory tract respond to and "express" infection. Therefore, it is not surprising that efforts to relate a single symptom or sign or even constellations of symptoms and signs to a specific etiologic agent is virtually impossible. Tonsillar or pharyngeal exudate is a good example of a sign of a URI which is of limited value in discriminating viral from bacterial infections. Exudate in a child under three is infrequently associated with streptococcal infections. Studies have shown that only 15-20% of children with exudate under 3 years of age have a streptococcal URI. However, in an older child where admittedly the probability of streptococcal infection is greater if exudate is present (40-60%), the sign is still of little value in making a clinical diagnosis of an individual child's URI.

Perhaps the most reliable clinical sign of a streptococcal URI is the typical exanthem of scarlet fever. For reasons not understood, scarlet fever is observed less often today than 20-30 years ago. The exanthem appears early in the course of the illness and is the result of an erythrogenic toxin produced by the streptococcus. The exanthem is an erythematous maculopapular eruption that is rough to the touch, often described as feeling like "goose-pimples on a patient with a sunburn." Typically the face is spared, the eruption is most intense in skin folds, and the skin desquamates. Although several immunologically distinct erythrogenic toxins are produced by Group A streptococci, scarlet fever rarely occurs more than once in the same individual. Antitoxin immunity is directed against the erythrogenic toxin and does not produce immunity to streptococcal infections per se.

Infections of the upper respiratory tract may occur without producing any symptoms at all or at least they're so mild that they will go unnoticed. This poses special problems in our efforts to prevent the non-suppurative sequelae of Group A streptococcal infections such as rheumatic fever. Unless children's throats are routinely cultured, how can a child receive prompt treatment for a streptococcal infection when the infection is not clinically evident?

A typical viral URI is characterized by rhinorrhea, obstructed nares, occasional sneezing, cough and pharyngeal irritation. Although this differs to some extent from the typical Group A streptococcal URI, which is commonly associated with more severe and prolonged pharyngeal discomfort, pain on swallowing, fever and less coughing and rhinorrhea, the information is of little practical importance to the clinician. It is simply not possible to distinguish, on clinical grounds, one type of URI from another in the individual patient.

3. DIAGNOSIS

Many URI's are self-diagnosed or, in the case of children, diagnosed by parents and older siblings. Furthermore, many URI's are managed at home in the absence of consultation with a health professional. However, children with upper respiratory infections still account for 25-30% of the total number of office visits made to pediatricians. Thus, the physician is still faced with the problem of diagnosis and management of many upper respiratory infections.

At present, the physician must rely upon a throat culture to determine if the streptococcus is the offending agent in an upper respiratory infection. This enables him to classify upper respiratory infections into streptococcal versus non-streptococcal (or presumably viral) etiologies. Although there are other treatable causes of URI's, e.g., Neisseria gonorrhea, and C. diphtheriae, these infections occur so infrequently in children today that it is not possible or practical to attempt to identify these agents in every child with an upper respiratory infection seen in the office or clinic. (See Chapter on Venereal Diseases for Management of N. gonorrhea infections.)

It is essential that proper technique for obtaining a throat culture is followed. First, there must be adequate exposure of the oropharynx. Second, the individual obtaining the culture must be certain to swab the pharynx and tonsils rather than the tongue or buccal mucosa. The throat culture swab should then be plated onto appropriate culture medium, or retained in a dry, sterile tube until it is convenient to plate the culture. Blood agar plates containing 5% sheep blood should be used. These plates are available from commercial sources or can be prepared in a clinical laboratory. Plates are incubated for approximately 18 hours at 37°C. and then examined for evidence of beta hemolytic colonies. Small, inexpensive incubators are available for use in physicians' offices, making the overall cost of a throat culture a very economical procedure.

In many clinics and offices, the number of colonies on the culture plate are quantitated and, provided an optimal culture has been taken, there is general agreement between the acuteness of the infection and the number of organisms recovered from the growing culture. The following is a convenient method for estimating the number of organisms present: 1+=10 colonies or less, 2+=10-50 colonies, 3+=more than 50 colonies, 4+=predominant or pure culture. Patients with 3+ or more cultures are the ones in whom a diagnosis of streptococcal pharyngitis can be made with greatest certainty. In contrast, the recovery of small numbers of beta hemolytic streptococci is less often associated with acute infection or the dangerous carrier state. It is well documented that children with 3+ or more cultures are more likely to show a rise in anti-streptolysin 0 or other streptococcal antibody titers and it is these children who are at greatest risk of developing non-suppurative complications. Unfortunately, it is impossible to always distinguish these patients from patients who have a positive culture but represent a transient or chronic carrier whose URI may be caused by a viral agent. Thus, although the presence of beta-hemolytic streptococci does not unequivocally indicate that the sore throat is streptococcal, it is most appropriate that if streptococci are identified, the physician managing that patient proceed with treatment on that basis.

It is also highly desirable to distinguish group A streptococci on the culture plate, from non-group A streptococci. The simple Bacitracin disc sensitivity method of Maxted is still the most reliable means of establishing that the organism is a presumptive group A streptococcus. These discs are also available from commercial sources. Over 95% of serologically proven group A streptococci are very sensitive to Bacitracin whereas most of the non-group A beta hemolytic streptococci are resistant.

A number of streptococcal antibody tests are available for documentation of streptococcal infections. However, the delay in streptococcal antibody response is such that routine use of antibody tests in the patient with a streptococcal upper respiratory infection is of limited value. Serial antibody titers may be helpful in evaluating a patient in whom the diagnosis of repeated streptococcal infections versus persistent carriage without infection is being considered and in those instances it would be advisable to obtain both an anti-streptolysin 0 titer as well as anti-DNase B and other antibody titers. These tests are essential in documenting antecedent streptococcal infections in patients with acute rheumatic fever or acute glomerulonephritis. It is in the evaluation of patients with these two conditions that streptococcal antibody tests are of greatest value to the clinician.

4. MANAGEMENT

4.1: Streptococcal URI's: Management of URI's becomes relatively simple given the fact that a throat culture is the only practical way to evaluate whether or not the patient has a streptococcal or a non-streptococcal URI. Because relatively few children under the age of three in the United States have streptococcal respiratory infections, one might seriously question whether or not every child with an URI needs a throat culture. Also, the pros and cons of treating without taking a culture have recently and succintly been summarized by Wannamaker (1976).

It is the practice in our clinic not to routinely culture children under 2 years of age simply because the probability of group A streptococcal infections is so low. The risk of rheumatic fever following a group A streptococcal infection in children living in the United States who are under 4 years of age is extremely remote, which also minimizes the need for routine throat cultures in very young children with upper respiratory infections.

Children who present in the office or clinic with URI's who are over two years of age should have a throat culture in an effort to identify group A beta-hemolytic streptococci. The principal reason for treating a patient with a streptococcal URI is to prevent both suppurative and non-suppurative complications. It is also possible that prompt treatment with antibiotics may modify the symptoms and shorten the course of the illness. However, because of the variability of the disease and its brief natural history if not treated at all, this rationale is subject to question. Beta-hemolytic streptococci should be identified by throat culture within 24 hours and based on the results of that culture the physician may elect to initiate therapy prior to obtaining the results of the Bacitracin disc sensitivity test. However, it is important that the latter confirmation be obtained.

The goals of treatment of streptococcal pharyngitis are threefold: 1. to eradicate the group A streptococcus from the upper respiratory tract; 2. to relieve symptoms and reduce morbidity; and, 3. to educate parents regarding the importance of recognizing and treating group A streptococcal infections (Dudding, 1976). Similarly, the goals of managing all upper respiratory infections should be to relieve symptoms and reduce morbidity and to educate parents about the importance of recognizing and treating group A streptococcal infections. The latter may be in part accomplished at the time the child is seen with an URI while explaining to the parents why a throat culture is necessary.

In most instances, it is practical to have the results of the throat culture prior to instituting appropriate antibiotic therapy. When the culture is found to be positive for beta-hemolytic streptococci, patients should be notified to return to the office to receive appropriate therapy and this may be accomplished within 24 hours after the culture has been taken. This approach minimizes the unnecessary use of antibiotics in patients who have viral or non-streptococcal URI's.

There are a number of antibiotics which effectively eradicate group A streptococci from the upper respiratory tract. However, the recommendations of the Committee on Infectious Diseases of the American Academy of Pediatrics as well as the recommendation of the American Heart Association, recognize only two antibiotics in the treatment of group A streptococcal infections - penicillin, and for individuals allergic to penicillin, erythromycin.

A single intramuscular injection of Benzathine Penicillin G is the preferred therapy for streptococcal pharyngitis, primarily because this form of treatment most likely assures patient compliance, it is probably the least inconvenient to the child and family, and in most instances costs less than other forms of therapy. Recently, a mixture of 900,000 units of benzathine penicillin G and 300,000 units of procaine penicillin G, have been used which reduced the incidence and severity of local reactions, and offered comparable therapeutic outcome when compared to 1.2 million units of benzathine penicillin (Bass, et al. 1976). A summary of the current recommendations of the American Academy of Pediatrics and the American Heart Association for patients with streptococcal pharyngitis is shown in Table 1-2.

4.2: Non-streptococcal URI's: Streptococcal upper respiratory infections are the only infections which require specific antibiotic treatment. Infants and children with non-streptococcal URI's need only be treated symptomatically and parents should be educated regarding the "commonness" of upper respiratory infections in the pediatric age group.

A number of studies have clearly documented the lack of efficacy of broad spectrum antibiotics in the management of upper respiratory tract infections in children. This topic was most recently reviewed by Soyka et al. (1975) and clearly documents the lack of the value of antibiotics in preventing complications of upper respiratory infections.

A recent article reviewing the role of oral decongestants in the management of URI's (Lambert, et al. 1975) concludes that "lacking convincing evidence, one cannot presently recommend on a rational basis, the routine use of decongestants in upper respiratory infections." Although no one questions the temporary relief from nasal congestion following instillation of phenylephrine nose drops, or perhaps even salt water nose drops, the efficacy of oral decongestants administered in the doses currently recommended is to be questioned. In another recent review regarding the use of antihistamines in patients with URI, the authors concluded that there was little rationale for their use in the management of these infections, and further, that there may be a number of hazards involved. (West, S. et al. 1975.)

The use of oral decongestants and antihistamines results in a tremendous expenditure annually in order to ameliorate the symptoms of upper respiratory infections, and the physician should seriously consider the cost of these preparations versus their benefits. Furthermore,

TABLE 1-2: ANTIBIOTIC THERAPY FOR STREPTOCOCCAL PHARYNGITIS

ANTIBIOTIC	DOSE	DURATION OF THERAPY
I. PENICILLINS		
Benzathine Penicillin G	Children <60 lbs., 600,000 units Adults and children >60 lbs., 1,200,000 units	1 dose, intramuscularly "
Phenoxymethyl Penicillin	Children <60 lbs., 500 mgm in two, three or four equal doses/day Adults and children >60 lbs. 1.0 gm in two, three or four equal doses/day	10 full days by mouth "
Buffered Penicillin G	Children and Adults, 1,000,000 units, in two, three or four equal doses/day	10 full days by mouth
II. ALTERNATIVE DRUG FOR PATIENTS WITH KNOWN OR SUSPECTED PENICILLIN ALLERGY		
Erythromycin	Children, 40 mgm/Kgm/day in four equal doses Adults, 250 mgm four times a day	10 full days by mouth

the therapeutic relief from home remedies such as honey and lemon
juice cough syrup, and in older children, salt water nose drops,
may be just as beneficial and certainly less costly than prescription
or proprietary "cold" preparations. It is appropriate to emphasize
to parents the necessity for good hydration during an upper respiratory infection, recommending fruit juices and other good tasting
liquids for the child. Also appropriate use of antipyretics and analgesics such as acetaminophen to reduce the temporary morbidity
associated with URI's is advised. However, the continued use of
expensive remedies such as antihistamines and oral decongestants
alone or in combination, is not recommended.

All parents want to have well children and to make them feel better
when they are sick. Parents have expectations that they want to do
something for the child who has a URI and often look to the physician
for help. Physicians can help by spending more time educating parents about the use of antibiotics and other drugs of questionable efficacy in the management of non-streptococcal upper respiratory
infections, emphasizing the commonness of these infections, the
brief duration of these illnesses, and the fact that symptomatic relief can often be obtained by relatively simple, safe and inexpensive
remedies.

REFERENCES

Bass, J.W., Crast, F.W., Knowles, C.R. and Onofer, C.N.:
Streptococcal Pharyngitis in Children, JAMA 235:1112, 1976.

Cassell, E.T., Lebowitz, M.D., Woller, D.W. and McCarroll,
J.R.: Health and the Urban Environment: IX: The Concept of the
Multiplex Independent Variable, Am J Pub Health 61:2348, 1971.

Cherry, J.D.: New Respiratory Viruses: Their Role in Respiratory
Illnesses of Children, in Advances in Pediatrics, Volume 20,
Irving Shulman, Ed., Year Book Medical Publishers, Inc., Chicago,
1973, pp. 225-290.

Cooney, M.K., Fox, J.P. and Hall, C.E.: The Seattle Virus Watch
VI; Observations of Infections with and Illness due to Parainfluenza,
Mumps and Respiratory Syncytial Virus and Mycoplasma Pneumoniae,
Am. J. Epidemiol., 101:532, 1975.

Dillon, H.C. and Dudding, B.A.: Streptococcal Infections in Brene-
mann's Practice of Pediatrics, Vol. 17, Ch. 6, Harper and Row,
New York, 1970, p. 1-15.

Dingle, J.H., Badger, G.F., Jordan, W.S.: Illness in the Home -
A Study of 25,000 Illness in a group of Cleveland Families, Western
Reserve University Press, Cleveland, 1964.

Dudding, B.A.: Streptococcal Pharyngitis in Current Therapy, Conn., H.F. Ed., W.B. Saunders Co., Philadelphia, 1976, pp. 50-52.

Lampert, R.P., Robinson, D.S. and Soyka, L.F.: A Critical Look at Oral Decongestants, Pediatrics 55:550, 1975.

Lebowitz, M.D., Cassell, E.J. and McCarrol, J.: Health and the Urban Environment XII. The Incidence and Burden of Minor Illness in a Healthy Population: Methods, Symptoms and Incidence, Am. Review of Respiratory Disease 106:824, 1972.

Loda, F.A., Glezen, W.P. and Clyde, W.A.: Respiratory Disease in Group Day Care, Pediatrics 40:428, 1972.

Soyka, L.F., Robinson, D.S., Lachant, N. and Monaco, J.: The Misuse of Antibiotics for Treatment of Upper Respiratory Tract Infections in Children, Pediatrics 55:552, 1975.

Wannamaker, L.W.: A Penicillin Shot Without Culturing the Child's Throat, JAMA 235:913, 1976.

West, S., Brandon, B., Stolley, P. and Rumriff, R.: A Review of Antihistamines and the Common Cold, Pediatrics 56:100, 1975.

::

1.2: CROUP SYNDROME

INTRODUCTION: The syndrome of "croup" implies inspiratory stridor, hoarseness, and cough, all secondary to varying degrees of laryngeal obstruction. The management of children with croup syndrome requires that the clinician differentiate among its many causes. Foreign body aspiration, acute epiglottitis, retropharyngeal abscess, angioneurotic edema, retropharyngeal and/or mediastinal tumors, trauma, neonatal hypocalcemic tetany, acute viral laryngotracheobronchitis (ALTB), and spasmodic croup may all give rise to the croup syndrome. Measles, diphtheria, and certain other bacterial infections (pneumococci, streptococci, hemophilus) may involve the glottis and subglottic areas giving rise to a severe, life-threatening croup syndrome requiring intubation or tracheostomy. A careful history is essential to the correct diagnosis of the child presenting with a croup syndrome. Historical facts and physical findings which may aid in establishing the etiology of a croup syndrome are noted in Table 1-3. For review purposes, this chapter will focus on three causes of the croup syndrome: acute epiglottitis, acute viral laryngotracheobronchitis (ALTB), and spasmodic croup.

TABLE 1-3: HISTORICAL AND PHYSICAL FINDINGS WHICH DIFFERENTIATE THE ETIOLOGIES OF THE CROUP SYNDROME IN CHILDREN		
ENTITY	HELPFUL HISTORICAL INFORMATION	PHYSICAL FINDINGS WHICH SUGGEST ETIOLOGY
Foreign Body Aspiration	Recent choking episode or coughing episode while eating; Recent intake of material likely to have been aspirated (nuts, small hard candy, tablets); Absence of any infectious prodrome (no history of fever, URI, malaise); May have history of hemoptysis.	Absence of fever; Wheezing may be present; Hemoptysis may be present; Direct or indirect laryngoscopy reveals presence of foreign body (radiograph may show radiopaque foreign bodies).
Acute Epiglottitis	Child usually 2-5 years old; Sudden onset of intense sore throat and hoarseness; Well 24 hours previously.	Child usually drools, refuses to swallow, hyperextends neck and refuses to recline; Child appears toxic and acutely ill and is highly febrile; Lateral neck radiograph reveals enlarged epiglottis; Characteristic "burgundy red," edematous epiglottis (SEE TEXT!) on exam.
Retropharyngeal Abscess	Child usually under three years old; May have history of high fever, drooling, refusal to swallow; Onset usually over several days.	Child usually hyperextends neck, sits up and refuses to recline; Cervical adenitis usually present; Bulging of posterior pharynx may be apparent; Lateral neck radiograph

		taken in inspiration usually diagnostic, revealing soft tissue bulge anterior to cervical spine.
Angioneurotic Edema	History of previous such episodes; History of allergies and/or acute allergic reactions (urticaria, sudden wheezing).	Externally obvious angioedema or urticaria may be present concurrently; Angioedema of uvula may be present; Usually responds rapidly to epinephrine; Direct or indirect laryngoscopy reveals supraglottic angioedema.
Retropharyngeal or Mediastinal Tumor	May have failed to gain weight; Low grade fevers may be present; Chronic cough, wheezing or dyspnea may have occurred.	Adenopathy may be present; Findings suggesting other diagnoses are absent; Chest or neck radiographs may reveal a tumor mass; Laryngoscopy may reveal tumor mass or extrinsic laryngeal compression.
Trauma	History of trauma; History of recent intubation or surgical procedure.	External evidence of trauma about head and neck or elsewhere; Exam of pharynx and mouth may reveal evidence of trauma.
Neonatal Hypocalcemic Tetany	Patient is a neonate; May have history of being jittery; May be low birth weight infant, infant of a diabetic mother; May have history of difficult delivery.	Jittery infant; Infant may convulse (NOTE: Carpopedal spasms rare in infants); Serum calcium is diagnostic.

TABLE 1-3 (Continued)

ENTITY	HELPFUL HISTORICAL INFORMATION	PHYSICAL FINDINGS WHICH SUGGEST ETIOLOGY
Acute Laryngotracheobronchitis (ALTB)	Child usually six months to two years of age; Usually has history of preceding URI; Onset over several days; May have had low grade fever; May occur during epidemic of ALTB.	May have low grade fever; Usually swallows easily; Findings are absent suggesting other diagnoses; Lateral neck radiograph reveals subglottic narrowing; Epiglottis is normal (SEE TEXT!) on exam.
Spasmodic Croup	Child usually 1-3 years old; Sudden onset in evening; No history of fever; History of previous such episodes (which resolved within several hours).	No significant findings; Usually much better by the time seen.
Measles Croup	History compatible with measles syndrome; Usually failed to receive measles immunization; Croup syndrome developed after rash.	Rash of measles present; Findings of coryza, conjunctivitis compatible with measles.
Diphtheritic Croup	Usually has been inadequately immunized against diphtheria; Insidious onset of malaise, sore throat, low grade fever.	Cervical adenopathy present (may be severe with "bull-neck" appearance); May be slightly febrile or highly febrile (NOTE: Laryngeal diphtheria usually occurs as an extension of tonsillopharyngeal diphtheria); Culture positive for

| Bacterial Croup | May have prodrome of URI, sore throat; History of fever, pain on swallowing. | diphtheria bacilli; Membrane of diphtheria may be present over tonsils and/or pharynx.

Toxic-appearing child; May have exudative tonsillopharyngitis; Leukocytosis may suggest bacterial etiology; Blood culture positive (or pharyngeal swab in the case of Group A Beta-Streptococci) suggests etiological agent. |

ACUTE EPIGLOTTITIS

In general, acute epiglottitis occurs in children between the ages of
two and five years. Pathologically acute epiglottitis is a disease in
which there occurs marked inflammation and edema of the supra-
glottic structures, thereby obstructing the airway. The disease
has a dramatic and sudden onset of symptomatology, is associated
with marked hoarseness, an intense sore throat, drooling, a refusal to swallow, and results in a toxic and acutely ill-appearing
and highly febrile child. One will note that such symptomatology
may also be seen in the child with a retropharyngeal abscess though
the abscess is usually seen in a younger child. Since both the examination of the epiglottis in patients with acute epiglottitis and the
manipulation of the pharynx in children with retropharyngeal abscesses have been associated with unexpected deaths, such manipu-
lations must be undertaken with considerable caution. It has been
shown by Poole et al. (1963) and Rapkin et al. (1972) that lateral
radiographs of the neck will determine the absence or presence of
significant epiglottal edema. Such radiographs, when taken in inspiration, will also reveal a retropharyngeal abscess, if present.
Therefore, when either acute epiglottitis or retropharyngeal abscess
is suspected, the child is manipulated as little as possible, and every attempt is made to avoid provoking anxiety in the child such as
might occur with parental separation or venipuncture. The child is
taken with his parents for a radiograph by a clinician skilled in the
techniques of endotracheal intubation and emergency tracheostomy
(the necessary equipment to perform these procedures accompanies
the child as well). An upright, lateral radiograph of the neck (re-
cumbency may result in airway obstruction) is then obtained. The
radiograph is taken during inspiration so that a retropharyngeal abscess may be ruled out. Films taken in expiration exaggerate the
soft tissue distance between the vertebral column and the esophagus
and trachea. If acute epiglottitis is suggested by the radiograph, the
child is taken to an appropriate facility where preparation is made
for both intubation and tracheostomy and a direct examination is then
performed. The diagnosis is confirmed by the presence of a bur-
gundy colored, edematous epiglottis, which on occasion appears as
a "hunk of raw meat" in the posterior pharynx. Next, the airway is
secured by intubation and/or tracheostomy, blood and epiglottal or
pharyngeal cultures and other desired laboratory studies obtained,
and intravenous antibiotics begun. The etiologic agent in most cases
(95%) of epiglottitis is Hemophilus influenzae, and therefore ampicillin or chloramphenicol administered intravenously is the drug of
choice. The detection of ampicillin resistant strains of H. influenzae
in one's geographic area of practice should result in the use of chloramphenicol in the treatment of serious H. influenzae infections. The
recommended dosage (see page 572) of either drug is that which is
currently recommended for serious H. influenzae infections. Response is rapid so that most children may be extubated by day three
or four.

In the past, most authorities have recommended tracheostomy for acute epiglottitis: Baxter (1967), Margolis, et al. (1972), Rapkin (1973), Johnson, et al. (1974). Since the advent of the soft poly-vinyl, endotracheal tubes, however, many authorities, Geraci (1968), Tos (1973), Milko, et al. (1974), Schuller, et al. (1975), Battaglia, et al. (1975), are utilizing prolonged endotracheal intuba-tion rather than tracheostomy for this disorder. Whether tracheos-tomy or intubation is optimal for the management of this disorder is unclear at the present, each method having its proponents. It seems most probable that both individual and institutional experience dic-tates which procedure is preferred. It would appear that since man-agement by prolonged intubation is a more recently developed thera-peutic mode, individuals and institutions having developed considerable expertise in performing and caring for tracheostomies will be some-what reluctant to switch management modes.

2. ACUTE VIRAL LARYNGOTRACHEOBRONCHITIS (ALTB)

The most common cause of the croup syndrome in children is viral infection of the respiratory tract. The infection may be isolated to the larynx (viral laryngitis), may extend to the trachea (viral laryn-gotracheitis), or may involve the larynx, trachea, and the bronchi (viral laryngotracheobronchitis or ALTB). Because it is clinically difficult and impractical to determine the extent to which the airway is involved, and because the management must assume that involve-ment extends to the bronchi, a discussion of ALTB suffices for viral laryngitis and viral laryngotracheitis.

ALTB occurs most frequently in children between the ages of six months and two years. The parainfluenza group of viruses, and less frequently the respiratory syncytial viruses and adenoviruses, are the primary etiological agents of viral croup. The illness commonly begins with the usual symptoms of the common cold, rhinorrhea, nasal congestion, and mild cough, and the child is usually afebrile. After two to three days of such symptomatology, the child's breath-ing acquires a "raspy" quality as inspiratory stridor develops, and the cough acquires a barking quality not unlike the bark of a seal. Many children will have only the above symptoms, while those in whom the stridor becomes more severe, may develop intercostal, subcostal, suprasternal, and supraclavicular retractions, tachypnea, and nasal flaring. Many may also develop a low grade fever, but rarely does the fever exceed $38.5^{\circ}C$. Histologically, it is edema of the true vocal cords and subglottic structures that gives rise to symptomatology, and it is the degree of edema which determines the severity of symptoms. As indicated previously, inflammation need not be limited to the larynx, but may extend to the trachea and bron-chi. On occasion, the fine, crepitant rales and the expiratory wheezes so characteristic of bronchiolitis are found coincidentally with viral croup, indicating even bronchiolar involvement. Szpunar et al. (1971) studying the airways of thirteen children who died of croup found inflammatory changes involving the trachea, bronchi,

and bronchioles in all thirteen. It is of interest that Newth et al.
(1973) found that of thirty-five children with croup studied, twenty-
nine were hypoxemic and nineteen hypercapneic. It is highly significant that they also found no useful clinical means to assess the degree of hypoxemia, thereby concluding that the hypoxemia "can be
assessed accurately only by determination of arterial blood gases."

The diagnosis of ALTB is established by the typical history and findings noted above, though care must be taken not to overlook the possibility of acute epiglottitis or retropharyngeal abscess or other
causes of the croup syndrome. When such diagnoses are considered
probable, an upright, lateral neck radiograph taken in inspiration is
obtained. When the radiograph is normal or reveals only subglottic
narrowing, or when other etiologies of the croup syndrome are considered improbable, the child's pharynx is examined and the epiglottis visualized. Caution should be exercised to perform as little
manipulation as is possible to avoid provoking agitation and subsequent laryngospasm. Once the examination reveals the absence of
the typical findings of acute epiglottitis and there is no evidence for
other disorders, the patient is assumed to have ALTB. Should the
child be highly febrile, bacterial involvement is questioned and
blood and nasopharyngeal cultures are obtained (the nasopharyngeal
culture is helpful only if it grows a pure culture of a pathogenic organism). Other evidence for bacterial infection (lobar pneumonia,
marked leukocytosis with polymorph predominance, exudative tonsillitis, or a septic-appearing child) may prompt initiation of antimicrobial therapy immediately after cultures are obtained; the absence of such additional evidence dictates awaiting culture results
before initiating such therapy. In the child who is afebrile or only
slightly febrile ($<38.5^{o}C$) a nasopharyngeal culture is not generally
obtained. The decision to manage the child in or out of the hospital
is based upon the severity of symptoms and the age and size of the
child. An assessment as to the severity of symptomatology must be
based on history as well as examination, for it is a well recognized
phenomenon that children with viral croup may have rapid resolution
of their symptoms upon sudden exposure to cool air as frequently occurs on the way to seek medical attention. Children with severe stridor are best hospitalized while those with moderate symptoms should
probably be hospitalized if very young and/or small (<6 months old/
<7 kg). Though arterial gases have not usually been utilized to determine the degree of severity in physicians' offices, clinics and
emergency rooms, such studies provide a more objective determination of those children with a croup syndrome at risk for a severe
course. Arterial blood gases are obtained on those children admitted
to the hospital to determine the necessity for providing supplemental
oxygen.

When children with ALTB are to be managed at home, it is common
practice to recommend increasing the humidity in the child's room by
utilization of a cool mist humidifier or a steam vaporizer. It should
be noted, however, that while the majority of clinicians recommend

humidity, good controlled studies related to the efficacy of such therapy in children with ALTB are sorely lacking. The addition of medications to the water utilized for humidification has not been shown to be of benefit. The usually recommended therapy, in addition to increasing humidity, consists of keeping the child well-hydrated, minimizing agitation or stress, monitoring temperature and the severity of symptoms, and explaining that exposure to cool, outside air or to a steam-filled bathroom (run shower hot water with bathroom door closed) may result in rapid improvement should acute exacerbation of symptoms occur. Parents are urged to call and/or return should symptoms worsen or additional symptoms develop. The child in mild to moderate distress who begins to refuse liquid intake warrants intravenous hydration.

The child with severe symptomatology or the young and/or small child with moderate symptomatology is generally hospitalized. Though manipulation does seem to exacerbate the disease, routine CBC and arterial blood gases are indicated in children admitted to the hospital with ALTB. The child who refuses to drink and the child for whom drinking provides excessive stress should receive intravenous hydration. Oxygen, when arterial gases dictate, is administered in concentrations which will maintain a $PaO_2 \geq 60$. Use of a high humidity tent seems to be of benefit in ALTB, though again controlled studies are lacking. Many children with ALTB seem to improve when calm and worsen when agitated, and it has been customary to sedate such children with drugs such as chloral hydrate or hydroxyzine. Because restlessness and agitation are well recognized reactions of the human organism to hypoxia, arterial blood gases are essential prior to the use of such sedation.

In most discussions of the management of infants and children with ALTB, little attention is given to the effect of body position on respiratory distress. Unfortunately, most young children receiving intravenous therapy must be restrained to maintain the intravenous line, and almost without fail, the child is restrained in the supine position on the horizontal plain. Children with ALTB who are not restrained and who are old enough to roll over do not elect that position, but rather choose to lie prone or to sit up. Marked improvement of symptoms upon turning a restrained child with ALTB from the supine to prone position has been noted frequently. When restraints are necessary, the child is preferably placed prone, and if placed supine, the bed should be placed in the reverse Trendelenburg position.

Routine antibiotic therapy of ALTB was not demonstrated to be of benefit in a controlled study by Tercero-Talavera et al. (1974), and such therapy is therefore not recommended. Antibiotics may, however, be indicated on such occasions as noted previously.

In 1971, Adair et al. introduced the treatment of ALTB with racemic epinephrine. Their protocol utilized a 1:8 dilution of 2.5% racemic

epinephrine administered per IPPB with a Bird Mark 7 respirator
for fifteen minutes. While this therapeutic modality has stimulated
controversy in recent years, it is recommended for hospitalized
children. Though patients so treated usually improve immediately,
they frequently have an exacerbation of symptomatology within hours
and require repeated treatments. Therefore, it does not seem pru-
dent to use this modality for outpatients who are treated and sent
home. While the use of racemic epinephrine does not seem to
shorten the course of ALTB, repeated treatments may well obviate
the necessity for endotracheal intubation and/or tracheostomy.

Corticosteroid therapy of ALTB remains somewhat controversial.
Eden et al. (1967, 1967a) have shown no benefit from steroid administration while James (1969) and Andreasson et al. (1971) have
suggested benefit. In view of the data regarding such therapy, it
appears unwarranted to recommend steroid therapy.

Downes et al. (1972) have derived criteria for assessing the degree
of respiratory distress in infants and children, and the use of their
criteria, which requires arterial blood gas measurement, is helpful in the management of ALTB. The criteria are summarized in
Table 1-4.

**TABLE 1-4: CRITERIA FOR ASSESSING DEGREE OF
RESPIRATORY DISTRESS IN INFANTS AND CHILDREN
per Downes et al. (1972)**

1. CLINICAL CRITERIA:

   1.1 Inspiratory Breath Sounds: decreased or absent
   1.2 Respiratory Effort: severe retractions and use of
         accessory muscles
   1.3 Skin Color: cyanosis in 40% oxygen
   1.4 Level of Awareness: decreased level of consciousness
         and decreased response to pain
   1.5 Muscle Tone: decreased

2. PHYSIOLOGIC CRITERIA:

   2.1 $PaCO_2 \geq 75$ mm Hg
   2.2 $PaO_2 \leq 100$ mm Hg in 100% oxygen

THE PRESENCE OF THREE CLINICAL AND ONE PHYSIOLOGI-
CAL CRITERIA CONSTITUTE ACUTE RESPIRATORY FAILURE
NECESSITATING IMMEDIATE ACTION.

As in the management of acute epiglottitis, endotracheal intubation
with a polyvinyl tube or tracheostomy is indicated when respiratory
failure occurs in ALTB (currently intubation seems to be preferred).
In some instances, particularly in small, exhausted infants, mechanical positive pressure ventilation will be required for a short
period of time.

It is noteworthy that the influenza viruses have been noted to cause
unusually severe ALTB. Howard et al. (1972) noted elevated titers
to influenza A2 virus (Hong Kong Flu) in eight children with a severe
croup requiring tracheostomy during an influenza epidemic in 1972.
During an influenza B epidemic, Goldstein (1975) found two boys,
ages nine and ten years, to have a croup syndrome identical to that
of acute epiglottitis (sudden onset, high fever, acute sore throat,
hoarseness, leukocytosis with polymorph predominance); viral titers were obtained on only one and were diagnostic of influenza B,
while blood and throat cultures revealed no pathogens in either.

3. SPASMODIC CROUP

No discussion of croup syndrome is complete without making mention of "spasmodic croup." The etiology of this condition is uncertain, and some authorities question its existence as an entity separate from viral croup. However, most clinicians caring for children
are familiar with children who undergo repeated attacks of stridor of
sudden night-time onset, unassociated with fever or other evidence
of infection, resolving in several hours. "Subemetic" doses of ipe-
cac have often been recommended for this entity, even though the
only consistently subemetic dose is none at all. Emesis in a child
with respiratory distress is to be avoided whenever possible, as
there is an increased risk of aspiration in such patients. Antihistaminics and combinations of antihistaminics and expectorants have
been suggested as being effective in spasmodic croup by others.
Little data has been published with respect to the management of
this entity and, therefore, therapy remains empiric and largely an-
ecdotal. It is probably best treated in the same manner as viral
ALTB.

4. COMPLICATIONS AND PROGNOSIS

Mediastinal emphysema, atelectasis, pneumothorax, and bronchopneumonia may complicate both ALTB and epiglottitis. Combined
pneumonia and atelectasis may ultimately result in bronchiectasis
and should therefore be treated aggressively. Complications associated with respiratory failure, respiratory arrest, and the procedures
of endotracheal intubation and tracheostomy must also be anticipated.
Cerebral edema, seizures, and seizure disorders may result from
severe hypoxic insult, and intubation and tracheostomy may be associated with hemorrhage or complicated by secondary airway damage.
Molteni (1976) revealed that of 72 cases of epiglottitis, 25% were

complicated by pneumonia and cervical lymphadenitis. Otitis media and exudative tonsillitis were the only other complications and were infrequent. Though 50% of the patients with epiglottitis were bacteremic, no cases of septic arthritis or meningitis occurred.

The prognosis for ALTB and epiglottitis depends on the severity of airway obstruction, the extent of infection, and the necessity for intubation or tracheostomy. In epiglottitis and in croup caused by certain influenza viruses, the rapidity with which the diagnosis is established and the airway secured seems to play a significant role in reducing mortality. H. influenzae epiglottitis has such a fulminant course that deaths have been reported as occurring within nine hours following the onset of inspiratory obstruction. On the other hand, most patients with ALTB have an uncomplicated course and seem to suffer few sequelae.

REFERENCES

Adair, J.C., Ring, W.H., Jordan, W.S., and Elwyn, R.A.: Ten-year experience with IPPB in the treatment of acute laryngotracheobronchitis, Anesth. Analg. 50:649, 1971.

Andreasson, L., Ingelstedt, S. and Rundcrantz, H.: Laryngitis with respiratory obstruction, Nord. Med. 85:133, 1971.

Battaglia, J.D. and Lockhart, C.H.: Management of acute epiglottitis by nasotracheal intubation, Am. J. Dis. Child. 129:334, 1975.

Baxter, J.D.: Acute epiglottitis in children, Laryngoscope 77: 1358, 1967.

Downes, J.J., Fulgencio, T., and Raphaely, R.C.: Acute respiratory failure in infants and children, Pediat. Clin. N.A. 19:423, 1972.

Eden, A.N., and Larkin, V.D.P.: Corticosteroid treatment of croup, Pediatrics 33:768, 1967.

Eden, A.N., Kaufman, A., and Yu, R.: Corticosteroids and croup, JAMA 200:133, 1967.

Geraci, R.P.: Acute epiglottitis management with prolonged nasotracheal intubation, Pediatrics 41:143, 1968.

Goldstein, N.: Unpublished data, 1975.

Howard, J.B., McCracken, G.H., and Luby, L.P.: Influenza A2 Virus as a cause of croup requiring tracheostomy, J. Pediat. 81: 1148, 1972.

James, J.A.: Dexamethasone in croup, Am. J. Dis. Child. 117: 511, 1969.

Johnson, G.L., Sullivan, L.L. and Bishop, L.A.: Acute epiglottitis, Arch. Otolaryngol. 100:33, 1974.

Margolis, C.Z., Ingram, D.L., and Meyer, J.H.: Routine tracheotomy in Hemophilus influenzae B epiglottitis, J. Pediat. 81: 1150, 1972.

Milko, D.A., Marshak, G., and Striker, T.W.: Nasotracheal intubation in the treatment of acute epiglottitis, Pediatrics 53:674, 1974.

Molteni, R.A.: Epiglottitis: Incidence of extraepiglottic infection: Report of 72 cases and review of the literature, Pediatrics 58:526, 1976.

Newth, C.J.D., Levison, H. and Bryan, A.C.: The respiratory status of children with croup, J. Pediat. 81:1068, 1973.

Poole, C.A., and Altman, D.H.: Acute epiglottitis in children, Radiology 80:798, 1963.

Rapkin, R.H.: The diagnosis of epiglottitis: simplicity and reliability of radiographs of the neck in the differential diagnosis of the croup syndrome, J. Pediat. 80:96, 1972.

Rapkin, R.H.: Tracheostomy in epiglottitis, Pediatrics 52:426, 1973.

Schuller, D.E. and Brick, H.G.: The safety of intubation in croup and epiglottitis: an eight-year follow up, Laryngoscope 85:33, 1975.

Szpunar, J., Glowacki, J., Laskowski, A., and Miszek, A.: Fibrinous laryngotracheobronchitis in children, Arch. Otolaryngol. 93: 173, 1971.

Tercero-Talanera, F.I., and Rapkin, R.H.: Antibiotic usage in the management of acute laryngotracheobronchitis (croup), Clin. Pediat. 13:1074, 1974.

Tos, M.: Nasotracheal intubation in acute epiglottitis, Arch. Otolaryngol. 97:373, 1973.

::

1.3: PERTUSSIS

INTRODUCTION: Pertussis, the disease resulting from infection with __Bordetella pertussis__, while less common than in years past, continues to produce its characteristic whoop. In 1975, there were 1,738 cases reported in the United States. The etiologic agent was first described in 1906, and routine immunization against the agent has been commonplace in the U.S. for the past 25 years. The disease spares no countries and no races and occurs in individuals of all ages; however, most cases occur in children under age five, and the greatest morbidity and mortality is in infants under one year of age. Females have been shown to have an increased morbidity and mortality from pertussis in many case series. In the United States, there is only minimal seasonal variation with a slightly greater number of cases occurring during the summer months.

Pertussis is spread by human to human contact, and patients developing the disease are considered to be capable of spreading the disease for a period of from one to three weeks after onset of coughing.

1. ETIOLOGY AND PATHOGENESIS

It has been appreciated for some time that Bordetella parapertussis and Bordetella bronchiseptica may also result in respiratory tract infections resembling pertussis. More recently, the adenoviruses have been implicated as etiological agents of a pertussis-like syndrome, and Klenk et al. (1972) and Nelson et al. (1975) have shown that pertussis occurs in many individuals in whom evidence is found for a combined Bordetella pertussis and adenovirus infection. Such evidence has led some to speculate that many of the complications seen in pertussis may in actuality be due to adenovirus infection.

The pathological changes occurring in patients with pertussis result from the Bordetella pertussis organisms, secondarily infecting organisms, and from bronchial plugging by cellular debris, mucus, and pus. The mucous membranes of the airways, from the nose to the bronchi, are inflamed early in the course of the disease. Changes in the lung include peribronchial infiltration and areas of emphysema and atelectasis. Microscopically, areas of necrosis of the bronchial epithelium are seen, often infiltrated with polymorphonuclear leukocytes. The pulmonary lesions may ultimately progress to constitute typical interstitial pneumonia with a mononuclear cell infiltrate and tracheal and peribronchial lymphadenopathy. Pulmonary hemorrhages occur early in the course of pertussis, while frank bronchiectasis may occur either during the course of disease or subsequently.

The brain, too, may exhibit changes, and most often those of edema and punctate hemorrhages occur. Plugging of the capillaries by cellular infiltrates and even cerebral cortical degeneration have been described in rare instances.

2. CLINICAL MANIFESTATIONS

Most children contracting pertussis develop symptoms within the first ten days following exposure to an infected individual. In fact, failure to develop symptoms two weeks following exposure is usually indicative of failure to contract the illness.

Traditionally, the symptomatology of pertussis is divided into the catarrhal, paroxysmal, and convalescent stages. The catarrhal stage begins with coughing, sneezing, coryza, and low grade fever, not unlike a common upper respiratory infection. The catarrhal stage lasts ten to fourteen days, and in contrast to a common cold, rather than subsiding, the cough becomes worse and begins to occur in paroxysms, thereby beginning the paroxysmal stage.

The cough begins to occur in sudden episodic bursts with episodes ultimately consuming all of expiration. During such an attack, the child's face becomes first reddened, then cyanotic, the eyes bulge, the tongue protrudes, and the child becomes a truly piteous sight to behold. The end of the episode is followed by a forceful inhalation as the child struggles to replenish his oxygen, and it is this rapid, sudden inspiration that results in the whooping sound so typical of pertussis in children beyond the first year of age. In infants, particularly those younger than six months of age, the whoop may not occur, and as a result the physician may fail to diagnose pertussis, even in the presence of paroxysms. The paroxysms of coughing are accompanied by profuse mucus production, and it is not uncommon to see the child's face covered with thick, tenacious mucus streaming from both nostrils and the mouth. The exertion of the paroxysm usually results in profuse sweating and is often followed by emesis, facial edema, and petechiae about the face. The attacks may be precipitated by exertion, eating or drinking, or may seem to begin without provocation.

The paroxysmal stage usually persists for five or six weeks, though it may extend for ten to twelve weeks, with the frequency of the paroxysms diminishing as the weeks pass. While mild cases may have five or six attacks a day, severe involvement may result in ten times that number of paroxysms each day.

The cessation of vomiting and whooping marks the beginning of the convalescent stage, though paroxysms which are less severe in intensity continue to occur. Subsequently, the cough becomes indistinguishable from that associated with a typical viral respiratory tract infection. The convalescent stage is usually concluded in two to four weeks, though children having had pertussis may experience exacerbations of their paroxysmal cough when subsequently contracting respiratory infections. Such paroxysms are frequently complete with whoop and emesis, and such episodes may recur over months and, in rare instances, years following the episode of pertussis.

2.1: Complications: The highest mortality from pertussis seems to occur in infants under six months of age developing the disease. Deaths occur primarily as a consequence of superimposed bacterial pneumonia or asphyxia secondary to the paroxysms and/or mucus obstruction. Epistaxis, petechiae about the face and neck, subconjunctival hemorrhages, melena, atelectasis (usually right upper lobe), subcutaneous emphysema, convulsions and weight loss in

infants are all well-known complications of pertussis. Pertussis
has long been implicated as a cause of bronchiectasis, but prospective studies showing a causal relationship are not available. Chronic
atelectasis, however, may lead to bronchiectasis, and it may become necessary to utilize bronchoscopy to remove mucus plugs
and to re-expand atelectatic areas of lung. In children under a year
of age, providing adequate caloric intake may be a major problem.
Rarely does severe malnutrition ensue, but it is often difficult to
achieve positive nitrogen balance in a child who constantly vomits,
uses excessive energy to cough, and who coughs whenever fed.

Intracranial hemorrhages are rare in pertussis, though they have
been reported and have been associated with death and paralysis.
Small, punctate hemorrhages may occur in the brain and may be
secondary to pressure changes and/or hypoxia resulting from the
paroxysms.

<h3 align="center">3. DIAGNOSIS</h3>

The clinical pertussis syndrome in its classical presentation of paroxysmal coughing, inspiratory whoop, and vomiting is rarely confused with other clinical entities. Obtaining a positive culture for
B. pertussis confirms the diagnosis of pertussis. However, it is
during the catarrhal stage that the organism is most easily cultured,
and during that stage little is present clinically to differentiate the
disease from a routine respiratory infection. Certainly, a history
of exposure to a known case of pertussis and a history of immunologic susceptibility (inadequate immunizations) should raise the possibility of pertussis in a child with a respiratory illness. It should
be noted, however, that fully immunized children may still contract
pertussis; thus, the diagnosis must be considered even in those fully
immunized.

Cystic fibrosis, foreign body aspiration, pneumonia, bronchiolitis,
and tracheal compression may all require differentiation from pertussis. Since most infants under six months of age are not fully immunized and will not have a whoop and since bronchiolitis is associated with cough and mucus production, infants with pertussis may be
misdiagnosed early in their course as having bronchiolitis.

Two methods for obtaining material for culture in pertussis have
been found useful and have replaced "cough plates." A nasopharyngeal swab is placed through a nostril and held in place with the tip in
the pharynx until the patient coughs. The swab is then removed and
used to inoculate a fresh plate of Bordet-Gengou media. An alternate method utilizes "auger Suction" which consists of inserting a
small rubber or plastic tube through a nostril into the nasopharynx
and aspirating mucus with a 20 cc syringe. The mucus obtained is
cultured in the same manner as the nasopharyngeal swab.

A fluorescent antibody staining method has been developed for the pertussis organism but is useful only as an adjunct in diagnosis. A false positive incidence of 30-40 percent has been noted in large scale attempts to apply the fluorescent technique.

Total and differential white blood cell counts (WBC) and chest radiographs may assist in establishing the diagnosis of pertussis. During the paroxysmal stage the WBC is likely to be >25,000 with most patients having a lymphocytosis of 60-80 percent. Infants under six months of age usually do not exhibit the characteristic WBC and differential. The chest X-ray will frequently reveal perihilar infiltrates which may surround the cardiac silhouette to such an extent that the term "shaggy heart sign" has been coined. Such changes are non-specific, however, and may be seen in other conditions.

4. MANAGEMENT

The treatment of children with pertussis is essentially the provision of good supportive care. It is generally recommended that children less than one year of age with pertussis be admitted because of the hazards of asphyxia in small children thus affected and because of the high frequency of complications in this age group. Those older than a year of age should be hospitalized if paroxysms are severe or if significant complications arise. It is also recommended that children under one year of age receive Human Immune Pertussis Globulin in a dose of 1.25 ml. IM on three successive days. It is unclear whether the administration of the globulin significantly alters the course of pertussis, though some studies have suggested that it does.

Antibiotics have not been shown to alter the course of pertussis once contracted, but numerous studies have shown various drugs to be effective in rendering culture positive patients culture negative. Bass et al. (1969) compared the antibiotic susceptibility of <u>Bordetella pertussis</u> to nine antibiotics. Erythromycin was the antibiotic to which the organisms seemed most sensitive and chloramphenicol, kanamycin, ampicillin, oxytetracycline, streptomycin, penicillin G, lincomycin, and cephalothin followed in order of decreasing susceptibility. Bass et al. (1969) then compared ampicillin, erythromycin, oxytetracycline, and chloramphenicol in patients with pertussis and found that none of the drugs altered the course when given well into the paroxysmal stage. All but ampicillin rendered culture positive patients culture negative. In addition, their results suggested that erythromycin may abort or attenuate pertussis when given in the very early paroxysmal stage and may prevent pertussis in exposed individuals. Other authors have disagreed as to the usefulness of ampicillin in effecting bacteriologic cure. It would, therefore, seem warranted, in view of the relative side effects of those drugs studied, to recommend erythromycin as the drug of choice with which to treat both contacts and those with pertussis. Because relapse of bacteriologic cure has been noted after both seven and ten day antibiotic courses but not after courses longer than ten days, such therapy is recommended for a duration of fourteen days.

While frequent and prolonged suction of the naso- and oropharynx may produce hypoxia and induce paroxysms in pertussis, mechanical suction immediately following paroxysms when the child appears "refractory" to being stimulated to cough is recommended. A large catheter is required to effect rapid removal of the copious and viscous secretions.

Arterial blood gas studies are lacking in patients with pertussis, though it is obvious that children becoming markedly cyanotic during a paroxysm are significantly hypoxic. Oxygen administration is therefore recommended for those children having severe paroxysms. In view of current studies of mist therapy in asthma and cystic fibrosis, mist cannot be recommended for the therapy of pertussis. In addition to a lack of data supporting its benefit, mist hides the patient, thereby interfering with optimal supportive care. Certainly, when oxygen is administered it should be moistened and when administered to small infants it should be warmed; there is, however, a difference between moist oxygen and the delivery of oxygen with mist.

When necessary to provide hydration and when feeding is impossible, intravenous fluids should be administered. In those infants for whom adequate oral nutrition becomes impossible for several weeks, parenteral hyperalimentation should be considered.

It is the goal of management in pertussis to support the child through acute illness preventing severe complications from asphyxia or secondary infections. The ultimate prognosis will then be determined by the small risk of subsequent bronchiectasis or central nervous system sequelae.

4.1: Prevention: Though immunity from pertussis vaccination is less than 100 percent effective and is of short duration, it is recommended routinely for children under age six years. In epidemic situations, children over age six years may be given booster doses. Recommended schedules and dosages for immunization are found elsewhere in this text.

Most studies of patients with pertussis have shown many of the affected individuals to have been inadequately immunized. A major objective in the control of this disease, therefore, should be the compulsive updating of the immunization status of all children seen by all health providers. Such prevention is especially critical when so little can be done to alter the course of the disease once it is contracted.

REFERENCES

Balagtas, R.C., Nelson, K.E., Levin, S., and Gotoff, S.P.: Treatment of pertussis with pertussis immune globulin. J. Pediat. 79: 203, 1971.

Bass, J.W., Klenk, E.L., Kotheimer, J.B., Linnemann, C.C., Smith, M.H.D.: Antimicrobial treatment of pertussis. J. Pediat. 75:768, 1969.

Bass, J.W., Crast, F.W., Kotheimer, J.B., and Mitchell, I.A.: Susceptibility of Bordetella pertussis to nine antimicrobial agents. Am. J. Dis. Child. 117:277, 1969.

Brooksaler, F. and Nelson, J.D.: Pertussis: a reappraisal and report of 190 confirmed cases. Am. J. Dis. Child. 114:389, 1967.

Connor, J.D.: Evidence for an etiologic role of adenovirus infection in pertussis syndrome. NEJM 282:390, 1970.

Islur, J., Anglin, C.S. and Middleton, P.J.: The whooping cough syndrome: a continuing pediatric problem. Clin. Pediat. 14:171, 1975.

Jernelius, H.: Pertussis with pulmonary complications: a follow-up study. Acta Paediatr. 53:247, 1964.

Klenk, E.L., Gaultney, J.V., and Bass, J.W.: Bacteriologically proved pertussis and adenovirus infection. Am. J. Dis. Child. 124: 203, 1972.

Krugman, S. and Ward, R.: Pertussis. Infectious Diseases of Children and Adults. The C.V. Mosby Company, St. Louis, 1973.

Linnemann, C.C., Partin, J.C., Perlstein, P.H., and Englender, G.S.: Pertussis: Persistent problems. J. Pediat. 85:589, 1974.

Nelson, J.D.: Antibiotic treatment of pertussis. Pediatrics 44: 474, 1969.

Nelson, K.E., Gavitt, F., Batl, M.D., Kallick, C.A., Reddi, K.T. and Levin, S.: The role of adenoviruses in the pertussis syndrome. J. Pediat. 86:335, 1975.

::

1.4: BRONCHIOLITIS

INTRODUCTION: Acute bronchiolitis is a disease of infancy and early childhood, commonly seen in winter and spring. Approximately 95% of cases occur in infants less than one year of age and the majority (65%) are less than 6 months of age (Table 1-5). The disease seems to occur twice as often in male infants as in female infants.

TABLE 1-5: DISTRIBUTION OF AGE AND SEX IN 296 CASES OF ACUTE BRONCHIOLITIS		
AGE (MONTHS)	MALE/FEMALE (%)	TOTAL (%)
0-3	68/32	33
4-6	60/40	32
7-9	68/32	14
10-12	58/42	8
13-18	67/33	9
19-24	50/50	4
25-30	75/20	1
Total	64/36	100

Modified from Leer, et al. (Am. J. Dis. Child. 117:495, 1969).

Bronchiolitis is characterized by a marked airway obstruction at the level of the bronchioles with air trapping. It has a dramatic clinical course with a rapid onset of progressive respiratory distress and a rapid clearance of the symptoms within 24 to 48 hours.

1. ETIOLOGY AND PATHOGENESIS

Acute bronchiolitis is primarily caused by viruses. Respiratory syncytial (RS) virus is the most important causative agent. Other offenders include parainfluenza, adenoviruses, influenza, rhinoviruses, and Mycoplasma pneumoniae. Hemophilus influenzae has also been suggested to play a causative role, but the evidence is equivocal.

The most prominent feature of acute bronchiolitis is the rapid development of hyperinflation (air trapping) of the lungs. This is the result of a partial obstruction of the bronchioles, which permits air to enter the alveoli on inspiration but prevents the air from leaving on expiration. Alteration of alveolar structure from overinflation (or emphysema) results in: 1) poor oxygenation of the blood leading to hypoxia, 2) impairment of CO_2 release, causing respiratory acidosis, and 3) increased resistance in the pulmonary circulation, adding a strain to the right heart.

The pathogenesis of bronchiolitis is not well defined. It has been suggested that immunologic responses (humoral and cellular) may be responsible for the severe disease (pneumonia and bronchiolitis) caused by RSV. This is based on the observation that RSV causes the most severe disease in young infants with high titers of maternal neutralizing antibody to RSV and in children previously immunized with killed RSV vaccine.

Infants who die of the disease usually show evidence of a diffuse respiratory tract inflammation, but the bronchioles are most severely affected. The walls of the bronchioles as well as the small and medium-sized bronchi are swollen and infiltrated with inflammatory cells. The lumina are often occluded, partially or completely, by the tenacious exudates containing mucus, leukocytes, and tissue debris. In areas where the lumina are partially occluded, the distal alveoli are severely distended resulting from air trapping. Atelectasis is also seen in distal areas where the bronchioles or bronchi are occluded completely, since no air enters or leaves the areas.

2. CLINICAL MANIFESTATIONS

The disease is characterized by a preceding history of upper respiratory symptoms such as rhinorrhea and slight cough for one to several days followed by the abrupt rapid, labored breathing. There is increasing inspiratory difficulty, manifested by intercostal, substernal, and suprasternal notch retraction. There is also expiratory difficulty with wheezing or grunting. The infant becomes restless and agitated because of hypoxia. The cough may be paroxsymal, like that of whooping cough, leading to vomiting and interfering with feeding, and eventually may result in dehydration. Cyanosis occurs if the airway obstruction continues, and the cyanosis is intensified by coughing or crying. Fever, usually of low grade, occurs in less than 50% of the patients.

The most important physical finding on auscultation is diminished breath sounds bilaterally, caused by hyperinflation of the alveoli and poor air exchange. Wheezes, rhonchi or fine rales may be heard later in the course of the disease. Tachycardia is common but signs of right heart failure occur infrequently. A mortality of 5.5% in 1230 cases was reported by Heycock (1962), but in most series the mortality is less than 1%. Infants with congenital heart defects or other anomalies are at a greater risk of death.

3. DIAGNOSIS

Acute bronchiolitis is easy to diagnose. The disease has several unique features: 1) age distribution (early infancy), 2) seasonal occurrence (winter-spring), and 3) characteristic history and physical findings.

Chest roentgenograms show the lung fields to be abnormally radiolucent. There is increased bronchovascular marking due to interstitial infiltration. Both diaphragms are depressed or flattened (Fig. 1.1).

The white blood cell count is often within normal limits. Arterial blood gas studies may show a low PO_2, high PCO_2 with a low blood pH.

Virologic studies to confirm the presence of the causative agent are usually not necessary. Tissue culture methods are needed for isolation of the viral agent from throat or nasopharyngeal swab specimens. Direct examinations of the swab smears by immunofluorescent antibody staining have been successfully used by some laboratories. Demonstration of antibody responses by various methods will also confirm the etiologic diagnosis.

4. MANAGEMENT

The management of acute bronchiolitis is primarily supportive, which includes mist, oxygen, and fluid.

The infant should be placed in an atmosphere enriched with high humidity and oxygen. The humidity will render the bronchial secretions less tenacious and sticky. Arterial blood gases need to be determined during the acute stage of the illness, since absence of cyanosis is an unreliable indication of a normal arterial oxygen tension. At least 40% of inspired oxygen concentration is needed to achieve a normal PO_2 in many infants with lower respiratory infection. Higher oxygen concentrations are necessary in severe disease. To use oxygen effectively it is essential to monitor the concentration in the oxygen tent.

In a small number of cases, satisfactory PO_2 levels may not be achieved even with high ambient oxygen concentration. Tracheal intubation with intermittent positive pressure breathing may be necessary.

An adequate fluid intake to avoid dehydration is important. Parenteral fluid therapy is often used in a sick infant with respiratory distress. Dehydration renders the bronchial secretions more tenacious.

If marked metabolic acidosis is present, intravenous administration of sodium bicarbonate is needed to improve the utilization of oxygen and myocardial function. Digitalization is useful for patients who develop signs of congestive heart failure (e.g. enlargement of liver, gallop rhythm, tachycardia, and lung edema).

Corticosteroids have been used by some clinicians on the hypothesis that their anti-inflammatory effect will reduce bronchiolar edema and inflammation, thus improving the airways. However, several

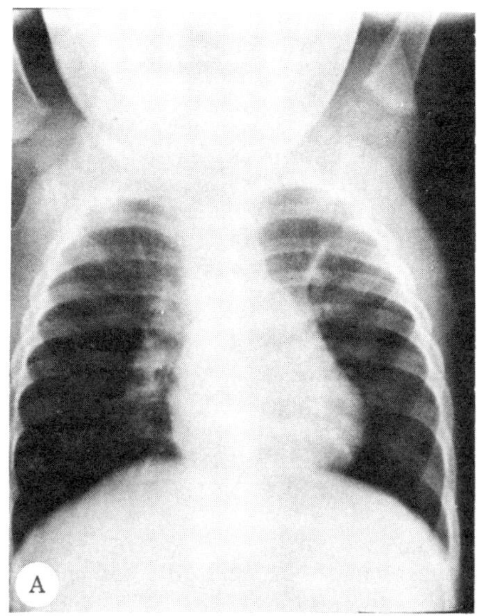

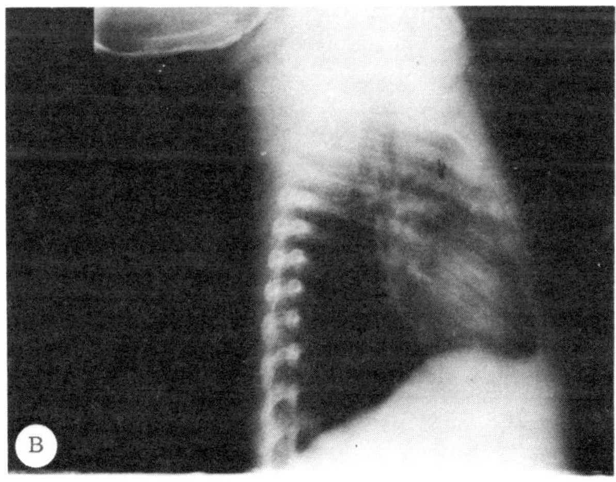

FIG. 1.1: Acute bronchiolitis due to respiratory syncytial
virus in a 4-month-old infant. Chest roentgenograms (A. anterio-posterior view and B. lateral
view) show a hyperinflation of both lung fields
with depressed diaphragms. There is an increased bronchovascular marking secondary to
interstitial infiltration.

controlled studies have indicated that corticosteroids offer little if any benefit in the general or routine treatment of acute bronchiolitis. In severely ill infants hydrocortisone may be given, but it is difficult to assess its value.

Routine use of prophylactic or therapeutic antibiotics in acute bronchiolitis is not indicated. However, since it is impossible to determine whether bacterial infection is present, broad spectrum antibiotics (such as ampicillin) may be used if the infant is gravely ill and the disease progresses in spite of the adequate supportive measures, or if there is roentgenographic evidence of pneumonic infiltrates.

In some cases epinephrine (0.1 ml of a 1:1000 solution injected subcutaneously) or aminophylline seem to improve the airway by relieving the spasm. In general, bronchodilators are not very effective, since bronchiolar muscles are not well developed.

REFERENCES

Elderkin, F.M., Gardner, P.S., Turk, D.C., and White, A.C.: Aetiology and management of bronchiolitis and pneumonia in childhood. Br. Med. J. 2:722, 1965.

Gardner, P.S., McQuillin, J. and Court, S.D.M.: Speculation on pathogenesis of death from respiratory syncytial virus infection. Br. Med. J. 1:327, 1970.

Glezen, W.P., and Denny, F.W.: Epidemiology of acute lower respiratory disease in children. NEJM 288:498, 1973.

Heycock, J.B., and Noble, G.C.: 1230 cases of acute bronchiolitis in infancy. Br. Med. J. 2:879, 1962.

Holdaway, D., Romer, A.C., and Gardner, P.S.: The diagnosis and management of bronchiolitis. Pediatrics 39:924, 1967.

Jacobs, J.W., and Peacock, D.B.: Respiratory syncytial and other viruses associated with respiratory disease in infants. Lancet 1: 7705, 1971.

Macasaet, F.F., Kidd, P.A., Bolano, C.R., and Wenner, H.A.: The etiology of acute respiratory infections. III. The role of viruses and bacteria. J. Pediatr. 72:829, 1968.

Mufson, M.A., Krause, H.E., Mocega, H.A., and Dawson, F.W.: Viruses, Mycoplasma pneumoniae and bacteria associated with lower respiratory tract disease among infants. Am. J. Epidemo. 91:192, 1970.

Parrott, R.H., Kim, H.W., Brandt, C.D., and Chanock, R.M.: Respiratory syncytial virus in infants and children. Preventive Medicine 3:473, 1974.

Phelan, P.D., and Stocks, J.G.: Management of severe viral bronchiolitis and severe acute asthma. Arch. Dis. Child. 49:143, 1974.

Ross, C.A., Pinkerton, I.W., and Assaad, F.A.: Pathogenesis of respiratory syncytial virus disease in infancy. Arch. Dis. Child. 46:702, 1971.

Simpson, H., Matthew, D.J., Inglis, J.M., and George, E.L.: Virologic findings and blood gas tensions in acute lower respiratory tract infections in children. Br. Med. J. 2:629, 1974.

Wohl, M.E.B., Stigol, L.C., and Mead, J.: Resistance of the total respiratory system in healthy infants with bronchiolitis. Pediatrics 43:495, 1969.

::

1.5: PNEUMONIA

INTRODUCTION: Pneumonia is a lower respiratory tract infection associated with an inflammatory reaction involving the bronchial and alveolar spaces. Diagnosis of pneumonia usually requires roentgenographic evidence of pulmonary infiltration. When the inflammation involves primarily the alveolar spaces, a lobar pneumonia, or a bronchopneumonia is diagnosed depending on the extent of the lung involvement. Interstitial pneumonia usually denotes the inflammatory changes involving the supporting interstitium. Different groups of microorganisms are often associated with each type of pneumonia which dictates different forms of antimicrobial therapy.

Although the lung is ordinarily free of demonstrable microorganisms, it is easily colonized by microorganisms from the patient's upper respiratory tract or from the surrounding environment. This is particularly true when host defense mechanisms such as the ciliary movement and mucous secretions of the respiratory epithelium are not functioning optimally. For infectious droplets to reach the terminal bronchioles and alveolar spaces, the aerosol particles should be less than 3 nm in size. Particles larger than 3 nm are usually trapped in the upper respiratory passages. Microorganisms also can enter the lungs by the hematogenous route associated with bacteremia or septic emboli. Medical management of such pneumonias should aim at treating and eradicating the primary infection. Aspiration pneumonia is due to inhalation of food or gastric contents in unconscious or chronically ill patients requiring tube feeding. Aspiration of foreign materials disrupts the normal pulmonary functional defense by irritation and obstruction which facilitates the growth of a mixture of microorganisms reaching the lungs from aspiration. Anaerobes are important organisms commonly found in lung abscess as a result of aspiration pneumonia.

Differentiation of bacterial and nonbacterial pneumonia is not always easy. However, certain guidelines may be useful (Table 1-6).

TABLE 1-6: DIFFERENTIATION OF BACTERIAL AND NONBACTERIAL PNEUMONIAS		
CHARACTERISTICS	BACTERIAL	NONBACTERIAL
1. Onset	Abrupt	Gradual
2. Cough	Productive; sputum may be bloody or purulent	Non-productive
3. Pleuritis	Common	Uncommon
4. X-rays vs. physical	Correlated	Not always correlated
5. Leukocyte count	>15,000 with left shift	>15,000 without shift
6. Sputum smear and culture	Neutrophils; bacterial pathogens	Mononuclears; no bacterial pathogens
7. Serologic tests	Not helpful	Helpful

In young infants and children, clinical signs and symptoms of infection of the lower respiratory tract may be quite non-specific. Not infrequently, pneumonia is found by roentgenographic examinations in infants who present only with upper respiratory infections or only tachypnea and fever. It is well established that viral agents are responsible for over 90% of the upper respiratory infections. The contribution of bacterial and viral agents in pneumonia is not precisely known.

The following types of pneumonias are discussed in this chapter:

I.   BACTERIAL PNEUMONIAS
    A.   Streptococcus pneumoniae
    B.   Staphylococcus aureus
    C.   Other bacterial pneumonias
        Group A beta-hemolytic streptococcus, Klebsiella
        pneumoniae.

II. NONBACTERIAL PNEUMONIAS
    A. Mycoplasmal pneumonia
    B. Viral pneumonias
    C. Other nonbacterial pneumonias

I: BACTERIAL PNEUMONIAS

Among all bacterial pathogens, pneumococcus and staphylococcus
are the most important causative agents both for primary pneumonias and secondary infections following viral diseases, such as epidemic influenza. Streptococcus and Hemophilus influenzae may
cause pneumonia but are uncommon. Gram negative bacilli are
rare etiologic agents for bacterial pneumonias in pediatric patients
except in the newborn period or in children with compromised host
defense (see Chapters 8 and 9).

A. STREPTOCOCCUS PNEUMONIAE

(1) Etiology and Epidemiology: Pneumococcal pneumonia is the
most common cause of bacterial pneumonia. In adults, pneumococcal pneumonia classically is lobar in type. In children and the aged,
it may also be seen as a patchy bronchopneumonia.

Streptococcus pneumoniae is a gram-positive nonmotile, encapsulated
lenticular shaped bacteria. Growth is facilitated in 5-10% CO_2 and
causes alpha hemolysis on sheep blood agar. With continued incubation, pneumococci undergo rapid autolysis and the convex colonies
collapse centrally resulting in a crater or double ring form: To
differentiate from other Streptococcus viridans, pneumococcus is
bile soluble and inhibited by Optochin (ethylhydrocupreine hydrochloride). Encapsulated pneumococci form smooth colonies and the capsule is composed of polysaccharides which are the virulent factors of
the pneumococcus. Using the Neufeld quellung reaction, 82 serologically distant types of pneumococci have been identified.

Pneumococci are normal inhabitants of the human upper respiratory
tract. Depending upon the season and environmental conditions, 5-
60% of the population may harbor these organisms.

Pneumococcal pneumonia occurs in all seasons but more commonly
in the winter and spring. In the U.S.A., influenza and pneumonia
rank as the fifth leading cuase of death and the first among infectious
diseases. Pneumococcal infections are seen in all age groups. In
children the highest attack rates are under 4 years. In adults, types
1,3,4,7 and 12 may account for 80% or more of all pneumococcal
pneumonias. The higher serotypes, 6,14,19 and 23 are more commonly seen in children. Paradoxically the serotypes causing illnesses bear little relation to the serotypes of pneumococci found in
carriers.

(2) <u>Pathogenesis</u>: Pneumococci gain entrance to the lung through droplet infection or aspiration of infected secretions. Prior damage of respiratory epithelial function and edema of alveoli following viral infection such as epidemic influenza may also facilitate growth of pneumococci. Transient bacteremia may be a common event at the beginning of pneumococcal pneumonia. However, in hospitalized patients, pneumococcal bacteremia may be detectable in only 25-30% of the cases.

Pneumonias begin commonly in the right lower, right middle or left lower lobes, the sites where respiratory secretions are more prone to be aspirated when supine during sleep. Rapid, acute inflammatory changes ensue with hyperemia, polymorphonuclear infiltration, exudation of edematous fluid with fibrin. This stage is characteristically termed red hepatization; this is followed by gray hepatization in which fibrin deposits are predominant and the polymorphonuclear phagocytosis of pneumococci is active. During the resolution stage, the consolidated exudate within the alveolar spaces is enzymatically digested and either absorbed or removed by coughing. In uncomplicated cases, lung morphology and physiology are restored to normal.

(3) <u>Clinical Manifestations</u>: Although many patients with pneumococcal pneumonia do give a history of a mild upper respiratory infection for several days, the onset of pneumonia is usually abrupt. Commonly there is an initial shaking chill and rigor, followed by fever, cough with purulent and bloody sputum and pleuritic pain. Multiple chills and rigor are rare occurrences for pneumococcal infection. If this appears, clinicians should be alert to look out for other etiologic diagnoses. Because of pleuritic pain, many patients have splinting of the affected side of the thorax during inspiration. Physical examination reveals dullness, increased tactile and focal fremitus, fine to medium rales, tubular and bronchial breath sounds and bronchophony. Chest roentgenogram usually shows pulmonary consolidations consistent with the physical findings.

In young children and infants, the clinical signs and symptoms may be variable with minimal pulmonary findings associated with fever, fretfulness, apprehension, and respiratory distress.

(4) <u>Diagnosis</u>: Leukocytosis of 15,000 to 30,000 cells/mm^3 with shift to the left is usually seen. When leukocytopenia is present ($<$4000 cells/mm^3), the prognosis is grave. Visualization of pneumococci on sputum smear and a positive sputum culture is helpful but may not be conclusive as pneumococci are common inhabitants in the nasopharynx. In adults, the blood culture is positive in about 25-30% of patients with pneumococcal pneumonia. The incidence of bacteremia accompanying pneumococcal pneumonia in children is less well documented but may vary from 10-30%. If the blood culture is positive, not only is the diagnosis certain but this alerts the physician to the possibility that extrapulmonary complications may occur. Although counterelectrophoresis has been used to detect pneumococcal

antigen in body tissue fluids such as CSF and blood, its practical usefulness and general availability in routine hospital laboratories need further study.

(5) <u>Prognosis and Complications</u>: In uncomplicated cases of pneumococcal pneumonia, the prognosis is very favorable particularly when appropriate antimicrobial therapy is started early. The mortality is probably less than 1% and persistent morbidity is negligible.

Although pleuritis is common, empyema as a complication of pneumococcal pneumonia occurred in 5-10% of patients during the pre-antimicrobial era and is a rare complication today. Direct extension of pneumococcal infection to the mediastinum and pericardium may occur. Distant metastatic lesions resulted in meningitis or osteomyelitis may be seen in bacteremic patients. In infants and young children, paralytic ileus causing abdominal distention may be a serious complication. Extrapulmonary complications such as meningitis, pericarditis, peritonitis and osteomyelitis may occur but are rare. When these complications occur, the patients require more prolonged and vigorous therapy. Overwhelming pneumococcal infection with a leukopenia is an ominous prognostic sign.

(6) <u>Treatment</u>: Penicillin G is the drug of choice for treatment. Practically all strains of pneumococci are susceptible to penicillin and no antibiotic testing is necessary. A dose of 25,000 to 50,000 units/kg/day of procaine penicillin G given as a daily single intramuscular injection initially, followed by oral penicillin (50,000 units/ kg/day) for a period of 7-10 days. In older children and adults, 600,000 to 1,200,000 units procaine penicillin is appropriate. Daily dosages in excess of 1.2 million units are rarely necessary. If the patient is allergic to penicillin, erythromycin or a cephalosporin may be used. Supportive therapy with oxygen for cyanosis and correction of fluid and electrolyte imbalances are important. If empyema is present, thoracentesis is necessary to remove the pleural fluid. Penicillin G solution 50,000 to 100,000 units may be instilled intrapleurally after thoracentesis every 2-3 days to help sterilize the pleural cavity and hasten the recovery. When extrapulmonary complications are present, more vigorous treatment is needed.

B. STAPHYLOCOCCUS AUREUS

(1) <u>Epidemiology</u>: Colonization of infants with <u>Staphylococcus aureus</u> is a predictable event occurring in almost 90% of infants during the neonatal period, chiefly in the nostril and on the umbilical stump. The nasal carrier rate drops during infancy and rises again beginning in childhood to about 40% in adult life. In the hospital environment, certain strains of staphylococcus identifiable by bacteriophage typing are prevalent. The mode of spread of staphylococci by hand contact is more important than other means in hospital environments particularly in the newborn nursery. The incidence of staphylococcal

pneumonia is more prevalent in winter months following viral upper respiratory infections such as epidemic influenza. Serious staphylococcal infections including pneumonia in the pediatric age group are more prone to occur in young infants under 1 year of age.

(2) <u>Pathology and Pathogenesis</u>: A variety of toxins and enzymes is produced by <u>Staphylococcus aureus</u>. Among them, hemolysin, leukocidin, coagulase, staphylokinase and an enterotoxin are well known. However, none of the toxins or enzymes has conclusively been shown to be the virulent factor in the pathogenesis of staphylococcal infections. There is good data to suggest that coagulase-positive staphylococci are more virulent and pathogenic than coagulase-negative organisms. In contrast to older children and adults, infants and newborn babies apparently do not handle staphylococcal infections well, permitting a superficial skin lesion to progress into septicemia and pneumonia. A confluent bronchopneumonia with multiple abscesses and hemorrhagic necrosis leading to cavitation is characteristic of staphylococcal pneumonia. Rupture of subpleural abscess often lead to formation of bronchopleural fistuli resulting in pneumothorax and empyema.

(3) <u>Clinical Manifestations</u>: Primary staphylococcal pneumonia occurs most commonly in young infants preceded by a history of upper respiratory infections or staphylococcal skin lesions. The strain of staphylococcus is likely to be hospital acquired. Staphylococcal pneumonia is a rapidly progressive disease with an abrupt onset. Tachycardia, grunting respirations, cyanosis, fretfulness, sternal and substernal retractions are common. The infant will appear toxic or lethargic.

Physical findings may be minimal in the early phase of pneumonia, consisting only of diffuse rhonchi and rales with diminished breath sounds. Chest x-ray may show patchy bronchopneumonia undifferentiable from other lower respiratory infections. Within a matter of hours the clinical picture may change quickly. The infant may show signs of toxicity and deterioration with increasing dyspnea. If pneumothorax and empyema occur from bronchopleural fistula formation, dullness on percussion and marked diminished breath sounds and vocal fremitus will be present. Roentgenography of the lungs may show "honey-combed" multiple abscesses and pneumotoceles as well as pleural fluid. If the pneumothorax is severe, shift of the mediastinum toward the unaffected side is noted.

(4) <u>Diagnosis</u>: Since staphylococcal pneumonia is a rapidly progressive disease carrying a high mortality and morbidity, early diagnosis is important. The clinician should be especially suspicious of an infant with a rapidly progressive pneumonia in the presence of skin infection and/or upper respiratory infection. In older infants, leukocytosis of $>15,000$ WBC/mm^3 and left shift are common. However, in young infants and newborns, the white counts may be within normal range. When empyema is present, aspiration of fluid by thoracentesis should be done. A smear of the aspirate should be examined

and if gram positive cocci in clusters are seen, the diagnosis is presumptive and should be subsequently confirmed by culture. When no pleural fluid is obtainable and since young infants do not cooperate to produce sputum samples, a gastric lavage for smears and culture may be helpful as purulent discharge from the respiratory tract may be swallowed. About 10% of infants with staphylococcal pneumonia will have positive blood cultures.

Although a typical case of staphylococcal pneumonia is easily recognized, often times it may not be readily differentiated from other bacterial pneumonias during the early phase of infection. Differential diagnoses should include pneumococcal, streptococcal, H. influenzae, tuberculosis; proper cultures and microbiological studies should be carried out for confirmation.

(5) Complications and Prognosis: Empyema and pyopneumothorax from bronchopleural fistula are commonly seen in staphylococcal pneumonia as a result of rupture of pneumatoceles. Hematogenous spread of the infection to distant sites may result in osteomyelitis, meningitis and multiple metastatic abscesses. Pericarditis may be a result of direct extension from the pulmonary focus.

Prognosis of staphylococcal pneumonia depends greatly on the early recognition and institution of appropriate antimicrobial therapy. Even with the availability of β-lactamase resistant antibiotics such as semi-synthetic penicillins and cephalosporins, the mortality has been reported still as high as 10-20%. On the other hand, the long-term morbidity in survivors is low. The pneumatoceles which are commonly seen in staphylococcal pneumonia are generally asymptomatic and resolve spontaneously. As a rule, children recovered from staphylococcal pneumonia have normal growth and development and normal pulmonary functions in their later lives.

(6) Treatment: Upon completion of diagnostic studies, antimicrobial therapy should be instituted immediately without delay once staphylococcal pneumonia is suspected. Since most staphylococcal strains are resistant to penicillin G, nafcillin 60-120 mg/kg/day should be given intravenously. Other semisynthetic penicillins in appropriate dosages may also be used. If the staphylococcus turns out to be sensitive to penicillin G, this agent in a dosage of 150,000 to 200,000 units/kg/day may be used. Duration of therapy depends on the clinical response. In general, 3-4 weeks of therapy may be required. Supportive therapeutic measures in terms of oxygen inhalation for relief of cyanosis, fluid and electrolytes replacement are important.

Development of empyema and pyopneumothorax demands surgical intervention with insertion of a large caliber chest tube and application of closed suction for drainage. Instillation of antibiotics and/or enzymes such as deoxyribonuclease into the pleural cavity to hasten healing and promote drainage is of doubtful therapeutic value and may even produce systemic toxic reactions.

C. OTHER BACTERIAL PNEUMONIAS

Group A Beta-hemolytic streptococcus usually causes upper respiratory infections and is a rare cause of pneumonia. Following
viral infections, such as measles or epidemic influenza, group
A streptococci may invade the lower respiratory tract giving rise
to bronchitis, or bronchiolitis advancing to pneumonia. Clinically, the
child who begins with an upper respiratory infection develops intermittent fever, cough and dyspnea. Physical findings may consist of
scattered rales and patchy dullness together with roentgenographic
evidence of bronchopneumonia. Pathologically, streptococcal pneumonia is quite hemorrhagic and empyema is common. For treatment, penicillin in the same dosage as in pneumococcal pneumonia
is recommended.

Nontypable strains of Hemophilus influenzae organisms are common
inhabitants in the nasopharynx of normal children and H. influenzae
type b is capable of producing serious infections in infants and young
children such as acute epiglottitis and meningitis. However, primary H. influenzae pneumonia is not a common event. Only 1 of
833 cases of pneumonia admitted to the Children's Hospital in Philadelphia between 1965-1970 was caused by H. influenzae. H. influenzae pneumonia is usually of lobar distribution simulating pneumococcal pneumonia but invariably is accompanied by empyema. The
antimicrobial agent of choice is ampicillin 100-200 mg/kg/day or
chloramphenicol 25 mg/kg/day for newborns and 50-100 mg/kg/day
for older children given parenterally.

Klebsiella pneumoniae (Friedlander's bacillus) as a cause of pneumonia is rare in children. Even in adults, the incidence is probably
less than 1% of all pneumonias and occurs primarily in alcoholics
or chronic debilitated individuals. Bulging of the interlobular fis-
sure by effusion is a common roentgenographic sign. There is a tendency for abscess formation and empyema. E. coli pneumonia may
be seen in newborns as a consequence of septicemia or aspiration of
contaminated amniotic fluid. For antimicrobial therapy, kanamycin
15 mg/kg/day or gentamicin 5-7 mg/kg/day in divided doses is given.

II: NONBACTERIAL PNEUMONIAS

Clinical manifestations of nonbacterial pneumonias are in general
less acute and less severe than those associated with bacterial pneumonias. However, the differences may be more elusive than real.
Viral pneumonias are usually preceded by a mild upper respiratory
illness and the common nonspecific respiratory manifestations of
fever, cough, headache, malaise, anorexia are present. An etiologic
diagnosis is difficult as cultivation of nonbacterial agents and serologic procedures require more refined and sophisticated laboratory
facilities and personnel.

A. MYCOPLASMA PNEUMONIA

(1) <u>Etiology</u>: Mycoplasma is a cell wall deficient genus of microorganisms. Several mycoplasmas are found in the respiratory tract but <u>Mycoplasma</u> pneumoniae is the only pathogenic mycoplasma consistently shown to cause clinical infections in man. Growth of <u>M.</u> pneumoniae requires enriched medium with added horse serum and yeast extract. Optimal growth occurs at 35-37°C under anaerobic or aerobic conditions. Lacking a cell wall, <u>M. pneumoniae</u> is resistant to β-lactum antibiotics but is suceptible to antimicrobials which are able to inhibit protein synthesis such as tetracyclines and erythromycins. <u>M. pneumoniae</u> colonies are small and require magnification (50-70X) for visualization.

(2) <u>Epidemiology</u>: Mycoplasmal pneumonia occurs sporadically in all seasons. Its spread is by close contact such as in families or barrack type living facilities. Older children 5-14 years of age and young adults are primarily affected and the organism rarely causes pneumonia in infants. In the community, the family is the major epidemiologic unit into which a school child introduces the infection and it then spreads to other family members over an extended period of time. The majority of infected individuals have a lower respiratory tract illness with 30-50% of infections manifesting as pneumonia.

(3) <u>Pathology and Pathogenesis</u>: <u>M. pneumoniae</u> grows on the surface near the ciliated border of respiratory epithelial cells. The ability of the organism to produce peroxide might contribute to cell damage. There is also suggestive evidence that clinical illness may be a result of hypersensitivity or antigen-antibody reactions as immunodeficient patients appear to have less severe pneumonia. Since the mortality from mycoplasma pneumonia is very low, only limited information regarding pathologic findings is available. The chest x-ray may show interstitial pneumonia, patchy or confluent bronchopneumonia or lobar involvement. Microscopically mononuclear cells are seen in alveolar exudates as well as in peribronchial areas. Bronchiolar respiratory epithelium is usually intact and bacteria are infrequently seen. As a rule, no pathological changes are seen in organs other than the lungs.

(4) <u>Clinical Manifestations and Diagnosis</u>: Mycoplasma infections result in nonspecific respiratory infections such as pharyngitis, tracheobronchitis and bullous myringitis. However, pneumonia is the most commonly recognized and best described syndrome. The incubation period is about 2-3 weeks. Onset of illness is generally insidious with fever, malaise and a dry nonproductive cough. The patient does not appear seriously ill and can usually continue to carry on routine activities or attend classes. The tympanic membranes may be inflamed and bullae may be present. Auscultation of the lungs may reveal wheezes, rhonchi or moist rales in affected lung areas. However, the roentgenographic findings may show little correlation with auscultatory findings or are out of proportion to physical findings.

Diagnosis of mycoplasmal pneumonia on clinical grounds relies primarily in exclusion of other bacterial and viral pneumonias. Isolation of M. pneumoniae from pharyngeal swabs and sputum can be done but is time consuming. Routine laboratory examinations such as leukocyte differential counts and urinalysis are usually not helpful. A rise in cold agglutinin titer is a helpful but not a discriminating diagnostic aid, since other viral infections may result in elevated cold agglutinins. Only about 50-60% of patients with mycoplasma pneumonia may show positive cold agglutination antibody titers and this seems to occur more often in severely ill patients. Other serologic procedures such as complement fixation and growth inhibition tests against M. pneumoniae organisms can be performed but may not be available in many community hospital laboratories.

(5) Course and Complications: The clinical course of mycoplasmal pneumonia is usually a self-limited one with gradual defervescence and subsiding malaise and cough over a period of 2-3 weeks. Mortality is extremely low and complications are few.

In patients with unusually high cold agglutinin titers, coating of patient's own blood cells with the anti-I antibody may lead to intravascular hemolysis. A variety of other clinical syndromes involving all organ systems has been reported to be associated with mycoplasma infections. This includes meningoencephalitis, radiculopathy, erythema multiforme, Stevens-Johnson's syndrome, pericarditis, myocarditis, thrombocytopenia, arthritis and Guillain-Barre syndrome.

(6) Treatment and Prevention: In most cases of mycoplasma pneumonia, no specific treatment is necessary. By the time a confirmatory diagnosis is made, the patient is on the road to recovery. In several clinical studies, tetracycline 250 mg or its equivalent, q. 6 h. or erythromycin 500 mg. q. 8 h. have shown to be effective in shortening the clinical course with earlier disappearance of fever, malaise, cough and pulmonary infiltrates. Total recommended duration of therapy is 6-10 days. Since mycoplasma pneumonia is much less commonly seen than pneumococcal pneumonia, the use of tetracycline or erythromycin as the initial antibiotic for treatment of undifferentiated pneumonia is not advisable because strains of pneumococci resistent to these two antibiotics are known to occur. Although development of a vaccine against M. pneumoniae has been under investigation, no effective prophylactic program is available.

B. VIRAL PNEUMONIAS

(1) Etiology: Well over 100 viral agents have been shown to be associated with respiratory illnesses and pneumonias (see Chapter on URI). Respiratory syncytial virus and parainfluenza viruses are the most important agents causing severe respiratory infections and pneumonias in young children and infants. Influenza virus can produce primary pneumonia but more often the pneumonia following

epidemic influenza is a secondary bacterial infection. Adenoviruses, variola, varicella and measles can also cause primary viral pneumonias in children and adults. Cytomegalovirus has gained importance in recent years as a pathogen for viral pneumonitis particularly in immunosuppressed hosts following renal transplantation and chemotherapy for malignant diseases.

(2) Epidemiology: In an 8-year longitudinal epidemiologic study of lower respiratory infections in pediatric practice in Chapel Hill, N.C., Glezen and Denny have shown the infection rate is higher, 240 per 1000 children per year, in young infants under 1 year of age, compared to only 34 per 1000 per year in older children and adolescents. As expected, the seasonal peak of illnesses was in mid-winter to early spring with infrequent illnesses during the summer and increasing numbers of infections in early autumn. Among the 4 pathogens most frequently associated with lower respiratory illnesses in children, respiratory syncytial virus produced yearly epidemics of bronchiolitis and pneumonia in infants. Parainfluenza type 1 virus produced biannual epidemics of croup that peaked in the autumn of even numbered years. Parainfluenza type 3 virus was less predictable but it was associated with substantial numbers of cases of pneumonia and bronchiolitis in infants. The agent also caused croup in children 1 to 3 years of age and tracheobronchitis in older children. Mycoplasma pneumoniae infection was more likely to occur in autumn and winter as pneumonia but may occur in any season in school age children.

(3) Clinical Course and Diagnosis: The onset is usually insidious preceded by an upper respiratory illness but sometimes the onset may be sudden. Like most respiratory illnesses in children, cough, fever, listlessness, or irritability, anorexia, malaise are common findings. Physical signs are quite variable. Fever may or may not be present and respiration may be normal. Chest findings may be minimal, limited to medium moist rales and slight impairment of percussion notes or breath sounds. Laboratory findings and bacteriological cultures are generally not remarkable. Detection of the presence of pneumonitis usually requires the aid of roentgenographic examinations. The clinical course is usually benign and complete recovery within 1-3 weeks is to be expected. Complications are few but deaths have been reported.

Etiologic diagnosis can only be made by isolation of the viral agent from respiratory secretions or tissues and/or serologic tests measuring rise of antibody titer against specific viruses. Immunofluorescent staining of smears containing infected respiratory cells can offer more rapid etiologic diagnoses and this technique has been successfully applied in infections due to influenza, parainfluenza and respiratory syncytial viruses.

(4) Treatment and Prevention: Viral pneumonias do not respond to antimicrobial treatment. Supportive therapy with moist air, oxygen

and fluids is important. However, since the differentiation of viral from bacterial pneumonias is often difficult and any severe lower respiratory infection in young children carries a significant morbidity and mortality, cautious use of antimicrobial therapy in certain cases is justified. Other than influenza and certain types of adenoviruses, no practical respiratory vaccines are available to prevent these infections.

C. OTHER NONBACTERIAL PNEUMONIAS

Coxiella burnetii, a rickettsia, is the cause of Q fever. With good sanitary control of cattle raising and dairy products, this form of pneumonia is rarely seen today.

Fungi as etiologic agents for nonbacterial pneumonia usually manifest themselves as granulomatous disease in the lungs. Histoplasmosis, coccidioidomycosis and blastomycosis can also lead to systemic infections with fatal outcome. Cryptococcosis in its serious form is usually a chronic meningitis. In normal individuals, these fungal diseases are usually self-limiting and patients recover spontaneously without specific therapy. In disseminated disease, particularly in immunosuppressed hosts, amphotericin B or other antifungal therapy is needed.

Pneumocystis carinii is considered to be a protozoa. It has become an important cause of nonbacterial pneumonia in immunosuppressed patients. A confirmatory diagnosis can only be obtained by examination of lung biopsy specimens. For treatment, pentamidine isothionate is the drug of choice. It is not generally available for use in the United States but the drug may be obtained from the Center for Disease Control in Atlanta, Georgia. The recommended treatment regimen is 4 mg/kg/day given as a single dose intramuscularly for 10-15 days. The total dose should not exceed 56 mg/kg. Bone marrow suppression and transient azotemia have been reported as adverse effects. More recently, the combination of trimethoprim and sulfamethoxazole taken orally has been reported to be an effective therapy.

REFERENCES

Macleod, C.M.: The pneumococci: In Dubos, R., and Hirsch, J. (eds.): Bacterial and Mycotic Infections of Man. 4th ed. J.B. Lippincott Company, Philadelphia, 1965, Chap. 16.

Smith, M.H C.: Pneumococcal pneumonia: In Kendig, E.L., Jr. (ed.): Disorders of the Respiratory Tract in Children. 2nd ed. W.B. Saunders Company, Philadelphia, 1972.

Austrian, R. and Gold, J.: Pneumococcal bacteremia with especial reference to bacteremic pneumococcal pneumonia. Ann. Intern. Med. 60:759, 1964.

Jay, S.J., Johanson,W.G., Jr., Pierce, A.K.: The radiographic resolution of Streptococcus pneumoniae pneumonia. NEJM 293:798, 1975.

Ceruti, E., Contreras, J. and Neira, M.: Staphylococcal pneumonia in childhood; long-term follow-up. Am. J. Dis. Child. 122: 386, 1971.

Kevy, S.V., and Lowe, B.A.: Streptococcal pneumonia and empyema in childhood. NEJM 264:738, 1961.

Honig, P.J., Pasquariello, P.S., and Stool, S.E.: H. influenzae pneumonia in infants and children. J. Pediat. 83:215, 1973.

Tillotson, J.R.: Bacillary, anaerobic and opportunistic pneumonias: In Reimann, H.A. (ed.): Acute Respiratory Tract Diseases. Medcom Press, 1975, Chap. 4.

Utz, J.P.: Mycotic pneumonias: In Reimann, H.A. (ed.): Acute Respiratory Tract Diseases. Medcom Press, 1975, Chap. 5.

Liu, C.: Nonbacterial pneumonia: In Hoeprich, P.D. (ed.): Infectious Diseases. 1st ed. Harper and Row, New York, 1972, Chap. 30.

Foy, H.M., Grayston, J.T., Kenny, G.E., Alexander, E.R. and McMahan, R.: Epidemiology of Mycoplasma pneumoniae infection in families. JAMA 197:859, 1966.

Denny, F.W., Clyde, W.A., Jr., and Glezen, W.P.: Mycoplasma pneumoniae disease: clinical spectrum, pathophysiology, epidemiology, and control. J. Infect. Dis. 123:74, 1971.

Murray, H.W., Masur, H., Senterfit, L.B., et al.: The protean manifestations of Mycoplasma pneumoniae infection in adults. Am. J. Med. 58:229, 1975.

Reimann, H.A.: Chest cold or viral pneumonia? How to tell the difference. Mod. Med. 42:47, 1974.

Chernick, V. and Macpherson, R.I.: Respiratory syncytial and adenovirus infections of the lower respiratory tract in infancy. Clinical Notes on Respiratory Diseases. Vol. IV, No. 2, p. 3, 1971.

Davis, S.D. and Wedgewood, R.J.: Antibiotic prophylaxis in acute viral respiratory diseases. Am. J. Dis. Child. 109:544, 1965.

Gardner, P.S., Turk, D.C., Aherne, W.A. et al.: Death associated with respiratory tract infections in children. Br. Med. J. 4:316, 1967.

Glezen, W.P. and Denny, F.W.: Epidemiology of acute lower respiratory disease in children. NEJM 288:498, 1973.

Chanock, R.M. and Parrott, R.H.: Acute respiratory disease in infancy and childhood. Present understanding and prospects for prevention. Pediatrics 36:21, 1965.

Rosen, P.P., Martini, N. and Armstrong, D.: Pneumocystis carinii pneumonia. Am. J. Med. 58:794, 1975.

Weller, T.H.: The cytomegaloviruses: ubiquitous agents with protean clinical manifestations. NEJM 285:203, 1971.

CHAPTER 2. EAR, SINUS, AND EYE INFECTIONS

2.1: ACUTE SUPPURATIVE OTITIS MEDIA

INTRODUCTION: Acute suppurative otitis media may be defined as
an infection of the middle ear which results in the accumulation of
purulent fluid from which bacteria, frequently, and viruses, rarely,
can be cultured.

The incidence of this infection varies from one population or ethnic
group to another and the variables which account for these variances
are poorly understood. For example, of 847 British children studied
over a five-year period, 19% had at least one attack of otitis media
and one third of these had more than one attack during this period
(Miller, 1960). Otitis media was diagnosed in 22% of 734 new patient visits made to the medical emergency clinic at the Children's
Hospital Medical Center in Boston in 1960. This was the most common diagnosis and 59% of the children were under three years of
age (Bergman, 1962). This is similar to the age incidence noted by
Howie et al. (1970) where he found in 858 episodes of acute otitis
media, 25% occurred in the first year of life, and 22% in the second.
In another study of 772 children followed from birth (early infancy)
through $7\frac{1}{2}$ to $13\frac{1}{2}$ years of age, the peak incidence of otitis media
occurred between 1 and 2 years of age (18%), but there was no other
significant difference in yearly occurrences during the first 6 years
of life (Brownlee et al., 1969). The peak months of occurrence were
November through March with the maximum daily incidence occurring in February and the minimum in July.

In contrast with the incidence obtained from British and U.S. studies,
a study of 489 Alaskan Eskimo children followed for ten years showed
that 41% had perforations or scars of the tympanic membranes
(Kaplan, et al., 1973). A high prevalence of purulent otitis media
also has been noted among some of the Maori of New Zealand (Tonkin,
S., 1970), the Aborigines of Australia (Jose, D.G. et al., 1967),
and the American Indians. In some areas of one Navajo reservation,
50% of children had chronically perforated ear drums (Mortimer,
1973). By contrast, in East Africa chronic purulent otitis media is
uncommon even among desperately malnourished infants with infections such as measles, pneumonia and tuberculosis (Manning, et. al.,
1974). Other factors which may also affect the incidence of otitis
media are prematurity (Bland, et. al., 1972; Warren et al., 1971)
and the supine position in which some infants are fed (Beauregard,
1971).

1. ETIOLOGY AND PATHOGENESIS

<u>1.1: Etiology</u>: Bluestone and Shurin (1974) summarized etiologic data of otitis media based on isolation of bacterial pathogens from numerous studies in children. <u>Diplococcus pneumoniae</u> was the organism most frequently encountered, accounting for 40% (average) of isolates (range 25-50%), followed by Hemophilus influenzae (average 20%, range 15-25%) and Streptococcus pyogenes, group A (average 10%, range 0.3-24%). Of significance is the average number of cases of otitis from which no organisms could be cultured (25%, range 13-50%). It is known that middle ear exudate from children with otitis media inhibits bacterial growth (Lahikainen, E.A., 1953). The fluid contains immunoglobulins, as well as phagocytic cells, which presumably can eliminate the pathogenic bacteria and render the fluid sterile at the time of tympanocentesis. Another reason for sterile cultures can be attributed to viruses such as influenza and respiratory syncytial virus which have been cultured from the middle ear during epidemics. In the newborn and young infants a wide variety of gram negative bacteria can be cultured from infected middle ears so that one must rely on tympanocentesis and culture to direct rational therapy, because the more commonly encountered organisms such as <u>D. pneumoniae</u> and <u>H. influenzae</u> seen in older children are unusual causes of otitis media in very young infants.

<u>1.2: Pathogenesis</u>: Swallowing occurs from 1,000-1,200 times a day, and this function serves to open the eustachian tube and thereby equalize pressure on either side of the tympanic membrane. This allows for an evaporative or drying effect to occur for fluid which might be present in the middle ear cavity, as well as provide for drainage of fluid which may be physiologically secreted into that space. The amount of time the tube is open is brief, and the majority of the time the eustachian tube remains closed and thereby protects the middle ear from aspiration of nasopharyngeal secretions. Therefore, the eustachian tube has three functions: 1) ventilation, 2) drainage, and 3) protection. Middle ear infections may result when any or all three of these activities fail to function properly.

A patient may develop an upper respiratory infection initially characterized by rhinorrhea, sneezing, nasal congestion, and fever. After three to four days the child may develop fever to 39ºC, ear pain, and a physician after taking a history and examining the patient may diagnose acute suppurative otitis media. The infection probably develops in the following manner: the inflammatory reaction, presumably caused by a virus, may result in edema of the eustachian tube which in turn causes a negative pressure build-up in the middle ear cavity. The resultant atelectasis produces a middle ear effusion. The effusion becomes secondarily infected with bacteria which, because of higher than usual negative pressure, are drawn in from the nasopharynx by sneezing or nose blowing. It is also postulated that bacteria may invade the middle ear from the blood stream and lymphatics. Continued obstruction of the tube, plus multiplication of bacteria in the middle ear with persistent effusion, produce the signs and symptoms of otitis media.

Eustachian tube "floppiness" or increased compliance can result in a chronically collapsed tube and thereby cause a functional obstruction. In these cases nasopharyngeal secretions might be aspirated into the middle ear cavity when ventilation occurs because of a high negative pressure "pulling" from the middle ear cavity. This particular type of eustachian tube dysfunction is frequently seen in children with a cleft palate. Furthermore, the problem of over compliance can be compounded by feeding the child in the supine position.

Children with imperfect host defenses, such as those with an immune deficiency or those receiving immunosuppressive agents, are obviously more predisposed to ear infections, as well as many other infections. On the other hand, there are a large number of "otitis prone" children in whom no mechanical, immune, allergic, etc. defect can be noted and who continue to have repeated bouts of otitis for reasons which are not clear (Howie and Ploussard, 1975).

2. CLINICAL MANIFESTATIONS

As noted above, children may frequently present with the signs and symptoms of a viral respiratory illness which progresses to otitis media. Other children may have an accompanying cough, suggesting the presence of both an upper and a lower respiratory tract infection. Some children present with vomiting and diarrhea as the only sign of otitis media, whereas in others the only presenting sign may be irritability. Fever is a variable sign and was absent in 33% to 57% of infants and children with bacteriologically proven otitis media (Rowe, 1975). In older children, the verbal complaint of earache may be an indication of otitis media, but otitis externa can also cause this symptom. Ear pulling or slapping at the ear in an infant or young child is not a reliable indication of otitis media. Some children pull on their ears out of habit, and it is uncommon to find ear manipulation to be associated with otitis media in the absence of other signs and symptoms. Hearing loss may also be a presenting symptom but rarely in the absence of a prior history of multiple infections.

Acute suppurative otitis media may resolve successfully in time without therapy of any sort. An unknown percentage of cases will undergo spontaneous rupture of the tympanic membrane due to ischemic necrosis, with subsequent drainage of pus and resolution of the process usually within a few weeks. Others may rupture but develop a chronic perforation and drainage which may progress to form a cholesteatoma. In other children the infection will resolve spontaneously without any evidence of perforation - they simply get well.

Perhaps the most commonly encountered complication is secretory or chronic serous otitis media which, if not dealt with adequately, can produce a conductive hearing loss. If the fluid is allowed to remain in the middle ear long enough, it will organize and produce a severe conductive loss secondary to immobilization of the middle ear ossicles. In Kaplan's study of Eskimo children (1973) significant hearing losses were present in 16% of patients studied. This figure jumps to approximately 50% in children and adults with a cleft palate. Although not a complication in the classic sense of the word, early recurrences (relapses) within two weeks to one month after initial successful treatment occur in 2%-5% of cases and later recurrences are more common. Furthermore, the bacteria which are cultured from middle ear aspirates during recurrences are often different from those isolated during the previous episode (Rowe, 1975).

Other complications include mastoiditis, lateral sinus thrombosis, brain abscess, and subdural empyema. However, since the antibiotic era, these latter complications have occurred with decreasing frequency to the point that they are now considered rare. Meningitis is also a complication of otitis, but it is not uncommon to have children present with both problems simultaneously and, under these circumstances, when the antecedent illness is limited to a few days and has the characteristics of an upper respiratory infection, it is difficult to say which preceded which or whether the two are causally related. Any suspicion of meningitis, even in a child with otitis media, warrants a spinal tap. This is especially true if the child is noted to be irritable rather than simply fussy.

3. DIAGNOSIS

The identification of acute suppurative otitis media, especially in the early stages, can often be difficult and perplexing, even to the experienced clinician. The child who presents with ear pain, fever $39.5^{\circ}C$, rhinorrhea, vomiting, and a bright red, bulging ear drum with loss of landmarks, is very easily identified as having acute suppurative otitis media. However, if the symptoms are minimal and the drum is inflamed but not bulging and the landmarks (light reflex, umbo, manubrium of the malleus, and short process) are present or only minimally altered or obscured, then one has difficulty deciding between an early otitis, myringitis, or myringitis with some degree of fluid in the middle ear.

If the child has myringitis alone, the ear drum may be red with an accentuation of the erythema around the annulus. There may be increased vascularization of the tympanic membrane and this is especially prominent on the manubrium of the malleolus. The drum may also be retracted and the short process is thereby made more prominent. Occasionally, the tympanic membrane takes on a blueish coloration and may have bullae on one or more areas of the drum. Since bacteria have been cultured from patients who present with bullous myringitis (Rowe. 1975), the presence of bullae is not a reliable sign of a nonbacterial or viral otitis. If the myringitis is accompanied by fluid in the middle ear, the condition may then be referred to as serous or secretory otitis media. It is not as common to encounter increased vascularization in this condition as it is in simple myringitis and, in serous otitis, bubbles or air fluid levels may also be present behind the drum. Neither myringitis nor serous otitis should be treated with antibiotics, but if bullae are noted on the drum, it is probably wiser to assume that a suppurative condition exists and treat with antibiotics, since more cases of bullae on the drum involve bacteria than do not.

Perhaps the best single criteria for diagnosing acute suppurative otitis media is bulging of the drum with loss of landmarks. It must be emphasized that erythema, like fever, need not be present. The use of the pneumatic otoscope and noting the degree to which the tympanic membrane moves when exposed to positive and negative pressure can give an indication of whether fluid is present in the middle ear, but it obviously cannot distinguish between sterile and purulent fluid. The electro-acoustic impedance bridge (tympanometer) is an electronic device which gives objective and quantifiable information regarding the compliance of the tympanic membrane, as well as the amount of positive or negative pressure which exists in the middle ear cavity. Both this device and pneumatic otoscopy would seem to have more use in following the resolution of acute suppurative otitis media, or in identifying cases of serous otitis following a bout of acute otitis, than it would in making the initial diagnosis of pus in the middle ear cavity.

In equivocal cases, tympanocentesis with culture of any fluid is the most reliable way to establish the diagnosis. But even this is not 100% effective because as noted above, host defense mechanisms can render previously infected middle ear fluid sterile. There are, however, patients in whom tympanocentesis is mandatory for diagnosis and proper management, and those are newborns and young infants up to the age of three months. As stated previously, these children have an unpredictable and wide variety of etiological organisms causing their disease. To treat without first identifying the agent puts the patient at the risk of having the wrong antibiotic prescribed and an increased incidence of complications or even death. Most authors would agree that otitis in the neonate and in the immunologically compromised host, as well as otitis that continues in the patient who is already receiving antibiotics, are absolute indications for myringotomy. Other less widely agreed upon indications are failure of medical management as defined by two ten-day courses of antibiotics with no resolution of the infection, the onset of severe pain unrelieved by analgesics, and suppurative complications.

To wait for two full courses of antibiotics before deciding that medical management has failed seems an unduly long period of time, causes the patient unnecessary morbidity, and possibly increases the risk of suppurative complications. The common practice of giving codeine or other analgesics to relieve the pain of a bulging drum rather than taking the few minutes to relieve the pressure with a needle or myringotomy knife seems at the very least not in the patient's best interest. Performing a myringotomy after a suppurative complication has occurred is similar to closing the corral gate after the horses have fled. Therefore, it is the opinion of this author that myringotomy or tympanocentesis should be used far more liberally than is currently the practice, and that this in turn may decrease the morbidity, complications, and lessen the need for multiple courses of antibiotics in patients with otitis media.

4. MANAGEMENT

The patient who presents with unequivocal signs and symptoms including a red bulging drum with loss of landmarks but no ear pain, should be treated with one of the following antibiotic regimens.

Ampicillin in a dose of 75-100 mg/kg per day in 4 divided doses for 14 days is recommended for children 6 years of age and under. However, if a patient develops recurrent episodes of otitis after consecutive courses with ampicillin, it is suggested that a course of erythromycin 50 mg/kg/day plus sulfisoxazole 100-150 mg/kg/day for 14 days be tried before the child is placed on any prophylaxis or before surgical intervention of any sort has been attempted. For children over 6 years of age, oral phenoxymethyl penicillin is recommended in a dose of 50 mg/kg/day for 14 days. A combination of phenoxymethyl penicillin and sulfisoxazole in the above mentioned doses is also acceptable therapy.

For the patient who presents with a "classically" appearing drum and also has ear pain, the author recommends that a myringotomy/tympanocentesis be performed immediately, the fluid cultured, and sensitivities determined. This has the advantage of affording the patient immediate and dramatic relief of pain and accurately directs the physician's prescribing of antibiotics should his initial choice prove to be ineffective against the organism cultured.

The patient who has equivocal signs of otitis media should ideally be treated conservatively with aspirin or acetaminophen for fever and/or fussiness, and seen again in 12 to 24 hours. After that period of time the physician may be in a position to act definitively. However, the ideal situation may be jeopardized by poor patient follow-up and poor compliance. Under these latter circumstances, pneumatic otoscopy and the use of an electro-acoustic impedance tympanometry may be of value in helping the physician decide whether he will or will not prescribe antibiotics.

If the patient is an infant in the first three months of life and has even equivocal signs of otitis, it is mandatory to perform a tympanocentesis and begin the child on antibiotics prior to return of the culture results.

Patient follow-up is important. Ideally the patient should be checked in two to three days and if there has been no resolution of the bulging and no return of at least a few of the landmarks, then a tympanocentesis/myringotomy should be performed and antibiotics prescribed on the basis of culture results. The patient should again be rechecked in two to three weeks unless the mother indicates the child's course is not going as predicted. In this case the drum should be reexamined and an attempt made to determine if fluid still remains in the middle ear. Here the pneumatic otoscope and the electro-acoustic impedence bridge have their greatest usefullness. If fluid is known to be present, then a change in antibiotics and/or tympanocentesis should be performed if not done previously.

If at the two to three week check the drum appears perfectly normal and moves readily on pneumatic otoscopy, then the child's acute infection is considered to have completely resolved. If, on the other hand, signs of infection are still present, prolonging the antibiotics for another week and rechecking the ear seems reasonable, with another examination afer completion of the antibiotics. If, on the other hand, the signs of infection have resolved and one notes or strongly suspects that fluid remains in the middle ear, then a two- to six-week course of a decongestant such as ephedrine or pseudoephedrine is recommended. Following this, if fluid still remains or is suspected, the patient should be referred to an ENT specialist for audiometric testing and consideration of placement of tympanostomy tubes. Some studies have shown minimal benefit and/or equivocal results when decongestants, with or without the addition of antihistamine, are used in treating the initial attack of acute suppurative otitis media. At present there is insufficient data to support the use of decongestants and antihistamines initially and their current usage should be confined to the management of serous or secretory otitis media. However, a recent study (Olson, 1976) of the use of Sudafed® demonstrated no benefit either in preventing the development of serous otitis media or in its treatment. Before decongestants and antihistamines are judged to be ineffective, other investigators should replicate Olson's findings with Sudafed and other drugs of this class and insure that therapeutic drug levels have been achieved.

Tonsillectomy is contraindicated for any type of otitis media - acute suppurative or serous/secretory (McKee, 1963). Adenoidectomy can be helpful if it is demonstrated that the adenoids are causing chronic obstruction of the eustachian tube. Adenoidectomy will not benefit children who preoperatively show reflux of contrast medium from the nasopharynx into the middle ear (Bluestone, 1922). In general adenoidectomy is not recommended until it has been demonstrated that adequate medical therapy has failed.

From the standpoint of prognosis, children with allergy and cleft palate are at a decided disadvantage from the standpoint of both repeated infections and hearing loss and, presumably, an increased incidence of suppurative complications. This would also apply to the immunologically compromised host. Other children, if managed as recommended, have a very low percentage of complications. Some children, although properly managed with each infection, have recurrent infections, e.g., six infections in one year. Sulfasoxazole prophylaxis 500 mg p.o. bid (Perrin, 1974) has been shown to be effective in reducing the rate of recurrence in these children.

REFERENCES

Beauregard, W.G.: Positional Otitis Media, Pediatr. Vol. 79, 1971, p. 294.

Bergman, A.B., Haggerty, R.J.: The Emergency Clinic, Am. J. Dis. Child, Vol. 104, July 1962, 36-44.

Bland, R.D., et al.: Otisis Media in the First Six Weeks of Life: Diagnosis, Bacteriology, and Management, Pediatrics, Vol. 49, 1972, p. 187.

Bluestone, C.D.: Eustachian Tube Obstruction in the Infant With Cleft Palate, Ann. Otol. Rhinol. Laryngol., Vol. 80, Suppl. 2, 1971.

Bluestone, C.D.: Prevalence and Pathogenesis of Ear Disease and Hearing Loss, In Cleft Palate: Ear Disease and Hearing Loss, Graham, M., ed., Charles C Thomas, Springfield, 1974.

Bluestone, C.D., et al.: Eustachian Tube Function as Related to Adenoidectomy for Otitis Media, Trans. Amer. Acad. Ophthal., Vol. 76, 1972, pp. 1325-1339.

Brownlee, R.C., et al.: Otitis Media in Children: Incidence, Treatment, and Prognosis in Pediatric Practice, J. Pediatr., Vol. 75, 1969, p. 636.

Howie, V.M., et al.: Otitis Media: A Clinical and Bacteriological Correlation, Pediatrics, Vol. 45, 1970, pp. 29-35.

Howie, V.M., Ploussard, J.H.: The "Otitis-Prowe" Condition, Am. J. Dis. Child., Vol. 129, June 1975.

Jose, D.G., et al.: A Survey of Children and Adolescents on Queensland Aboriginal Settlements, 1967, Aust. Pediatric Journal, Vol. 5, 1969, p. 71.

Kaplan, G.J., et al.: Long-term Effects of Otitis Media: A Ten Year Cohort Study of Alaskan Eskimo Children, Pediatrics, Vol. 52, 1973, p. 577.

Lahikainen, E.A.: Clinical-Bacteriologic Studies on Acute Otitis Media: Aspiration of Tympanum as Diagnostic and Therapeutic Method, Acta Otolaryng. Suppl. 107, 1953, p. 1.

Manning, P., et al.: Purulent Otitis Media: Differences Between Populations in Different Environments, Pediatrics, Vol. 53, No. 2, February 1974, p. 135.

McKee, W.J.E.: The Part Played by Adenoidectomy in the Combined Operation of Tonsillectomy With Adenoidectomy: Second Part of a Controlled Study in Children, British J. Prev. Soc. Med., Vol. 17, 1963, pp. 133-140.

Miller, F.J.W., et al.: Growing Up in Newcastle Upon Tyne London, published for the Nuffield Foundation by the Oxford University Press, 1960, p. 219.

Mortimer, E.A.: Indian Health: An Unmet Problem, Pediatrics, Vol. 51, 1973, p. 1065.

Olson, A., Klein, S., Charney, E., Mac-Whinney, J., McInerny, T., Miller, R., and Nazarian, L.: Prevention and Therapy of Serous Otitis Media by Oral Decongestant: A Double Blind Study in Pediatric Practice. Presented at the Sixteenth Annual Meeting of the Ambulatory Pediatric Association, April 1976.

Perrin, J.M., et al.: Sulfisoxazole as Chemoprophylaxis for Recurrent Otitis Media: A Double-Blind Crossover Study in Pediatric Practice, NEJM, Vol. 29, No. 13, September 26, 1974.

Roddey, O.F., et al.: Myringotomy in Acute Otitis Media, A Controlled Study, JAMA, Vol. 197, pp. 849-853.

Rowe, D.S.: Acute Suppurative Otitis Media, Pediatrics, Vol. 56, No. 2, August 1975.

Tonkin, S.: Maori Infant Health: II Study of Morbidity and Medico-Social Aspects, New Zealand Medical Journal, Vol. 72, 1970, p. 229.

Warren, W.S., et al.: Otitis Media in Low-Birth Weight Infants, J. Pediatr., Vol. 79, 1971, p. 740.

:::

2.2: SINUSITIS

INTRODUCTION: Sinusitis, or the infection of the cranial sinuses, is a disease not frequently diagnosed in infancy or childhood, partly because it is probably overlooked on occasion. An understanding of sinusitis in childhood requires a review of the developmental anatomy of the cranial sinuses.

During gestation the lateral walls of the nasal cavities divide to form the ethmoid and the maxillary sinuses. These paranasal sinuses form as evaginations of the mucous membranes and are lined by a continuation of the respiratory epithelium of the nasal cavities.

Development of the maxillary sinus begins at 3 months gestation as an outpouching from the lateral wall of the ethmoid infundibulum. At birth, it measures 3-4 mm laterally, 8-10 anteroposterior, and 3-5 mm vertically. Its growth is proportional to the body of the maxilla, and by 9 yrs. it measures 25 x 18 x 18 mm.

The ethmoidal sinus is always present at birth and ethmoidal sinusitis can occur in early infancy. Development is six to seven months gestation when definite spaces arise from recesses in the lateral walls of the middle, superior, and supreme meatuses.

The sphenoidal sinus also appears at 3 mo. gestation as an outgrowth of the posterosuperior part of the spheno-ethmoidal recess. At birth it has no clinical significance and grows slowly in the first 4-5 years, reaching adult size during adolescence. It is important to remember its intimate relationship with the ophthalmic and maxillary nerves.

Arising from the frontal recess or the anterosuperior extension of the middle meatus of the nose is the frontal sinus. Development begins around the third to fourth fetal month. This sinus is rarely recognizable at birth and may not be present until two to three years of age. The frontal sinus is commonly absent or underdeveloped. Frontal sinusitis rarely occurs before five to six years of age and usually not until ten to twelve years of age.

1. ETIOLOGY AND PATHOGENESIS

Acute purulent sinusitis is not likely to occur prior to two to three years of age, and most infections occur in school-age youngsters. Predisposing factors include an imperforate choana, a deviated nasal septum, allergic rhinitis, polyps, foreign bodies and tumors. Individuals who are debilitated or have poor resistance are candidates for infection. Swimming and diving, particularly jumping feet first into the water, may also be a predisposing factor. An acute upper respiratory infection is a precipitating factor, as can be fractures in the area of the sinuses followed by secondary infection. Nasal allergy is thought to play a major role in some children. Finally, enlarged adenoids are a common, predisposing factor because they trap nasal and sinus secretions which then stagnate and become infected. Contrary to sinusitis in adults, infected teeth are rarely a cause of sinusitis in children! Sinusitis has also been shown to be more common in children with cyanotic congenital heart disease, in association with bacterial endocarditis and brain abscess. (Rosenthal and Fellows, 1973) Also, ethmoidal and/or frontal sinusitis are commonly associated with orbital cellulitis (Haynes and Cramblett, 1967).

Sinuses become contaminated with bacterial pathogens usually by direct spread from the nasal cavity to the mucous membranes of the sinus. The ostium of the sinus may become obstructed because of the edema around it. The edema, plus a change in the pH, lead to decreased activity of the cilia resulting in stagnation of the secretions. Early changes consist of an inflammatory exudate with edema of the mucous membranes, marked hyperemia, and perivascular infiltration of polymorphonuclear leukocytes. There is also hyperemia of the mucous glands. Later, areas of hemorrhage may appear. If the infection is resolved early, there is usually little permanent damage. If not, ulceration and ultimately scarring of the surface epithelium may occur. Moreover, the periosteum may become involved, leading to bone necrosis and soft tissue abscesses.

Common pathogens in sinusitis during childhood include alpha- and beta-hemolytic streptococci, Diplococcus pneumoniae, Staphylococcus aureus, Hemophilus influenzae, and rarely Escherichia coli. Data regarding the incidence of infection caused by various etiologic agents in children are not available. However, in Axillson's study of maxillary sinusitis in adults, he found pneumococci in 35%, H. influenzae in 17%, anaerobic streptococci in 6% and no growth in 25%, with staphlococci being found as a normal flora (1973).

2. CLINICAL MANIFESTATIONS

Early sinusitis may be clinically indistinguishable from acute purulent rhinitis. Commonly, one sees a purulent nasal drainage, nasal obstruction, coughing and sneezing. The nasal discharge may be associated with epistaxis. The patient may develop fever, sore throat, leukocytosis, and signs and symptoms of acute otitis media, or acute laryngotracheobronchitis may be present.

Older children with maxillary sinusitis may complain of pain in the cheek referable to the teeth, or of headache on the affected side. The cheek may be flushed and swollen with tenderness over the antrum.

Before five years of age, infection of the frontal sinus is rare. However, in older children, the symptoms of frontal sinusitis are the same as in an adult. The patient complains of tenderness on pressure of the forehead overlying the sinus, a severe headache during the day with decreased intensity at night, and a fullness or heaviness with increased pain upon coughing or nose-blowing.

There are, unfortunately, no localizing symptoms in ethmoiditis in the younger child, while older children may complain of pain over one side of the nose and behind the eye. The presence of orbital cellulitis should always alert the clinician to the possibility of frontal or ethmoidal sinusitis.

Sphenoidal sinusitis in pediatric patients is extremely rare.

3. DIAGNOSIS

Upon examination of the patient, the nasal mucosa appears red and swollen, and a mucopurulent discharge may be present. Pus in the middle meatus is suggestive of paranasal sinus disease. Transillumination of the paranasal sinuses is unreliable in children less than twelve years old. The roentgenogram is a useful diagnostic aid, especially in maxillary, frontal and sphenoidal sinusitis and may be used to assess the initial extent of involvement and in following the response to therapy (Kogutt M.S. and Swischuk, L.E., 1973).

Complications of sinusitis do not occur as frequently since the advent of the antibiotic era. However, the child with sinusitis may develop lower respiratory disease such as chronic bronchitis, bronchopneumonia, and bronchiectasis. Associated infections include otitis media, osteomyelitis, and an orbital soft-tissue infection. Other complications or associated infections include pneumonia, acute bronchitis, lung abscess, acute pharyngitis, acute laryngitis and pyelitis, phlyctenular conjunctivitis, uveitis, panophthalmitis, and optic neuritis. Rarely, extradural, subdural, or cerebral abscesses, thrombosis of venous sinuses or meningitis may occur.

4. TREATMENT

Most authors strongly advocate a conservative approach to management of sinus infections in childhood. Bed rest in a well humidified room is recommended, with aspirin for fever but no other analgesics. Decongestants, both systemic and topical, such as phenylephrine, ephedrine and oxymetazoline may be useful. The nasal discharge should be aspirated prior to application of topical decongestants and the child should be upright. Topical decongestants such as phenylephrine should not be used for more than three or four days because of the possibility of rebound phenomenon. In older children, the nostrils may be packed three times a day with cotton soaked in a vasoconstrictor. The packs should be placed in the middle meatus. A dry heat lamp for 10 minutes, three to four times a day, may also be of benefit.

An appropriate antibiotic should be administered, the choice being based on culture and sensitivity whenever possible. Cultures may be obtained by sampling the middle and inferior meatuses. If antibiotics are begun before the culture is obtained, ampicillin in doses of 50-100 mg/Kg/day is the drug of choice.

The resolution of acute purulent sinusitis will usually take place with simple, conservative treatment. However, once in a while, either because of a failure to recognize and treat or a lack of response to therapy, a child will develop chronic sinusitis. If the problem persists past the acute stage, irrigation of the maxillary sinus may be indicated. However, surgery is to be avoided if at all possible, and is never indicated in acute sinusitis.

The symptoms of the chronic sinusitis include nasal discharge and obstruction with usually no complaint of pain or headache. Associated findings may include cough, hoarseness, cervical lymphadenitis, chronic dacryocystitis and conjunctivitis, weight loss, irritability, epistaxis, apathy, and dullness in schoolwork. Diagnosis is made from the history, findings on nasal examination and roentgenograms. If there is fluid in the maxillary sinus, a diagnostic puncture may be done. Again, therapy is conservative. The membranes in the area of the natural sinus openings should be shrunk. The antrum may need to be washed once or twice, and Proetz displacement may be indicated. Parenteral antibiotics are the treatment of choice and surgery is to be undertaken only as a last resort.

With adequate therapy, most sinusitis in children will resolve with little or no damage to the sinuses, and prognosis for recovery is excellent.

REFERENCES

Axelsson, A. and Brorson, J.E.: The Correlation Between Bacteriological Findings in the Nose and Maxillary Sinus in Acute Maxillary Sinusitis, Laryngoscope 83:2003-2011, 1973.

Bernstein, L.: Pediatric Sinus Problems, Otolaryng. Clin. N.A., February 1977, pp. 127-142.

Evans, F., Syndor, J.B., Moore, W., et al.: Sinusitis of the Maxillary Antrum, NEJM 293:735-739, 1975.

Friedberg, J.: Maxillary Sinus Disease in the Pediatric Patient, Otolaryng. Clin. N.A., February 1976, pp. 163-172.

Haynes, R.E. and Cramblett, H.: Acute Ethmoiditis, Am. J. Dis. Child. 114:261-267, 1967.

Hoshaw, T. and Nickman, N.: Sinusitis and Otitis in Children, Arch. Otolaryng. 100:194-195, 1974.

Kogutt, M.S. and Swischuk, L.E.: Diagnosis of Sinusitis, Pediatrics 52:121-124, 1973.

Rosenthal, A. and Fellows, K.E.: Acute Sinusitis in Cyanotic Congenital Heart Disease, Pediatrics 52:692, 1973.

:::

2.3: CONJUNCTIVITIS

INTRODUCTION: Conjunctivitis is defined as inflammation of the conjunctiva, the delicate membrane that lines the eyelids (palpebral conjunctiva) and covers the exposed surface of the eye (bulbar or ocular

conjunctiva). Conjunctivitis is a common problem during infancy
and childhood. There are two broad categories of conjunctivitis -
infectious and noninfectious. Included in the latter group are physical and chemical causes such as exposure to acids, lye, aerosol
spray, etc.; neoplasms (carcinomas, melanomas, and rhabdomyo-
sarcomas); and, finally, allergic causes. Allergic conjunctivitis,
along with bacterial and viral infections, comprise the majority of
cases of conjunctivitis in infants and children.

Accurate diagnosis and proper therapy are dependent upon obtaining
a complete history and performing a thorough examination of the
entire anterior segment of the eye. Ideally, two smears of conjunctival epithelial cells should be made, staining one with gram stain
for microorganisms and the other with Wright or Giemsa stain for
cytology. A predominance of neutrophils may indicate a bacterial
infection, whereas mononuclear cells are more likely indicative of
a viral infection, and eosinophils or basophils are found in association with allergic conjunctivitis.

1. NEONATAL CONJUNCTIVITIS

True ophthalmia neonatorum is caused by Neisseria gonorrhoeae, although chlamydial and staphylococcal organisms may also cause infectious conjunctivitis in the neonatal period (Armstrong, J.A. et
al., 1976). Gonococcal ophthalmia is usually acquired upon passage
through the birth canal and manifests by the second or third day of
life. It is an acute process producing a profuse, purulent discharge
from the eyes, marked lid edema and hyperemia. The bacterial
toxins are capable of destroying and perforating the cornea, resulting in blindness. The diagnosis is made by scrapings and culture.
Treatment with systemic penicillin should be instituted immediately.
Adequate prophylaxis can be achieved with instillation of a 1% solution of silver nitrate (Crede method) just after delivery. However,
this procedure is not infallible and it is estimated that even with silver nitrate prophylaxis, the risk of gonococcal ophthalmia neonatorium
is still slightly less than 2% for infants born of infected mothers.

The most common cause of conjunctivitis during the neonatal period,
occurring usually between the 5th and 9th day of life, is Chlamydia
occulogenitalis. Like gonococcal ophthalmia, this infection is contracted upon passage through the birth canal. The symptoms are a
purulent, papillary conjunctivitis with a sterile discharge and scrapings. The diagnosis is made when cytoplasmic inclusion bodies are
seen in the conjunctival scrapings. Topically applied sulfonamides
are most effective in treating chlamydial ophthalmia.

The majority of the time the etiology of conjunctivitis during the neonatal period remains uncertain (44% of cases in Armstrong and colleagues' study, 1976). Staphylococcus aureus was thought to be the
cause of approximately 10% of the cases in their series, and a variety
of other bacterial species were isolated from conjunctival cultures.

2. BACTERIAL CONJUNCTIVITIS

Although there is no specific incidence data available, staphylococcal conjunctivitis is thought to be the most common cause of bacterial conjunctivitis in children. In the acute form, there may be a purulent discharge with scaling of lid margins with a yellow crust, and congested blood vessels. Fissuring and ulceration of the skin about the orbit are common, and marginal corneal ulcerations can occur. Staphylococcus aureus infections of the eye, especially associated with blepharitis, may also lead to a chronic conjunctival inflammatory process, with styes, meibomitis, trichiasis, marginal corneal infiltrates, ulcers and epithelial keratitis. Topical antibiotics are recommended for children with blepharitis and suspected staphylococcal infections in order to reduce the risk of chronic infections.

Diplococcus pneumoniae is a common cause of "pink eye" seen in school age children. The inflammatory process is characterized by hyperemia with petechial and subconjunctival hemorrhages. The cornea is usually unaffected and the infection responds well to topical applications of sulfonamides.

The Koch-Weeks bacillus, also known as Haemophilus aegyptius, is a cause of conjunctivitis in warm, tropical climates, most commonly in the spring and fall months. It can produce severe conjunctivitis with a mucopurulent discharge, lid edema, photophobia and blepharospasm. The treatment of choice for this infection is topical application of 0.1% polymyxin B sulfate.

Other bacterial organisms rarely associated with conjunctivitis are Streptococcus pyogenes, group A, Neisseria meningitidis and Corynebacterium diphtheriae.

3. VIRAL CONJUNCTIVITIS

Adenoviruses are throught to be the most common cause of viral conjunctivitis in infants and children. Infection is most commonly manifest by a mild, follicular conjunctivitis, unaccompanied by systemic manifestations. This conjunctivitis will clear spontaneously in 7 to 10 days unless a secondary bacterial infection becomes superimposed. Most of the adenovirus types causing disease in children have been implicated in this condition. Adenoviruses also produce conjunctivitis in association with pharyngoconjunctival fever. This infection is characterized by the triad of fever, pharyngitis and follicular conjunctivitis. Although associated with Type 3 adenovirus, other types have been shown to produce a similar condition in children and young adults. A third type of conjunctivitis produced by adenovirus is the so-called epidemic keratoconjunctivitis, which is generally associated with Type 8 adenovirus. Epidemics in the western world have usually originated in a physician's office, clinic or dispensary (Dawson, G. and Darrell, R., 1963). The infection is characterized by hyperemia and edema of the conjunctiva along with photophobia and profuse tearing, which lasts for approximately 48 hours. Thereafter, a follicular conjunctivitis appears which sometimes leads to membrane formation (membranous conjunctivitis). The cornea can become affected, studded with epithelial lesions and sub-epithelial infiltrates, which disappear and reappear over a period of weeks to months.

A follicular conjunctivitis also occurs with Herpesvirus hommis, Types I and II infections. However, the importance of these viruses relates not to the conjunctivitis which they can produce, but to the keratitis resulting in punctate erosions or dendritic figures in the epithelium overlying the cornea. Prompt recognition of corneal infections is mandatory, and fluorescein should be applied to the eye in suspicious cases in order to demonstrate areas of denuded epithelium, which will stain green. Treatment of herpes keratitis includes debridement of infected epithelium, use of topical iododeoxyuridine (IDU) every two hours and IDU ointment at night, cycloplegics to control iridocyclitis, and sometimes the addition of steroids for iritis. Patients with herpes infections are best managed by an ophthalmologist.

Two common exanthems of childhood are associated with conjunctivitis. Along with the telltale exanthem and Koplik's spots of measles, a child may develop a catarrhal conjunctivitis with a mucopurulent discharge. Conjunctivitis may be especially prominent during the prodromal period. When accompanied by photophobia, the cornea may be involved. However, no therapy is usually required. During varicella, vesicles may form on the lid margins, but the cornea is rarely involved. In both instances, topical sulfonamides may be used to prevent secondary infection.

Another group of viruses, the so-called psittacosis-lymphogranuloma-trachoma or PLT group, are frequently associated with conjunctivitis and other types of eye infections. Trachoma is seen widely in the Orient but is uncommon in the U.S., except in areas of the Southwest, on Indian reservations, and in Arizona and New Mexico. One study of Navajo Indians revealed that about 50% of adults showed signs of past or present infection. Also there is an increased incidence in the 14-19 year old age group, predominantly in females, suggesting eye cosmetics as a possible source of contamination. The causal agent is a virus-like organism belonging to the PLT group intermediate between rickettsiae and true viruses. Although most infections are mild, the disease can involve progressive stages of acute catarrhal conjunctivitis with the development of follicles, papillary hypertrophy and corneal involvement with vascular invasion. This results in cicatricial changes and total corneal vascularization. Scrapings of epithelium demonstrate cytoplasmic inclusion bodies, while follicle material shows large macrophages and lymphoblasts. The treatment includes systemic sulfonamides for two weeks, with topical antibiotics four times daily for 6 weeks.

Another PLT agent is thought to be responsible for "swimming pool conjunctivitis." This is an inclusion conjunctivitis with a follicular conjunctival response. This infection responds to topical sulfonamides.

It is probable that another agent from the PLT group causes Cat Scratch Disease. This is often associated with a minimal conjunctival erythema and purulent exudate. However, granulomatous lesions can occur in the conjunctiva and are associated with preauricular adenopathy on the affected side. Antibiotics and steroids are of no value. Like the conjunctivitis of Cat Scratch Disease, Parinaud's conjunctivitis is also unilateral and associated with preauricular adenopathy and tenderness on the same side. This conjunctivitis may be catarrhal or follicular, and ptosis of the upper lid may be present. The conjunctiva may in time become granulomatous, and the parotid gland is usually enlarged. A variety of etiologic agents have been implicated in this condition and at present it is probably best recognized as simply a clinical entity associated with conjunctivitis, preauricular adenopathy and parotid gland enlargement.

Conjunctivitis is also a complication of vaccinia, occurring in approximately 1 out of 40,000 vaccinations. Lesions may appear on the lids as white, umbilicated pustules surrounded by edema and redness, accompanied by preauricular adenopathy. Conjunctival lesions are usually excavated ulcers with a white necrotic center near the semilunar fold or the caruncle. Hyperimmune vaccinia globulins are indicated in the management of these patients. Finally, conjunctivitis may be part of Stevens-Johnson Syndrome, which includes erythema, multiform lesions of the skin and involvement of the mucous membranes of the mouth, conjunctiva and urethrogenital areas. The ocular involvement may be catarrhal, purulent, or severely pseudomembranous with marked swelling of the lids and profuse discharge. The cornea may ulcerate and perforate. This disease can last for several weeks and therapy is aimed at the prevention of secondary infection.

4. MANAGEMENT - GENERAL COMMENTS

The list of causes of conjunctivitis in infants and children are considerable. A careful history, thorough examination of the eye, and laboratory studies are of help in making the correct diagnosis and implementing appropriate therapy. Some principles common to the management of all patients with conjunctivitis should be kept in mind:

4.1: The eye, when covered with a discharge, should be irrigated with sterile saline or water in order to minimize crusting and closure of the lids.

4.2: When antibiotics are applied topically, they should be administered at frequent intervals - at least every two hours during the day. An ointment may also be applied at bedtime.

4.3: When using an eye dropper, care should be taken not to contaminate the dropper by touching the lashes, and parents should be reminded that good hand-washing techniques are important in reducing spread of the infection to other family members.

4.4: Although steroids are useful in managing patients with allergic conjunctivitis, they should be used with great care in treating infectious conjunctivitis of any cause. Not only may they mask the effects of drug toxicity in the eye, but they are contraindicated in the treatment of conjunctivitis due to herpes viruses.

4.5: Compresses, warm or cold, may be a useful therapeutic adjunct. Often a person who has not responded to multiple topical medications may benefit from discontinuation of all drops and the application of lukewarm compresses three to four times a day.

REFERENCES

Armstrong, J.H., Zacarias, F., and Rein, M.F.: Ophthalmia Neonatorum, A Chart Review, Pediatrics 57:884, 892, 1976.

Buchta, R.M.: Membranous Conjunctivitis due to Adenovirus Type 7 Infection, Clin. Pediatr. 13:232-234, 1974.

Dawson, C. and Darrell, R.: Infections due to Adenovirus Type 8 in the United States, I. An Outbreak of Epidemic Keratoconjunctivitis Originating in a Physician's Office, NEJM 268:1031-1034, 1963.

Harley, Robinson D.: Pediatric Ophthalmology, W.B. Saunders Co. Philadelphia, 1975.

Mund, Michael L.: The Pediatrician and the Eye, Pediatric Conferences (From the Children's Hospital of Newark), Vol. 17, pp. 1-17, 1974.

CHAPTER 3. ACUTE EXANTHEMATOUS DISEASES

3.1: MEASLES

INTRODUCTION: Measles is typically an acute febrile exanthem of
childhood associated with significant morbidity and a high attack
rate in susceptible persons. The availability of an effective live-
virus vaccine has markedly reduced the prevalence of disease in
immunized populations; the fact that measles is probably a strictly
human pathogen offers promise that this infectious disease can be
eventually eradicated. Nevertheless, until universal immunization
has been accomplished, measles will continue to be encountered. In
addition, several unusual features of the clinical expressions of such
infections have provided insight into some general features of virus-
host interaction for these and other viruses.

1. CLINICAL FEATURES

Measles is primarily an infection of the respiratory tract and, as
such is transmitted via infectious aerosols. Infection is primarily
initiated in the upper respiratory tract and perhaps also in the conjunctiva. It is important to bear in mind that such infections occur
in a substantial portion of all exposed persons whether they are susceptible or immune (Stokes, et al., 1961). Immunity as the result
of natural or artificial (vaccine) infection protects the individual
against disease, but the individual remains epidemiologically important in his inability to reliably interrupt transmission. Virus replication in the immune host is, however, presumably limited to the
upper respiratory tract and is asymptomatic.

In the susceptible person, the interval between the initial infection
and the development of clinical symptoms is typically 10-11 days,
although this incubation period has been reported to range from 7-21
days. The onset of disease is characterized by nonspecific constitutional signs such as fever and malaise, followed within a day by
the so-called "prodrome." The latter is regularly a feature of measles and in fact helps to distinguish this condition from other febrile
exanthems. Symptoms consist of cough, coryza and conjunctivitis
(the three C's of measles). The cough is dry and irritative and the
conjunctivitis is diffuse and may be accompanied by annoying photophobia. These symptoms as well as the fever each become progressively more pronounced and are present for some 3-4 days before
the typical exanthem appears. On careful examination, however, an
enanthem is present during the last day or so of the prodrome.
The enanthem is one of the few pathognomonic signs in medicine and
as every student of infectious disease learns, is present on the buccal
mucosa and are referred to as Koplik spots. However, it should be

noted that the enanthem has been observed on multiple mucosal surfaces, such as the conjunctivae and the vaginal mucosa. They have been observed in the colon mucosa as well (Hobson, 1940). The lesions are minute bluish-white dots surrounded by an erythematous zone; they are so small that they never photograph well and illustrations usually exaggerate their size and are misleading. Koplik spots on the buccal mucosa typically first appear opposite the upper molars and at first are few in number. They rapidly spread in extent and become more numerous but frequently are no longer visible once the skin rash appears. While Koplik spots are apparently associated with other virus infections on rare occasions (Schaffner, et al., 1968) their presence at the very least should strongly suggest measles.

Although the pathogenesis thereof is not at all understood, it is fortunate that many of the infectious exanthems express very characteristic lesions, and do so in a distinctive order of appearance. Measles is no exception to this. The rash begins on the upper part of the body, is maculopapular in nature and appears progressively downward over the body. The rash typically appears first behind the ears and upper forehead. It is then noted in sequence downward over the face, trunk and limbs (Fig. 3.1). At first the lesions are

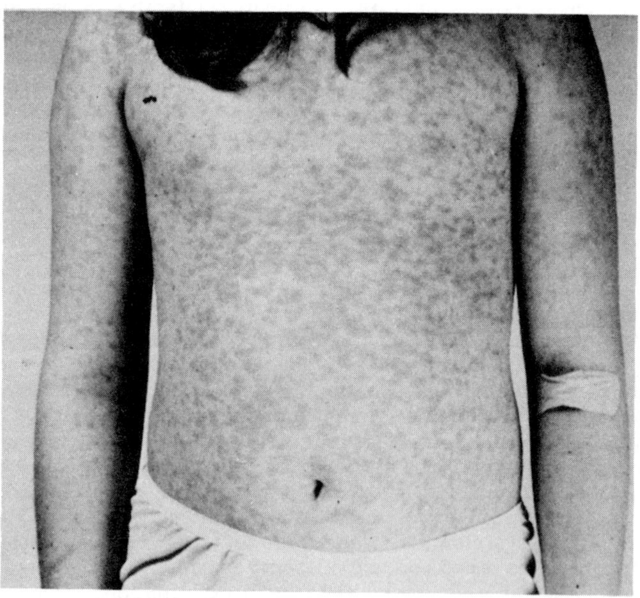

FIG. 3.1: Generalized maculo-papular rash due to measles virus.

discrete, dark red macules and maculopapules but once they have
been present in an area for a time, enlarge, become bright red
and frequently coalesce. From the first appearance of the rash until the entire body is covered generally requires 1-3 days. By the
latter stage the child is most acutely ill; the respiratory symptoms
have usually continued to worsen and the fever may have reached
104°-105°F. This represents the peak of severity and is shortly
followed by defervescence and fading of the rash. The rash fades
first on the face and thence in the same order by which it prog-
ressed. Frequently after the erythema has disappeared, a residual light pigmentation (staining) persists for a week or so to be followed by a fine desquamation, especially on the trunk and extremities.
Recovery by this time is complete.

The patient with measles is probably most infectious for others during the respiratory phase of the prodromal disease. Virus excretion from the respiratory tract ceases shortly after the rash appears
although measles virus may be present in the urine for a number of
days thereafter (Llanes-Rodas and Liu, 1966).

1.1: Complications: A number of complications may develop in the
patient with measles, either as an untoward effect of the infectious
process itself or as the result of bacterial superinfection. However, it must be emphasized that the uncomplicated infection alone
is a severe disease and the physician must refrain from treating
suspected complications unless they are adequately documented.

Severe involvement of the respiratory tract may result in specific
syndromes becoming predominant. For example, laryngeal inflammation may lead to significant stridor and occasionally measures
may have to be taken because of the ensuing respiratory embarrass-
ment (see Viral Croup in Chapter 1). Otitis media usually is a part
of measles infection and is rarely symptomatic. Bacterial invasion
of the middle ear may occur, a situation which is seen much less
frequently than formerly. In fact, mastoiditis was a common sequelae of measles in the early part of this century, usually as the
result of group A streptococcal infections. Additionally, rare complications of measles, such as idiopathic thrombocytopenic purpura,
enteritis, and myocarditis, have been recorded.

The lower respiratory tract is another site where significant complications of measles may occur. In some patients, particularly
those suffering concurrent disorders of which immunodeficiencies
are a part, extensive pathology may result from virus infection of
the lung. This is essentially an acute interstitial pneumonitis; as it
is characterized by the typical cytopathology associated with measles virus, it is referred to as giant cell pneumonia. Its significance will be discussed in more detail below. In other patients the
virus infection seem to predispose to bacterial infection of the lung.
The causative organisms are typically the extracellular invasive
bacteria such as the pneumococcus, streptococcus, Haemophilus

influenzae or rarely the staphylococcus. Whereas leukopenia characterizes uncomplicated measles infections, bacterial complications are usually accompanied by leukocytosis. Demonstration of the latter in a patient with a compatible clinical picture and appropriate chest x-ray findings would be sufficient justification to institute antibiotic therapy.

It is in the central nervous system that the most serious consequences of infection with measles virus are apt to occur (Bell and McCormick, 1975). Indeed, electroencephalographic abnormalities are commonly observed in measles (Gibbs, et al., 1959), and these are most striking around the time the rash first appears. They are, however, transient and recovery is usually complete. In addition, convulsions are not an uncommon occurrence during measles in children predisposed to febrile seizures. The severe form of neurologic complication, as with many other kinds of virus infection, is post-infectious encephalitis. This complication is found approximately once per thousand cases of measles and typically is first manifest in a child apparently recovering from the disease. The onset is abrupt and is frequently heralded by the sudden onset of convulsions or coma. In other patients, the condition may begin more insidiously. Again, electroencephalographic abnormalities will be displayed. The cerebrospinal fluid demonstrates a moderate lymphocytic pleocytosis and a somewhat elevated protein content. This condition is essentially an acute demyelinating encephalomyelitis. Its etiology is suggested by the striking similarity to the pathology of experimental allergic encephalomyelitis. The isolation of measles virus from brain tissue in this disorder may indicate that the pathogenesis of the inflammatory demyelination depends on more than a simple autoimmune process. In any event, up to one-third of patients with post-measles encephalitis die; of the survivors half may be left with significant neurologic abnormalities (Tyler, 1957).

Two other central nervous system disorders appear to be causally related to measles virus infection but only after an interval of many years. The first is subacute sclerosing panencephalitis (SSPE). This condition begins an average of five years after the patient experienced the typical measles infection, and occurs in approximately one per million children. It is a chronic, progressive and invariably fatal disease with well-recognized stages. These are usually classed, in order of appearance, as lethargic, regression of intellectual functioning, development of myoclonus and finally, cerebellar abnormalities. Thereafter the course is one of progressive deterioration until demise. Typical EEG findings are present (Ibrahim and Jeavons, 1974), and the diagnosis may be confirmed by demonstrating elevated measles antibody titers in the CSF. That this disorder is etiologically associated with the presence of measles virus is firmly established; the pathogenesis is unclear but possible mechanisms will be discussed in the section of Pathogenesis and Immunity.

Certain epidemiological features of SSPE, such as the higher incidence in the southeastern states compared to other regions of the U.S.,
and its more frequent occurrence in rural areas, remain unexplained (Jabbour, et al., 1972).

The other chronic disease of the central nervous system which may
be related to measles virus is multiple sclerosis (Black, 1975).
Here the relationship is only tenuously established and it appears
that host factors such as a genetic predisposition to the condition
(Alter, et al., 1976) may be major determinants.

2. ATYPICAL MEASLES

The usual course of measles virus infection may be greatly altered
in patients with impaired host defense mechanisms. This is most
striking in patients with immune deficiency states, particularly those
in which cellular immune mechanisms are impaired. The latter
contrasts sharply to the normal clinical disease following exposure
seen in children with congenital agammaglobulinemia.

In patients with combined immunodeficiencies or occasionally in
those suffering severe underlying disorders such as leukemia,
Letterer-Siwe disease or cystic fibrosis it appears that the virus infection is not normally controlled. Instead, the patient may continue
to be febrile for months, active virus-induced pathology continues to
develop and virus has been isolated many weeks after the onset of
disease. The infection is usually fatal in such cases, most often as
the result of progressive giant cell pneumonia. The patient may not
develop antibody to measles virus during the course of the infection,
and diagnosis may be complicated by the fact that a skin rash may
not develop.

The immunodeficiency state that accompanies malnutrition may similarly explain the severe morbidity and high mortality rates that are
seen in children living in some underdeveloped areas of the world.
Conversely, "virgin soil" epidemics could not be attributed to such
factors. These represent epidemics of measles in populations which
have not had experience with the virus for many years. These epidemics are explosive and attended by high mortality rates in individuals of all ages and who were previously healthy.

A different sort of atypical disease has been seen in persons acquiring natural infection who were previously immunized with killed virus
vaccine. In these individuals, pneumonia with pleural effusion and
edema and a petechial rash of the extremities were prominent features (Nader, et al., 1968).

3. PATHOGENESIS AND IMMUNITY

The respiratory tract is obviously a favored site for many viruses as
it is readily accessible to the initiation of infection. Further, the

infectious process elicits rhinorrhea, cough and sneezing, each of
which ensures continued dissemination of infectious virus to new
susceptible hosts. Measles virus additionally possesses certain
characteristics which allow the virus to spread beyond the respiratory tract, attributes which are ultimately responsible for the rash
and certain other features of the clinical syndrome. It seems likely
that a major virulence determinant in this regard is the predilection
of measles virus to infect and replicate in leukocytes. Thus, an
early event in measles infection is spread from the primarily infected site of the upper respiratory tract to local lymphoid tissue.
Active replication continues in these tissues and soon results in a
primary viremia. While virus replication persists in the upper respiratory tract, it is likely that this takes place in occult sites. The
infected individual is not demonstrably infectious for others during
the early incubation period.

As a consequence of the primary viremia virus is disseminated to
multiple sites, a process perhaps facilitated by clearing of the virus
by reticuloendothelial tissues which in turn become infected. However, continual viremia is readily demonstrable for some time during the asymptomatic incubation period (Gresser and Chany, 1963).
This observation implies that host factors contribute to the pathogenesis of disease. Considerable evidence suggests that such is indeed
the case.

First, cell lysis is not the usual fate of measles virus-infected cells.
Rather, cell morphology is either altered or syncytial cells are
formed. The latter probably represent large aggregates of infected
cells in which fusion has been induced as a consequence of virus-
induced surface membrane alteration (Cascando and Karzon, 1965).
In infected tissues these are referred to as Warthin-Finkeldey giant
cells; they are wide-spread during measles infection, especially in
reticuloendothelial tissues. An additional feature in the intact host
is local inflammation represented primarily by infiltrates of mononuclear cells. From this latter it may be inferred that the cellular
immune response is of paramount importance in the recovery from
measles infection. This concept is further reinforced by the clinical
course of measles in children with immune deficiency disorders referred to previously. Humoral immunity is not without benefit,
however.

The induction of anti-viral antibody is of value in three respects.
First, the presence of secretory antibody in the respiratory tract
(Bellanti, et al., 1969) would protect the individual against reinfection by neutralizing inhaled virus before the virus had opportunity to
infect cells. The fact that reinfection locally is a common phenomenon, however, suggests either that local immunity is either short-
lived or is inefficient. Second, circulating antibody probably serves
as a barrier to dissemination of virus from the respiratory tract; this
system is apparently quite effective and would explain the life-long

immunity to clinical disease and protection offered by passive immunization. Third, immunoglobulins may also participate in the immune destruction of infected cells. The reaction of antibody with virus antigens on the surface of the infected cell activates complement leading to the lysis of infected cells (Joseph and Oldstone, 1975).

Ordinarily, the contribution of the cellular immune mechanisms is for the detection and destruction of infected cells. The ability of measles virus to replicate in T lymphocytes (Sullivan, et al., 1975), an essential mediator of these immune reactions, has interesting implications. First, the intracellular location of virus in these circulating cells provides a means by which virus may disseminate in the presence of humoral antibody; the viremia of measles is in fact primarily leukocyte-associated (Grasser and Chany, 1963). Second, it might be anticipated that infection would interfere with leukocyte function and it has been demonstrated that T cell helper function is impaired in experimental measles infection (McFarland, 1974). The clinical correlate of this may be the regular observation that measles infection or immunization induces temporary anergy with loss of delayed hypersensitivity to antigens to which the patient had previously responded. The significance of this in terms of human disease is uncertain; measles may or may not be detrimental to the course of tuberculosis, for example.

Ultimately, however, immune destruction of infected cells occurs, probably via both humoral and cellular mechanisms, and clinical recovery follows. It is probable that the skin rash is at least in part a consequence of the immune destruction of infected cells and the resultant inflammatory reaction.

Two observations have suggested that measles virus is not eradicated during the course of infection but merely controlled. One is the recurrence of active infection many years after initial infection as the disease state SSPE; the other is the life-long immunity to disease and persistence of humoral antibody decades after the initial antigenic experience with the virus. It has been suggested that periodically, limited sub-clinical recurrence of virus replication serves as endogenous antigenic stimuli to maintain continuing immunity.

The mechanisms involved in "slow" measles virus infections (SSPE or multiple sclerosis) are of obvious interest. Two main hypotheses have been advanced to explain these phenomena. One is that the infection involves mutant or recombinant virus (Burnstein, et al., 1974). As a result the virus replicates intracellularly, alters the surface membrane and elicits an anticellular immune response. The other explanation involves the immune response itself. Joseph and Oldstone (1975) have proposed that the central nervous system is a relatively immunologically protected site, especially with regard to the availability of complement for complement-mediated lysis of infected cells. The effect of antibody alone is to result in disappearance

of membrane-associated virus antigens from the infected cell either
by internalization ("capping") or by sloughing these complexes from
the cell surface. Consequently cell lysis does not occur, intracellular virus replication continues and virus antigens are regener-
ated. Presumably the consequences of chronic infection is eventual
disruption of cell function. Both mechanisms would account for the
chronic progressive character of SSPE. Additional data are required for the final elucidation of the mechanisms of the disease
process in SSPE, but both hypotheses offer a framework for future
studies.

4. TREATMENT

Uncomplicated measles need be treated only symptomatically. Antipyretics should be given to control fever, and the patient is more
comfortable in a quiet darkened room. Bed rest need not be forced,
particularly in that the acutely ill child will satisfactorily regulate
his own activities.

Complications of superinfections rarely occur, but the physician
must be alert for the possibility of suppurative otitis media or pneumonia. Prophylactic antibiotics should not be given, however;
Weinstein (1955) has demonstrated that not only do such drugs not
reduce the incidence of bacterial complications but the incidence
actually increases and involves resistant organisms which are more
difficult to treat. If complications do occur the responsible organi-
isms should be determined, insofar as possible, and treated with
the appropriate choice of drugs.

Measles encephalitis can also only be treated symptomatically as
for most other viral encephalitides. There is currently no antiviral
drug that appears to be effective in measles.

4.1: Prevention: Live virus vaccine as it is currently supplied offers promise as an instrument potentially capable of eradicating
measles. Since the institution of measles immunization, the incidence of this disease and its complications have declined dramati-
cally (Barkin, 1975).

The current recommendation for routine immunization is to administer live attenuated measles vaccine not before 15 months of age.
Administration to younger children will result in a certain proportion being unsuccessful, apparently because of the persistence of
passively acquired maternal antibody which interferes with replication of vaccine virus. A child who has not been immunized at any
age (up to child-bearing age for girls) should be immunized against
measles after completion of diphtheria-pertussis-tetanus and poliovirus primary series. Prior to administration of measles virus skin
testing for tuberculosis should be done for two possible reasons:
1) measles virus, live or attenuated, may potentially cause exacerbation of tuberculosis infection, and 2) measles vaccine will

temporarily abrogate delayed hypersensitivity skin responses to mycobacterial antigens and thus otherwise deprive the physician of a valuable means of case finding during this period should it be necessary.

A child between 6-15 months of age, or an older child who has never been immunized and who is exposed to measles should be given immune serume globulin; 0.04ml/kg, and live measles vaccine (Edmonston B) in a separate site. This regimen will supply passive immunization to ameliorate natural measles which the patient might be incubating and which would not be affected by immunization alone. Careful follow-up is necessary in these patients as their immunity is by no means ensured, and they should be routinely reimmunized at a later date (not before age 15 months nor within two months) with live virus vaccine.

The use of live virus vaccine in immunodeficient patients is contraindicated, as it is for those patients receiving immunosuppressive drugs, pregnant patients and persons with active tuberculosis.

The long-term protection offered by measles vaccine and whether routine reimmunization is advisable has received considerable attention recently. Presently it appears that live further attenuated virus vaccine (Schwartz and Moraten) induces serum antibody comparable in duration to natural measles (Krugman, 1977). Infection in previously immunized individuals has been noted, and usually occurs in one of the following groups of patients: those immunized with live virus before 15 months of age; those immunized with Edmonston B and concurrent immune serum globulin; and, as previously noted, in patients who had received killed virus. For persons not in one of these groups immunization is about 98% effective. Consequently, during outbreaks of measles reimmunization should be carried out specifically in those individuals in one of the three identifiable high risk groups and, of course, persons not previously immunized. Admittedly, however, historical information as to age and type of immunization may not be immediately available. In such cases a decision wil have to be made as to who should be immunized. Routine reimmunization has its adherents (Bass, et al., 1976); there does not appear to be a risk to the patient who is reimmunized.

REFERENCES

Alter, M., Harshe, M., Anderson, V.E., Emme, L., and Yunis, E.J.: Genetic association of multiple sclerosis and HL-A determinants. Neurology (Minneapolis) 26:31, 1976.

Barkin, R.M.: Measles mortality; A retrospective look at the vaccine era. Am. J. Epidem. 102:341, 1975.

Bass, J.W., Halstead, S.B., Fischer, G.W., Podgore, J.K., Pearl, W.R., Schydlower, M., Wiebe, R.A., and Ching, F.M.: Booster vaccination with further live attenuated measles vaccine. JAMA 235:31, 1976.

Bell, W.E., and McCormick, W.F.: Neurologic infections in children. Major Prob. Clin. Ped. XII: 167, 1975.

Bellanti, J.A., Sanga, R.L., Klutinis, B., Brandt, B., and Artenstein, M.S.: Antibody responses in serum and nasal secretions of children immunized with inactivated and attenuated measles virus vaccines. NEJM 280:628, 1969.

Black, F.L.: The association between measles and multiple sclerosis. Prog. Med. Virol. 21:158, 1975.

Burnstein, T., Jacobsen, L.B., Zeman, W., and Chen, T.T.: Persistent infection of BSC-1 cells by defective measles virus derived from subacute sclerosing panencephalitis. Infect. Immun. 10: 1378, 1974.

Cascardo, M.R., and Karzon, D.T.: Measles virus giant cell inducing factor. Virology 26:311, 1965.

Gibbs, F.A., Gibbs, E.L., Carpenter, P.R., and Spies, H.W.: Electroencephalographic abnormality in "uncomplicated" childhood diseases. JAMA 171:1050, 1959.

Gresser, I. and Chany, C.: Isolation of measles virus from the washed leukocytic fraction of blood. Proc. Soc. Exper. Biol. Med. 113:695, 1963.

Hobson, F.G.: Koplik spots in colon. Lancet 2:134, 1940.

Ibrahim, M.M., and Jeavons, P.M.: The value of electroencephalography in the diagnosis of subacute sclerosing panencephalitis. Develop. Med. Child. Neurol. 16:295, 1974.

Jabbour, J.T., Duenas, D.A., Sever, J.L., Krebs, H.M., and Horta-Barbosa, L.: Epidemiology of subacute sclerosing panencephalitis (SSPE). A report of the SSPE registry 220:959, 1972.

Joseph, B.S., and Oldstone, M B.A.: Immunologic injury in measles virus infection. II. Suppression of immune injury through antigenic modulation. J. Exper. Med. 142:864, 1975.

Krugman, S.: Present status of measles and rubella immunization in the United States: A medical progress report. J. Pediat. 90:1, 1977.

Llanes-Rodas, R., and Liu, C.: Rapid diagnosis of measles from
urinary sediments stained with fluorescent antibody. NEJM 275:
516, 1966.

McFarland, H.F.: The effect of measles virus infection on T and
B lymphocytes in the mouse. J. Immunol. 113:1978, 1974.

Nader, P.R., Horwitz, M.S., and Rousseau, J.: Atypical exanthem following exposure to natural measles: Eleven cases in children previously inoculated with killed vaccine. J. Pediat. 72:22,
1968.

Schaffner, W., Schluederberg, A.E.S., and Byrne, E.B.: Clinical
epidemiology of sporadic measles in a highly immunized population.
NEJM 279:783, 1968.

Stokes, J., Reilly, C.M., Buynak, E.B., and Hilleman, M.R.:
Immunologic studies of measles. Am. J. Hyg. 74:293, 1961.

Sullivan, J.L., Barry, D.W., Lucas, S.J., and Albrecht, P.:
Measles infection of human mononuclear cells. I. Acute infection
of peripheral blood lymphocytes and monocytes. J. Exper. Med.
142:773, 1975.

Tyler, H.R.: Neurological complications of rubeola (measles).
Medicine 36:147, 1957.

Weinstein, L.: Failure of chemotherapy to prevent the bacterial
complications of measles. NEJM 253:679, 1955.

::

3.2: RUBELLA

INTRODUCTION: Rubella emerged as a significant infection after
Gregg's (1941) description of some of its teratogenic associations.
During the epidemic year of 1964 the serious consequences of congenital rubella were confirmed when about 30,000 children developed
rubella-associated birth defects. Shortly thereafter the attenuated
rubella virus vaccine was introduced.

The widespread use of rubella vaccine has reduced significantly the
childhood incidence of rubella. The expectations from vaccination
were based on provision of diminishing risks to adults by interruption
of childhood transmission. This goal may have been accomplished,
except for the fact that recruitment of susceptibles during rubella
outbreaks is not all-or-none, but rather in-between, thus leaving
non-immune reservoirs particularly among older children and adults.

POST-NATAL RUBELLA: Rubella virus is found in pharyngeal secretions; the available evidence indicates person-to-person respiratory

transmission. The incubation period averages about 17 days with a range of 14 to 23 days. Risks of infection depend on a continuum of exposure. In closed populations the majority of susceptible become infected, some without evidence of skin eruption (Krugman, et al., 1953). But, in various populations-at-risk, rates of recruitment differ widely; serologic evidence of immunity may be absent in from 10 to 60 percent of young adults.

The ratio of inapparent (rubella without rash) and apparent infections during childhood approximates 2:1, among adults the ratio is variable ranging from 1:1 to 6:1 (Berno, et al., 1969). A much higher rate is found among vaccinees.

CONGENITAL RUBELLA: Rubella virus has a catastrophic effect on the developing embryo resulting in fetal wastage or organogenic handicaps present at birth (Dudgeon, 1975). Many infants born with the congenital rubella syndrome are chronically infected (Rawls, 1968). Such infants are sources of infectious virus for personnel attending their care, for they have an abundance of virus in pharyngeal secretions, urine, feces, and other body fluids.

POST-VACCINAL RUBELLA: Rubella virus may be detected in pharyngeal secretions following vaccination. Spread of vaccine virus from person-to-person occurs infrequently, if at all. Vaccinated individuals are susceptible and may be involved in silent reinfection.

1. ETIOLOGY AND PATHOGENESIS

Rubella virus is propagable in cell cultures in vitro (Weller and Neva, 1962; Parkman, et al., 1962). The virus is a moderately large particle with an overall diameter of 500-700A^O. The outer envelope is acquired by a budding process involving host-cell membranes. The nucleoid is composed of RNA. Rubella virus possesses hemaglutinin, complement-fixing and precipitating antigens.

1.1: Post-Natal Rubella: The site of primary implantation of rubella virus is in the pharynx. Both wild-type and vaccine viruses are found in pharyngeal secretions. Wild-type virus is detectable in the pharynx midway during the incubation period, and persists through the eruptive phase and for several days thereafter. At its peak, a pharyngeal swab may yield 1,000 infectious viral particles. Lymphadenopathy suggests an early involvement of these tissues in virus replication; these nodes probably switch later to cellular release of antibodies. Viremia develops before onset of rash, almost coincidental with pharyngeal replication. Quantitative patterns of viremia are not well defined; it is known that $\geq$100 viral particles have been found in unit volumes of blood. The stage of viremia ends with the onset of rash. Antibodies develop within the ensuing fortnight. Rubella virus has been recovered from maculopapular skin lesions (Heggie, 1971). There are controversies about whether or not the evolution of the rash is generated by rubella virus or by virus-antibody complexes.

1.2: Congenital Rubella: When rubella intervenes during the first trimester of pregnancy, circulating virus may injure the vascular endothelium of decidua and placenta. Tondury (1962) noted tissue changes indicating that the fetus is infected by embolization from bits of necrotic endothelium. Primary sites of virus multiplication in the fetus, are in all probability, within endothelial cells in view of visible angiopathies. Practically all organs are involved eventually in fetal infections. Surviving infants, in addition to the florid syndrome, may become chronically infected; rubella virus may persist in various tissues and body secretions during the first year of life or longer. The antibody responses as recounted later in the chapter differ from that raised during natural infection.

1.3: Post-Vaccinal Infection: Attenuated rubella virus multiplies in non-immune vaccinees. Virus may be recovered in pharyngeal secretions from the 7th to 14th days and occasionally longer after inoculation. The concentrations of virus are said to be less than in the natural disease. Communicability has not been demonstrated. Viremia has been detected in young adults but not in children. Vaccine virus has been recovered from synovial fluid (Hildebrandt and Maassab, 1966) and from uterine and fetal tissues (Vaherie, et al., 1972; Modlin, et al., 1976). Antibodies may follow the intranasal instillation of the Ra27/3 rubella attenuated virus vaccine (Ogra, et al., 1971).

2. CLINICAL FEATURES

2.1: Post-Natal Rubella: During childhood the rash may be the only signal of disease. Prodromal complaints are seldom mentioned. Adults may develop myalgia, headache and mild pharyngeal irritation a day or two before appearance of rash. Post-auricular, suboccipital and cervical lymphadenopathy may appear midway in the incubation period. These large tender lymph nodes attain maximal size just before the skin lesions appear and recede over the next 10 days. A transient enanthem (Forchheimer spots) may be noted just prior to the rash. These discrete, pinpoint rose-spots may coalesce and extend onto the mucous membranes of the fauces. The spleen may be enlarged.

The rash appears first on the face, neck and scalp, and spreads within hours over the trunk and extremities. The discrete, red, slightly elevated lesions, rose-pink in color, may coalesce, particularly on the trunk and sometimes on the face. The rash is apt to be more intense on the flexor surfaces of the extremities. Lesions are present on palms and soles. The rash fades rapidly in the order of appearance, disappearing within a day, or persisting for as long as 4 days. Desquamation is usually trivial.

2.2: Congenital Rubella Syndrome: The variable clinical features of infection involving the fetus after a natural infection in the mother have been described in detail (Cooper, 1968; Krugman and Ward, 1973). The florid disease in surviving infants encompasses intra-uterine growth retardation, purpuric and petechial lesions of skin and mucous membranes, hepatosplenomegaly, cataracts, glaucoma, retinopathy, congenital heart disease and meningoencephalitis. About 25 percent of affected infants die. Surviving infants may develop interstitial pneumonia, deafness, recurrent infections, and gastrointestinal disturbances. There may be leukopenia, thrombo-cytopenia and hypogammaglobulinemia. Survivors may or may not be mentally retarded.

The timing of fetal infection affects the outcome. The first 6 weeks after conception, when organogenesis is at its nadir, is a most vul-nerable period regarding risks to eyes and heart. Fetal infection is not all-or-none, however; some infants escape, presumably because the virus has not crossed the placental barrier. By the 16th week risks of chronic infection subside and such infants are often born with fewer stigmata, or they may entirely escape infection.

2.3: Infection From Vaccine Virus: A modified illness has been noted occasionally among children, and with greater frequency among women given attenuated rubella vaccine. Macular rashes, lymph-adenitis, arthralgias and peripheral neuropathies may develop 8 to 21 days after vaccination. These signs abate in a manner similar to the natural disease. Such illness may have occurred more frequently with vaccine prepared in dog kidney cultures; they have been encoun-tered, however, with other vaccine preparations.

Rubella vaccine virus has been inoculated into women during early pregnancy, either knowingly (with the women's consent) or inadver-tently. The data regarding fetal risks following intrauterine infec-tion are based on small numbers. Based on these figures the risks of intrauterine infection appears to be about 23 percent, and of dem-onstrated fetal infections about 3 percent. No infant born of these women had florid congenital rubella. Thus, the overall risk of fetal infection would seem to be much less than the 10 percent to 50 per-cent risks following wild-type rubella virus (Fox, et al., 1976).

3. COMPLICATIONS

Complications following post-natal and post-vaccinal rubella are relatively uncommon. Among them are: (1) arthropathies, (2) poly-neuropathies, (3) hemorrhagic manifestations, and (4) encephalitis. All of these complications may be encountered in post-natal rubella; only the first two have been noted in post-vaccinal infections.

Arthritis may follow either natural rubella or vaccination (Austin, et al., 1972); Modlin, et al., 1975). Adults are involved more often

than children. Onset in the natural disease occurs 5 to 6 days after
the rash; the arthralgias last about 10 days (range 2 to 14 days).
Small joints of the hands and wrist, of the feet and ankle are involved more than others; occasionally arthralgias develop in larger
joints. The arthralgias may be characterized as (1) vague and fleeting with or without (2) associated stiffness and (3) joint swelling.
On the other hand, onset of arthralgia may be delayed for as long
as 2 months following vaccination. Synovial fluids contain macrophages, mononuclear and synovial cells. The synovial membranes
are hyperplastic and infiltrated with inflammatory cells. Rubella
virus may be recovered from synovial fluid.

Polyneuropathies take two forms (Kilroy et al., 1970). In the first,
children are awakened at night with pain and paraesthesias involving
arms, wrists and hands. These signs cease during the day only to
recur nightly over a period of days. Nerve conduction velocities
are slowed. In the second form, children on getting out of bed have
popliteal pain and difficulties in arising upright; they squat in a
crouched position (catcher's crouch) or reluctantly walk with a
crouching gait. Onset of these neuropathies may be delayed for one
or 2 months or even longer after vaccination.

Hemorrhagic manifestations are rarely encountered. Purpura may
develop in association with thrombocytopenia. Periorbital and pala-
tine ecchymosis and skin petechiae may appear, or there may be
gastrointestinal or genitourinary bleeding, or hemorrhages within
the CNS. Bleeding time is prolonged and capillary fragility may be
increased. Non-thrombocytopenic forms of purpura occur also.

Encephalitis (risk ~ 1:6000) when it intervenes it generally does so
during the eruptive period. Headache, vomiting and nuchal rigidity
may be followed by convulsions, coma and respiratory failure. Clinically, the course may be like that of Reye's syndrome or of acute
toxic encephalopathy. Widespread neuronal injury of non-specific
nature precedes death (Kinney, et al., 1965). The mortality is about
20 percent. In those who survive, recovery is almost always
complete.

4. DIAGNOSIS

4.1: Post Natal Rubella: Clinical recognition is not difficult during
outbreaks of rubella. But the sporadic case either in children or
adults is not always clearly differentiable from some other exanthematous diseases. Textbooks generally list modified rubeola, exanthem
subitum and infectious mononucleosis among differentiable masquer-
aders; to these should be added rashes associated with enteroviruses
(see Section on Enteroviruses).

4.2: Congenital Rubella: The segregation may not be easy, for many
of the signs present at birth may mimic those of congenital syphilis,
toxoplasmosis, cytomegalovirus and herpesvirus infections.

<u>4.3: Post-Vaccinal Rubella (sine rash)</u>: The major problems relate to recognition of late onset arthritis or polyneuronitis following vaccination.

Rubella virus can be detected in pharyngeal secretions during infections acquired after birth, and in these and in other body fluids during congenital rubella. The virus is unlikely to be recovered in blood after the onset of the rash in the natural disease. The serological test most often used for the diagnosis of rubella is the hemagglutination-inhibition antibody test. Such antibodies appear within one or 2 days following the rash and reach maximal levels within 2 weeks. For delineation of rubella infection in the pregnant woman it may be necessary to determine whether the early antibody is IgM (due to a primary response) or IgG due to preexistent and recall antibodies. The newborn infant infected in utero presents a different pattern of antibody development. Antibodies are derived from the infant and the mother. The infant contributes specific IgM and the mother provides passively acquired IgG. In contrast to normal infants, the rubella baby has elevated IgM antibodies that persist up to a year after birth.

Other serological methods include complement fixation, indirect fluorescent antibody, neutralization and precipitin tests.

5. TREATMENT

None is generally required. Arthralgias may be treated with aspirin. Bed rest is often helpful. The polyneuropathies may be vexsome and at times perplexing. The severe encephalopathies are treated in an intensive care unit containing the supportive facilities necessary to sustain life. Transfusions and corticosteroids may be required to counteract loss of blood.

The management of the serious disturbances of the infant with congenital rubella is beyond the scope of this chapter. However, it should be pointed out that these infants shed virus in pharyngeal secretions, urine and elsewhere, and that susceptible adults on exposure are likely to acquire infection. Personnel working in intensive care nurseries should either be sero-positive for rubella, or at least aware of their seronegative status.

6. PREVENTION AND CONTROL

<u>6.1: Vaccination: Active Immunization</u>: Three live attenuated virus vaccines are available: the Cendehill strain was grown in rabbit kidney cells, the HPV-77 strain prepared in duck embryo cell cultures (DE-5) and the RA27/3 virus propagated in a human diploid cell line. The latter vaccine should soon be licensed for use in the U.S.A. The vaccine is given subcutaneously, either as a unit stock or in combination with attenuated mumps and rubeola virus. The RA27/3 vaccine

(Plotkin, et al., 1973); Schiff and Linneman, 1974) may have advantages in providing an immunity more closely resembling natural rubella.

Currently live rubella virus is recommended for boys and girls between the ages of one year and puberty. In the United Kingdom the vaccine is available to prepubertal girls and to seronegative women during the post-partum period. The routine immunization of seronegative sexually mature females has attendant risks because of unrecognized early pregnancies. The rule is the avoidance of pregnancy for at least 2 months after vaccination. In certain areas of the U.S.A., immunization of sero-negative women has been recommended. Seronegative males might be included also (see below).

Specific antibodies are engendered in children following immunization. The titers with current vaccines are 4 to 8-fold lower than those following natural rubella. Horstmann (1975) observed that 8 percent of children given DE-5 vaccine within 3 to 5 years had lost detectable HI antibody. These were children mainly with weak post-vaccinal antibody rises. Others have noted a slight decay of antibodies during the first 2 years post-vaccination, and that the pattern of antibody decline follows that of natural rubella, albeit at a lower level (Krugman and Katz, 1974).

6.2: Gamma Globulin: Passive Immunization: Standard gamma globulin has little value in the prevention of rubella. The rash may be averted, but infection can be demonstrated by the antibody rise. Very likely viremia intervenes even when gamma globulin is given early in the incubation period. Reliance on such protection against infection, particularly in the exposed pregnant woman, appears unwarranted.

7. OTHER CONSIDERATIONS WITH RESPECT TO CONTROL OF RUBELLA AND RISKS TO THE FETUS

Over the past several years a number of disquieting observations have followed the use of rubella vaccine. These relate largely to the efficacy of the vaccine in providing solid immunity to reinfection and no risk of viral injury to the fetus. Several studies (Horstmann, 1975; Wilkins, et al., 1969) indicate reinfection rates of 80 percent or more among vaccinees exposed to wild rubella virus; in contrast, reinfection rates among those naturally immune varies between 0.8 to 10.0 percent. During these reinfections virus appears to remain localized to the respiratory tract, with apparently little shedding and risks to susceptible human beings.

Outbreaks of rubella among clusters of susceptible children and adults signal the limitations of the current vaccine program to eradicate the disease (Klock and Rachelefsky, 1973). Carriers exist and provide an available source of virus. A primary concern, not entirely resolved, relates to the pathogenicity of wild-type rubella virus during modified infections developing after vaccination. Will rubella virus multiply only locally and will viremia occur, however transient, to threaten the fetus? Or will localized infections propitiously reinforce immunity and further reduce the risk of fetal injury? These questions cannot be answered completely, but should the last proposition apply, significant "herd" immunity could become operative in rubella.

REFERENCES

Austin, S.M., Altman, R., Barnes, E.K., and Dougherty, W.J.: Joint reactions in children vaccinated against rubella. Am. J. Epidem. 95:53, 1972.

Berno, A.L., Spence, L.P., Stewart, J.A., and Casey, H.L.: Rubella in Trinidad. Sero-epidemiologic studies of an institutional outbreak. Am. J. Epidem. 89:74, 1969.

Cooper, L.Z.: A preventable cause of birth defects. Birth Defects. Original Article Series. Vol. IV. No. 7. pp. 23-35. Intrauterine Infections. The National Foundation, 1968.

Dudgeon, J.A.: Congenital rubella. J. Pediat. 87:1078, 1975.

Fox, J.P., Rainey, H.A., Hall, C.E., Ray, C.G. and Patterson, M.J.: Rubella vaccine in postpubertal women. Experience in Western Washington State. JAMA 236:837, 1976.

Gregg, N.M.: Congenital cataracts following German measles in the mother. Trans. Ophthal. Soc. Aust. 3:35, 1941.

Heggie, A.D.: Pathogenesis of the rubella exanthem. Isolation of rubella virus from the skin. NEJM 285:664, 1971.

Hildebrandt, H.M., and Maassab, H.F.: Rubella syndrome in a one-year-old patient. NEJM 274:1428, 1966.

Horstmann, D.M.: Rubella: Problems and perspectives. Ann. Int. Med. 83:412, 1975.

Kilroy, A.W., Schaffner, W., Fleet, W.F., Lefkavitz, L.B., Karzon, D.T., and Fenichel, G.M.: Two syndromes following rubella immunization. Clinical observations and epidemiological studies. JAMA 214:2287, 1970.

Kinney, F.M., Michaels, R.M., and Davis, K.S.: Rubella encephalopathy. Am. J. Dis. Child. 110:374, 1965.

Klock, L.E., and Rachelefsky, G.S.: Failure of rubella herd immunity during an epidemic. NEJM 288:69, 1973.

Krugman, S., Ward, R., Jacobs, K.G., and Iga, M.: Studies on rubella immunization. I. Demonstration of rubella without rash. JAMA 151:285, 1953.

Krugman, S., and Ward, R.: Rubella (German measles). Chapter 21, pp. 236-253, 5th ed. In: Infectious Diseases of Children and Adults. C.V. Mosby & Co., St. Louis, 1973.

Krugman, S., and Katz, S.L.: Rubella immunization: A five-year progress report. NEJM 29:1375, 1974.

Modlin, J.F., Brandlin-Bennett, A.D., Witte, J.J., Campbell, C.C., and Meyers, J.D.: A review of five years experience with rubella vaccine in the United States. Pediatr 55:20, 1975.

Modlin, J.F., Herrman, K., Brandling-Bennett, A.D., Eddins, D.L., and Hayden, G.F.: Risk of congenital abnormality after inadvertent rubella vaccination of pregnant women. NEJM 294:972, 1976.

Ogra, P.L., Kerr-Grant, D., Umana, G., Dzierba, J., and Weinstraub, D.: Antibody response in serum and nasopharynx after naturally acquired and vaccine-induced infection with rubella virus. NEJM 285:1337, 1971.

Parkman, P.D., Buescher, E.L., and Artenstein, M.S.: Recovery of rubella virus from army recruits. Proc. Soc. Exp. Biol. Med. 111:225, 1962.

Plotkin, S.A., Farquhan, J.D., and Ogra, P.L.: Immunologic properties of RA27/3 rubella virus vaccine. A comparison with strains presently licensed in the United States. JAMA 225:585, 1973.

Rawls, W.E.: Congenital rubella: The significance of virus persistence. Prog. Med. Virol. 10:235, 1968.

Schiff, G.M., Linneman, C.C.: Evaluation of RA27/3 rubella vaccine. J. Pediat. 85:379, 1974.

Tondury, G.: Embryopathies. The mode of action (route of infection and pathogenesis) of viruses in the human embryo. Springer-Verlag, Berlin, 1962.

Vaherie, A., Vesikari, T., Oker-Blom, N., Seppala, M., Parkman, P.D., Veronelli, J., and Robbins, F.C.: Isolation of attenuated rubella-vaccine virus from human products of conception and uterine cervix. NEJM 286:1071, 1972.

Weller, T.H., and Neva, F.A.: Propagation in tissue culture of cytopathic agents from patients with rubella-like illnesses. Proc. Soc. Exp. Biol. Med. 111:215, 1962.

Wilkins, J., Leedom, J.M., Portnoy, B., and Savatore, M.A.: Reinfection with rubella virus despite live vaccine induced immunity. Am. J. Dis. Child. 118:275, 1969.

::

3.3: EXANTHEM SUBITUM (ROSEOLA INFANTUM)

INTRODUCTION: Exanthem subitum represents one of the first major febrile cutaneous exanthems of infancy and childhood. Infants less than 6 months of age are usually spared, suggesting modulation of infection by passively acquired maternal antibodies. Breese (1941) observed roseola in 11 of 70 (16 percent) infants followed during the first year of life. Susceptibility to disease is greatest between the 6th and 24th months of life, and has an equal sex distribution. Seasonal clustering has been noted during late winter and spring months, and again in the autumn months. The incubation period ranges from 5 to 15 days with a mean of 12 days.

Subclinical infections <u>may</u> exceed the overt disease, thereby accounting for widespread immunity among children and adults. Institutional outbreaks rarely occur; when such outbreaks occur, as many as 45 percent may develop roseola (Barenberg, et al., 1939; James and Freier, 1949). The infectious agent may be found in the nasopharynx. Presumably, the agent is spread from person to person by pharyngeal droplets. However, the mode of transmission, and evidences of widespread covert infection during infancy must await the availability of the etiologic agent and its use in age-specific antibody development.

1. ETIOLOGY AND PATHOGENESIS

Kempe et al. (1950) reproduced the clinical disease in a 6-month-old infant using serum from an affected donor. Hellstrom and Vahlquist (1951) confirmed the experimental transmissibility from infant to infant. The available evidence suggests a filterable virus as the causative agent. Thus far, the agent has not been cultivated in cell cultures, chick embryos, or rodents. Non-human primates may be susceptible to infection.

The pathogenetic aspects of the disease remained unresolved. Pathological data are not extant; deaths during the disease are rarely recognized.

2. CLINICAL FEATURES

Sudden onset of unexplained fever is the initiating feature of infection. Generally intermittent, sometimes remitting, fever ranges from 39 to 41°C for 3 to 5 days. Excepting restiveness, affected infants are more often than not alert and playful; sometimes associated respiratory signs intervene, possibly signaling coincidental pharyngeal

infection; a few may have filamentary, white tonsillar exudates.
Midway during the febrile period suboccipital and posterior auricular lymph nodes enlarge moderately; they remain firm, non-tender and freely movable. Usually fever ends abruptly (crisis) or subsides occasionally over several days (lysis).

The exanthem develops with **defervescence.** Characteristically pale pink macules appear first on the neck, behind the ears, and on the trunk, particularly on the back. The rash may spread onto the buttocks, thighs and shoulders. The face and the distal parts of the extremities are generally spared. Sometimes faint and transient, the rash may be missed; otherwise, it may be florid and last several days. Most infants have rashes intermediate between these extremes.

The rash is generally macular (macules 2 to 4 mm in diameter), occasionally papular, but is never vesicular. Clemens (1945) described pre-eruptive erythematous specks and streaks on the soft palate; others have not recounted such an enanthema. The skin eruption fade rapidly, often within hours, and rarely lasts for several days.

Sequelae are rarely encountered. Convulsions may intervene during the pre-eruptive period of the disease. These may be associated with transient hemiplegia; rarely residual neuronapathies follow the disease. These include persisting paresis, seizure disorders and mental retardation (Burnstine and Paine, 1959).

Nuchal rigidity is not uncommon. The cerebrospinal fluid examination, entirely normal in this disease, is made to rule out meningitis. Rarely young children may develop significant abdominal pain, suggesting the possibility of appendicitis.

3. DIAGNOSIS

Recognition of the syndrome rests on the characteristic clinical pattern and the development of rash (Zahorsky, 1910; Berenberg et al., 1949; Letchner, 1955). Unexplained fever during infancy often raises the suspicion of the pediatrician. The leukocyte patterns may provide further support. At the onset of fever there is often leukocytosis, followed by leukopenia and relative lymphocytosis midway ($\sim$ the 3rd day) in the febrile period. With the appearance of the rash the leukocyte pattern returns to normality for age (Clemens, 1945).

The differential diagnosis includes a number of viral infections, principally those caused by selected enteroviruses (see item 3.5), occasionally by adenoviruses, and possibly in other parts of the world by some arboviruses. Rubeola, rubella, infectious mononucleosis, scarlet fever and rickettsiosis may be excluded based on: (1) histories of exposures, (2) clinical desiderata, and (3) use of methods for either detecting the specific agents or antibodies raised against them. Drug-associated eruptions and various dermatoses may require differentiation.

4. MANAGEMENT AND TREATMENT

Management is entirely supportive. High fever may be controlled
by: (1) appropriate usage of aspirin or acetaminophen, or both,
(2) tepid sponges, or (3) cooling mattresses. Infants and children
with prior history of febrile seizures are generally already on phe-
nobarbital; the dosage may be increased appropriately during episodes of unexplained high fever. Fluid intake should be regulated
in relation to the increased metabolism. Antimicrobial agents are
only useful during intervening bacterial infections.

REFERENCES

Barenberg, L.H., and Greenspan, L.: Exanthem subitum (roseola
infantum). Am. J. Dis. Child. 58:983, 1939.

Berenberg, W., Wright, S., and Janeway, C.A.: Roseola infantum
(exanthem subitum). NEJM 241:253, 1949.

Breese, B.B., Jr.: Roseola infantum (exanthem subitum). N.Y.
State J. Med. 41:1854, 1941.

Burnstine, R.C., and Paine, R.S.: Residual encephalopathy following roseola infantum. Am. J. Dis. Child. 98:144, 1959.

Clemens, H.H.: Exanthem subitum (roseola infantum). Report of
80 cases. J. Pediat. 26:66, 1945.

Hellstrom, B., and Vahlquist, B.: Experimental inoculation of
roseola infantum. Acta Paediat. 40:189, 1951.

James, U., and Freier, A.: Roseola infantum. Arch. Dis. Child.
24:54, 1949.

Kempe, C.H., Shaw, E.G., Jackson, J.R., and Silver, H.K.:
Studies on the etiology of exanthem subitum (roseola infantum).
J. Pediat. 37:561, 1950.

Letchner, A.: Roseola infantum: A review of fifty cases. Lancet
2:1163, 1955.

Zahorsky, J.: Roseola infantilis. Pediatrics 22:60, 1910.

::

3.4: ERYTHEMA INFECTIOSUM (THE FIFTH DISEASE)

INTRODUCTION: Erythema infectiosum, sometimes called the
"fifth" disease, is a specific nosographic clinical entity often misdiagnosed by the uninitiated physician. The eponym "fifth" is derived from a succession of eruptive fevers, namely scarlet fever,

measles, rubella and Duke's (the fourth) disease. Duke's disease remains a medical curiosity! Other names given to erythema infectiosum are epidemic megalerythema and ringelrothein (ring rubella).

Periodically, erythema infectiosum emerges in community epidemics, largely involving the elementary school-age population. The peak age incidences encompass 5 to 14-year-old children. Attack rates are greater among females. Multiple cases may occur in affected families; usually multiplicity relates to children but adults may acquire the disease. The epidemiologic pattern suggests close intimate contact for transmission, thereby resembling some other respiratory transmissible infections. Subclinical cases, however, cannot be identified and their frequency is unknown. There can be little doubt of silent infection, but until recognition becomes possible it must be said that the mode of transmission remains unknown. Additionally, the precise incubation period is uncertain. The study by Ager et al. (1966) provided an incubation period of about 9 days (range 7 to 11 days), whereas Balfour (1969), based on secondary familial incidence, suggested a 16-day interval.

1. ETIOLOGY AND PATHOGENESIS

Many attempts have been made to recover the infectious agent believed to be responsible for the disease (Wenner and Low, 1963); none has been found. Several studies (Werner et al., 1957); Wilcox and Evans, 1958; Wenner, unpublished) have observed suggestive, but inconstant evidence of cytopathogenicity in inoculated cell cultures. Balfour (1972) recovered rubella virus from a fraction of patients with erythema infectiosum; he inoculated a strain of rubella virus into adult volunteers who developed a rash more resembling erythema infectiosum than rubella. No further details of the disease are known. Whether or not Balfour co-cultivated the virus of erythema infectiosum in addition to rubella is as yet unresolved.

The pathogenesis of the disease is also unknown. Presumably, if acquired by the respiratory route, the agent multiplies and follows the pathways of other viruses, causing cutaneous disease. But there may be compelling reasons, namely recrudescence, arthralgias, etc., (see below) for associating the rash with emerging antibody-antigen complexes accountable for the cutaneous lesions. The histology of the skin lesion is essentially non-specific, consisting of epidermal swelling and cleavage spaces between epidermis and cutis. Histiocytes are present in the cleavage spaces. Capillary endothelial cells appear swollen. Small blood vessels are cuffed by mononuclear cells (Grimmer, 1959).

2. CLINICAL FEATURES

There are few, if any, prodromal signs preceding the appearance of the rash in children. Adults may have low-grade fever, pharyngitis, and malaise.

The nature of the rash suggests the diagnosis. Noted first on the face, the cheeks present a symmetrical rose-red hue. This is referred to as a slapped cheek appearance. The overlying skin is hot and swollen, but remains non-tender and blanches with pressure. Usually the nose is spared; there is circumoral pallor. During the next day or two maculopapules appear on the trunk, extremities, buttocks and, slightly later, on the hands and feet. The eruption on the extremities generally develop proximally and move distally, involving lateral and posterior-lateral surfaces of the skin until it eventually involves the dorsum of the hands and feet. The typical appearance is a rash consisting of annular red marginations with paler centers, with a lace-like or net-like appearance. The rash on the trunk may be quite sparse or on the buttocks, intense and blotchy.

The rash on the face fades within the next few days (1 to 4) while remaining on the trunk and extremities for about a week longer in the average case. Recrudescences with repeat staging of the cutaneous lesions may occur. Occasionally these prevail for a month or longer. A number of factors appear to be responsible for the prolonged repeating expressions of the rash, namely exposure to sunlight, exercise, and emotional stress. Occasionally, itching may be bothersome. Post-eruptive desquamation is unrecognized.

The evolution of the rash through several stages is distinctive enough to provide the diagnosis. The waxing and waning of the "butterfly" facial erythema and the reticulated contours of the rash on the extremities are the major clinical criteria for differentiating the disease from other maculopapular eruptions.

Children have few complaints during the illness. Myalgia and arthralgia may occasionally be noted in children, but are encountered more often among adults ($\sim$ 60 percent). The wrists and knees are common sites of pain and occasional swelling. Mucosal lesions have been reported, consisting of tiny dark red or grayish papules on the palate and pharyngeal mucosa. Their presence has not been noted consistently.

Virtually all patients recover without complication. Singular instances of encephalitis (2 cases), pneumonitis and hemolytic anemia have been associated with erythema infectiosum (Wadlington and Riley, 1968).

3. DIAGNOSIS

Recognition is based entirely on the clinical features of the disease. Isolated infections are often unrecognized; during outbreaks recognition is easier. Almost all of the common eruptive fevers, particularly rubella, enter the diagnosis list. Infectious mononucleosis and acquired toxoplasmosis may be included. Patients presenting with the peculiar rash of erythema infectiosum and arthralgia have been misdiagnosed as lupus erythematosis and rheumatoid arthritis. The prolonged rashes noted in a few patients with erythema infectiosum may be a cause of physician anxiety with respect to an underlying collagen disease expression.

The leukocyte count and the leukocyte ratios are within the normal range. Specific laboratory tests for erythema infectiosum are not available; appropriate tests for differentiation of some other eruptive fevers are of value only in their exclusion

4. MANAGEMENT AND TREATMENT

Ordinarily no specific therapy is required for this benign disease. Analgesics may be given for discomforting myalgias and arthralgias.

Our experience indicates that by the time an outbreak in the community is recognized, many affected children have been in attendance at school, and their subsequent quarantine has no appreciable bearing on the course of the epidemic. Such children, in our opinion, should remain in the classroom unless their physicians, for other reasons, decide otherwise.

REFERENCES

Ager, E.A., Chin, T.D.Y., and Poland, J.D.: Epidemic erythema infectiosum. NEJM 275:1326, 1966.

Balfour, H.H., Jr.: Erythema infectiosum (fifth disease): clinical review and description of 91 cases seen in an epidemic. Clin. Pediat. 8:721, 1969.

Balfour, H.H., Jr., May, D.B., Rotte, T.C., Phelps, W.R., and Schiff, G.M.: A study of erythema infectiosum: recovery of rubella virus and echovirus-12. Pediatrics 50:285, 1972.

Grimmer, H., and Joseph, A.: An epidemic of infectious erythema in Germany. Arch. Dermatol. 80:283, 1959.

Wadlington, W.B., and Riley, H.D., Jr.: Arthritis and hemolytic anemia following erythema infectiosum. JAMA 203:473, 1968.

Wenner, H.A., and Low, T.Y.: Virus diseases associated with cutaneous eruptions. Prog. Med. Virol. 5:219, 1963.

Werner, G.H., Brackman, P.S., Ketler, A., Scully, J., and Rake, G.: A new viral agent associated with erythema infectiosum. Ann. N.Y. Acad. Sci. 67:338, 1957.

Wilcox, K.R., and Evans, A.S.: Erythema infectiosum. Wisc. Med. J. 57:107, 1958.

3.5: ENTEROVIRUSES ASSOCIATED WITH CUTANEOUS ERUPTIONS

INTRODUCTION: The enteroviruses comprise 71 serotypes; among these are the polioviruses, coxsackieviruses and echoviruses (enteric cytopathic human orphan [echo] viruses). This family of viruses is responsible for a variety of clinical syndromes including muscular weakness and paralysis, aseptic meningitis, pleurodynia, respiratory illnesses and an assortment of rashes involving the skin and mucous membranes. Depending on the serotype and host, the rash may be the solitary clinical expression (e.g., coxsackievirus A16) or an expression associated with meningitis (e.g., echovirus, type 9).

The enteroviruses are ubiquitous inhabitants of the alimentary tracts of human beings. Found among all races around the world, they emerge periodically in confined community outbreaks or occasionally in broader epidemics. Clinical disease expressions often occur during summer and autumn months. Infants and children are primary targets; adults are usually spared but there are exceptions, recounted below.

Infants and children are purveyors of virus. Spread is from person to person; the fecal-oral route is a major mode of transmission; droplet spread from respiratory secretions very likely occurs. In the family setting the majority of susceptibles become infected, although not all develop recognizable disease. Following infection, enteroviruses are excreted in the feces. These viruses are recoverable also from pharyngeal secretions. Virus concentrations in feces may reach $10^5 TCID_{50}/gm$ during the first week of infection; for some (e.g., echovirus, type 9) concentrations in the pharyngeal secretion may be as great, although usually lesser quantities prevail. The duration of the carrier state varies from a few days to several weeks.

Enteroviruses are found in raw sewage; they may not be inactivated by primary and secondary sedimentation procedures. The usual concentration of chlorine used in water treatment plants may not inactivate some of these viruses.

1. ETIOLOGY AND PATHOGENESIS

The human enteroviruses are classified among the picornaviruses. The group consists of small viruses (15-30 mm in diameter) containing ribonucleic acid cores. Lacking lipid, they are insensitive to ether. Structurally, they have cubic symmetry of icosohedral type.

Most of the enteroviruses multiply in primate cell cultures producing gross cytopathic effect. Some are refractory initially, but can be adapted to grow in cell cultures. Some others have been recovered only after inoculation into mice.

Pathogenic strains appear to use common pathways in infected human beings. Primary viral implantation is in the mucosa of the pharynx and intestine. The available evidence suggests early invasion of local lymphatic tissues, particularly the tonsils and/or Peyer's patches, among others. After a cycle(s) of replication, virus can be detected in the blood stream, and is transported thereafter to susceptible target organs such as the central nervous system, skin, pancreas and testis, among others. Viremia, prevailing during the incubation period, ends with onset of clinical disease. At this time, antibodies are detectable and continue to increase over the next 10 to 20 days (Wenner and Behbehani, 1968).

2. CLINICAL FEATURES

Skin and mucosal lesions associated with enteroviruses are occasionally specific enough that the diagnosis is unmistakable (e.g., hand, foot and mouth syndrome); otherwise, they are so alike (maculopapular rashes) that clinical separation is impossible. The clinical variability should become clearer in the following discussions relating to two subgroups of the enteroviruses and the rashes associated with them (Wenner and Lou, 1973; Wenner, 1973).

3. THE COXSACKIEVIRUSES

3.1: Herpangina: This is a specific febrile illness recruiting children during late spring and summer (Zahorsky, 1924). Following an abupt onset of fever ($\leq$ 40.6 C) associated with headache, myalgia, pharyngeal discomfort and dysphagia, examination reveals clusters of vesicles or shallow ulcers on the soft palate, pillars of the fauces, tonsils and pharynx. The number of lesions varies from a few to as many as 30. The fever subsides within 3 days. General and local symptoms abate within 3 to 5 days. Healing is usually complate within a week from onset.

At least 9 Group A coxsackieviruses are definitely associated with herpangina. Other enteroviruses have been encountered sporadically.

3.2: Hand, Foot and Mouth Syndrome: This distinctive syndrome features vesicular and ulcerative lesions involving the oropharynx, hands, feet and buttocks. Onset of illness is associated with moderate fever, sore mouth or throat. At this time, or shortly thereafter, lesions like those of herpangina can be seen. The distribution may differ from classical herpangina by their presence on buccal mucous membranes and tongue; macules, vesicles and shallow ulcers develop in rapid sequence over a day or two. Vesicles surrounded by a red areola sometimes coalesce, yielding shallow ulcers measuring 1 to 2 cm in diameter.

The exanthem develops in concert with the enanthem or within hours afterward; maculopapular lesions present on the hands, and feet

undergo vesiculation. Maculopapular lesions may be present elsewhere on the body, particularly on the buttocks of infants, where
they may coalesce. These lesions fade without vesiculation.

The eruption is not profuse; only a few vesicles may appear, or
several large blister-like lesions may develop (3 to 10 mm). Such
vesicles are found most often on the dorsum of fingers and toes and
on the lateral margins of the feet. When lesions develop on palms
and soles they have been numerous, deep-seated and resembled
grains of rice.

The incubation period ranges from 3 to 6 days. The lesions persist
from 1 to 6 days. Recovery is complete without sequelae. About
80 percent of hand, foot and mouth disease occur in children under
9 years of age. Adults are not totally immune.

The serotypes associated with the syndrome include A5, A10 and
A16 (Robinson et al., 1958) coxsackieviruses. Virus may be recovered from vesicle fluid.

3.3: Other Coxsackieviruses and Rashes: An assorted variety of
rashes have been associated with other coxsackieviruses. In general Group A, type 9 is associated with maculopapular eruptions;
these rashes may occur in association with aseptic meningitis. A9
virus is also associated with vesicular lesions developing during an
illness characterized by fever, sore throat and suboccipital adenopathy. The rash, first visible on the face, extends to the trunk and
extremities. Healing without crusting occurs in 3 to 5 days, differentiating the rash from varicella.

Localized and generalized vesicular rashes have been described also
for several Group A (A4 and A7) and Group B (B1, B2, B3 and B5)
coxsackieviruses. Clusters of such infections may be encountered;
more often they are sporadic clinical encounters. They may remain
unrecognized or confused with insect bites, varicella, rubella or
even scarlet fever. These kinds of rashes have been discussed in
greater detail by Cherry (1969).

4. THE ECHOVIRUSES

4.1: Echovirus, Type 9: Widespread outbreaks during the 50's
brought this theretofore unknown disease into clinical perspective.
Infants and young children develop rash more often than older individuals. In Milwaukee, the majority of those developing the rash
were under 3 years of age (Sabin et al., 1958).

The incubation period averages about 6 days (range 2 to 10 days).
Among adults, onset of illness is abrupt and prostrating. Headache,
myalgia, photophobia, nausea, vertigo and stiffness of the neck and
back are common complaints. Children are similar affected.

The rash usually develops within a day or two after onset of illness.
Macules and papules (1-3 mm in diameter) develop on the face,
trunk and lateral surfaces of the limbs, as well as on the palms
and soles. In the Milwaukee outbreak the rash was noted to be generalized in more than half the patients; it remained confined to the
face in 25 percent, to the face and neck in 11 percent, and to the
face, neck and chest in 8 percent of children. Petechial lesions
and purpuric lesions may resemble the cutaneous lesions of meningococcemia. A white or gray enanthem may appear on the buccal
mucosa opposite the upper molars; small vesicules and ulcers may
appear on the tongue. The rash may fade in a day, or last 4 to 5
days. There is no desquamation. Biphasic and rarely triphasic
febrile episodes intervene, each with recrudescence of rash. During E9 epidemics meningitis without rash, rash without meningitis,
meningitis with rash and abortive febrile illnesses may be encountered. Recovery is almost always complete. Rarely encephalomyelitis may develop.

Echovirus type 9 can be recovered from blood, cerebrospinal fluid
(CSF), oropharyngeal secretion and feces. Viremia has been found
up to 5 days before onset of illness.

4.2: Echovirus, Type 16: The Boston Exanthem: In 1951 an epidemic of an unusual exanthematous disease was eventually associated with echovirus type 16 (Neva et al., 1954). Broad communicability has been noted among familial associates. All children and
one or both parents may contract the disease. The incubation period is about 5 days with a range of 3 to 7 days.

The rash is the last clinical manifestation of infection. Prior to its
appearance the disease is characterized by an abrupt onset of fever
($\leq 39^{\circ}$ C), shaking chills, headache, myalgia and burning or painful
eye sensations. These symptoms are more pronounced in adults and
subside less quickly than in children. In most, but not all cases the
rash appears within 24 to 48 hours after the fever subsides, and lasts
from 1 to 4 days. A discrete salmon-pink macular eruption appears
on the face, neck and chest. Usually scanty, occasionally confluent,
the rash may involve the extremities, including the palms and soles.
An enanthem characterized by small raised red or yellow-white lesions may be found on the soft palate, fauces and uvula. When present, the enanthem serves to distinguish this rash from that of exanthem subitum. Recovery occurs without any sequelae.

Echovirus type 16 may be recovered readily from feces and oropharyngeal secretions.

4.3: Other Echoviruses and Rashes: Only a few of the echovirus
infections have not been associated with rashes. A large number
have indefinite association whereas others (e.g., types 2, 4, 5, 6,
11, 18, 25 and 30) have definite associations. Marked variations

exist not only in the frequency of occurrence in relation to other signs of infection (e.g., aseptic meningitis) but also with respect to the nature of the rash, even within the same serotype. Rashes vary from maculopapular (types 2, 4, 5, 11 and 30) to scarlatiniform (type 14) to vesicular (types 9, 11, 16, 17 and 25) to petechial (types 14 and 32).

5. DIAGNOSIS

At this point it should be clear that clinical differentiation of rashes etiologically related to many of these viruses is difficult, if not often impossible. Many of the above rashes may resemble exanthem subitum, rubella, insect bites and/or drug eruptions, especially in the sporadically involved patient. Clinical laboratory data are seldom helpful. The virus laboratory is the only resource for providing the needed studies. Samples apt to be helpful include: (1) vesicle fluid, (2) feces, and (3) pharyngeal secretions. When there is associated meningitis a sample of CSF may provide the diagnosis.

Antibodies develop quickly during the course of these infections. These may be detected by hemagglutination-inhibition, complement fixation, fluorescence-antigen labeling or neutralization tests. Since there are 71 specific enterovirus serotypes, and none of them sharing common antigens, it is a practical impossibility to search for a type-specific antibody response.

In evaluating laboratory data the clinician should recall that the singular recovery of an enterovirus from feces may not signal the true etiology of the exanthem. Human beings may acquire and excrete virus in "silent" infections of the gastrointestinal tract, and such may be unrelated to the presenting disease (Melnick and Wenner, 1969).

6. MANAGEMENT AND TREATMENT

Except for the polioviruses, no practical means are available for preventing the diseases caused from other enteroviruses. The efficacy of gamma globulin is doubtful even when administered early in the incubation period. Treatment is entirely supportive and directed toward alleviation of the associated discomforts.

Nomenclature: Because of some overlapping biological properties, it is no longer possible to classify the enteroviruses as coxsackie or echoviruses. A new numbering system has been developed ranking all enteroviruses from 1 to 71. We have retained the familiar but outdated nomenclature. The reader may refer to the current serotype classification (Rosen et al., 1970).

REFERENCES

Cherry, J.D.: Newer viral exanthems. Advances in Pediatrics. Vol. 16. pp. 233-286. Year Book Medical Publishers, Inc., Chicago, 1969.

Melnick, J.L., and Wenner, H.A.: Enteroviruses in Diagnostic Procedures for Viral and Rickettsial Infections. Chapter 17. Am. Pub. Health Assoc., Inc., New York, 1969.

Neva, F.A., Feemster, R.F., and Gorbach, I.J.: Clinical and epidemiological features of an unusual epidemic exanthem. JAMA 155:544, 1954.

Robinson, C.R., Doane, F.W., and Rhodes, A.I.: Report of an outbreak of febrile illness with pharyngeal lesions and exanthems. Toronto, summer 1957 - isolation of group A Coxsackie virus. Canad. Med. Assoc. J. 79:615, 1958.

Rosen, L., Melnick, J.L., Schmidt, N.J., and Wenner, H.A.: Subclassification of enteroviruses and ECHO virus type 34. Arch. ges. Virusforsch. 30:89, 1970.

Sabin, A.B., Krumbiegel, E.R., and Wigand, R.: ECHO type 9 virus disease. Am. J. Dis. Child. 96:197, 1958.

Wenner, H.A., and Behbehani, A.M.: ECHO viruses. Virol. Monographs. Vol. 1., pp. 1-72, Springer-Verlag, Wien, 1968.

Wenner, H.A., and Lou, T.Y.: Virus diseases associated with cutaneous eruptions. Prog. Med. Virol. 5:219, 1963. See also Wenner, H.A.: Prog. Med. Virol. 16:269, 1973.

Zahorsky, J.: Herpangina (a specific disease). Arch. Paediat. 41: 181, 1924.

::

3.6: VARICELLA AND HERPES ZOSTER

INTRODUCTION: Varicella is a common contagious disease with a distinctive generalized rash. In contrast, the less commonly encountered eruption of herpes zoster is localized to segmental areas of the skin and mucous membranes. Both diseases are caused by Herpesvirus varicellae (Weller, 1976).

Varicella develops in susceptible individuals following exposure to an infected person. The period of communicability ranges from one to 4 days before and up to 5 days after the rash appears. The available evidence suggests airborne transmission of virus emanating from the pharynx, but factually this has not been demonstrated (Nelson and St. Geme, 1966). The incubation period averages about 15 days with a range of 11 to 20 days.

The endemicity of varicella and its periodic slow moving epidemicity in the U.S.A. are well recognized (Fig. 3.2). The phenomenon relates largely to variable recruitment of susceptible children in an otherwise largely immune population. Infection provides solid immunity; second attacks of clinical varicella are unlikely. Silent reinfection probably occurs based on antibody rises recognized following exposure to varicella-zoster (VZ) virus (Brunell et al., 1975).

In this country, attack rates from varicella are greatest among children, especially in age groups attending elementary school. Overall attack rates among susceptible children in hospitals range from 68 to 75 percent; about 60 percent of susceptible siblings acquire varicella when the disease is introduced in the family unit. Such exposures in large families generally recruit all susceptibles; sometimes a sibling(s) escapes the first exposure only to develop the disease at a later interval (tertiary case). Most adults have had the disease; outbreaks of varicella are rarely recognized among military recruits.

Herpes zoster is a sporadic disease. The incubation period is unknown. Most zoster patients have no known exposure to varicella or zoster. The prevailing evidence indicates reactivation of VZ virus lying latent in neural ganglia having arrived therein from an earlier attack of varicella. There may be exceptions, namely the development of zoster in infancy, if congenital infection can be excluded (Frey et al., 1977). On the other hand, varicella has been contracted by children following exposure to herpes zoster.

1. ETIOLOGY AND PATHOGENESIS

The VZ virion contains a central core of DNA lying within capsids surrounded by a bilaminar envelope. VZ virus is recovered readily from vesicle fluid producing, in cultured cells, focal lesions which enlarge by peripheral extension directly involving adjacent cells; intranuclear inclusions develop within infected cells (Weller et al., 1958). These inclusions are found within epithelial cells of vesicles developing in both varicella and zoster. The infectious nature of the virus particles in vesicle fluid has been established by experimental infection of children.

The site(s) of primary implantation of VZ virus in varicella is thought to be in the pharynx, even though virus cannot be recovered readily from pharyngeal secretions. Viremia occurs (Feldman and Epp, 1976). The cellular components contributing to viremia, whether they be in lymph nodes, spleen, endothelial cells or leukocytes remain unknown. Virus in the blood stream is transported to the skin

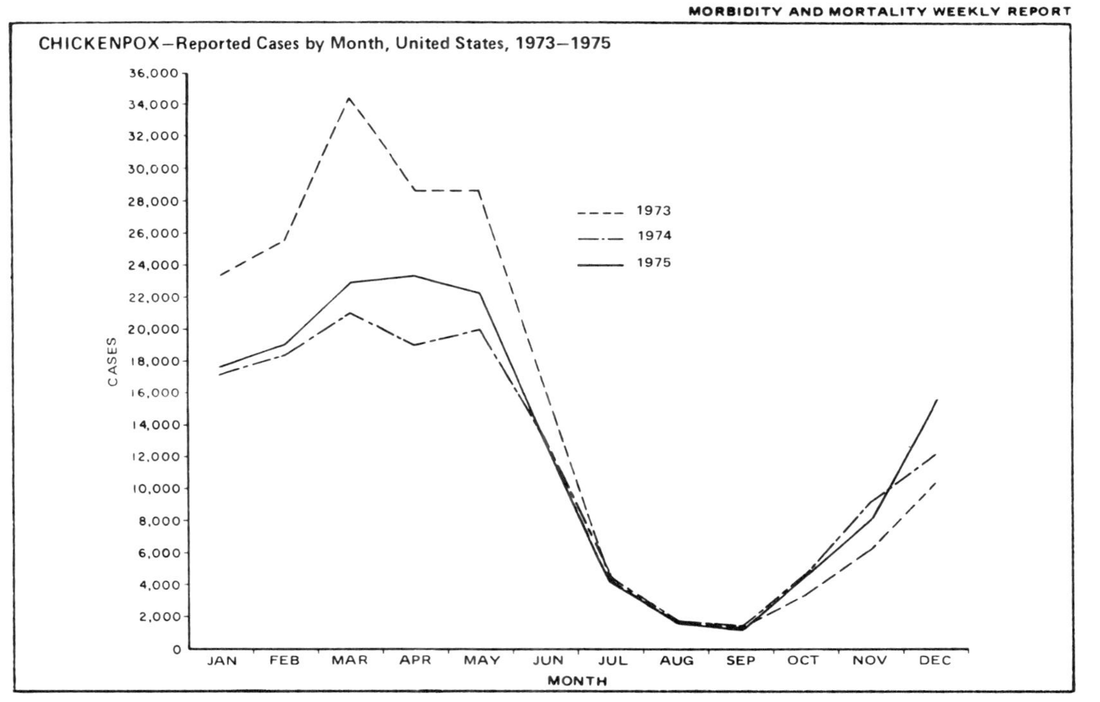

FIG. 3.2: Seasonal variation of chickenpox.

and mucous membranes. The initiation of the dermal lesion is primarily a virus effect. Antibodies, developing just before or at onset of rash may engender further cellular injury by complexing with VZ virus abundantly present in vesicle fluid.

Virus in skin lesions is transported to the central nervous system (CNS) by moving inward along sensory nerve fibers. Reaching neural ganglia, the virus may remain dormant therein for the lifetime of the individual. Otherwise, with activation, the virus may move outward along neurones to involve the skin in development of zoster, or inward into the spinal cord with the development of either leptomeningitis, or paralysis from involvement of anterior horn cells. VZ virus has been found in cerebrospinal fluid (Luby, 1973) spinal ganglia (Shibuta et al., 1974) and CNS tissues (McCormick et al., 1969). Whether or not encephalitis is a consequence of viral action remains unclear. Current concepts generally consider encephalitis a response of immunologic injury.

2. CLINICAL FEATURES

During childhood the eruption may be the first sign of infection. Prodromal signs may precede the rash by several days. These consist of low-grade fever ($\leq 38^\circ$ C), listlessness, headache, backache and abdominal pain, in any of several combinations.

At its onset, the exanthem may resemble scarlet fever. Usually such erythema preceding the development of macules and papules lasts only a few hours. The papular lesions commonly appear first on the back, then on the rest of the trunk and, within hours, on the face and scalp. Sometimes they are first seen above the neck. Macular lesions may be distributed sparsely on the buccal and pharyngeal mucosa. The skin of the extremities is involved last, with most lesions distributed on proximal surfaces. Small "dew drop" vesicles develop in the center of papules.

The skin lesions develop in a series of crops as a rule. After a day or 2 all classes of lesions ranging from macules, papules and vesicles may be found. Pustulation is not usually much in evidence. Vesicles may quickly crust over. One to 5 crops may develop during the ensuing several days. The number of pocks varies from several to many hundreds.

The cyclic emergence of vesicles may go on for 5 days. Vesiculation usually ceases by the 2nd or 3rd day; as a rule the transition from vesicle to crust lasts 24 to 36 hours. The earliest lesions may have crusted before the last vesicles develop. By the end of the first week, and certainly by the second, all crusts have fallen away.

Vesicles may appear on the conjunctivae. Occasionally, lesions, usually seen as shallow ulcers, involve the mouth, pharynx, larynx, and trachea; a croup-like syndrome may be associated with involvement of the latter tissues. Esophagitis may develop. Typical lesions may develop on vulval mucosa and on vaginal epithelium.

Leukopenia, thrombocytopenia and relative lymphocytosis may precede onset of rash. After onset of rash leukocytosis and absolute lymphocytosis may follow.

3. COMPLICATIONS

Generally, complications are few; they may occasionally compromise the life of the patient. Among these are pyodermas, bleeding manifestations, pneumonia and a variety of neurologic disorders.

3.1: Pyodermas: Superimposed pyogenic bacteria, principally Group A hemolytic streptococci and invasive staphylococci may lead to cellulitis and suppurative lymphadenitis. Bullous lesions may develop from VZ virus, but suggest toxic epidermal necrolysis from staphylococci (Fig. 3.3). Gram stain and cultures may be helpful in differential diagnosis.

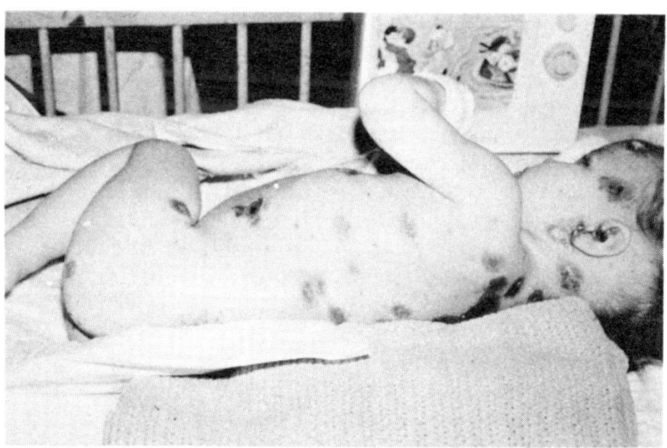

FIG. 3.3: Secondary staphylococcal skin infection in a
child with chickenpox.

3.2: Bleeding Manifestations: In uncomplicated varicella an occasional vesicle may contain blood. These may relate to minor angiopathy. A transient benign thrombocytic purpura involving a variable number of vesicles develops in a few patients (~2 percent). Postinfectious thrombocytic purpura develops later during the crusting stage; the outcome is favorable although bleeding (i.e., nose bleeds, gastrointestinal oozings) may occur intermittently for several months. Rarely, malignant forms of bleeding develop, involving the skin and subcutaneous tissues (purpura fulminans). There may be significant loss of blood from the genitourinary and gastrointestinal tracts (Hallersley, 1970).

3.3: Pneumonia: Adults may develop varicella pneumonia within one to 6 days after onset of the rash. Onset is sudden with cough, chest pain, dyspnea, occasional cyanosis and hemoptysis. Roentgenograms reveal nodular pulmonary infiltrates often peribronchial in distribution. These may calcify. Pneumonia complicating varicella of children is more likely of bacterial origin; however, varicella pneumonia does occur infrequently in apparently normal children, and somewhat more often in the immunologically handicapped. Respiratory epithelial cells may be found to contain intranuclear inclusions.

3.4: Neurological Disorders: Cerebellar ataxia, leptomeningitis, encephalitis, myelitis, acute ascending spinal paralysis, polyneuritis and optic neuritis may complicate varicella. The incidence is about 0.5 percent. About a third of the neurological sequelae relate to cerebellar ataxia.

Involvement of the CNS may occur before, during or after the eruption and has no relationship to the clinical severity of varicella. At the outset there are classic signs of neuronal irritation. A mild CSF pleocytosis mainly lymphocytic is usually found; spinal fluid protein is elevated. The course is variable. Complete recovery may be anticipated with cerebellar ataxia. For other CNS involvement, the course is less benign. The overall mortality rate is about 5 percent; for the encephalopathies the risk of death approaches 40 percent. About 80 percent recover completely; a fraction (~15 percent) have residual neuromuscular sequelae including mental retardation and blindness.

3.5: Other Problems: Varicella may be associated with glomerulonephritis. Some renal injury relates to superimposed infection from Group A streptococci; some may be related to injury by varicella antigen-antibody complexes. Carditis and orchitis have been encountered in young adults. Appendicitis may be related to mucosal lesions in the gut.

Reye et al. (1963) recognized a syndrome consisting of hypoglycemia (not always a feature), encephalopathy and fatty degeneration of liver and kidney; sometimes this ominous syndrome develops during varicella (Jenkins et al., 1967).

A transient anergy to tuberculin has been noted during the eruptive and immediate eruptive period. Tuberculin sensitivity is restored usually within 2 weeks.

3.6: Neonatal Varicella: Infants born of mothers developing varicella at the end of pregnancy may develop varicella. The risks of serious disease in the neonate can be related to the time of appearance of varicella in the mother and her baby. The onset of varicella in the mother within 4 days of delivery will not allow for the development of maternal antibodies for placental transfer. These babies then may develop varicella within 5 to 10 days after birth. Late onset varicella carries an estimated mortality of 20 percent due to generalized varicella (Meyer, 1974).

On the other hand, should maternal varicella develop 10 to 20 days prior to delivery and the baby acquires early onset varicella (within 4 days after birth), then the disease is almost always benign, due in a large part to maternally derived antibodies.

3.7: <u>Congenital Varicella</u>: There is evidence that women developing varicella or zoster early in pregnancy may deliver a deformed infant. The infants present with cicatrices along dermatomes, limb atrophy of an affected part, eye defects, consisting of microphthalmia and chorioretinitis and sometimes cortical atropy (Frey et al., 1977).

3.8: <u>Herpes Zoster</u>: Zoster is characteristically a localized lesion. The vesicular eruption usually is restricted to an area of the skin supplied by sensory nerves of a single or neighboring group of dorsal-root ganglia. In childhood, the principal sites are on the trunk or proximal parts of extremities. The naso-lingual branch of the fifth nerve may be involved (zoster ophthalmicus) as may the geniculate ganglion (zoster of the external ear) with accompanying paralysis of the seventh nerve. A generalized vesicular rash indistinguishable from varicella may immediately precede or follow (by several days) the appearance of the localized lesions.

The eruption in children is often painless; it develops and heals faster than in adults. Mild fever and malaise are present at the outset. Local lesions develop as papules which quickly vesiculate, increasing in numbers over 2 or 3 days. Outcropping is less well defined than in varicella; the crops are fewer and evolution of lesions sometimes faster. Drying begins in a few days; scab formation continues up to 2 weeks. Regional lymphadenitis is an accompanying feature of the infection. The prognosis is for full recovery.

Post-herpetic neuralgia does not usually develop. Rarely there is involvement of CNS tissues related very likely to inflammatory lesions of contiguous motor nerve nuclei, anterior horn cells, or neuronitis of peripheral mixed motor and sensory nerves.

Factors predisposing to development of herpes zoster include diseases involving the lymphatic (Hodgkin's disease, etc.) and hematopoietic (leukemia) systems.

Immunologically handicapped children, either genetically determined (e.g., Nezelof's syndrome) or disease-acquired (e.g., Letterer-Siwe's disease), are at risk of fatal dissemination of VZ virus, whether from varicella or zoster. Other adverse factors relate to radiation and cytolytic therapies directed toward control of the disease processes mentioned above.

4. DIAGNOSIS

Recognition of varicella is seldom difficult. Rickettsial pox may resemble mild varicella when the vesicles appear on erythematous papules. The course is atypical for varicella; a search should be made for the papular eschar caused by the bite of the infected mite. Other cutaneous lesions include those caused by insect bites, and by other viruses, namely herpes simplex, variola and vaccinia.

Zoster-like lesions during infancy may be caused by herpes simplex virus (Music et al., 1971).

VZ virus can be grown in a variety of cell cultures, principally of human origin. The virus is readily recovered from vesicle fluid; it is less readily recovered from blood, CSF and other body fluids. In the disseminated disease the virus can be rescued from visceral organs. Identity is established by the cytopathic characteristics, and by direct fluorescence of viral antigen using appropriately labeled antisera. Scrapings from the base of the vesicle provide multinucleate giant cells containing intranuclear inclusions. Viral particles can be seen by microscopy, but it is impossible to differentiate VZ from other herpesviruses.

Antibody development may be determined by complement fixation, fluorescent microscopy, or neutralization tests. The procedures used will depend upon the facilities available locally or in regional public health laboratories. Complement-fixing antibodies develop 5 or 6 days after onset of varicella, and often earlier in zoster. In both diseases there is progressive antibody rise during the ensuing month and, thereafter, progressive fall with total loss over a period of months up to 2 years. Varicella antibody rises may occur during primary herpes simplex virus infection. The fluorescent antibody membrane antigen (Williams et al., 1974) test and the neutralization tests are not only more sensitive but provide means of measuring both transient (IgM) and persistent antibody (IgG).

5. MANAGEMENT AND TREATMENT

Varicella developing in the normal child requires only supportive care, if any. Cleanliness, and paring of fingernails are all that are generally needed. Itching may require lotions or pruritic (Benadryl) medications. Pain and paraesthesias from zoster may require analgesics or sedatives for a brief time. For localized pyodermas, starch baths and bacitracin ointment applications may be helpful. In more severe pyodermas and cellulitis appropriate cultures (skin lesions and blood) should reveal the offending bacteria; and thereafter from the antimicrobial sensitivity patterns, the appropriate therapy.

Severe infections, particularly those associated with varicella pneumonia or with risks of progressive dissemination in persons with immunological deficiencies require prompt therapy. Zoster immune globulin (see below) is not apt to be helpful. Leukocyte transfusions may be helpful. At this time such individuals should receive adenine arabinoside, a purine nucleoside now available for such usage. This compound is less toxic and more effective than cytosine arabinoside. The current dosage is 10 mg/kilo/24 hrs given as a 6-hour infusion daily for 5 days. The trial studies with this drug have been encouraging; the drug is now available for selected usage (Johnson et al., 1975).

Additionally, it is important to maintain water and electrolyte balances and to meet the nutritional needs of the few patients developing severe VZ infections or their complications.

6. PREVENTION

6.1: __Immunoglobulins__: The clinical course of varicells can be either modified, or aborted with the use of appropriate immune globulin. Ordinary Red Cross gamma globulin, even in large doses (0.6 ml/kilo) does not prevent but will modify the disease (Ross, 1962). Zoster immune globulin (ZIG) is effective (Brunell et al., 1969; Judelson et al., 1974). ZIG is the gamma globulin fraction of sera obtained from convalescent zoster patients.

ZIG can be obtained through the auspices of regional consultants or from the Center for Disease Control, Atlanta, Georgia (see Red Book, American Academy of Pediatrics). ZIG is reserved for use in __prevention__ of VZ infection in patients at risk of developing disseminated disease. ZIG is __ineffective in the treatment__ of either varicella or zoster. ZIG dosage is weight-related and distributed in 1.25 ml vials (see Table 3-1).

TABLE 3-1: ZIG* DOSAGE SCHEDULE ACCORDING TO WEIGHT OF RECIPIENT		
BODY WEIGHT	DOSE	
Kilograms	Ml.	No. Vials
0-9[#]	1.25	1
10-19	2.50	2
20-29	3.75	3
$\geq$ 30	5.00	4

* ZIG - zoster immune globulin

\# From Center for Disease Control, 1973.

ZIG provides transient immunity. Risks of re-exposure should be reassessed in the family setting where secondary and even tertiary cases develop.

6.2: Vaccine: An approved VZ virus vaccine is not available. An apparently attenuated virus preparation has been developed and studied in Japan (Asano et al., 1977). The Japanese group report protection in a small group of hospitalized and familial contacts. The risks associated with an attenuated virus vaccine for susceptible compromised persons is as yet unknown.

REFERENCES

Asano, Y., Nakayama, H., Yazati, T., Kato, R., Hirose, S., Tsuzuki, K., Ito, S., Isomura, S., and Takahashi, M.: Protection against varicella in family contacts by immediate inoculation with live varicella virus. Pediatrics 59:3, 1977.

Brunell, P.A., Gershon, A.A., Uduman, S., and Steinberg, S.: Varicella zoster immunoglobulins during varicella, latency and zoster. J. Infect. Dis. 132:49, 1975.

Brunell, P.A., Ross, A., Miller, L.H., and Kuo, B.: Prevention of varicella by zoster immune globulin. NEJM280:1191, 1969.

Center for Disease Control: Zoster immunoglobulin program. Mortality and Morbidity Weekly Report 22:62, 1973.

Feldman, S., and Epp, E.: Isolation of varicella-zoster virus from blood. J. Pediat. 88:265, 1976.

Frey, H.M., Bialkin, G., and Gershon, A.A.: Congenital varicella: Case report of a serologically proved long-term survivor. Pediatrics 59:110, 1977.

Hallersley, P.G.: Purpura fulminans. Am. J. Dis. Child 120:467, 1970.

Jenkins, R., Dvorak, A., and Patrick, J.: Encephalopathy and fatty degeneration of the viscera associated with chickenpox. Pediatrics 39:769, 1967.

Johnson, M.T., Luby, J.P., Buchanan, R.A., and Milulec, D.: Treatment of varicella-zoster virus infections with adenine arabinoside. J. Infect. Dis. 131:225, 1975.

Judelson, R.G., Meyer, J.D., Ellis, R.J., and Thomas, E.K.: Efficacy of zoster immune globulin. Pediatrics 53:476, 1974.

Luby, J.P.: Varicella-zoster virus. J. Invest. Dermatol. 61:212, 1973.

McCormick, W.F., Rodnitzky, R.L., Schochet, S.S., Jr., and McKee, A.P.: Varicella-zoster encephalomyelitis. A morphologic and virologic study. Arch. Neurol. 21:559, 1969.

Meyer, J.D.: Congenital varicella in term infant. Risks reconsidered. J. Infect. Dis. 129:215, 1974.

Music, S.I., Fine, E.M., and Togo, Y.: Zoster-like disease in the newborn due to herpes simplex virus. NEJM 284:24, 1971.

Nelson, A.M., and St. Geme, J.W., Jr.: On the respiratory spread of varicella-zoster virus. Pediatrics 37:1007, 1966.

Reye, R.D.K., Morgan, G., and Baral, J.: Encephalopathy and fatty degeneration of the viscera. Lancet 2:749, 1963.

Ross, A.H.: Modification of chickenpox in family contacts by administration of gamma globulin. NEJM 267:369, 1962.

Shibuata, H., Ishikawa, T., Hondo, R., Aoyama, Y., Kurata, K., and Matumoto, M.: Varicella virus isolation from spinal ganglion. Arch. ges. Virusforsch. 45:582, 1974.

Weller, T.H.: Varicella-herpes zoster virus. Chapter 21. In: Viral Infections of Humans: Epidemiology and Control. A.S. Evans, ed., Plenum Medical Book Co., N.Y., 1976.

Weller, T.H., Witton, H.M., and Bell, E.J.: The etiologic agents of varicella and herpes zoster: I. Isolation, propagation, and cultural characteristics in vitro. J. Exp. Med. 108:843, 1958.

Williams, V., Gershon, A., and Brunell, P.A.: Serologic response to varicella-zoster membrane antigens by indirect immunofluorescence. J. Infect. Dis. 130:669, 1974.

GENERAL REFERENCES - NOT CITED

Burgoon, C.F., Jr., Burgoon, J.S., and Baldridge, G.D.: The natural history of herpes zoster. JAMA 164:265, 1957.

Gordon, J.E.: Chickenpox: an epidemiologic review. Am. J. Med. Sci. 244:362, 1962.

Krugman, S., and Ward, R.: Varicella-zoster infection. Chapter 31. 5th ed. In: Infectious Diseases of Children and Adults. C.V. Mosby Co., St. Louis, 1973.

Taylor Robinson, D., and Caunt, E.: Varicella virus. Virology Monograph No. 12. Springer-Verlag, N.Y., 1972.

Wesselhoeft, C.: The differential diagnosis of chickenpox and smallpox. NEJM 230:15, 1944.

::

3.7: POXVIRUSES

1. VARIOLA

INTRODUCTION: Smallpox has almost been eradicated as one of the scourges once widely prevalent in the world-at-large. The global vaccination program of the World Health Organization launched 10 years ago has eradicated the disease in all but a few of the remaining endemic areas. Ethiopia remains one of the last strongholds.

North America and Europe became free of smallpox about 40 years ago; such freedom has been maintained by local containment of the disease (quarantine and vaccination) following arrival of an infected person from an endemic area. The impact of vaccination on the disappearance of smallpox in the U.S.A. and the United Kingdom is not precisely known. But it is known that the hazards associated with vaccination are greater currently than those that ordinarily follow imported smallpox.

Smallpox is a disease of human beings. Man is the natural reservoir; the disease is transmissible from person to person. The incubation period is about 12 days. Communicability is greatest within families, in hospitals, and by crowding and unhygienic conditions during war and other catastrophes. In endemic areas children have maximal incidence; in virgin populations no age group is exempt.

Smallpox virus is transmitted <u>initially</u> in droplets expelled from the pharyngeal mucosa. An infected person begins to shed virus just prior to the eruption when local lesions in the pharynx are developing. An abundance of virus develops in vesicles and persists in dermal lesions through the stage of crusting. Dermal crusts and infected squames contain virus available for aerosol, or possible intradermal transmission.

Monkeys may acquire infection from a closely related pox-virus; their importance as either viral reservoirs or as transmitters of virus to human beings is not yet fully understood. Human infections from monkeypox virus simulate smallpox.

1.1: ETIOLOGY AND PATHOGENESIS: Variola and vaccinia viruses are members of the poxvirus group. They are among the largest viruses measuring 230 x 500 mμ. Like other virions of the group, they contain a DNA genome coated by proteins and enveloped by lipoproteins. These viruses are extremely stable; they may survive in dessicated crusts for over a year. The elementary bodies in vesicle fluid can be seen by light microscopy, and their characteristic mulberry-like contour delineated by electron microscopy. Variola and vaccinia viruses have similar antigens; hence they have closely related immunologic properties.

The available evidence indicates viral entry and penetrance in cells of the upper respiratory tract. After local multiplication within susceptible cells the virus enters regional lymph nodes whereupon it undergoes further replication. Although the precise movement of variola virus is unknown, the forthcoming viremia preceding the eruption suggests either: (1) another multiplication cycle in secondary target organs (e.g., Kupffer cells or hepatocytes), or (2) in endothelial cells. Following onset of viremia variola virus reaches the tertiary target organs, namely skin and mucous membranes (Downie, 1965).

Vaccinia virus, particularly in the compromised host, may use similar pathways; viremia arising from vaccinia virus is usually not detectable in the uncompromised host.

1.2: CLINICAL FEATURES: On about the 12th day after exposure there is sudden onset of fever ($\leq 40^{\circ}$C) with accompanying headache, myalgia and photophobia. Between the 2nd and 4th day of illness a few faint macules develop on the face, back, chest or forearm. At this stage the fever abates and the patient feels better. An erythematous blush may appear in the groins, axillae and on the abdomen. The fever again mounts and new macules rapidly develop in fairly orderly progression on the face, back, forearms, hands, and spread thence to the chest, legs and feet. The earliest lesions may be seen in the mouth and pharynx. Papules quickly vesiculate (12 to 24 hours). There is a gradual change in the density of the lesions; the majority are located on the upper face and on the arms and legs and a minority on the trunk. Multiloculated, pearly vesicles pustulate within hours. Pustules encrustate about the 8th day; by the 14th day the crusted scales begin to fall away proceeding centrifugally over the next 8 or 10 days.

This description applies to the classical benign semi-confluent type of smallpox described by Dixon (1962). He has classified smallpox into 9 types from malignant (purpura variolosa) to abortive (variola sine eruptione) forms. The mortality rates vary, averaging about 30 percent for the confluent types of illness. Superimposed bacterial infections do not account for the risks of dying; the risks relate, it would seem, to the consequences of viral replication in critical visceral target organs, and to multifactorial sequences involving the respiratory mucous membranes, the skin, the bone marrow, the cardiovascular and the gastrointestinal systems.

Variola minor differs from classical variola in its milder clinical expression and much lower risk of death. Prodromal features of infection and the evolution of the rash are similar to those of classical varicella, excepting that the rash in the minor variant usually is not confluent. Toxic manifestations are not as great; secondary fever may not develop, and the disease is not as prolonged. On the other hand, both the classical and minor variants may be equally severe.

Modified smallpox may develop in previously vaccinated individuals. Such infections are clinically quite different from those noted above. While the distribution of lesions is characteristic, the rash is apt to resemble chickenpox. In the abortive form (no rash) the only signs are those of a prodromal grippe-like syndrome. Kempe (1975) has pointed out that risks of exposure and contracting smallpox are unrelated to the severity of the clinical disease in an index case.

1.3: DIAGNOSIS: Physicians in the U.S.A. and elsewhere in nonendemic areas of the world may not recognize smallpox. The earliest lesions may be mistaken for varicella, erythema multiforme, meningococcemia, typhus fever, etc. Hence, several features of pox exanthema should be carefully noted, namely the pre-eruptive fever, the rapid progression of a singular crop of papules, and the centrifugal distribution of the lesions, all of which suggest the possibility of smallpox. A history of travel into the remaining endemic areas, and of known exposure to smallpox, should be ascertained.

Suspected cases should be reported to local health authorities. Appropriate laboratory studies will quickly confirm (or rule out) the diagnosis. These include studies of cutaneous lesions and their contents, and of blood and serum. Viral particles in vesicular fluids are visible by electron microscopy; viral antigens can be readily detected in the vesicle or pustular fluid and even in the crusts. The virus can be propagated in chick embryos or in cell cultures. Antibodies appearing between the 5th and 10th day after onset of illness can be defined. A reference laboratory can confirm the diagnosis within a few hours.

1.4: MANAGEMENT AND PREVENTIVE MEASURES: Specific antiviral drugs effective in the treatment of smallpox are not currently available. Treatment is entirely supportive and directed toward prevention or treatment of superimposed bacterial complication, and maintenance of cardiovascular and metabolic homeostasis. Prevention: Vaccinia immune globulin and methisazone (N-methylisatin β-thiosemicarbizone) have been recommended following recognized exposure. The use of these substances and other applicable control measures have been described in a very nice synopsis by Kempe (1975).

2. VACCINIA

INTRODUCTION: Vaccinia virus is closely related to variola and monkeypox viruses. It has the same size, stability and complex morphology of other numbers of the mammalian subgroup. The origin of many stocks of vaccinia virus used for vaccination is obscure. Vaccination against smallpox is protective but such immunity is not absolute. Protection declines with time, although modulation of infection may persist for years.

The recommended procedure for vaccination, revaccination and the anticipated responses therefrom have been discussed also by Kempe (1975) and need not be recapitulated here.

Data accumulated in several studies (Lane et al., 1967; Dick, 1971) indicate an appreciable morbidity following vaccination. Undesirable complications considered along with the currently reduced risks of acquiring smallpox in this country, and the capabilities of limiting spread following importation of smallpox, have all been influential in the discontinuation of routine vaccination. Thus, in the U.S.A., vaccination is recommended only for selected persons, namely those traveling into endemic areas, those working in health-related fields, and members of the Armed Forces.

Vaccination is contraindicated in infants and children with defects in cell-mediated immunity, and in persons with malignant diseases involving bone marrow, lymph nodes and the thymus.

2.1: CLINICAL FEATURES: Ordinarily vaccinia virus evokes only the local lesion and the relatively trivial consequences of vaccination. Occasionally however, given the right circumstances, complications may intervene. These are: 1) Vaccinia gangrenosa: This progressive form of generalized vaccinia is rarely encountered. The vaccinal pustule, instead of receding by the 14th day, continues an indolent erosive burrowing eventually reaching deeply into subcutaneous tissues. New satellite cutaneous lesions may appear locally or new lesions may develop on other parts of the body (e.g., nostrils, groin, and in visceral organs) following viral metastasis. In untreated patients these ulcerative lesions progress, often over several months, and the patient dies. 2) Generalized vaccinia: By definition, the uncomplicated form pertains to persons with an intact skin. At about the second week following primary inoculation, vaccinal lesions erupt over a period of 4 to 6 days elsewhere on the body. The development and resolution of these lesions follow the course of the primary reaction. Generalized vaccinia develops more often among children and adults than among infants. The mortality rate is probably about 7 percent or less. 3) Eczema vaccinatum: Individuals with skin eruptions (eczema) may develop a widely disseminated eruption by translocation of virus from the primary vaccinal source elsewhere to their skin. These persons are at risk of generalized infection since viremia upsurges during maturation of the many local lesions. Primary lesions emerge rapidly within a week and are followed by new crops involving part or all of the integument. Mortality rates in untreated patients range from 10 to 20 percent.

4) <u>Accidental vaccinia</u>: Solitary or multiple vaccinal lesions may appear elsewhere on the body on about the 12th day following primary vaccination. Such lesions may occur anywhere but are commonly found on the lip, tongue, genitalia and eyelid. These lesions develop from autoinoculation. 5) <u>Roseola vaccinia</u> (erythema multiforme-like eruptions): This dermal reaction encompasses a macular, brilliant red rash appearing 7 to 14 days following primary vaccination. The rash, sometimes most intense around the vaccination site, may involve the entire body. The rash may be papular, vesicular or urticarial. The vesicular form must be distinguished from generalized vaccinia; their courses differ. Roseola vaccinia evolves and disappears within a week. 6) <u>Encephalitis</u>: This rare complication intervenes at about the time the vaccinal reaction is at its nadir, that is, about day 12 (range 5 to 15 days). The case fatality in the U.S.A. approaches 25 percent.

2.2: DIAGNOSIS: The complications noted above usually intervene during the evolution of the primary vaccinal lesion; the associated events provide the diagnosis as a rule. Biopsy of the dermal lesion reveals characteristic cytoplasmic inclusions (Guarnieri bodies). Vaccinia virus is readily propagated, and its identity revealed from virus recovered in cell cultures or in chick embryos.

Differentiation of eczema vaccinatum and eczema herpeticum present particular challenges. Herpesviruses produce intranuclear inclusions; they are readily propagated in cell cultures or in chick embryos, and are easily identified.

2.3: MANAGEMENT AND TREATMENT: Children with eczema should not be vaccinated with the standard vaccinia virus vaccines. They should not be exposed to individuals, particularly siblings, who have been recently vaccinated. The uncomplicated generalized vaccinia, the acquired local variety from autoinoculation, and the roseola vaccinia generally require only vigilant observation. Most patients are engendering antibodies when these complications intervene; hence most recover quite quickly.

Human vaccinia immunoglobulin is effective in the prevention and treatment of eczema vaccinatum. In vaccinia gangrenosa, methisazone and vaccinia immune globulin should be used simultaneously. The resource aids in effective diagnosis and treatment schedules are summarized in Kempe's resume (1975).

3. OTHER POXVIRUS INFECTIONS

3.1: <u>Monkeypox</u>: Monkeypox virus infections are very similar to experimental variola. There is a close relationship of these viruses (Cho and Wenner, 1973). Infections simulating variola have been observed in African children.

3.2: Yaba Tumor Virus: Subcutaneous noncapsulated tumors of
histocytic origin have been linked with a specific poxvirus infection
in monkeys. Human volunteers inoculated with Yaba tumor virus
develop similar tumors, as do laboratory workers after accidental
inoculations.

3.3: Tanapox: Observed in Africa (Downie et al., 1971), this poxvirus infection is associated with prodromal signs similar to those
of variola. During the primary fever a papule develops on the upper
arm, face, neck or trunk. The papule develops into a raised umbilicated vesicle. Evolution thereafter into a large firm lesion, without further outcrops of lesions, distinguishes the disease from variola and vaccinia.

REFERENCES

Cho, C.T., and Wenner, H.A.: Monkeypox virus. Bacteriol. Rev.
37:1, 1973.

Dick, G.: Routine smallpox vaccination. Brit. Med. J. 3:163, 1971.

Dixon, C.W.: Smallpox. J. & A. Churchill, Ltd., London, 1962.

Downie, A.W.: Smallpox. In: Viral and Rickettsial Infections of
Man. 4th ed. Horsfall, F.L., Jr., and Tamm, I., eds. J.B.
Lippincott Co., Philadelphia, 1965.

Downie, A.W., Taylor Robinson, C.H., Caunt, A.E., Nelson, G.S.,
Manson-Bahr, P.E.C., and Matthews, T.C.H.: Tanapox: a new
disease caused by poxvirus. Brit. Med. J. 1:363, 1971.

Kempe, C.H.: Variola and vaccinia. In: Textbook of Medicine.
Vol. 1. Chapter 21. Beeson, P.B. and McDermott, W., eds.
W.B. Saunders Co., Philadelphia, 1975.

Lane, J.M., Ruben, F.L., Neff, J.M., and Millar, J.D.: Complications of smallpox vaccination, 1968: National surveillance in the
United States. NEJM 281:1201, 1969.

CHAPTER 4. SKIN AND SOFT TISSUE INFECTIONS

4.1: IMPETIGO

INTRODUCTION: Superficial infections of the skin due to bacteria
are common in children, especially under six years of age. These
infections are usually described within the broad category of pyodermas and include two major clinically recognized forms of impetigo: streptococcal impetigo (also called impetigo contagiosa) and
staphylococcal impetigo (frequently referred to as bullous impetigo).
Group A beta hemolytic streptococci and staphylococci are the two
bacteria generally responsible for the vast majority of these infections. The only other causal agent of significance is Corynebacterium diphtheria, which may be isolated from children with impetiginous lesions in those sub-tropical parts of the United States where
C. diphtheria is endemic (Belsey et al., 1969).

Table 4-1 lists the salient epidemiological features of streptococcal
impetigo. Within the 2-5 year old age group, pure staphylococci
impetigo is much less frequent, and is known to occur in sporadic
outbursts in newborn nurseries and within families. Transmission
of staphylococcal impetigo, like streptococcal impetigo, is thought
to occur by direct contact. However, careful studies of the sequence
of spread of streptococcal and staphylococcal organisms in children
with impetigo suggest that whereas streptococci are isolated from
normal skin prior to development of impetigo, with colonization of
the upper respiratory tract following later, staphylococci are first
recovered from the upper respiratory tract, then from normal skin
and, finally from the impetiginous lesion (Ferrieri, P., et al., 1972;
Dajani, A.S., et al., 1972). C. diphtheria skin infections also occur most frequently in younger children and the seasonal pattern is
similar to that of streptococcal impetigo. Other epidemiologic simi-
larities include the role of minor trauma, transmission by direct
contact, and importance of the carrier-state (Belsey, M.A., et al.,
1969).

1. ETIOLOGY AND PATHOGENESIS

Group A streptococci are the most common cause of impetigo. Although many studies have shown that cultures of impetiginous lesions
most commonly yield both Group A streptococci and staphylococci
(50-70%) and less frequently pure group A streptococci (20-30%), the
studies of Dajani, et al., 1972 demonstrated the subsidiary role of
the staphylococcus in these infections. Group A streptococci with or
without staphylococci account for 80-90% of all impetigo seen in children living in the United States.

TABLE 4-1: EPIDEMIOLOGY OF STREPTOCOCCAL IMPETIGO	
FEATURE	IMPETIGO
Age	Young children (2-5 years)
Sex	Equal incidence
Climate/Geography	Tropical - Temperate - Cool
Season	Late summer, early fall in cool and temperate climates
Transmission	Probably by direct contact; insects may be mechanical vectors
Carrier State	Organisms found on normal skin prior to development of lesions
Preceding Trauma	May predispose to natural or experimental infection
Socio-economic Status	Incidence related to hygiene

There are over 60 distinct Group A streptococcal serotypes (based
on M protein antigen typing). In general, the higher number serotypes have been more frequently associated with skin infections and
the lower numbered serotypes with respiratory infections. Pure
staphylococcal impetigo may be associated with a variety of phage
types of S. aureus. However, bullous impetigo is most often caused
by Group 11 phage types including types 3A, 3B, 3C, 55 and 71.
These are the same types often associated with generalized separation of the intra-epidermal layer of skin seen in toxic epidermal
necrolysis ("scaled skin syndrome").

Experimental studies of streptococcal impetigo in the hamster model
showed that 4-6 hours following intradermal inoculation of streptococci, a papular, erythematous area appeared which rapidly prog-
ressed into a small vesicle by 6-8 hours after inoculation (Dajani
and Wannamaker, 1970). By 12-16 hours the vesicles had disappeared and the lesions became crusted over, the crusted stage lasting 4-6 days. The crust gradually became thinner and the base of
the crust dry. Complete healing occurred with little or no scar
formation. Concomitant histopathological studies revealed a typical inflammatory cell response shortly after inoculation in the epidermal and subepidermal adipose layers, with vesicles arising later
directly beneath the horny layer. Although polymorphonuclear cells
were in abundance in the vesicle fluid, there was a paucity of organisms seen on gram stain. The addition of foreign bodies to the streptococcal inoculum greatly potentiated the infection. These studies
suggest that minor trauma from insect bites, poison ivy, and foreign

bodies (dirt) may all be contributing factors in the pathogenesis of human impetigo, not only in the sense of inoculating the streptococcus residing on top of the normal epidermal layers, but also in potentiating the infectious process following inoculation.

2. CLINICAL MANIFESTATIONS

Table 4-2 modified from Wannamaker, 1970, illustrates the major differences in the clinical appearance of streptococcal impetigo and staphylococcal impetigo. The transient vesicular stage of streptococcal impetigo, previously described as lasting but a few hours in experimental infections in hamsters, is infrequently observed clinically. However, the crusted stage persists for several days. When the lesion is caused by S. aureus, the vesicular stage persists and there is little crusting.

TABLE 4-2: COMPARISON OF STREPTOCOCCAL AND STAPHYLOCOCCAL IMPETIGINOUS LESIONS		
FEATURE	STREPTOCOCCAL IMPETIGO*	STAPHYLOCOCCAL IMPETIGO**
Vesicular State	Transient-often not seen	Persistent purulent bullae
Crusted Stage	Thickened, amber or honey colored crusts-persistent	More transient; varnish-like, white or gray-colored
* pure streptococcal or mixed streptococcal and staphylococcal lesion		
** usually phage Group II		

Other clinical aspects of these two forms of impetigo also differ. Bullous impetigo tends to have a more abrupt onset, with lesions occurring with similar frequency on the face, trunk and extremities. Streptococcal impetigo tends to be more indolent, with lesions persisting and new ones developing over several weeks, primarily involving exposed parts of the body, especially the arms and legs. An exception to the latter distribution pattern are the honey-colored crusted lesions located about the nose and mouth in the patient with a streptococcal upper respiratory infection.

Regional lymphadenopathy is a common feature of streptococcal impetigo, occurring in 92% of the patients reported by Dillon (1968). Lymphadenitis and cellulitis, though less frequent suppurative complications (8%), were not reported in any patient with bullous (staphylococcal) impetigo.

The role of streptococcal impetigo in the subsequent development of acute glomerulonephritis (AGN) is well established in a number of studies (Dillon, 1970). Furthermore, the serotypes of streptococci that cause AGN following impetigo differ from those serotypes that cause AGN following streptococcal respiratory infections, just as the serotypes causing the two primary infections also differ.

In general, epidemiologic features of AGN following impetigo parallel the epidemiologic features of impetigo in terms of seasonal occurrence, age group, geographic distribution, etc. The attack role of AGN following infection due to a nephritogenic strain is estimated to be 10-15%, and the latent period between infection and AGN is approximately 3 weeks, the latter differing considerably from the latent period of 10-12 days for AGN following streptococcal upper respiratory infections. The occurrence of subclinical cases of AGN among family members following impetigo is frequent, as determined by low serum complement levels. Recurrences are unusual and the prognosis is generally favorable.

3. DIAGNOSIS

In many instances, the clinical appearance of streptococcal or staphylococcal impetiginous lesions is so typical, that bacteriological confirmation of the cause of infection may not be warranted. In the patient with one or two lesions, it is doubtful that results of a culture of a skin lesion will influence the therapy prescribed or the outcome. However, a culture of the skin lesion is indicated: 1) when multiple family members possibly are infected, 2) when there is considerable risk in spreading infection to other siblings, 3) when extensive infection is present, or 4) when the clinical diagnosis is in slightest doubt. As a general rule, any patient who requires parenteral or oral antibiotics for treatment of impetigo should probably have a culture taken of one lesion prior to the initiation of therapy.

Skin lesions are best cultured by removing the crust or the top of the pustule or vesicle with a sterile needle. Extensive cleansing of the lesion prior to obtaining the culture is unwarranted and may interfere with bacterial growth on the culture medium. Also, in the early stages of streptococcal impetigo, it is important to culture the moist base of the lesion because of the paucity of organisms in the vesicular fluid. Swabs should be placed on 5% sheep blood agar plates. Staphylococci may be isolated along with streptococci, but when the plates are streaked properly, even in the presence of large numbers of staphylococci, it is possible to isolate and identify beta-hemolytic streptococci. Subsequent confirmation of beta-hemolytic organisms as group A streptococci by the bacitracin disk sensitivity method of Maxted is highly desirable.

4. MANAGEMENT

In the patient with one or two suspected streptococcal impetiginous lesions on the extremities, systemic antibiotic therapy is probably

not warranted. Simple removal of the crust with or without application of a topical antibiotic ountment, such as bacitracin, is often
therapeutic. However, the patient with one or two lesions about the
nose or mouth should have cultures of the lesion and/or upper respiratory tract and, following confirmation of a beta-hemolytic infection by culture, should be treated in the same manner as any
other child with a streptococcal respiratory infection.

Patients with extensive streptococci impetigo or bullous (staphylococcal) should receive systemic antibiotic therapy which may be
initiated while awaiting culture confirmations. Antibiotic therapy
is indicated, not only to prevent suppurative complications but also
to reduce spread of infection to siblings and other children in the
immediate environment (e.g. day care center, nursery school,
etc.). Treatment regimens for streptococcal impetigo are similar
to those previously recommended for streptococcal respiratory infections (see Chapter 1). Penicillin alone, given orally or parenterally, has been shown to be highly effective in treating patients
with pure streptococcal impetigo or with mixed lesions containing
either penicillin resistant or penicillin sensitive staphylococci in
addition to the streptococci. In children with extensive streptococcal
impetigo, requiring treatment with systemic antibiotics, there is no
added advantage in using topical antibiotic ointments, which is both
laborious and messy. Nor will daily scrubbing of the lesion with
hexachlorophene soap hasten recovery (Ruby and Nelson, 1973).

Patients with pure staphylococcal impetigo should be treated with a
penicillinase resistant penicillin. In patients with a few lesions who
can be safely managed at home, dicloxacillin (12.5-25 mg/Kg/24
hours in 4 doses for 5-7 days) is recommended. However, staphylococcal impetigo in newborns, very young infants, and in children
with debilitating chronic diseases where host defenses are compromised, should possibly be treated in the hospital with a parenteral
antibiotic such as nafcillin or oxacillin in doses of 200-300 mg/Kg/
24 hours in 4 equally divided doses for 7-10 days.

::

4.2: SOFT TISSUE INFECTIONS

INTRODUCTION: Soft tissue infections in children are not uncommon and include lymphadenitis, cellulitis, and omphalitis, in addition to secondary infections of wounds and burns. The three organisms most commonly found in these infections are <u>Streptococcus
pyogenes</u>, group A, <u>Staphylococcus aureus</u>, and <u>Hemophilus influ-
enzae</u>, group B. Omphalitis is discussed in the chapter entitled
"Neonatal Infections."

1. LYMPHADENITIS

Acute suppurative lymphadenitis is caused by group A Streptococci
or S. aureus (Barton, L. and Feigin, R., 1974). Rarely, gram

negative rods, mycobacterium, anaerobic organisms and fungi
cause lymphadenitis in children. The differentiation between lymphadenopathy and lymphadenitis is not always easy. The clinical findings of warm, tender lymph nodes, with or without overlying erythema, are indicative of lymphadenitis. The nodes are usually
moveable and firm, although superficial nodes may be fluctuent.
The etiologic diagnosis is confirmed by aspirating the node and obtaining a gram stain and culture of the aspirate. If no fluid is obtained initially, 0.5-1.0 ml of sterile saline should be injected into
the node and reaspirated for culture. If the child has or has recently had a URI, a throat culture may reveal the presence of group
A streptococci. Treatment should be initiated with penicillin pending results of the culture of the needle aspirate. In the event that
the culture yields S. aureus, resistant to penicillin, dicloxacillin
is the drug of choice.

2. CELLULITIS

Although streptococci and staphylococci are the major causes of
cellulitis, Hemophilus influenzae group B cellulitis occurs in young
children (usually under 3 years of age) and deserves special comment. In general, cellulitis is associated with the classic signs of
inflammation - heat, redness, and tenderness. Fever, chills and
other constitutional signs and symptoms may be present in severe
cases, and such patients will often have positive blood cultures
(Fig. 4.1). Streptococcal cellulitis will show a well-demarcated
advancing border and the red streak of lymphangitis is a common
associated finding, since these organisms spread via lympatics.
Streptococcal cellulitis most usually occurs on the extremities but
can occur elsewhere, including the anus. Peri-anal cellulitis in a
child, manifested by pain on defecation and/or soreness, may be
associated with streptococcal infections of the upper respiratory
tract (Amren and Wannamaker, 1966). Streptococcal cellulitis on
the face (erysipelas) has virtually disappeared in the past 30 years.
Cellulitis may occur in the absence of an obvious portal of entry, or
result from a small blister or puncture wound some distance from
the cellulitis.

H. Influenzae group B cellulitis commonly occurs in young children
(3 months to 2 years of age) and is characterized by high fever and
typical findings of cellulitis (see Fig. 4.2). Although it was previously thought that a purplish or violaceous discoloration of the skin
was pathogenetic of H. influenzae cellulitis, recent studies have
shown this to be a variable finding (Granoff and Nankervis, 1976),
for it can occur in cellulitis caused by other organisms. Unlike
streptococcal cellulitis, H. influenzae cellulitis commonly occurs
on the face (cheeks, peri-orbital area), is unilateral, and is seen
less frequently on the extremities (Smith, 1976). Many of these patients have associated H. influenzae infections of the ipsilateral middle ear or para-nasal sinuses, and because of the propensity of the
organism for hematogenous dissemination, meningitis can also occur.

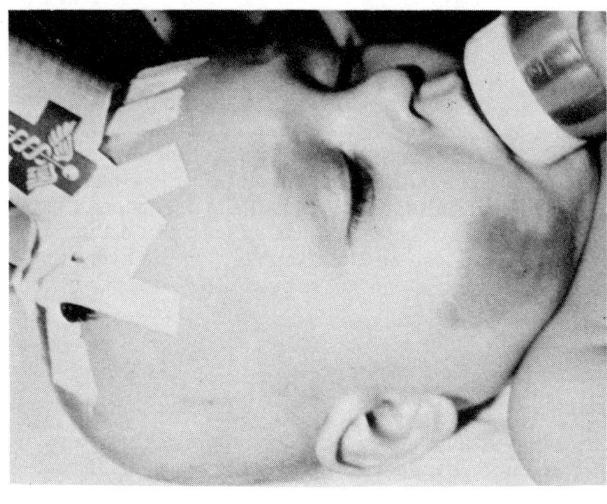

FIG. 4.2: _Hemophilus influenzae_ cellulitis on the cheek of an infant. Note poorly marginated borders.

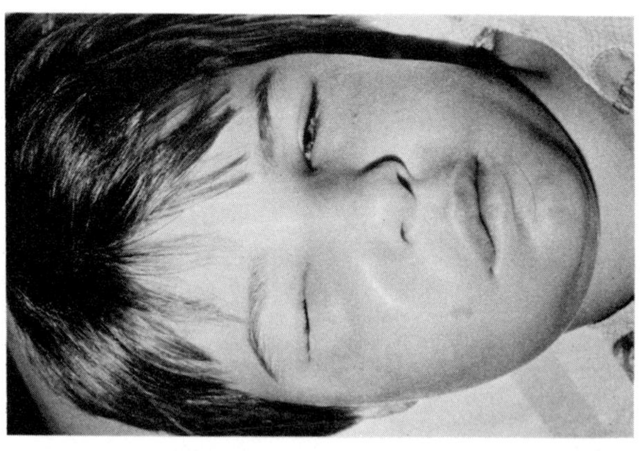

FIG. 4.1: Facial and orbital cellulitis associated with _staphylococcus aureus_.

The etiologic diagnosis of cellulitis must be established by culture. It is relatively simple to obtain a needle aspiration of the cellulitis at the advancing margin for culture, and this should be done in most instances. Other cultures, especially blood cultures, are also useful in establishing the diagnosis in suspected cases of H. influenzae cellulitis, wherein 80% may be positive.

Treatment of cellulitis usually requires parenteral antibiotics, although in early cases when the infection is well localized and there is no evidence of systemic toxicity, oral antibiotics may be used. These patients require prompt attention and treatment should be initiated just as soon as the cultures have been obtained. Children with streptococcal cellulitis who manifest systemic toxicity should be treated with benzathine penicillin G in doses used for treating streptococcal upper respiratory infections (see Chapter 1). Severely ill patients may require procaine penicillin (600,000 units q. 12 h IM) and should be followed closely. In the hospitalized patient who is apt to be monitored more closely than the child at home, it is well to remember that the cellulitis will continue to advance for 6-12 hours after treatment has begun. Thus sufficient time should pass before evaluating the efficacy of therapy.

Patients with extensive staphylococcal cellulitis are best hospitalized and treated with intravenous nafcillin or oxacillin (200-300 mg/Kg/day in 6 doses). For milder infections, dicloxacillin doses of 25-50 mg/Kg/day, in 4 divided doses, may be given orally.

The patient with suspected H. influenzae cellulitis should be hospitalized and treated with ampicillin in doses of 200-300 mg/Kg IV in 4 divided doses. In some centers, chloramphenicol has replaced ampicillin as the drug of choice for H. influenzae because of ampicillin resistant strains. Infants and young children with orbital cellulitis should be started on both a penicillinase-resistant penicillin and with ampicillin or chloramphenicol. Therapy of these infections should be continued for 7-10 days.

In addition to antibiotics, application of local heat (warm compresses) several times daily and, when feasible, elevation and immobilization of the affected extremity, are useful in the management of patients with cellulitis.

REFERENCES

Amren, D., Anderson, A., and Wannamaker, L.: Perianal cellulitis associated with group A streptococci. Am. J. Dis. Child. 112:546-552, 1966.

Barton, L. and Feigin, R.: Childhood cervical lymphadenitis: A reappraisal. J. Pediatr. 84:846-852, 1974.

Belsey, M.A., Sinclair, M., Roder, R.: Corynebacterium diphtheriae skin infections in Alabama and Louisiana. NEJM 280:135-141, 1969.

Dajani, A. and Wannamaker, L.: Experimental infection in the hamster simulating human impetigo. I. Natural history of the infection. J. Infect. Dis. 122:196-204, 1970.

Dajani, A., Ferrieri, P. and Wannamaker, L.: Natural history of impetigo. II. Etiologic agents and bacterial interactions. J. Clin. Invest. 51:2863-2871, 1972.

Dillon, H.C., Jr.: Impetigo contagiosa: Suppurative and non-suppurative complications. Am. J. Dis. Child. 115:530-541, 1968.

Dillon, H.C., Jr.: Streptococcal skin infections and acute glomerulonephritis. Postgrad. Med. J. 46:641-652, 1970.

Ferrieri, P., Dajani, A., Wannamaker, L.: Natural history of impetigo. I. Site sequence of acquisition and familial patterns of spread of cutaneous streptococci. J. Clin. Invest. 51:2851-2862, 1972.

Granoff, D. and Nankervis, G.: Cellulitis due to Haemophilus influenzae Type B. Am. J. Dis. Child. 130:1211-1214, 1976.

Ruby, R. and Nelson, J.: The influence of hexachlorophene scrubs on the response to placebo or penicillin therapy in impetigo. J. Pediatr. 52:854-859, 1973.

Smith, D.: Haemophilus influenzae cellulitis. Am. J. Dis. Child. 130:1193-1194, 1976.

Wannamaker, L.W.: Differences between streptococcal infections of the throat and of the skin. NEJM 282:23-31, 1970.

CHAPTER 5. BONE AND JOINT INFECTIONS

5.1: OSTEOMYELITIS

INTRODUCTION: The incidence of osteomyelitis has decreased gradually during the past 30 years based upon data reported in recent reviews by Waldvogel et al. (1970) and Dich et al. (1975). Similarly, the mortality rate has also declined markedly from 15-20% to less than 2% since the advent of the antibiotic era. In Dich's recent review of 163 cases, there was no mortality reported. However, certain other epidemiologic characteristics have remained relatively constant during this period:

Age: Osteomyelitis occurs most commonly in children between 2 and 10 years of age, accounting for over 60% of all cases reported in infants and children.

Sex: Osteomyelitis is far more common in boys than girls, with the majority of studies citing a 2:1 male to female sex ratio.

History of Preceding Trauma: A history of trauma is reported in over one-third of cases in most instances, but the trauma is often remote to the site of infection. Since osteomyelitis is rare following significant bony trauma, e.g., a simple fracture, the predisposing relationship of trauma to osteomyelitis is unclear.

History of Preceding Infection: In 20-30% of cases, a history of a preceding infection is obtained, usually involving either the respiratory tract or the skin.

Seasonal Occurrence: In several studies, osteomyelitis has occurred more often in the late summer and early fall, at the same time that pyogenic skin infections occur with greatest frequency.

1. ETIOLOGY AND PATHOGENESIS

For the past 40 years, Staphylococcus aureus has been the predominant etiological agent causing osteomyelitis in infants and children. Although the number of cases in which S. aureus is implicated has varied from series to series, this organism still causes two-thirds or more of all cases of osteomyelitis reported in the pediatric age group. In the remaining one-third of cases, streptococci - usually group A, Hemophilus influenzae, Streptococcus pneumoniae and various gram negative bacilli, account for the vast majority. Mixed infections have been reported, as have infections due to organisms not usually pathogenic such as Staphylococcus epidermitis. Salmonella organisms have been associated specifically with osteomyelitis in children with sickle cell disease and possibly other hemolytic anemias.

In younger children and infants with osteomyelitis, the etiologic agents seem to be more variable and, in a recent study (Dich et al., 1975), S. aureus accounted for less than one-third of the cases in children under 2 years of age. Within this same age group were 4 or 5 reported cases of osteomyelitis due to H. influenzae. Ten of 14 cases due to Streptococci occurred in patients 5 years of age or younger, which substantiates earlier studies that reported the occurrence of beta-hemolytic streptococcal osteomyelitis in the younger children.

Optimal management of the patient with osteomyelitis is based on the knowledge of the pathogenesis of this infection. Early investigators (Johnson, 1927) demonstrated the significance of the blood supply to the long bones in osteomyelitis. The nutrient artery supplies 50-70% of the long bone. Its terminal branches curve sharply like a hairpin in the metaphysis and open into venous capillaries which drain into the venous sinusoides of the marrow cavity. The infectious organism usually lodges in the venous capillary, presumably because of decreased flow and turbulence in this area. It is also possible that phagocytosis might be less active in the metaphysis than in the diaphysis, and that this could be an additional factor favoring localization of the bacteria there. Once the focus of infection is established, an inflammatory reaction occurs with hyperemia and thrombosis of the arterial side of the terminal portions of the nutrient artery, which in turn causes congestion and formation of an exudate (Starr, 1922; Larsen, 1938; Trueto, 1960). At this point, the inflammatory exudate in the metaphysis may spread in several directions, but most often follows lymphatics along the epiphyseal plate to the periosteum, then into cortical bone and the medullary cavity via the Haversian canals. Subperiosteal pus accumulates and may rupture into the soft tissue, forming a soft tissue abscess. As infection spreads down the diaphysis it also strips away the periosteum. Since periosteal vessels supply the outer one-half of the cortical bone, and when this blood supply is compromised by detachment of the vessels as the pus moves down the diaphyseal shaft, ischemic necrosis occurs in the outer part of the cortex. When the joint capsule is attached at the epiphyseal plate, secondary joint involvement is rare, but in the hip and shoulder this is more frequently seen since the periostem is attached below the epiphysis. Once infection has spread into the medullary cavity, the problem of bone necrosis is enhanced by the ischemia produced by increased intramedullary pressure.

Differences in the pathogenesis of acute osteomyelitis in infants and in older children should also be considered. In infancy, the metaphyseal vessels are not limited by an avascular epiphyseal plate, and this explains why suppurative arthritis and epiphysitis occur more frequently in this age group. Also, the complications may be more severe since damage to the epiphyseal side of the growth plate is irreparable. Also, due to the increased vascularity, large amounts of sequestrum form which are more quickly reabsorbed, and remodeling of the damaged bone is more rapid than in older children.

In childhood, the inflammatory exudate is limited by the avascular epiphyseal plate, and complications of epiphysitis and arthritis occur less frequently, but with two exceptions: 1) when the focus of infection is in the head of the femur, or 2) head of the humerus. Then, joint infection (septic arthritis) may occur since the synovial capsules reach beyond the epiphyseal growth plate, thus permitting the infection to spread by rupturing into the joint through the bony cortex. However, subperiosteal and soft tissue abscesses are more frequent due to the relatively loose adherence of the periosteum early in life. After cessation of skeletal growth, epiphysitis is more common since by this time there are many anastomoses between the metaphyseal and epiphyseal vessels associated with closure of the epiphyses. Also, little sequestra is formed and subperiosteal abscesses are less frequent, since the periosteum is quite firmly attached to the bone later in life.

2. CLINICAL MANIFESTATIONS

The child or infant with osteomyelitis usually presents with fever, accompanied in the majority of cases by localized (point) tenderness, and swelling overlying the infected portion of bone. Decreased range of motion, localized erythema, and drainage may also be present. Invariably, symptoms are present for several days prior to establishing the correct diagnosis. Since morbidity associated with this infection may be reduced considerably by prompt institution of appropriate therapy, it is essential that physicians consider this diagnosis whenever an infant or child presents with the constellation of symptoms and signs noted above. Occasionally, pseudoparalysis of an arm or leg may be the only sign of bone or joint infections in infancy (Yuille, 1975).

3. DIAGNOSIS

In a patient in whom a diagnosis of osteomyelitis is suspected on clinical grounds, the following studies are indicated to further substantiate the diagnosis:

3.1: White Blood Count and Differential: Although an elevated white blood cell count with $>5\%$ band forms may provide additional support for the diagnosis of osteomyelitis, this laboratory test may not be helpful. In a recent study, only 14% of children with osteomyelitis had WBC's of 20,000/cu. mm., and fewer than one-third of patients had $>5\%$ band forms on differential cell count.

<u>3.2: Erythrocyte Sedimentation Rate (ESR)</u>: Contrary to the WBC, an ESR may be helpful, not only in helping to establish the diagnosis but also in following the patient after therapy has begun. Only 4 of 88 patients had normal ESR's on admission in the series reported by Dich et al. For all patients, the mean ESR rate was 69.7 mm/hr. Further, in patients with uncomplicated osteomyelitis, ESR's decreased over time in relation to the days of treatment.

<u>3.3: Radiographic Studies</u>: In most instances, the diagnosis of osteomyelitis will be confirmed by roentgenographic techniques. However, the earliest changes seen on x-ray (destruction of bone and periosteal new bone formation) are not seen for at least 7 to 10 days following onset of symptoms. In some instances, loss of soft tissue planes adjacent to the affected bone may be visible within 3 to 4 days, but this finding is not constant or reliable. Recently, scintigraphy techniques have been used in an effort to demonstrate infection prior to the changes seen on x-ray (Treves, et al., 1976). Early osteomyelitis was visualized on the scintigram as discrete areas of increased radioactive uptake (using Technetium (Tc)99 m diphosphorate) in the absence of bony changes on routine x-ray. Although further studies are needed to conclusively demonstrate the value of this technique, the results of initial studies are encouraging.

<u>3.4: Bacteriologic Studies</u>: Bacteriologic confirmation of infection and an etiologic diagnosis can be expected in over 85% of cases of osteomyelitis, provided cultures are obtained from all available sources. Blood cultures should be routinely obtained and will yield the etiologic agent in over 50% of cases. More often, blood cultures will be obtained in conjunction with cultures of a needle aspirate of bone, pus obtained at the time of surgical drainage, joint fluid and wound drainage. Every attempt should be made to obtain cultures prior to institution of antibiotic therapy.

4. MANAGEMENT AND PROGNOSIS

Certain aspects of the management of the patient with osteomyelitis are controversial but clearly involve three major areas: 1) supportive therapy (IV fluids, immobilization, nursing care, etc.); 2) antibiotics; and 3) surgical drainage which encompasses everything from a simple needle aspiration of the bone to incision and drainage by drilling holes into the medullary cavity.

Most aspects of suppurative care during the early phase of treatment are obvious and need little consideration. The only point which might be disputed concerns the need for and duration of immobilization. Currently, most authors strongly advocate immobilization in the early phase of treatment, presumably because the affected limb is more comfortable at rest and, in the active child, a pathological fracture may be prevented. However, in view of the need for optimal blood supply to the infected area, both to carry antibiotics and to promote healing, unnecessary or prolonged immobilization should perhaps be avoided.

There is little controversy, if any, about the use of antibiotics in the treatment of acute osteomyelitis. Beginning with penicillin, there was a marked drop in the mortality of this disease. Today it is the morbidity associated with this disease that is of primary concern. Although this too has been markedly reduced by the use of antibiotics, the incidence of chronic osteomyelitis following the acute disease is still 15-25%, regardless of the types of therapy used.

The efficacy of antibiotics in this disease depends upon several factors: choice of antibiotics, timing of therapy in relation to onset of symptoms, dosage and duration of therapy.

4.1: Choice and Dose of Antibiotics: Initial antibiotic therapy should be based upon the results of the gram stain. However, if no fluid or pus is obtained, but the clinical diagnosis is strongly suspected, methicillin in a dose of 200-300 mg/Kg/day should be given intravenously in 4 divided doses initially until the results of the cultures are known. The majority of cases are caused by S. aureus. Since 40% or more of these organisms will be resistant to penicillin, a penicillinase resistant penicillin (e.g. nafcillin) should be used until penicillin sensitivity studies of the organism are available. Several authors suggest using both phenoxymethyl penicillin G (in doses of 10 million units/M^2/day in 4 divided doses) and methicillin until culture results and in vitro susceptibility of the organism are known.

4.2: Timing of Antibiotic Therapy: Few studies of osteomyelitis have examined the relationship between the timing of antibiotic therapy and outcome. However, when this variable has been considered, a direct relationship between the early institution of antibiotic therapy and morbidity is apparent. The value of early treatment is obvious from the previous discussion of pathogenesis. If an effective antibiotic is given early enough, ischemic bone necrosis and subsequent sequestration can be prevented. The studies of Bremner (1954), Neligan (1965) and Hall and Silverstein (1963), all indicate that delay in institution of appropriate antibiotic therapy (7 days or more after onset of symptoms) results in significant increase in complications and morbidity.

4.3: Duration of Antibiotic Therapy: The recent study of Dich et al. points out the important role that duration of parenteral antibiotic therapy plays in the final outcome of the disease. Only one treatment failure occurred in children with S. aureus osteomyelitis who were treated parenterally for longer than 3 weeks. In children receiving briefer courses of parenteral antibiotics followed by oral antibiotics (regardless of the duration of the latter), there was a treatment failure rate of 19%. Although other variables will no doubt influence outcome (e.g. timing and extent of surgical intervention), the duration of parenteral antibiotic therapy remains an important aspect of management and should continue for 4 weeks.

The question of surgical intervention (needle aspiration vs. open drainage) remains controversial. However, whenever osteomyelitis is suspected, needle aspiration for subperiosteal and then intramedullary pus should be undertaken, if for no other reason than to establish their presence or absence and provide material for a gram stain and culture. This degree of surgical intervention may alone have some therapeutic value. In the event that pus is obtained by needle aspiration, further surgical drainage is indicated. During the first 24 to 48 hours, close observation of the patient is essential. If no pus is obtained initially by needle aspiration but the patient is improving on antibiotic therapy, further surgical drainage is probably not indicated. However, if no improvement has occurred, needle aspiration should be repeated and surgical drainage carried out if pus is found.

For chronic or recurrent osteomyelitis, primary treatment is surgical removal of sequestrum. The choice of antibiotic is based on culture results and sensitivity patterns. Prolonged oral antibiotic therapy of 3 to 6 months or longer is often needed.

In summary, early diagnosis is the key factor in reducing morbidity from osteomyelitis. Following appropriate diagnostic studies, including needle aspiration of bone, parenteral antibiotic therapy should be instituted without delay and continued for a minimum of 3 weeks, or until clinical and laboratory findings warrant its discontinuance. Surgical drainage should be carried out whenever pus is obtained by needle aspiration and/or whenever the patient fails to improve after a reasonable period of antibiotic therapy.

REFERENCES

Bremner, A.E., Neligan, G.A. and Warrick, C.K.: Surgical treatment of acute osteomyelitis in childhood. Lancet 1:953, 1954.

Dich, W.Q., Nelson, John D., and Hattalin, K C.: Osteomyelitis in infants and children. Am J. Dis. Child 129:1273, 1975. (An excellent review of 163 cases over a 15-year period in the modern antibiotic era.)

Hall, J.E. and Silverstein, E.A.: Acute hematogenous osteomyelitis. Pediatrics 31(6):1033, 1963. (A review of 100 cases at the Hospital for Sick Children (Toronto), emphasizing the importance of early treatment.)

Johnson, R.W., Jr.: A physiological study of blood supply of the diaphysis. J. Bone and Joint Surg. 9:153, 1927.

Larsen, R.M.: Intramedullary pressure with particular reference to massive diaphyseal bone necrosis. Ann. Surg. 108:127, 1938.

Neligan, G.A. and Elderkin, F.M.: Treatment of acute hematogenous osteitis in children assessed in a conservative series of selected cases. Brit. Med. J. 1:1347, 1965.

Starr, C.: Acute hematogenous osteomyelitis. Arch. Surg. 4:567, 1922.

Treves, S., Khetty, J., Broker, F.H., Wilkinson, R.H. and Watts, H.: Osteomyelitis: Early scintigraphic detection in children. Pediatr. 57:173, 1976.

Trueto, J. and Morgan, J.P.: The vascular contribution of osteogenesis. J. Bone and Joint Surg. 42-B:97, 1960.

Waldvogen, F.A. Medoft, G. and Swartz, M.N.: Osteomyelitis: A review of clinical features, therapeutic considerations and unusual aspects. NEJM 282:198-206, 260-266, 316-322, 1970. (A thorough, comprehensive review of osteomyelitis, including 62 cases of hematogenous osteomyelitis in children and adults.)

Yuille, T.D., Limb infections in infancy presenting with pseudoparalysis. Arch. Dis. Child. 50:953, 1975.

::

5.2: SEPTIC ARTHRITIS

INTRODUCTION: Septic arthritis is primarily a disease of childhood with the peak incidence in the under 2 age group. Within this 2-year span, it is most commonly seen between 0-3 months and 9-24 months (Borella et al., 1963). Although the incidence of septic arthritis has remained fairly constant over the past 30 years, the clinical picture has changed markedly during the antibiotic era. Prior to availability of antibiotics, septic arthritis was associated with a mortality rate as high as 60% (Smith, 1874); today the mortality rate is less than 1%. If treated promptly with appropriate therapy, the morbidity varies from less than 10% to up to 30%. The important variables affecting morbidity are the specific joint involved and the time lag between onset of symptoms and initiation of appropriate therapy.

The predominant etiologic agents associated with septic arthritis appear to be changing, with the gram-positive cocci dominating the studies reported through the early 1960's (Borella et al., 1963; Samulson et al., 1958), and with later reports showing an increased incidence of H. influenzae infections (Almquist, 1970; Nelson and Kootnz, 1966). One author (Almquist) found a 90% predictability of the etiologic organisms by looking at age alone. In the 7 months to 4 year group H. influenzae predominated, and in children 5 years of age and older, the staphylococcus accounted for over 90% of the cases. In the 0-6 months age group the etiologic agents were variable but gram negative bacilli were often involved.

1. ETIOLOGY AND PATHOGENESIS

Organisms gain access to joints by: 1) hematogenous seeding - the source of the blood-borne organisms may be any infection such as pneumonia, otitis media, meningitis and skin infections, 2) spread from contiguous infected areas, such as osteomyelitis, and 3) direct puncture wounds, such as femoral venipuncture; in some cases no source can be found. Any pathogenic organism can cause septic arthritis. The most common are staphylococcus, H. influenzae and streptococcus. The complete list, however, includes pneumococcus, coliforms, pseudomonas, meningococcus, gonococcus and, rarely, such organisms as Salmonella, Yersinia, and Moraxella.

Joint infection due to the tubercle bacillus is today rare in children and usually associated with a chronic arthritis. Diagnosis frequently requires synovial biopsy. Other mycobacteria, fungi - especially candida, and filariasis, rarely cause septic arthritis.

The synovial membrane is not an intact sac, but a 1-3 cell layer that is contiguous with the articular cartilage and metaphyseal bone periosteum. As such it is not continuous (as are endothelial membranes) and is very vascular. This situation lends itself to easy seeding. It has been shown that particles and/or organisms gain access more easily to synovial fluid than CSF, vitreous humor, or urine. The presence of inflammation increases the permeability and hence augments passage of plasma proteins (Kushner and Somerville, 1971); this in turn enhances the synovial fluid as a culture medium for pathogenic organisms. The synovial fluid can be considered a dialysate of plasma, with the exception of hyaluronic acid which is produced locally by the lining cells. Normal synovial fluid contains approximately one-third the serum protein concentration (approximately 2 grams) and usually less than 200 cells/mm^3, primarily mononuclear cells.

2. CLINICAL MANIFESTATIONS

The majority of children with septic arthritis present with toxic manifestations of fever, malaise, joint pain and swelling. The pain is often acute and excruciating, in contrast to that seen in other types of inflammatory arthritis. A child may simply refuse to walk or bear weight at all. Many have antecedent or concurrent infections such as otitis media, pneumonia, skin infections, omphalitis as in neonates with indwelling umbilical catheters.

On examination, the joints show increased warmth, varying degrees of effusion, tenderness and limitation of range of motion. Of all joint involvement, hip involvement in the neonate is most easily missed. These infants frequently have other serious associated problems and do not manifest the usual systemic signs (Borella, 1963). However, if examined carefully, there is evidence of limited hip motion.

The pattern of joint involvement is usually monarticular, affecting the large, weight-bearing joints. The knees are most frequently affected, followed by hips, elbows, shoulders and ankles (Borella, 1963), but any joint can be affected. The involvement of more than one joint does not exclude septic arthritis. One large series reported up to 4 joints involved in an individual patient (Nelson and Koontz, 1966). Polyarticular disease is seen more frequently with gonococcal and streptococcal infections (Nelson and Koontz, 1966, Fink, 1965). Gonococcal infections frequently have a migratory polyarthalgia with later localization in one joint.

3. DIAGNOSIS

A high index of suspicion is important in the early diagnosis of septic arthritis. Any child who presents with acute pain and swelling of a joint should be presumed to have septic arthritis until proven otherwise. The most helpful diagnostic tool in making a definitive early diagnosis is joint aspiration and synovianalysis. This procedure should be carried out immediately so that appropriate antibiotic therapy can be instituted. A negative aspiration (no fluid) does not rule out septic arthritis unless one is certain the joint space has been entered.

The fluid should be cultured aerobically and anerobically and a gram stain made. The gram stain and chemical determinations of synovial fluid glucose and protein are especially important because cultures of purulent synovial fluid are negative from 30% to 50% of patients (Almquist, 1970; Nelson and Koontz, 1966). Negative cultures are obtained primarily in patients who previously received antibiotic therapy, but not always. Pus itself is inhibitory to bacteria. The majority of negative synovial fluid cultures (69%) in Almquist's study were in the 7 month to 4 years age group and were presumably associated with H. influenzae infections. This organism is fastidious and more difficult to grow than the gram-positive cocci.

WBC counts in synovial fluid of greater than 100,000 cells/mm^3 and a glucose determination of less than 20 mg% are seen almost exclusively in septic arthritis. However, WBC counts between 2,000 - 100,000 cells/mm^3 can be seen in a variety of inflammatory arthridites: juvenile rheumatoid arthritis, systemic lupus erythematosus, rheumatic fever, as well as septic arthritis. The same is true for synovial glucose values ranging from greater than 20 mg% to values nearly equal that of blood glucose. The mucin clot is poor or friable in an inflammatory arthritis - septic or not.

An important adjunct to synovial fluid culture is repeated blood cultures. The blood culture is positive in 40-50% of septic arthritis (Nelson and Koontz, 1966) and the combination of blood cultures and synovial fluid cultures produce an etiologic agent in from 60-80% of cases (Nelson and Koontz, 1966; Almquist, 1970; Russell and Ansell, 1972).

In addition to these essential diagnostic procedures, the patient should obviously be examined carefully for other sources of infection and appropriate cultures obtained. Blood should be drawn for antinuclear antibodies, rheumatoid factor, C-reactive protein, and sedimentation rate. X-rays should be ordered of the chest and the involved joint. TB skin test should be applied, and urethral smear should be done when appropriate.

The differential diagnosis list is long and includes systemic lupus erythematosus, juvenile rheumatoid arthritis, rheumatic fever, arthritis associated with bowel disease, viral arthritis, osteomyelitis with a sympathetic effusion (note: this effusion may have a non-inflammatory fluid, <2000 WBC/hpf, good mucin clot, normal glucose and protein), "toxic synovitis," and leukemia. However, one must remember that septic arthritis is the first concern in any patient with acute arthritis.

Radiographic changes are not particularly helpful early in the course. Only soft-tissue swelling is seen. Ideally, the diagnosis and treatment would be completed without significant radiographic abnormalities. However, as the time lag increases to greater than 48 hours between onset of symptoms and initiation of therapy, radiographic changes become apparent, i.e. subchondral bone loss, periostitis, and then 7-10 days later gross bone destruction. By the time the diagnosis can be confirmed radiographically, irreversible damage has occurred.

4. MANAGEMENT AND PROGNOSIS

The goals of management are: 1) prompt treatment of the infection, 2) relief of pain and discomfort, and 3) prevention of deformities.

Initial antibiotic therapy should be guided by the age of patient and gram stain results. If the initial gram stain is negative, a penicillinase-resistant penicillin and kanamycin or gentamicin should be used in infants under 1 year of age. In patients 1-5 years of age, ampicillin in combination with a penicillinase-resistant penicillin should be used, and over 5 years of age a penicillinase-resistant penicillin alone is probably adequate initial therapy. Antibiotic therapy can be modified within the next 2 or 3 days pending culture results. In patients with a history of penicillin allergy, cephalothin or clindamycin may be used. The antibiotics should be administered intravenously every 4-6 hours for a two to three week period and may be followed by oral therapy for another 3-6 weeks, depending on the patient's response, the organism involved and overall course. It has been shown that antibiotic concentrations in septic joint effusions are equal to or exceed blood levels for ampicillin, methicillin, penicillin, cephalothin (Nelson, 1971) and are adequate for gentamicin and clindamycin. Therefore, intra-articular antibiotics offer no additional benefits and indeed may be harmful, causing a chemical synovitis.

Adequate drainage of the affected joint is also important. There is general agreement that surgical drainage should be carried out initially when the hip is involved, as repeated aspiration is technically difficult and if drainage is inadequate, hip dislocation is likely. Surgical drainage should also be employed on any other joint when closed aspiration is inadequate. This latter situation is generally considered to exist when the patient evidences a poor clinical response after 3-4 days of appropriate antibiotics and daily closed aspirations. However, many joints, especially the knee, can be treated adequately with repeated closed aspirations. One recent study involving adults and children (Goldenberg et al. 1975) showed fewer sequelae in the closed aspiration group vs. the surgical drainage group. Children represented approximately 20% of each treatment group.

The involved joint should be splinted in mild (5-10°) flexion and, after the first few days, passive range of motion done.

Complications of septic arthritis include avascular necrosis, dislocation of the hip, a spectrum of degenerative changes from mild sclerosis to ankylosis, and growth disturbances. The growth disturbances are most significant in the hip, where loss of the capital femoral epiphysis may lead to a severe leg length discrepancy. In one study (Borella et al., 1963) all cases of pathologic dislocation of the hip led to destruction of the capital femoral epiphysis.

Generally, complications are directly related to the time lag between onset of symptoms and institution of appropriate therapy. In the above study (Borella et al., 1963), 77% of all complications were in children in whom therapy was not instituted for 7 days or more after onset of symptoms.

Osteomyelitis is associated with approximately 10% of septic arthritis and may precede, occur concurrently or follow septic arthritis. The last situation occurs particularly in infants under two years of age. Other complications include chronic joint effusion and joint flexion contracture.

The prognosis is directly related to the time interval between the onset of symptoms and initiation of appropriate antibiotic therapy. When that time interval is greater than 7 days, the prognosis for normal joint function is poor. Other factors associated with a poor prognosis include dislocation of the hip and associated osteomyelitis.

In most studies, the joint with the poorest prognosis is the hip. Most likely this occurs because of greater delay in diagnosis in infants and the difficulty of adequate drainage.

The infecting organism appears to be of less importance in determining outcome than the above factors. The staphylococcus has been thought to be the most destructive organism, but one recent study (Almquist, 1970) indicates that H. influenzae is just as destructive.

REFERENCES

Almquist, E.E.: The changing epidemiology of septic arthritis in children. Clin. Orthop. 68:96, 1970.

Borella, L., Goobar, J.E., Summitt, R.L. and Clar, G.M.: Septic arthritis in childhood. J. Pediatr. 62:742, 1963.

Fink, C.W.: Gonococcal arthritis in children. JAMA 194:237, 1965.

Goldenberg, D.L., Brandt, K., Cohen, A.S. and Cathcart, E.S.: Treatment of septic arthritis. Arthritis Rheum. 18:83, 1975.

Kushner, I. and Somerville, J.: Permeability of human synovial membrane to plasma proteins. Arthritis Rheum. 14:560, 1971.

Nelson, J.D.: Antibiotic concentrations in septic joint effusions. NEJM 284:349, 1971.

Nelson, J.D., and Koontz, W.C.: Septic arthritis in infants and children: A review of 117 cases. Pediatrics 38:966, 1966.

Samilson, R.L., Bersani, F.A., and Watkins, M.B.: Acute suppurative arthritis in infants and children. Pediatrics 798, 1958.

Smith, Sir T.: On the acute arthritis of infants. St. Bart's Hosp. Rep. 10:189, 1874.

CHAPTER 6. INFECTIONS OF THE CENTRAL NERVOUS SYSTEM

INTRODUCTION: During the past few decades, significant progress has been made in our understanding of the etiology, mode of prevention and management of many central nervous system (CNS) infections. Although a large number of microbial agents responsible for CNS infections have been discovered, there are still many clinical syndromes in which the role of infectious agents requires further documentation (e.g. Reye's syndrome, multiple sclerosis, Guillian-Barre syndrome, acute cerebellar ataxia, febrile seizures, etc.). Application of prophylactic measures has reduced the mortality and complications of diseases such as polio, measles, tetanus, and tuberculosis; however, in less privileged populations these diseases continue to occur with a disturbing frequency. Antimicrobial therapy has also greatly altered the outcome of CNS infections. It is well recognized that early diagnosis and prompt antibiotic therapy are the most important factors in reducing mortality and morbidity in infants and children with bacterial meningitis.

In this chapter CNS infections will be considered in two broad categories: 1) generalized infections (meningoencephalitis - acute and subacute); and 2) focal infections (brain abscess, empyema, cerebellar ataxia, anterior horn cell disease, nerve root disease, and neuromuscular disease). For more comprehensive reviews of CNS infection in infants and children, the reader is referred to Swartz and Dodge (1965) and Bell and McCormick (1975).

6.1: ACUTE MENINGOENCEPHALITIS

INTRODUCTION: Diffuse infections of the brain and its lining have been theoretically divided into two clinical syndromes: (1) meningitis in which the meninges are infected causing headaches and stiff neck (meningismus), and; (2) encephalitis in which the brain substance is infected causing decrease in consciousness, seizures or focal deficits. Bacteria, which can multiply extracellularly in the subarachnoid space, are frequently the cause of "meningitis," and viruses, which multiply intracellularly in the brain substance, are frequently causes of "encephalitis." In fact it is rare for any pathogen to affect either the meninges or brain substance without affecting the other. Thus, meningoencephalitis is a more accurate description of the actual clinical presentation of these infections.

EPIDEMIOLOGY: Epidemiological factors are important in diagnostic consideration of CNS infections in infants and children. These factors include age, season, geography, and socio-economic status.

<u>Age</u>: In patients from 2 months to 4 years, <u>Hemophilus influenzae</u> is the most common bacterial agent in childhood CNS infections. In fact 90% of all Hemophilus CNS infections occur before the age of 5 years. <u>Streptococcus pneumoniae</u> (pneumococcus) is the second most common bacterial agent in this age group; 50% of pneumococal CNS infections occur before 1 year of age. <u>Neisseria meningitidis</u> is the third most common agent in this age group. Over 5 years of age the incidence of bacterial meningitis (especially <u>H. influenzae</u>) decreases markedly, presumably because of the development of immune "factors" after subclinical infections. For the same reason immunoglobulins, transferred passively from the mother, make these three agents extremely uncommon as causes of meningitis in neonates. Thus, an entirely different group of bacterial agents must be considered in the neonate: i.e. <u>E. coli</u>, streptococcus group B, and gram-negative organisms (proteus, pseudomonas, klebsiella) (see Chapter 8).

<u>Time of year</u>: Enteroviruses have peak incidence in late summer, influenza virus in winter, mumps in winter-spring, arboviruses in summer (Fig. 6.1).

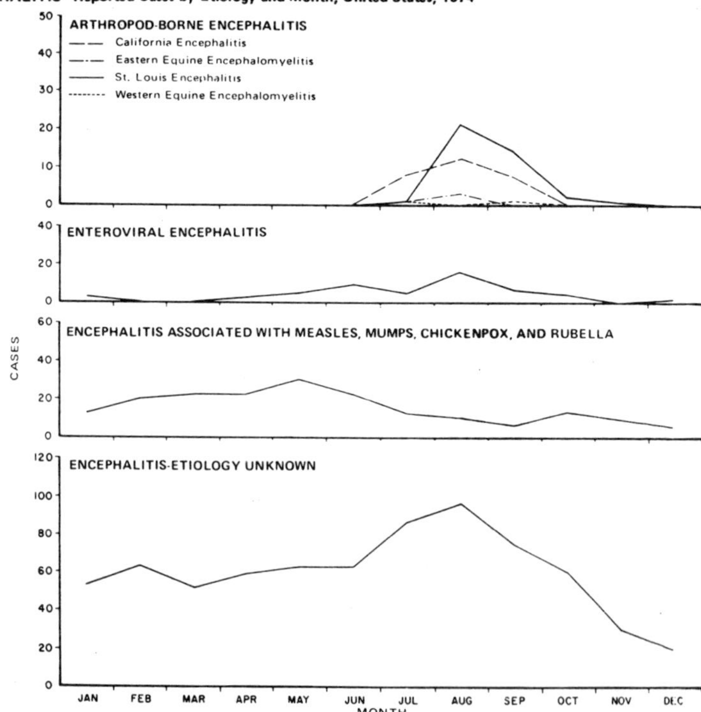

FIG. 6.1: Seasonal variations in incidence of viral encephalitis.

Geography: Geography is helpful in establishing the degree of suspicion for agents (especially arboviruses) limited to certain areas because of vectors: Eastern equine, western equine, St. Louis equine (see 4.6: Arboviruses).

Socio-economic status: Socio-economic status of the patient may affect the susceptibility of the host. For example, patients living in crowded conditions with poor hygiene, and who are also malnourished, are more susceptible to tuberculosis.

1. ETIOLOGY

As previously cited, bacterial meningitis in infants and children over two months of age is generally caused by H. influenzae type B, S. pneumoniae, or N. meningitidis. Other organisms, both pathogenic and non-pathogenic, may establish an infection when there is an alteration of mechanical and immunologic factors (Table 6-1). Recurrent meningitis is rare and is usually seen in the following conditions: (1) congenital defects (e.g. meningomyelocele, neurenteric cysts, or midline dermal sinus), (2) head trauma, (3) parameningeal foci of infection (e.g. chronic mastoiditis, sinusitis, brain abscess, subdural empyema, or epidural abscess of the spine) and (4) defects in immune system.

TABLE 6-1: PATHOGENESIS AND TYPE OF BACTERIA INVOLVED IN MENINGITIS BEYOND TWO MONTHS OF AGE	
MECHANISM OF SPREAD	COMMON TYPE OF BACTERIA
1. Blood stream invasion	H. influenzae B, S. pneumoniae, N. meningitidis
2. Direct spread from otitis media, mastoiditis, paranasal sinusitis	S. pneumoniae, H. influenzae, S. aureus, S. pyogenes
3. Trauma, anatomic defects or compromised host*	S. aureus, S. pneumoniae Klebsiella, E. coli, Pseudomonas
* Less common bacteria are Proteus mirabilis, H. parainfluenzae, Herellea vaginicola, Mima polymorpha, Serratia marcescens, N. catarrhalis, etc.	

Viral meningoencephalitis (or aseptic meningitis) is commonly caused by mumps, coxsackie, ECHO, and arboviruses. Other viruses such as measles, chicken pox, rubella, herpes simplex, cytomegalovirus, E-B virus, lymphocytic choriomeningitis, encephalomyocarditis, adenoviruses, rhinoviruses, louping ill, pseudolymphocytic meningitis, hepatitis, etc. may also cause viral meningitis syndrome. Approximately 70% of viral meningoencephalitis does not have a known cause.

2. PATHOGENESIS

2.1: <u>Bacterial Meningitis</u>: The majority of bacterial meningitis is probably the result of hematogenous spread of bacteria in the meninges. Colonization of infection of the upper respiratory tract (nasopharynx) often precedes meningitis, particularly when caused by <u>N. meningitidis</u>. Other less common routes of infection include direct extension of bacteria from localized infections such as otitis media, mastoiditis, paranasal sinusitis, or from trauma or anatomical defects of the CNS (e.g. open skull fractures, basilar skull fractures, penetrating wounds, surgery, meningomyelocele, encephalocele, dermal sinus).

Both mechanical and immunologic factors are considered important in defense against CNS infections:

<u>Mechanical factors</u>: Normally the CNS is protected from the environment by formidable mechanical barriers - the skin, subcutaneous tissue and bone. The only "weak point" is in the nasopharynx where the subarachnoid space follows the olfactory nerve fibers to the submucosa (the only site in the body where the subarachnoid space is separated from the environment by a thin layer of cells).

<u>Immunologic factors</u>: Specific immunologic defenses against CNS infections are probably mediated by both humoral and cellular factors. The mechanisms of action in preventing CNS infection of these resistance factors are known only in part. Transplacental antibodies against <u>H. influenzae</u> appear to afford protection during the first three months of life. Patients with immunodeficiency disorders or altered host resistance are found to be more susceptible to CNS infections. It is important to recognize that most patients with bacterial meningitis do not have detectable defects in their mechanical barriers or immunologic defense mechanisms.

2.2: <u>Viral Meningoencephalitis</u>: Virus can affect the CNS in two ways: (1) by direct invasion and (2) by post infectious, autoimmune, or allergic processes. Most acute viral meningoencephalitides occur as the result of viremia (e.g. arboviruses, enteroviruses) or by direct invasion along neural pathways (e.g. <u>Herpesvirus hominis</u>). In the viremic mode of spread, viruses first infect non-neural tissues where a site for multiplication is established. From this site the virus enters the blood, either by multiplying faster than it can be cleared, or by adsorbing to the red blood cells or the infected phagocytes. The virus penetrates the blood brain barrier and enters the CNS. The choroid plexus is an ideal site for penetration because it lacks a dense basement membrane. The endothelial cells of the choroid plexus lack tight junctions, and its location provides direct access to the spinal fluid. Once in the spinal fluid and subarachnoid space, there is no barrier to keep the virus from brain tissue. In general, the viremic phase is very brief and terminates at the time when circulating interferon and specific humoral antibody appear.

Studies in experimental animals have shown that H. hominis enters
the CNS along the neural pathways. Such a route of invasion is also
likely to occur in humans. The pathogenesis of post-infectious and
autoimmune encephalitides is largely unknown at this time.

3. PATHOLOGY

3.1: Bacterial Meningitis: Characteristic findings in bacterial
meningitis include vascular congestion of the meninges with accumulation of inflammatory exudate (polymorphonuclear leukocytes, fibrin, bacterial clumps, and red blood cells). The exudate or pus
accumulate in the sulci and basilar cisterns, and eventually fill the
entire subarachnoid space and extend along the Virchow-Robin
spaces where vasculitis and thrombosis develop. This may lead to
hypoperfusion of brain tissue, ischemic cortical softening, and
edema. Cerebral edema occurs in varying degrees, and herniation
may develop in severe cases. The inflammatory process may also
be seen in the ventricular system and on the ependymal surface, but
these sites are rarely involved to the same degree as the subarachnoid space.

The inflammatory exudate may involve the cranial nerves (especially
III, VI, VIII) and may result in transient or permanent blindness,
palsies, or deafness. The combined effect of vasculitis, thrombosis, and reduced blood flow to the brain substance may also impair
cerebral metabolism, and when this occurs during the first two
years of life, when the brain is growing and maturing, significant
neurologic sequelae may result.

3.2: Viral Meningoencephalitis: Information on the pathologic findings in patients with uncomplicated viral meningitis is incomplete.
The changes in viral infection are less severe than those seen in
bacterial meningitis. The vascular congestion in the meninges and
inflammatory response (predominantly lymphocytic) is much less
severe, and grossly there may be edema. Microscopic examination
reveals that viruses, an obligate intracellular organism, cause destructive changes in the cells they infect. Neurons will show nonspecific degenerative or necrotic changes. Some, but not all, viruses will form inclusion bodies in the nucleus or cytoplasm (e.g.
H. hominis, varicell-zoster, cytomegalovirus, and measles). During the healing phase, dead neurons are phagocytized and the microg-
lia and astrocytes proliferate causing glial nodules, the equivalent
of scarring. Inflammatory changes are variable and usually manifested by infiltration of perivascular lymphocytes. The white matter
is not spared and myelin breakdown may occur primarily or secondary to neuronal deaths.

Although virus invasion of the cerebrum is usually diffuse, some viruses have focal predilections (e.g. herpes in the temporal lobes,
varicella in the cerebellum, and polio in the anterior horn cells).

Involvement of the motor neurons of the brain stem and spinal cord
is characteristic of enteroviral infections. Herpesvirus hominis
tends to cause a profound focal hemorrhagic necrosis. Arboviruses
may cause actual necrosis of the brain tissues and mumps virus
tends to produce leptomeningitis.

4. CLINICAL MANIFESTATIONS

In a child over two months of age, symptoms of meningoencephalitis
include irritability, vomiting, lethargy, confusion or seizures (focal or generalized). The older child may complain of headache or
a stiff neck. There may be a history of antecedent infection involving the upper respiratory tract, ear, or gastrointestinal tract.

Signs of meningoencephalitis include fever, bulging fontanelle (in
patients young enough to have an "open" fontanelle), impaired level
of consciousness and evidence of meningeal irritation (stiff neck,
Kernig's sign, Brudzinski's sign). To elicit Kernig's sign, the supine patient's hip is flexed so the thigh is perpendicular to the trunk
and the knee is extended. The test is "positive" if the knee cannot
be extended and causes pain in the back or neck. Brudzinski's sign
involves passive flexion of the neck of the patient in supine position,
and is "positive" when spontaneous flexion of the lower extremities
occurs. These signs of meningeal irritation will disappear as the
patient improves, but will also disappear if the patient deteriorates
and becomes comatose.

Focal neurologic deficits can occur but are not usually present early
in the course of the infection; their presence should bring to mind
the possibility of abscess, hematoma or neoplasm. Focal neurologic
signs should also raise suspicion of specific virus infections: temporal lobe signs (herpes), cerebellar signs (varicella), anterior horn
cells or brain stem nuclei (enteroviruses).

The differential diagnosis in the patient older than two months with
this syndrome is limited. Subarachnoid hemorrhage can mimic
meningoencephalitis but is fortunately rare in childhood. Cervical
adenitis can cause a stiff neck, but the nodes are painful to palpation.
Children with rheumatoid arthritis involving the cervical spine have
symptoms that may mimic a CNS infection. A posterior fossa tumor
can cause a stiff neck which usually has a gradual onset with either
cranial nerve deficits or ataxia and papilledema. However, if hemorrhage into the tumor occurs, all the signs of meningoencephalitis
can develop acutely, and in such case, lumbar puncture can lead to
fatal tonsillar herniation.

4.1: Hemophilus Influenzae: Approximately 20,000 to 30,000 cases
of meningitis due to H. influenzae occur each year in the United
States. The incidence in children is estimated to be 1 case per
2,000 children per year. It is more common in winter months. The

non-specific meningoencephalitis syndrome may develop over hours. Rash is an uncommon manifestation but petechiae may occur. Subdural effusions are common as manifested by bulging fontanelle, positive transillumination, increasing head size in infants, persistent fever or progressing neurologic deterioration. Other complications include pericarditis, pneumonia and shock. Currently, the mortality rate is 5-8%, but serious sequelae are seen in additional 10-30% with only 40-60% of the patients having a completely normal neurologic examination at follow-up.

Sequelae include mental retardation, seizures, cranial nerve dysfunction (especially II, VII, VIII) and, rarely, hydrocephalus.

4.2: Streptococcus Pneumoniae: Pneumococcal meningitis usually presents with the non-specific meningoencephalitis syndrome. Its course may be more rapid, death may occur within several hours after onset of the syndrome. It is commonly seen between two and twelve months of age. Otitis media, upper respiratory infection or pneumonitis is likely to be present. Certain patients have a predisposition for pneumococcal meningitis, e.g. patients whose spleen has been removed, patients with sickle cell disease, histiocytosis X and immunodeficiencies. Subdural effusions are seen less frequently than in H. influenzae meningoencephalitis, but because the exudate is more purulent, hydrocephalus and cranial nerve dysfunctions are seen more commonly. The mortality rate approximates 20%.

4.3: Neisseria Meningitidis: Meningococcal meningitis is seen less commonly, but unlike H. influenzae and pneumococcal meningitis, meningococcal disease can occur in epidemics. In recent years, the incidence of meningococcal meningitis in the United States has been 1-2 cases/100,000 population per year. In addition to the nonspecific clinical manifestations of meningoencephalitis, 50-60% of patients will have a petechial rash, especially over the lower extremities. A similar rash can be seen in rickettsial, as well as in other bacterial or viral infections (ECHO viruses and adenoviruses). Complications are numerous, and these include myocarditis, pneumonitis, and shock. The mortality rate is less than 10%. Of surviving patients, approximately 20% have neurologic abnormalities, including mental retardation, seizures and cranial nerve dysfunction.

4.4: Enteroviruses: Enteroviruses are small RNA viruses and include coxsackie, ECHO and polioviruses.

(a) Coxsackie viruses, especially group B, appear to be the most frequent cause of "aseptic meningitis." Involvement of the brain substance can be extensive. In addition to the nonspecific meningoencephalitis syndrome, these viruses can occasionally cause an erythematous macular rash. Myocarditis or myalgia are complicated but morbidity and mortality rates are very low. The viruses can also affect the anterior horn cells and cause a "polio-like syndrome" with asymmetric flaccid paralysis. This agent characteristically produces a more benign infection than poliovirus and rarely affects bulbar nuclei.

(b) ECHO viruses cause 10-20% of "aseptic meningitis" cases. The clinical feature, similar to coxsackie virus infections, is usually mild and runs a benign course. About 10% of patients may have an erythematous maculopopular rash which rarely becomes petechial. Asymmetric limb weakness caused by anterior horn involvement can also occur.

(c) Poliovirus infections are seen much less frequently but still occur and are characterized by more severe asymmetric involvement of bulbar or anterior horn cells.

4.5: Mumps: Mumps infection of the central nervous system, commonly develops in patients with clinically apparent parotitis, occurring perhaps in more than 60% of the cases and is usually quite mild. Furthermore, it is estimated 50% or more cases of CNS mumps infections occur in the absence of clinically evident parotitis. Sequelae are correlated with degree of brain substance involvement, and are rare.

Recent animal studies and isolated case reports suggest that mumps virus has an affinity for ependymal structures and may be a causative factor in aqueductal obstruction.

4.6: Arboviruses: The clinically important arboviruses in the United States are transmitted by mosquito vectors.

California encephalitis virus is seen in northern midwestern states (LaCrosse strain) with a peak incidence in 4-10 year old children. The acute illness may be quite severe, with more than 50% developing seizures. Morbidity and mortality rates are low.

St. Louis encephalitis virus is usually seen in midwestern states and west of the Mississippi River. It is more likely to infect adults and have a 20% mortality rate; when children are infected the mortality rate is about 6%.

Eastern equine encephalitis virus is fortunately rare and usually seen on the eastern coast, but also occurs along the Gulf coast. This is the most severe arbovirus infection in children in the United States and has a mortality rate of 70%, with frequent complications seen in more than 90% of survivors. This may be related to a predilection for infection in younger children (25% of infections occur in children less than one year of age).

Western equine encephalitis virus occurs primarily in California and Texas; it has an intermediate severity with a mortality rate of approximately 10%. About 20-30% of all affected patients are less than one year of age.

Venezuelan equine encephalitis virus is rare in the United States,
but cases have been reported in Florida, Texas and California.

4.7: Herpes Simplex Virus (Herpesvirus hominis):

(a) Herpes simplex virus type I ("oral" type) causes a hemorrhagic
     encephalitis in children and produces focal signs in almost 80%
     of the cases in older children. There is a clear preference for
     the temporal lobe and orbitofrontal cortex, which causes fre-
     quent psychological disturbances, hallucinations, temporal lobe
     seizures or hemiparesis. Mortality is high (up to 70%) and
     sequelae are common. Only rarely will gingivostomatitis or
     vesicular lesions be present. The diagnosis is suspected if
     the brain scan or computerized tomography reveal a focal
     temporal lesion.

(b) Herpes simplex virus type 2 (genital type) is responsible for
     most cases of neonatal herpes infections. In addition to CNS
     infection, other organs are often affected. Vesicles, conjunc-
     tivitis, hepatosplenomegaly with abnormal bleeding, jaundice,
     lethargy and irritability can be seen. The mortality rate may
     exceed 90% in disseminated disease with CNS involvement
     (Chapter 7).

4.8: Varicella-Zoster: Varicella-zoster virus encephalitis usually
begins 4 to 6 days after the rash appears and it is usually manifested
by the nonspecific meningoencephalitis syndrome. The incidence of
encephalitis is less than 1 per 1000 cases of varicella. The mortality rate varies from 5 to 20%. Acute cerebellar ataxia may occur
5-10 days following appearance of the rash. It is not proven whether
this is caused by a localized infection or by a post-infectious "auto
immune" process. Complete recovery usually occurs (Chapter 3).

4.9: Epstein-Barr Virus: Infectious mononucleosis, probably caused
by E-B virus, may be complicated by meningoencephalitis in 1 to 5%
of cases. Findings vary from the nonspecific meningoencephalitis
syndrome to hemiparesis, ataxia or cord involvement (Chapter 17).

4.10: Rabies Virus: Rabies virus meningoencephalitis has become
a rare disease in the United States. The major reservoirs for this
virus are dogs, skunks, foxes, bats, racoons, etc. Since the virus
travels from the site of inoculation to the brain in peripheral nerves,
the incubation period is usually 2 to 6 weeks, but may vary from 15
days (from the face) to 2 years (from extremity bites). Dysfunction
of the peripheral nerve (paresthesia) is the first sign, followed by
excitability, and muscular spasm with difficulty swallowing. Once
the encephalon is involved, death has been almost universal.

5. DIAGNOSIS

Acute bacterial meningitis generally produces more severe clinical symptoms than those caused by viruses. However, in the early course of bacterial infections, the symptoms and signs may be simulated by viral infections. Therefore, the exact etiologic agent of acute meningoencephalitis syndrome cannot be diagnosed based on clinical grounds alone, and requires the aid of the laboratory.

Lumbar puncture is the most useful diagnostic test. The character- istic CSF findings of various forms (bacterial, viral, and mycobac- terial) of meningitis are shown in Table 6-2. The opening pressure

TABLE 6-2: CEREBRO-SPINAL FLUID FINDINGS IN CNS DISEASES			
DISEASE	NO. OF CELLS	GLUCOSE LEVEL	PROTEIN LEVEL
1. Acute bacterial meningitis	↑ (PMN)	↓	↑
2. Tuberculous meningitis	↑ (lymphocytes)	↓	↑
3. Aseptic meningitis	↑ (lymphocytes)	N	↑ or N
4. Brain abscess or tumor	N or ↑ (lymphocytes)	N	↑
5. Lead enceph- alopathy	N or ↑ (lymphocytes)	N	↑
6. Meningismus	N	N	N

Adapted from Krugman, S. and Ward, S., Infectious diseases of children and adults, C.V. Mosby Company, St. Louis, 1973.

of CSF may be elevated or normal, the color of the fluid may be cloudy or clear. Pleocytosis is usually observed. Presence and persistence of polymorphonuclear (PMN) leukocytes suggest a bac- terial infection. In contrast, a mononuclear pleocytosis is usually seen in viral or mycobacterial infections, or in partially treated acute bacterial meningitis. PMN pleocytosis may be seen during the early course of acute viral meningitis, but mononuclear cells quickly become the predominant cell type. Gram stain and cultures of CSF for bacteria are mandatory. Diagnosis of acute bacterial meningitis can usually be confirmed within 24 to 48 hours. In addi- tion to the gram stain and bacterial cultures, some laboratories also use counterimmunoelectrophoreses (CIE) to detect the bacterial antigens in CSF for rapid diagnosis or for diagnosis of partially treated bacterial meningitis.

Virus isolation techniques and serologic methods are used when virus infection is suspected. Viruses may be isolated from the CSF or from the feces (enteroviruses), urine (mumps), throat washings (enteroviruses, H. hominis), and saliva (mumps, H. hominis). Rapid diagnosis can be achieved by detection of viral antigens, using immunofluroescent staining method in H. hominis encephalitis (Fig. 6.2). Serologic methods commonly used in determining antibody response include complement fixation (CF), hemagglutination-inhibition (HI), and serum neutralization (SN).

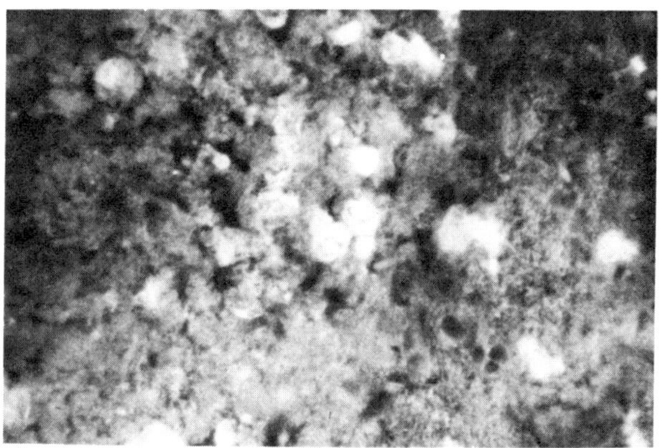

FIG. 6.2: A newborn infant with Herpesvirus hominis encephalitis. The viral antigens are shown in the brain biopsy specimen by immuno-fluorescent staining method.

6. MANAGEMENT

Management of bacterial meningitis is a medical emergency. If the clinical and CSF findings are compatible with acute bacterial meningitis, antibiotic therapy should be initiated immediately. The initial therapy is dependent upon: 1) the presumed etiologic agent based on the age of the patient; and 2) the presence or absence of an underlying disease. Current approach to antibiotic therapy for bacterial meningitis is shown in Table 6-3.

Selection of antibiotic is primarily based on the sensitivity of the organism and the ability of the antibiotic to penetrate the blood brain barrier. Bacterial resistance to antibiotics is changing constantly (e.g. meningococci to sulfa drugs, H. influenzae to ampicillin).

TABLE 6-3: ANTIBIOTIC THERAPY OF CENTRAL NERVOUS SYSTEM INFECTIONS	
CLINICAL CONDITION	**INITIAL THERAPY** (dose/kg/day)
1. Meningitis, under 2 months of age:	
Unknown etiology	Ampicillin 100-200 mg. I.V. in 2-3 doses and gentamicin 5-7 mg. I.V. in 2-3 doses
Escherichia coli	Ampicillin and gentamicin, as above
Group B streptococcus	Penicillin G, 100,000-200,000 units in 2-3 doses
Listeria monocytogenes	Ampicillin, as above
Pseudomonas aeruginosa	Carbenicillin 400 mg. I.V. in 4 doses and Gentamicin, as above
2. Meningitis, beyond 2 months of age:	
Unknown etiology	Ampicillin 200-400 mg. I.V. in 4-6 doses and Chloramphenicol 100 mg. I.V. in 3 doses
H. influenzae	Ampicillin or Chloramphenicol (depend upon sensitivity test)
Pneumococcus	Penicillin G 250,000 units I.V. in 6 doses
Meningococcus	Penicillin G, as above
3. Patients with anatomic or immunologic defects:	Nafcillin 100-200 mg. I.V. in 4 doses and chloramphenicol 100 mg. I.V. in 3 doses (pending culture results)

Chloramphenicol and sulfonamides easily enter the CNS tissues and CSF in both infected and uninfected tissues. Most other antibiotics depend upon the degree of meningeal inflammation. Penicillin and ampicillin can achieve the therapeutic concentrations by high doses given parenterally, whereas kanamycin, gentamicin, streptomycin, polymyxin B, and cephalosporins produce a low or very low CSF concentration.

A combination of ampicillin and chloramphenicol is currently used as initial antibiotics for bacterial meningitis in infants and children beyond two months of age who have no underlying disease. Single antibiotic may be used when the bacterial agent is identified and the antibiotic sensitivity pattern is known. Therapy should be given for 10 to 14 days in most patients. Duration of therapy is considerably longer if arthritis, osteomyelitis, mastoiditis, or brain abscess are present. Antibiotic dosage is generally not reduced as the patient improves, because antibiotic penetration into the CSF is significantly reduced when the acute inflammation has subsided. Intrathecal administration of an antimicrobial agent is seldom needed, unless pseudomonas meningitis exist.

Persistent or recurrent fever is generally due to phlebitis, drugs, subdural effusion, or concurrent respiratory viral infection.

Chloramphenicol alone may be used as a therapeutic agent for a patient who is allergic to penicillin and who has pneumococcal meningococcal or hemophilus meningitis.

Patients with anatomic defect (such as hydrocephalus with ventriculoperitoneal shunt) are often infected with unusual bacteria. Successful therapy depends upon the isolation of the bacterial agent and the antibiotic sensitivity pattern. Removal of the infected shunt is often required if the organism is to be eradicated.

Shock may occur in some patients with acute bacterial meningitis and must be corrected if present. Otherwise, fluid restriction (e.g. 2/3 maintenance) is applied to reduce cerebral edema.

At the present time, there is no satisfactory chemoprophylaxis for meningococcal meningitis. Rifampin is currently recommended for close contact (e.g. family member). Minocycline alone or minocycline plus rifampin have also been used in adults. Sulfonamide is useful if the epidemic strain is sulfonamide-sensitive. Careful observation of the contacts is of prime importance.

Most of the viral meningitis is benign and self-limited. Management is entirely symptomatic and supportive. Most patients recover completely within a few days; some patients may require weeks. Residual neuromuscular weakness needs follow-up and rehabilitation therapy. H. hominis encephalitis is a severe disease associated with high incidence of mortality and sequelae. Adenine arabinoside is currently under study for the treatment of this infection.

In the management of viral meningitis it is important to rule out: 1) partially treated bacterial meningitis, 2) early tuberculous meningitis, or 3) other obscure meningitis. History of illness and its preceding antibiotic therapy are important. If bacterial meningitis cannot be excluded, antibiotic therapy may be initiated until the bacterial culture results become available.

::

6.2: SUBACUTE MENINGOENCEPHALITIS

INTRODUCTION: The majority of infectious agents causing an encephalitis syndrome produce a rapid progression of symptoms and signs; only few infectious agents cause a subacute form of meningoencephalitis and these are primarily mycobacteria and fungi. Subacute meningoencephalitis, though less common, continues to be a cause of serious morbidity and mortality. Only the CNS involvement due to mycobacteria and fungi is discussed here, and additional information can be found in mycobacteria (Chapter 17) and fungi (Chapter 15).

1. TUBERCULOUS MENINGITIS

In the early 1900's, as much as two-thirds of bacterial meningitis in children under 3 years of age was caused by Mycobacterium tuberculosis. In the 1960's, less than 10% of bacterial meningitis was due to that organism. Tuberculous meningitis occurs primarily in children between 6 and 24 months of age. In the United States, those segments of the population with inadequate nutrition, crowded living conditions, and poor health care are more likely to be affected.

The respiratory tract is the site of primary infection. Spread to the CNS is presumably by the hematogenous route. A significant number of patients with tuberculous meningitis have miliary tuberculosis. The pathologic findings include an inflammatory response consisting of lymphocytes, plasma cells, and giant cells; arteries and veins which traverse the exudate develop adventitial swelling which may be so profound as to cause infarction. The cellular response produces a thick exudate which is most severe along the brain stem in the basilar cisterns. The exudate may be so thick as to cause obstruction of CSF flow resulting in communicating hydrocephalus (Fig. 6.3).

Clinically, fever, headache, restlessness and irritability are the first signs. The level of consciousness may decline gradually, nuchal rigidity, Kernig's sign, and vomiting develop later. Papilledema, rarely seen in acute encephalomyelitis, is frequently observed

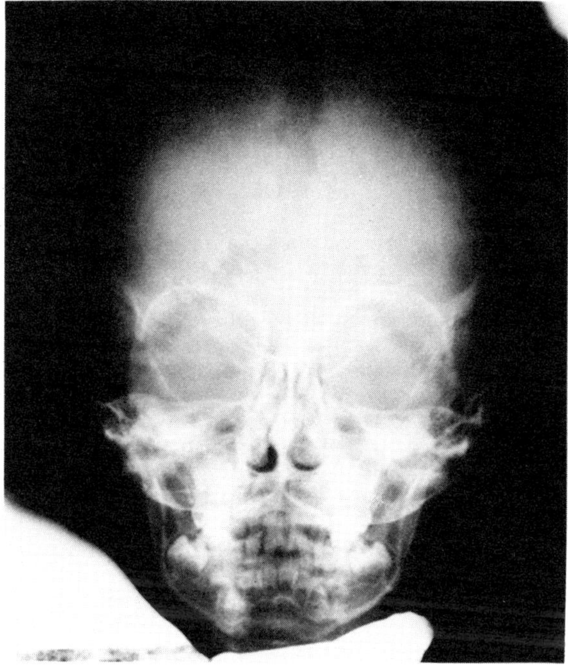

FIG. 6.3: A child with tuberculous meningitis showing signs of increased intracranial pressure (separation of sutures).

either because of cerebral edema or communicating hydrocephalus.
Tubercules may rarely be seen in the choroid on funduscopic examination. The disease is usually fatal in 3 to 5 weeks if untreated.
Even with chemotherapy, the mortality rate may approach 40%.
Complications include subdural effusions, communicating hydrocephalus, cranial nerve involvement (II, III, IV, VII, or VIII), mental retardation (in up to 50% of survivors) and seizures. Approximately 20-25% of survivors have neurologic deficits. Rare
complications include hypothalamic damage resulting in diabetes
insipidus, precocious puberty, pituitary insufficiency, and development of tuberculomas, which clinically resemble brain tumors, especially in the posterior fossa.

Approximately 15-20% of patients with CNS tuberculosis have spinal
cord involvement. It may be primary or associated with vertebral
infection (tuberculous spondylitis). Approximately 5-20% of patients
with vertebral involvement (usually in the lower thoracic vertebrae)
develop paraplegia (Pott's disease) which occurs most commonly in
patients over 2 years of age.

Examination of the spinal fluid will confirm the diagnosis. Lumbar puncture should be preceded by an emergency brain scan or computerized tomography if focal neurologic signs are present. Lumbar puncture reveals an elevated pressure, cloudy fluid, elevated protein (as high as 400 mg/dl); an acid fast stain may reveal bacilli, although cultures are difficult and may be positive in only 60-70% of cases. Chest x-ray may show typical changes of pulmonary tuberculosis. The tuberculin skin test is positive in 85% of cases, but can be negative if the patient is anergic.

Chemotherapy should be started when the diagnosis is strongly suspected. Combined use of three drugs (isoniazed, streptomycin and rifampin) is generally recommended (see page 405). In the past, para-aminosalicylic acid (PAS) was used in place of rifampin. Streptomycin is given for 4 to 8 weeks, whereas other medications are given for two years. Experience with ethambutol and ethionamide in infants and children is limited to date. Pyridoxine (25-50 mg/ day) is used. Steroids, although not proven effective, are frequently used if the patient is severely lethargic or has cerebral edema. M. tuberculosis resistant to isoniazid and streptomycin occurs in 3 to 6% of cases.

2. CRYPTOCOCCAL MENINGITIS

Meningoencephalitis caused by Cryptococcus neoformans, the most common fungal meningitis, is rare in the first decade of life, with 80-85% of cases occurring between 20 and 60 years of age. Approximately 10 to 30% of children with this infection have predisposing factors, such as Hodgkin's disease, leukemia, diabetes mellitus or chronic steroid therapy.

Cryptococcus is found in the trachea and bronchi of asymptomatic patients. Spread to the nervous system is presumably by the hematogenous route. Cellular reaction (perivascular lymphocytes and macrophages) is minimal, and the characteristic histologic finding is the organism itself (5-10 micron oval or round encapsulated organisms) in cystic spaces in the brain or Virchow-Robin spaces.

Clinical manifestations of cryptococcal meningitis are similar to those of tuberculous meningitis. About 40% of patients develop optic atrophy or papilledema. More rarely, the infection is localized to a single expanding mass lesion. Before chemotherapy, 90% of patients died within one year; with appropriate therapy, 70-80% survive.

Laboratory diagnosis is accomplished by lumbar puncture. The pressure is elevated; the fluid may be clear to cloudy, protein is usually elevated (up to 350 mg/dl), glucose is normal to low (to 10 mg/dl) and pleocytosis up to 1000 WBC/mm^3, predominantly lymphocytes. India ink preparation may yield encapsulated yeasts which are diagnostic, but these are found in less than 60% of patients. The fluid should also be submitted for culture. Antibodies to Cryptococcus neoformans may be detected in serum by complement fixation, latex agglutination or other methods.

Treatment consists of intravenous amphotericin B therapy (see page 360). Intrathecal amphotericin B is also frequently used. 5-Fluorocytosin (see page 355) has also been used alone or in combination with amphotericin B. After cessation of therapy, patients must have periodic examinations of spinal fluid for at least two years in order to detect relapses.

3. COCCIDIOIDES IMMITIS

Clinical manifestations of CNS infection due to Coccidioides immitis are indistinguishable from cryptococcal meningitis, but should be suspected in those patients with subacute meningoencephalitis following respiratory tract infections who live in hot, arid desert regions.

Laboratory tests are similar to those for cryptococcal CNS infections, except encapsulated yeasts are not seen in India ink preparations. Coccidioidin skin test and antibody studies (CF, precipitin) in serum and CSF are helpful. Amphotericin B is the drug of choice.

4. CANDIDA ALBICANS

This is the most common fungal meningocencephalitis in immunosuppressed patients or in infants receiving prolonged intravenous nutrition. A nonspecific meningoencephalitic syndrome is present and frequently overshadowed by the patient's underlying disease. The condition is frequently suspected because of other signs of systemic candidiasis. Treatment usually consists of intravenous amphotericin B.

5. ASPERGILLUS SPECIES

Aspergillus infection involving the CNS can occur by hematogenous spread from pulmonary lesions in patients with leukemia, from infected heart valves after cardiac surgery, in immunosuppressed patients or rarely, in patients who were previously in good health.

Clinically, the patient may develop a nonspecific meningoencephalitis syndrome, or perhaps more likely, signs of single or multiple mass lesions.

A brain-scan or computerized tomography might help localize focal lesions but will be nondiagnostic. Lumbar puncture is less likely to be abnormal than in cryptococcal meningoencephalitis and the organism is not usually cultured from CSF. Amphotericin B is used in therapy.

6. HISTOPLASMA CAPSULATUM

Although pulmonary infection with H. capsulatum is common in the
northeast United States and the Mississippi, Ohio, and lower Missouri river valleys, disseminated disease is rare, occurring in
less than 1 in 1000 infected patients. Disseminated disease usually
occurs in infants and in immunosuppressed or debilitated patients.
Some of the patients with disseminated disease develop a nonspecific
meningoencephalitis syndrome or multifocal neurologic dysfunction,
but this is usually overshadowed by the disseminated disease.

Spinal fluid findings are similar to those found in cryptococcal meningitis, and the culture is frequently sterile. Cultures of blood or
bone marrow aspirates may be helpful. Amphotericin B is used in
therapy.

7. MUCORMYCOSIS (PHYCOMYCOSIS)

Although rare, this group of fungi causes a distinct clinical syndrome. It occurs most commonly in diabetic patients with ketoacidosis, but has been reported in patients with leukemia, immunosuppression, and burns, as well as in narcotic addicts.

The initial site of infection is the upper airway, especially sinuses.
The characteristic cerebral lesions are caused by the profuse growth
of hyphae into arterial lumens (such as the cartoid), causing thrombosis and cerebral infarction or mycotic aneurysm.

Typically, the patient with ketoacidosis develops unilateral and painful proptosis; cranial nerves II, III, IV, and VI become involved.
A bloody nasal discharge may be present. The brain usually becomes involved within days due either to vascular thrombosis and
cerebral infarction or to direct extension. Manifestations may include headache, hemiparesis, convulsions, and cerebral edema.
Death may occur in one to two weeks.

Skull or sinus x-rays may show lytic bone lesions. Carotid angiog-
raphy may show vascular narrowing or occlusion. The fungus may
be seen and cultured from biopsy of the involved sinus tissues. Amphotericin B intravenous therapy is the drug most generally used in
treating this infection.

Other fungi, such as Blastomyces dermatitis, Sporotrichum
schenckii, Penicillium and Chaldosporium trichoides, are extremely
rare causes of subacute meningoencephalitis, but almost all reported cases have been adults.

::

6.3: SUBACUTE SCLEROSING PANENCEPHALITIS

INTRODUCTION: Subacute sclerosing panencephalitis (SSPE) occurs
worldwide. Over 200 cases were reported between 1965-1970. In
the United States, SSPE has been diagnosed most frequently in the
southeast and central states. Males are affected 3 to 5 times more
frequently than females and the clinical onset of the disease is usually between 2 and 20 years of age (with the extremes of 2 months
and 32 years). Children from rural environments are more often
affected than those from urban areas. Approximately 85% patients
with SSPE have a previous history of clinically typical measles,
and that they were at least 3 years younger than nonaffected children when they developed measles. Among SSPE patients, 25% developed measles under 1 year of age and 50% under 2 years of age.
SSPE becomes clinically apparent on an average of 5 years after the
measles infection. SSPE has also developed after measles vaccination, although this is rare and the latent period may be somewhat
shorter than when SSPE occurs following the natural measles infection.

1. ETIOLOGY AND PATHOGENESIS

Although the pathogenesis of SSPE is not completely understood at
this time, an association with measles (rubeola) virus is evident.
Para-myxovirus-like nucleocapsides have been demonstrated in the
brains of affected children by electron microscopy. The children
have elevated titers of measles antibody in blood and CSF. Measles
virus has been isolated from brain tissues of SSPE patients by co-
cultivation methods. Finally, measles-like virus has been transmitted to experimental animals, causing an encephalitis syndrome
with a prolonged incubation. Several theoretical possibilities for
the causal relationship of measles virus and SSPE have been suggested and are summarized as follows:

1) the virus is incomplete or a mutant, which allows it to lie
   dormant for long periods (slow virus);

2) the host's immune mechanisms may be abnormal, as suggested
   by measles infection at an age when the host's immune mechanisms are not mature;

3) the brain may be a "privileged site," with its absence of
   lymphatics and "blood-brain barrier" allowing survival after
   the virus is eradicated elsewhere;

4) an additional "helper virus" (papova virus-like structures
   have been reported in cells from SSPE patients) or other agent
   may alter the natural course of the infection;

5) a combination of the above.

Rubeola virus may not be the only pathogen involved in SSPE, since rubella virus has also been implicated in rare cases.

Pathological findings in SSPE are not specific. Lymphocytes, plasma cells, neuronophagia and neuron loss with gliosis and glial nodules are all nonspecific changes seen in viral infections. The 2-10 micron eosinophilic inclusions are best seen in oligodendroglia early in the course of the disease.

2. CLINICAL MANIFESTATIONS

Initial changes are subtle and gradual, consisting of decrease in school performance, amnesia, irritability and clumsiness. Within weeks to months the child develops myoclonus. Sudden flexion of the entire body occurs frequently, induced by sudden loud noises. The patient then develops various other neurologic dysfunctions, depending on the part of the brain most prominently affected. For example, spasticity, ataxia, nystagmus, parkinsonism, choreoathetosis or tremor may occur. Many patients develop a macular chorioretinitis which can cause decreased visual acuity. The final stage is one of complete amentia with posturing.

Although the course of the disease is usually 5-12 months, it may progress over weeks or years, and temporary arrests in progression or improvement can be seen. Rarely, the disease progresses extremely rapidly and can present with increased intracranial pressure and papilledema.

3. DIAGNOSIS

Patients with SSPE generally have high titers of complement fixation antibodies against measles virus in serum (1:64 to 1:2048) and in CSF (1:8 to 1:64). Measles CSF antibodies are not detectable in individuals without SSPE. Patients with SSPE also have an increased gamma globulin (20 to 50%) in the CSF when tested by protein electrophoresis, but total CSF proteins are only moderately elevated in the range of 50 to 80 mg/dl.

The electroencephalogram is often abnormal even early in the course of SSPE. The pattern is characterized by "burst-suppressions" with spike-slow wave burst appearing periodically, followed by very low voltage activity.

4. TREATMENT

There is no recognized treatment for SSPE, although various drugs are being used in experimental protocols. Standard anticonvulsants have little effect.

::

6.4: BRAIN ABSCESS AND EMPYEMA

INTRODUCTION: Focal infections of the central nervous system are much less common than the diffuse meningoencephalitis and occur in two areas: 1) in the brain parenchyma (<u>brain abscess</u>), or 2) in the epidural and subdural spaces (<u>empyema</u>).

BRAIN ABSCESS

1. ETIOLOGY AND PATHOGENESIS

Unlike meningoencephalitis, which occurs in previously normal brain tissue, abscess formation usually occurs in brain tissue which is previously damaged by trauma or infarction. Animal studies suggest that unless preceding damage has occurred, bacteremia will not cause an abscess. In children, the most common cause of initial brain damage is microinfarction caused by hypoxia and poly-cythemic hyperviscosity seen in patients with cyanotic heart disease. Damage can also be caused by embolization (septic emboli from subacute bacterial endocarditis "SBE," pulmonary abscess, pneumonia, bronchiectasis), thrombophlebitis (especially in veins bridging the meninges which become infected from mastoiditis, sinusitis, infections of the face and scalp), or direct penetrating head wounds (intracranial surgery, head injury). The necrotic tissue provides an excellent "culture medium" which is protected from the body's cellular and humoral defense mechanisms because of the reduced or absent blood supply to the damaged area.

The organisms, presumably by producing toxins, induce changes in the surrounding normal brain tissues, resulting in: (1) hyperemia, (2) edema, and (3) breakdown of the "blood brain barrier." The hyperemia is protective because it allows increased exposure to the body's circulating defense mechanisms. The edema and breakdown of the "blood brain barrier" causes dysfunction of the nerve tissue and may compress capillaries, preventing delivery of circulating humoral and cellular defense mechanisms. Both hyperemia and edema allow the focal collection of intravenously injected radionucleotides, and cause a focal "positive" brain scan. The edematous tissue is less dense than normal tissue and can cause a region of decreased density, as determined by computerized tomography which "enhances" when intravenously injected contrast material leaks across the damaged "blood-brain barrier" and accumulates at the abscess site. If the initial bacterial inoculum is large enough to establish rapid growth, or the body's response is inadequate (because of hypoxia, poor flow or thrombosis), the organisms will continue to invade normal tissue at the periphery, the center will be deprived of blood supply as well as nutrients, and this area will become an inactive accumulation of "pus." This causes the characteristic "doughnut sign" in the brain scan: an active rim of positive uptake surrounding a negative uptake "hole." This nonvascularized necrotic center also renders systemic antibiotic administration inadequate because the antibiotic is simply not delivered to the center of the lesion.

The most common agents responsible for brain abscesses are anaerobic bacteria (peptostreptococcus, fusobacterium, bacteroides, etc.) and aerobic cocci (Staphylococcus aureus, Streptococcus pneumoniae, Streptococcus pyogenes group A, Streptococcus viridans). Mixtures of anaerobes and/or aerobes are not infrequent. Other less frequent causes include H. influenzae, H. aphrophilus, E. coli, proteus, pseudomonas, corynebacterium, mycobacterium, Nocardia asteroides, candida, aspergillus, leptothrix, cryptococcus and Entamoeba histolytica.

2. CLINICAL MANIFESTATIONS

A predisposing history of cyanotic heart disease, trauma or focal infection (mastoiditis, otitis media, sinusitis) is usually present. The initial infarct is usually too small to cause neurologic symptoms, but as edema develops and the lesion enlarges, focal neurologic lesions develop depending on the site, e.g., motor strip (hemiparesis), optic radiation (hemianopsia), cerebellum (ataxia, stiff neck or "head tilt"), brain stem (cranial nerve deficits and "crossed paralysis" e.g. left VII paresis and right hemiparesis), frontal lobes (silent areas), If the lesion becomes large enough, it can cause cerebral herniation which, if untreated, will be fatal or, if the lesion occludes CSF flow (e.g. cerebellum or brain stem), it can cause noncommunicating hydrocephalus with headache and papilledema.

Fever may not be present; only 30% of patients may have fever above 38.5°C. Other nonspecific manifestations of brain abscess include drowsiness, confusion, stupor, generalized or focal seizures, nausea, vomiting and leukocytosis. Fatal complications include cerebral herniation, hemorrhage into the necrotic tissue, and rupture of the pus into the ventricular or subarachnoid space.

3. DIAGNOSIS

Lumbar puncture is a potentially dangerous diagnostic procedure in patients with brain abscess. This procedure should be done only if meningitis is strongly suspected, because such procedure can cause rupture of abscess or cerebral herniation, both complications being potentially fatal. About 10% of patients with brain abscess have normal CSF examination. However, the majority have increased pressure, moderately elevated protein level and clear fluid with small numbers (10 to 100/mm^3) of white blood cells (lymphocytes or PMN's). The fluid is usually sterile and thus cultures do not help in choosing appropriate antibiotic therapy.

The most helpful laboratory study is a brain scan or computerized
tomography. A "positive" focal uptake or "doughnut" sign in the
brain scan occurs in 30% of patients with brain abscess. Such signs
may also be seen in brain tumors. It may be difficult to detect a
posterior fossa abscess by this test. Computerized tomography is
much better in delineation of lesions than brain scan. Cerebral arteriography is indicated if the brain scan is positive and computerized tomography is unavailable. Pneumoencephalography is needed
if computerized tomography is unavailable and posterior fossa
lesions are seen on brain scan or suspected clinically. The EEG is
useful in a superficial abscess which can produce a slow wave (delta)
focus, but the test may be normal with deep or posterior fossa abscesses. Skull x-rays are less helpful, are usually normal and,
although they may show generalized increase in intracranial pressure ("split sutures"), rarely is gas seen in abscess cavity. In
some adolescents or adults, if the pineal body is calcified, it can
be shifted away from midline suggesting a mass lesion.

3.1: Differential Diagnosis: The following lesions may cause similar symptoms and signs and they should especially be considered if
no "predisposing history" of focal brain damage is present:

(1) Neoplasm: In childhood, two-thirds of brain tumors are in the
posterior fossa and patients are usually afebrile with gradual onset of focal signs. But if hemorrhage into the tumor occurs, the
onset can be sudden. If blood leaks into the subarachnoid space,
the patient may be febrile with nuchal rigidity and contrast studies may be quite similar; definitive diagnosis may be made only
at surgical exploration.

(2) Vascular accident: Embolization of any type can cause focal deficits and/or focal seizures. The onset is usually sudden and patient is afebrile but the course can be gradual ("stuttering"). A
brain scan should be normal for the first 3-5 days after onset.

(3) Trauma: Although acute trauma causing a cerebral contusion or
epidural hemorrhage should be easily recognized on the basis of
history and physical examination, subacute or chronic subdural
hematomas may present with headache, focal deficits and/or
seizures, and the history of trauma is denied or forgotten. A
brain scan should be helpful, and computerized tomography or
cerebral arteriography are diagnostic tests.

(4) Congenital malformation: Anomalies, such as subarachnoid cysts
or porencephalic cysts, usually are not confused with cerebral
abscess because the focal deficit is chronic. However, if the
deficit is minor and patient initially presents with focal seizures,
the brain scan should be negative and computerized tomography
should be diagnostic.

4. TREATMENT

Management of patients with brain abscess include the following:

(1) Anticonvulsant for seizures.

(2) Restriction of fluid is indicated if cerebral edema is present. If edema becomes life threatening with signs of early herniation, mannitol 1 gm/kg, I.V. or steroids may be considered. It should be pointed out that mannitol can cause heart failure in patients with heart disease.

(3) Antibiotics in high doses should be given before surgery. Generally antibiotics consist of a penicillin (penicillin G, ampicillin, methicillin, or nafcillin) plus chloramphenicol.

(4) Surgical exploration, as soon as the patient is stabilized, and studies document the lesion. Gram stain and cultures (aerobic, anaerobic and fungal) of the abscess material must be obtained at the time of surgery. Antibiotic therapy should be revised if an unsuspected pathogen is discovered. Therapy must be maintained for prolonged periods (two to four weeks or longer). Longer periods of therapy may be required for patients with associated extracranial foci or bacteremia.

EMPYEMA

Empyema refers to a collection of pus in a body cavity, whereas an abscess is a collection of pus within an organ. However, epidural and subdural "empyemas" are frequently referred to as "abscesses."

Empyema occurs as a result of direct extension of a contagious non-nervous system infection (e.g. osteomyelitis of the spine, sinusitis, or mastoiditis); or it may occur by hematogenous spread from a distant site (cutaneous furuncles, pyelonephritis, pneumonia, dental abscess, etc.). Spinal empyema usually occurs in the mid-thoracic or lower lumbar regions where there is more areolar tissue in the epidural space. Spinal epidural abscesses have been reported following blunt trauma to the back, but it has not been proven that this is not coincidental. The most common agent causing empyema in the CNS is the staphylococcus.

Children with chronic sinusitis may develop headache, fever, and seizures which are very difficult to control. Differentiation from cerebral abscess may be impossible on clinical grounds. The first symptom of spinal epidural abscess is usually back pain which rapidly becomes severe and is worsened by percussion, flexion of the spine or coughing. Fever is usually present and radicular pain, stiff neck and vomiting may occur. If the infection is in the lumbar region, sensory and motor loss in a nerve-root distribution, with areflexia in the legs, will develop; if in the thoracic lesion, cord compression syndromes with Babinski's sign may develop. Prognosis for recovery of function is generally poor, and complete recovery is unlikely if paralysis is present for 48 hours or longer.

Diagnostic laboratory studies may include brain scan, computerized tomography, EEG, spine roentgenogram, and lumbar puncture.

Intracranial empyema may show: (1) a positive uptake over the convexity of the brain by brain scan, and (2) a decreased voltage and/or seizure discharges on the affected side by EEG. Spinal lesions may show osteomyelitis by roentgenograms. Lumbar punctures must be done with care because complete penetration of lumbar epidural empyema can spread infection to the subarachnoid space causing meningoencephalitis. The tap should be prepared in the radiology department so that myelography can be performed. The needle should be inserted slowly, stopping at intervals to remove the stylet and gently aspirate. If pus is obtained, the needle should not be advanced any further and the pus should be cultured. If xanthochromic fluid is obtained, a myelogram should be performed.

Diseases which may be confused with epidural empyema are epidural neoplasms, epidural hematoma, spondyloarthritis, and Guillain-Barre syndrome.

6.5: OTHER FOCAL INFECTIONS

INTRODUCTION: Many infectious agents do not cause a meningoencephalitis syndrome, but limit their effect to small segments of the central or peripheral neuromuscular system. These agents may cause disease by direct invasion, by toxins, by induction of self-destructive immune reactions or by mechanisms not yet understood. Included among these kinds of infections are acute cerebellar ataxia, lower motor neuron diseases, nerve root diseases, and tetanus. Botulism is discussed elsewhere (Chapter 9).

1. ACUTE CEREBELLAR ATAXIA

Infectious diseases involving the cerebellum occur most commonly in children between 1 and 5 years of age. Since the condition is usually not fatal, knowledge of the pathogenesis is limited. Some data suggest direct viral invasion, while others invoke toxins or immune-mediated mechanisms. Associated infectious agents include varicella, infectious mononucleosis, enteroviruses (polio, ECHO, coxsackie) and Mycoplasma pneumoniae.

Clinically, at least half of the patients have a nonspecific upper respiratory infection a week or two before the onset of neurologic dysfunction; others have specific infections such as varicella, infectious mononucleosis, or mycoplasma. The patient develops truncal ataxia and/or dysarthria; hypotonia and diminished deep tendon reflexes may also be seen. A minority develop nuchal rigidity, nausea, vomiting, hyper-reflexia and cranial nerve dysfunction.

Laboratory studies may include: 1) antibody studies (acute and convalescent sera) for specific agents, and 2) examination of spinal fluid. The CSF may be normal or show a mild pleocytosis. If the patient has a posterior fossa mass, lumbar puncture can be fatal and is contraindicated. If papilledema is present, the procedure should be deferred until after other tests (brain scan, computerized tomography, or arteriography) have ruled out a mass lesion.

Differential diagnosis includes the following:

1) <u>Tumor</u>: peak incidence is in somewhat older children and astrocytomas usually cause lateralized symptoms and signs. Medulloblastoma can cause an identical syndrome.
2) <u>Trauma</u>: cerebellar contusion or posterior fossa subdural hematoma.
3) <u>Intoxication</u>: many drugs can cause a similar syndrome-alcohol, dilantin, sedatives, etc.
4) <u>Metabolic</u>: intermittent maple syrup urine disease, Hartnup's disease cause intermittent ataxia.
5) <u>Idiopathic</u>: benign paroxysmal vertigo consists of brief (seconds to minutes) episodes of vertigo and ataxia which are recurrent but self-limited.

Treatment is symptomatic and supportive.

2. LOWER MOTOR NEURON DISEASES

Although infectious agents which affect cranial nerve nuclei and anterior horn cells may also cause a meningoencephalitis, the motor neuron involvement is frequently severe enough to equal or eclipse the generalized signs and symptoms. Enteroviruses have a predilection for lower motor neurons. Poliovirus type 1 has been the most frequent cause of lower motor neuron infection in the United States in recent years, but coxsackie A (4,7,9), coxsackie B (2,3,4,5), and ECHO viruses (2,3,11) are now recognized to cause a similar but milder disease. Active immunization against poliomyelitis has drastically reduced the incidence, but this disease continues to occur in poorly immunized populations.

The hallmark sign is asymmetric flaccid weakness with areflexia and no sensory deficit develop after several days of a nonspecific meningoencephalitis syndrome. Involvement of neurons which control swallowing and breathing is most likely to cause fatal complications. Poliovirus is more likely to cause irreversible neuron destruction than the other enteroviruses. Approximately 45-50% of paralytic poliomyelitis cases are predominantly spinal, 15% bulbar and 15% bulbospinal form.

Laboratory confirmation is made by examination of CSF which shows mild pleocytosis with mildly elevated or normal proteins and normal sugar. CSF and stool cultures for viruses, and antibody studies on acute and convalescent sera, will provide proof for the diagnosis.

Treatment is supportive; artificial support of respiration and/or nutrition may be life-saving.

3. NERVE ROOT DISEASES

Occasionally lesions of the sensory and motor nerve roots and proximal peripheral nerves develop shortly after certain viral infections or vaccinations. The incidence is about 1-2 cases/100,000/year. Occurrences under 2 years of age is rare and there is a higher incidence between 2 and 10 years of age.

The symptoms develop one to three weeks after exposure to vaccinations (typhoid, tetanus, mumps, rubella, smallpox, influenza and rabies) or infections (varicella, coxsackie, ECHO, E-B, mycoplasma, cytomegalovirus). The pathogenesis is not clear. Rootlet edema occurs in the first few days followed by axonal edema. Patients with Guillain-Barre syndrome often have increased numbers of circulating atypical basophilic lymphocytes. Many of these patients have a circulating factor which is toxic to myelin in vitro. Although the current theory is that the antigens provoke an immune response whose target is the nerve roots, much remains to be proven.

The classic syndrome begins with asymmetric weakness in the legs and ascends up the trunk to varying extent. Some patients develop paresthesias which the patient may not complain of unless specifically questioned. Maximum weakness usually occurs in one to two days but it may progressively worsen for two or three weeks. The patient has an areflexic and flaccid weakness which may overshadow any minimal sensory deficits. Some patients develop bilateral seventh cranial nerve weakness. Other cranial nerves are rarely involved. Others may develop ataxia (Fisher syndrome) which can progress to lethargy. Papilledema, of uncertain etiology, can also develop. Involvement of automatic nerve roots can cause fleeting rashes or blood pressure instability. If the condition rises to the cervical cord, respiratory failure ensues, which can be fatal. With modern care, death rates of less than 10% are reported. Most patients recover completely, and even those with permanent disability (weakness, areflexia) may continue to improve over one to two years.

Laboratory studies are often inconclusive. The CSF may show
normal protein level initially, but after days or weeks the protein
is elevated in over 90% of patients. The cell count is usually normal resulting in a dissociation of cell count and protein level. Isolation of infectious agent and determination of antibody responses
may confirm the etiologic diagnosis.

Differential diagnosis includes: 1) infections (such as poliomyelitis-
asymmetric flaccid weakness, and botulism-lower cranial nerve involvement), 2) toxins (mercury neck paralysis) and 3) neoplasm
(spinal cord tumor).

Treatment is generally supportive. Usefulness of steroids is debated. Respiratory support is needed if respiratory failure occurs.

4. TETANUS

Approximately 100 cases of tetanus are reported each year in the
United States. Mortality occurs primarily in the newborn and in
the elderly.

Clostridium tetani produces an exotoxin which induces neuromuscular dysfunction (muscle spasms). Most studies suggest the toxin
produced at the site of an infected wound migrates along nerves and
interrupts synaptic function. Some suggest the toxin may act on the
muscle itself or spread to the CNS by the hematogenous route.

Although a grossly contaminated wound is the usual source of infection, tetanus has occurred after minor scratches, intramuscular
injections, or even middle ear infections. The incubation period is
usually 3 days to 3 weeks. The longer the incubation period, the
milder the illness. Muscular stiffness is the first symptom, especially of the paraspinal or abdominal musculature. Trismus or
spasm of the masseter muscles is common. The spasm becomes
generalized and can cause spinal fractures or respiratory failure.
The autonomic nervous system may also be involved, causing hyper-
or hypotension. Sometimes the spasm is entirely focal. The patient's mental status is normal if the patient is adequately ventilated.
The fatality rate may be as high as 80% in the neonate and 60% in
older children. Survivors may have persistent irritability, myoclonus or sleep disturbances.

Tetanus can be prevented by active immunization (Chapter 25).
Booster immunizations should be given at 10-year intervals. Management of patients with clinical tetanus should include: 1) cleaning
and debridement of the wound, 2) tetanus immune globulin (human)
3,000 to 6,000 units given intramuscularly, 3) antimicrobials (penicillin for 10 to 14 days), and 4) sedation and muscle relaxants (e.g.
Diazepam).

REFERENCES

BACTERIAL MENINGITIS

Artenstein, M.S.: Prophylaxis for meningococcal disease. JAMA 231:1035, 1975.

Chartrand, S.A. and Cho, C.T.: Persistent pleocytosis in bacterial meningitis. J. Pediatr. 88:424, 1976.

Davis, S.D., Hill, H.R., Feigl, P., and Arnstein, E.J.: Partial antibiotic therapy in Hemophilus influenzae meningitis. Its effect on cerebrospinal fluid abnormalities. Am. J. Dis. Child. 129:802, 1975.

Greenfield, S. and Feldman H.A.: Familial carriers and meningococcal meningitis. NEJM 277:497, 1967.

Mathies, A.W., Jr. and Wehrle, P.F.: Management of bacterial meningitis in children. Pediatr. Clin. N.A. 15:185, 1968.

McLaurin, R.L.: Infected cerebrospinal fluid shunts. Surg. Neurol. 1:191, 1973.

Naidoo, B.T.: The cerebrospinal fluid in the healthy newborn infant. S. Afr. Med. J. 42:933, 1968.

Neva, F.A.: Amebic meningoencephalitis - a new disease? NEJM 282:450, 1970.

Rapkin, R.H.: Repeat lumbar punctures in the diagnosis of meningitis. Pediatr. 54:34, 1974.

Salmon, J.H.: Ventriculitis complicating meningitis. Am. J. Dis. Child. 124:35, 1972.

Schoenbaum, S.C., Gardner, P., and Shillito, J.: Infections of cerebrospinal fluid shunts: epidemiology, clinical manifestations, and therapy. J. Infect. Dis. 131:543, 1975.

Sell, S.H.W., Merrill, R.E., Doyne, E.O., and Zimsky, E.P.,Jr.: Long-term sequelae of Hemophilus influenzae meningitis. Pediatr. 49:206, 1972.

Shackelford, P.G., Campbell, J., and Feigin, R.D.: Countercurrent immunoelectrophoresis in the evaluation of childhood infections. J. Pediatr. 85:478, 1974.

Shenkin, H.A. and Bouzarth, W.F.: Clinical methods of reducing intracranial pressure. Role of the cerebral circulation. NEJM 282:1465, 1970.

Shurtleff, D.B., Foltz, E.L., Weeks, R.D., and Loeser, J.: Therapy of Staphylococcus epidermidis: infections associated with cerebrospinal fluid shunts. Pediatr. 53:55, 1974.

Smith, D.H., Ingram, D.L., Smith, A.L., Gilles, F., and Bresnan, M.J.: Bacterial meningitis. A symposium. Pediatr. 52:586, 1973.

Stiehm, E.R. and Damrosch, D.S.: Factors in the prognosis of meningococcal infection. J. Pediatr. 68:457, 1966.

Swartz, M.N. and Dodge, P.R.: Bacterial meningitis: A review of selected aspects. NEJM 272:725-787, 842, 898-902, 954-960, 1003-1009, 1965.

Taber, L.H., Yow, M.D., and Nieberg, F.G.: The penetration of broad-spectrum antibiotics into the cerebrospinal fluid. Ann. N.Y. Acad. Sci. 145:473, 1967.

Whitecar, J.P., Reddin, J.L., and Spink, W.W.: Recurrent pneumococcal meningitis. A review of the literature and studies on a patient who recovered from eleven attacks caused by five serotypes of Diplococcus pneumoniae. NEJM 274:1285, 1966.

Widell, S.: On the cerebrospinal fluid in normal children and in patients with acute abacterial meningoencephalitis. Acta Paedtr. 47:(Suppl. 115), 1-102, 1958.

VIRAL MENINGOENCEPHALITIS

Balfour, H.H., Jr., Siem, R.A., Bauer, H., and Quie, P.G.: California arbovirus (LaCrosse) infections. 1. Clinical and laboratory findings in 66 children with meningoencephalitis. Pediatr. 52:680, 1973.

Bell, W.E. and McCormick, W.F.: Neurologic Infections in Children. W.B. Saunders Co., Philadelphia, 1975.

Center for Disease Control: Neurotropic viral disease surveillance annual summary - aseptic meningitis (May 1976) encephalitis (August 1976), U.S. Public Health Service.

Feigin, R.D. and Shackelford, P.G.: Value of repeat lumbar puncture in the differential diagnosis of meningitis. NEJM 289:571, 1973.

Grose, C., Henle, W., Henle, G., and Feorino, P.M.: Primary Epstein-Barr-virus infections in acute neurologic diseases. NEJM 292:392, 1975.

Herzon, H., Shelton, J.T., and Bruyn, H.B.: Sequelae of Western Equine and other arthropod-borne encephalitis. Neurol. 7:535, 1957.

Johnson, R.T. and Mims, C.A.: Pathogenesis of viral infection of the nervous system. NEJM 278:23-30, 84-91, 1968.

Lepow, M.L., Carnver, D.H., Wright, H.T., Woods, W.A., and Robbins, F.C.: A clinical, epidemiologic and laboratory investigation of aseptic meningitis during the four-year period, 1955. NEJM 266:1181, 1962.

Liu, C. and Llanes-Rodas, R.: Application of immunofluorescent technique to the study of pathogenesis and rapid diagnosis of viral infections. Am. J. Clin. Pathol. 57:829, 1972.

McGowan, J.E., Jr., Bryan, J.A., and Gregg, M.B.: Surveillance of arboviral encephalitis in the United States, 1955-1971. Am. J. Epiderm. 97:199, 1973.

Myer, H.M., Johnson, R.T., Crawford, I.P., Dascomb, H.E., and Rogers, N.G.: Central nervous system syndrome of "viral" etiology. Am. J. Med. 29:334, 1960.

Nogen, A.G. and Lepow, M.L.: Enteroviral meningitis in very young infants. Pediatr. 40:617, 1967.

Olson, L.C., Buescher, E.L., Artenstein, M.S., and Parkman, P.D.: Herpesvirus infections of the human central nervous system. NEJM 277:1271, 1967.

Wenner, H.A. and Behbehani, A.M.: The ECHO viruses. Monogr. Virol. 1:1-72, 1968.

BRAIN ABSCESS

Brewer, N.S., MacCarty, C.S., Wellman, W.E.: Brain abscess: A review of recent experience. Ann. Intern. Med. 82:571, 1975.

Hoffman, H.J., Hendrick, E.B., and Hiscox, J.L.: Cerebral abscesses in early infancy. J. Neurosurg. 33:172, 1970.

Matson, D.D. and Salam, M.: Brain abscess in congenital heart disease. Pediatr. 27:772, 1961.

Wright, R.L. and Ballantine, H.T.: Management of brain abscesses in children and adolescents. Am. J. Dis. Child. 114:113, 1967.

TUBERCULOUS MENINGITIS

D'Souza, B.J., Lansky, L.L., and Cho, C.T.: Tuberculous meningitis developing after six months of treatment of pulmonary tuberculosis: A complication of infection with a drug-resistant strain. Pediatrics 14:729, 1975.

Steiner, P. and Protugaleza, C.: Tuberculous meningitis in children. A review of 25 cases observed between the years 1965 and 1970 at the Kings County Medical Center of Brooklyn, with special reference to the problem of infection with primary drug-resistant strains of M. tuberculosis. Am. Rev. Resp. Dis. 107:22, 1973.

Sumaya, C.V., Simek, M., Smith, M.H.D., Seidemann, M.F., Ferriss, G.S., and Rubin, W.: Tuberculous meningitis in children during the isoniazid era. J. Pediatr. 87:43, 1975.

SLOW VIRUS DISEASES

Hotchin, J., ed.: Slow virus diseases. Prog. in Med. Virol. 18: 1-350, 1974.

Modlin, J.F., Jabbour, J.T., Witte, J.J., and Halsey, N.A.: Epidemiologic studies of measles, measles vaccine, and subacute sclerosing panencephalitis. Pediatrics 59:505, 1977.

Proceeding of the Conference of Cellular Immunity and SSPE. Arch. Neurol. 32:488, 1975.

Zeman, W. and Lennette, E., eds.: Slow virus diseases. Williams and Wilkins, Baltimore, 1974.

MISCELLANEOUS

Carter, S. and Gold, A.P.: Acute infantile hemiplegia. Pediatr. Clin. N.A. 14:851, 1967.

Cherington, M. and Snyder, R.D.: Tick paralysis. Neurophysiologic studies. NEJM 278:95, 1968.

Gelfand, H.M.: Oral vaccine: Associated paralytic poliomyelitis, 1962. JAMA 184:948, 1963.

Klastersky, J., Cappel, R., Sroeck, J.M., Flament, J., and Thiry, L.: Ascending myelitis in association with Herpes-simplex virus. NEJM 287:182, 1972.

Lerer, R.J. and Kalavsky, S.M.: Central nervous system disease associated with Mycoplasma pneumoniae infection: Report of five cases and review of the literature. Pediatrics 52:658, 1973.

Magoffin, R.L., Lennette, E.H., and Schmidt, N.J.: Association of coxsackie viruses with illness resembling mild paralytic poliomyelitis. Pediatrics 28:602, 1961.

Manning, J.J. and Adour, K.K.: Facial paralysis in children. Pediatrics 49:102, 1972.

Markland, L.D. and Riley, H.D., Jr.: The Guillain-Barre syndrome in childhood. A comprehensive review, including observations on 19 additional cases. Clin. Pediatr. 6:162, 1967.

Thomas, F.B., Perkins, R.L., and Saslaw, S.: Paralytic mumps infection in two sisters. Arch. Intern. Med. 121:45, 1968.

CHAPTER 7. CONGENITAL INFECTIONS

INTRODUCTION: The important known causes of chronic congenital infections in the United States include rubella virus, Toxoplasma gondii, cytomegalovirus, herpes simplex virus, and Treponema pallidum. These infections often manifest similar clinical features and are difficult to diagnose on clinical grounds alone. Laboratory confirmation, either by isolation or demonstration of the agent and/ or detection of specific antibodies (presence of IgM or persistence of IgG), is required in establishing a diagnosis. Because they share a common diagnostic problem, Nahmias (1974) termed these agents as "the TORCH complex," T for toxoplasma, R for rubella, C for cytomegalovirus, H for herpes simplex, and O for "others."

The approximate frequency of some of these infections are listed in Table 7-1. Cytomegalovirus is the most common and does not seem

TABLE 7-1: APPROXIMATE FREQUENCY OF VIRUS INFECTIONS IN THE MOTHER DURING PREGNANCY AND IN THE NEWBORN INFANT

INFECTION	APPROXIMATE FREQUENCY	
	Mother No./1000 preg.	Neonate No./1000 live birth
Cytomegalovirus	30-50	6-15
Rubella	1-22	0.7-7
Herpesvirus hominis	0.5-25	Uncommon*
Coxsackie B	90	Uncommon*
Mumps	1.0	Rare*
Varicella-zoster	0.5	Rare*
Rubeola	0.06	Rare*

* Insufficient data to permit numerical estimates. (J. Pediatr. 77:315, 1970.)

to vary in frequency from year to year. In contrast, rubella tended to occur in epidemics. Prior to the extensive use of rubella vaccine in 1969, epidemics occurred every 6 to 9 years and a large number of infants with congenital rubella infection accompanied each epidemic. The peak of rubella occurs during the spring and is lowest in the fall.

The pathogenesis of most of these congenital infections is poorly defined. Possible routes of infection and fetal outcomes are shown in Table 7-2. Clearly this group of agents causes an undefinable

TABLE 7-2: PATHOGENESIS OF CONGENITAL INFECTIONS AND FETAL OUTCOME	
ROUTE OF MATERNAL INFECTION	FETAL OUTCOME
1. Placental (via blood)	1. Normal fetus
2. Amniotic (via vagina)	2. Infected fetus ($\pm$ disease)
3. Ova (?)	3. Fetal death (abortion, still birth)
	4. Malformation ($\pm$ death)

number of abortions, stillbirths, neonatal deaths, and permanent
cellular damage. Rubella, cytomegalovirus, herpesviruses, and
toxoplasma are all known to produce congenital anomalies. The
types of anomalies produced by some of these agents are listed in
Table 7-3.

TABLE 7-3: VIRAL INFECTIONS WHICH PRODUCE CONGENITAL MALFORMATIONS IN MAN	
VIRUS	MALFORMATIONS
Rubella	Congenital heart disease, cataracts, microphthalmia, deafness, microcephaly, psychomotor retardation.
Cytomegalovirus	Microcephaly, chorioretinitis, deafness, psychomotor retardation.
Herpesvirus	Vesicular lesions, microcephaly, intracranial calcification, psychomotor retardation.

Recent information indicates that some of the low grade, chronic,
and latent infections of pregnancy have the potential to inflict continued injury to the offspring. The extent to which asymptomatic
congenital infections contribute to neurologic dysfunction in later
life needs to be defined. The possibility that congenital infections
initiate malignancy and immunological dysfunction also requires further study.

As indicated above, the TORCH agents often produce indistinguishable clinical features in infants. The most common clinical signs
include a low birth weight, hepatosplenomegaly, and jaundice (Table
7-4). Certain congenital anomalies are more often associated with

TABLE 7-4: MANIFESTATIONS OF SYMPTOMATIC CONGENITAL RUBELLA, CYTOMEGALIC INCLUSION DISEASE AND TOXOPLASMOSIS			
MANIFESTATION	RUBELLA	CID	TOXO
Low birth wt. (<2500)	+++	+++	++
Hepatomegaly	+++	+++	++
Splenomegaly	+++	+++	++
Jaundice	+	+++	++
Pneumonia	+	++	+
Microphthalmia	+	±	±
Corneal opacity	+	±	±
Glaucoma	+	±	±
Cong. heart disease	++++	+	±
Cataracts	++	±	+
Bone lesions	++	±	±
Microcephaly	±	++	+
Anemia	+	+++	+++
Petechiae	+++	+++	+
Retinopathy	+	+	++++
Cerebral Calcif.	±	+	++
Hydrocephaly	±	±	+

Frequency: (± = Rare or less than 1%, + = 1-25%, ++ = 26-50%, +++ = 51-75%, ++++ = 76-100%).

Modified from J. Pediatr. 77:315, 1970.

specific infections; for example, congenital heart disease, cataracts, and bone lesions accompany rubella; microcephaly, anemia and petechiae are seen in CMV infections; and retinopathy, cerebral calcification and hydrocephaly are associated with toxoplasmosis.

The precise contribution of infectious agents to congenital infections and their long-term effects on human development are far from clear. This chapter will deal primarily with the clinical aspects of congenital infections caused by cytomegalovirus, herpes simplex virus, and toxoplasma. Rubella infection is discussed in Chapter 3 and syphillis is discussed in Chapter 12. Other viral agents affecting the fetus or newborn and their effects are presented in Table 8-2 (Chapter 8).

7.1: CYTOMEGALOVIRUS INFECTION

INTRODUCTION: The disease caused by cytomegalovirus (CMV) has been described under a variety of names, e.g. protozoan cell disease, toxoplasma syndrome not due to T. gondii, salivary gland virus disease, inclusion body disease, cytomegalovirus inclusion disease, etc. Prior to 1950, the disease was not recognized clinically during life. M.G. Smith in 1956 isolated the virus in tissue culture and thus provided the means for making a specific diagnosis. At the present time, host-parasite relationship of this disease is still not well defined.

CMV infections are worldwide in distribution. Few humans escape infection during life. Most persons acquire the disease in an inapparent form. Although CMV is widely distributed in the population, there is marked variation in the incidence of infection in different socio-economic groups. In the United States there is evidence that infection is acquired at an earlier age by children of low economic status than by those better off, and by blacks earlier than whites. About 50-70% of women, upon entering the child bearing years, have previously experienced CMV infection. The remaining 30 to 50% of women have no antibodies and are presumably susceptible to infection. Inapparent infection, primary or secondary, during pregnancy is not uncommon. About 4% of all pregnant women excrete CMV in the urine and 10-15% excrete the virus in the cervix.

Intrauterine CMV infection is the most common congenital infection, occurring in approximately 0.5 to 1% of all live birth as evidenced by the presence of viruria during the first few days of life. CMV causes a wide range of clinical syndromes ranging from asymptomatic infection to severe, even fatal, disease. Most (95%) congenital CMV infections are asymptomatic; the classical syndrome of congenital cytomegalic inclusion disease (CID) is, in fact, very rare. Approximately 5 to 15% of infected infants, including some of those who were symptom-free, are subsequently found to be mentally retarded, or to have some learning disabilities. The long-term outlook for asymptomatic infants and the social impact of this infection needs further evaluation.

1. ETIOLOGY AND PATHOGENESIS

Cytomegalovirus belongs to the herpesvirus family, primarily because of its morphological and physiochemical characteristics. Many laboratory animals have their own specific CMV and are not susceptible to infection with CMV of humans. Human CMV is species specific and man is the only known reservoir of the virus. Cultured human fibroblasts are necessary for isolation and propagation of the virus. Viral multiplication in cell cultures is noted by development of characteristic focal cytopathic effect and large intranuclear inclusions.

The virus has been isolated from urine, throat swab, saliva, milk, cervical secretions, semen, feces, and peripheral leukocytes. The possible sources of infection are listed in Table 7-5. The mode of

TABLE 7-5: SOURCE OF PRIMARY CMV INFECTION	
PRENATAL:	a. Transplacental b. Intrauterine transfusion
PERINATAL:	a. Cervical secretions
POSTNATAL:	a. Contact infected urine, saliva, milk, feces (?), tears b. Iatrogenic: transfusion; organ transplantation

transmission is unknown in most instances. Congenital CMV infection appears to be transmitted transplacentally from a latently infected mother to her fetus. Primary maternal infection, mostly asymptomatic, often results in fetal infection. However, transmission may terminate at the placenta (not affecting the fetus) in a certain number of cases. The congenitally infected infant is often, though not invariably, the first born of a young woman. Therefore, one hypothesis suggests that congenital transmission reflects viremia associated with a primary maternal infection. It is now known that previous CMV infection in the mother may not afford full protection during future pregnancies. Consecutive infection of fetuses in subsequent pregnancies has been seen 3 months to 3 years following delivery of the first infected newborn.

Perinatal transmission may occur as a result of exposure to infected cervical secretions at the time of delivery or by ingestion of the virus containing breast milk. Infection through exposure to contaminated cervical secretions is probably common, particularly among population in low socio-economic conditions. Infants who acquire infection at birth usually do not have viruria during the first few days of life, but begin to excrete virus at 1 to 3 months of age or at some longer interval. Nosocomial infection acquired via contact with actively infected infants or nursery personnel remains an unproven possibility.

Beyond the newborn period, acquired infections have occurred in recipients of large quantities of fresh (but not stored) citrated blood, especially after open heart surgery, suggesting transmission by blood transfusion. Although the incubation period is from 3 to 5 weeks following blood transfusion, in most instances the incubation period is unknown. Based on serologic responses in recipients, it has been estimated that 5-12% of blood donors were carriers (Henle et al., 1970), and the risk of CMV infection was correlated with the number of units of blood transfused (Prince et al., 1971). Direct evidence that blood is the source of CMV was reported by Diosi et al. (1969), who isolated CMV from peripheral leukocytes of 2 of 35 asymptomatic nonviruric donors. Although blood has been strongly implicated as a vehicle of CMV transmission, it is suspected that CMV infection in the transfused patients might also result from reactivation of latent endogenous infection or from exogenous nosocomial sources unrelated to blood products. The events involved in latency, reactivation, and reinfection of CMV are poorly understood. Some of the factors associated with activation of latent infection are shown in Fig. 7.1.

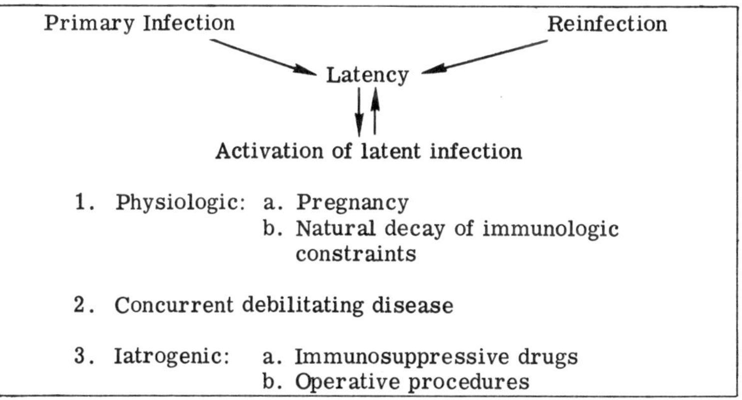

FIG. 7.1: Natural history of human CMV infection.

A high mortality rate is associated with CMV infection in patients with bone marrow transplants (Nieman et al., 1973). The deaths seem to be caused by interstitial pneumonitis that appears as a late complication, often in recipients who have survived crises with bacterial and fungal infections.

The pathological lesion of CMV infection consists of necrosis and characteristic alterations of the cells. The infected cells are enlarged (cytomegalic) and contain large eosinophilic intranuclear inclusions. The cytoplasm may be swollen and vacuolated, and may have basophilic inclusions which contain DNA and polysaccharide.

Severe CNS sequelae of congenital infections during easly gestation probably result from inflammation, necrosis or from destruction of dividing or migrating neural cells. Infection during late gestation might not cause obvious pathological lesions but might interfere with the development of dendritic ramifications and synaptic connections resulting in minor deficits in higher cortical function.

2. CLINICAL MANIFESTATIONS

The clinical manifestations of CMV infections vary with the age of the infant at the time of infection.

2.1: <u>Congenital Infection:</u> The spectrum of congenital infection varies from asymptomatic infection reflected only by viruria to severe disease incompatible with life. The majority of infected infants are asymptomatic; only 5% are symptomatic at birth. The disease may range from involvement of an isolated organ to multiple organ dysfunction, such as the classic cytomegalic inclusion disease. The later disease is manifested by a small, microcephalic, jaundiced neonate with hepatosplenomegaly, purpuric lesions, and CNS involvement (Fig. 7.2). Evidence of pneumonitis, myocarditis,

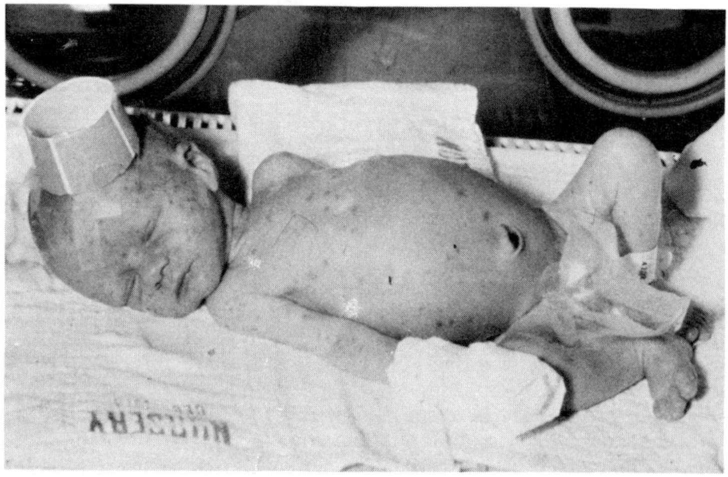

FIG. 7.2: Severe congenital cytomegalovirus infection in a malnourished 2-day-old baby with petechiae, jaundice, hepatosplenomegaly, low birth weight, and microcephaly.

a disseminated intravascular coagulaopathy may also be present.
Some patients fail to thrive, or have repeated respiratory infections.
The teratogenic potential of CMV has been well recognized (Hanshaw, 1969); defects in virtually every organ system have been
noted, particularly inguinal hernia, clubfoot, strabismus, microcephaly, deafness, and congenital heart disease.

There is considerable overlap of clinical manifestations between
congenital CMV infection and the chronic intrauterine infections
caused by other agents, therefore laboratory confirmation is necessary in all cases.

Most infants with symptomatic disease have some degree of encephalitis as evidenced by the frequent development of microcephaly
and/or other neurologic dysfunction in the early months of life.
Mental retardation, spastic diplegia, seizures, optic atrophy, blindness, and sensorineural deafness are often seen. Such defects may
also develop later in life in children who show no evidence of CNS
involvement at birth. Lesser degrees of handicaps such as defects
in perceptual skills, learning disability, minor incoordination, and
emotional lability have also been recognized and may indeed become
more apparent as more children are followed into the competitive
arena of the classroom.

Follow-up of infants with clinically inapparent CMV infection have
shown a significant number with sensorineural hearing loss. CMV
may cause endolymphatic labyrinthitis resulting in high frequency
hearing deficits.

2.2: Acquired Infection: Perinatal infections acquired via contact
with cervical secretions or by other routes are generally not associated with acute morbidity. In contrast to the frequent CNS involvement in congenitally infected infants, such involvement occurs
less frequently in children and adults with acquired infections.

CMV mononucleosis: Klemola et al. (1965) described a group of
patients with illnesses compatible with infectious mononucleosis but
lacking tonsillopharyngeal involvement who had heterophile-
antibodies. This syndrome was also seen later in patients undergoing open-heart surgery perfused with fresh blood, an entity previously termed "post-perfusion syndrome."

Target organs: 1) Minor degrees of liver involvement are now accepted as characteristic of acquired CMV infection. Hepatitis,
icteric or anicteric, is a common manifestation. 2) Hemolytic anemia may be a feature of both the congenital and the acquired form.
3) Interstitial pneumonitis is commonly found at autopsy in children
or adults who succumb to concomitant debilitating disease or after
immunosuppressive therapy. 4) Myocarditis and pericarditis are
not infrequent in acquired CMV mononucleosis. 5) In CMV mononucleosis vertigo and otoneurologic symptoms may be prominent.

In the Guillain-Barre syndrome, peripheral neuropathy, and poly-
neuropathy have been associated with CMV infection. 6) Although
CMV is most frequently isolated from the urine, lesions in the kidney have not as yet been associated with symptoms or progressive
pathological changes.

3. DIAGNOSIS

Diagnosis of CMV infection is best confirmed by isolation of the virus in cell culture of human fibroblasts. Urine is the best source
for virus isolation, although virus is recoverable from throat swab,
saliva, rectal swabs, and white blood cells. Transport of specimens is best accomplished by packing in wet ice.

Isolation of CMV during the first few days of life indicates congenital
infection. Acquisition of virus at birth or soon afterward may result in shedding as early as 3 weeks and usually by 8 weeks. Therefore, the isolation of CMV is less specific for intrauterine infection
with advancing age of the patient.

Cytologic examination of the urine sediment has the advantage of
relative simplicity and availability, but its value is considerably
decreased because of the high rate of false negatives even among
neonates with severe disease. The presence of large, intranuclear
inclusion bearing cells is presumptive evidence of infection especially in the neonatal period. Similar types of inclusions may also
be seen in adenovirus infection. Thus, confirmation by virus isolation or serial antibody tests is still required.

Elevation of levels of IgM in cord blood or baby's blood is suggestive of congenital infection. Serologic confirmation of overt neonatal infection can usually be obtained by demonstrating the presence
of CMV specific IgM antibodies in cord blood or baby's blood. Neonates with inapparent infection may not have such antibodies. At
present, technical difficulties severely limit the general availability
of this test. Serial examinations of the patient's serum for persistence of IgG antibodies by other serologic tests (e.g. CF) may be
useful. In the absence of intrauterine or perinatal infection, maternally derived antibodies will disappear from the infant's serum
by 6 months of age. Persistence of antibody beyond 6 months of
age, in most cases, suggest intrauterine or perinatal infection.

4. MANAGEMENT

No specific methods of prevention or treatment of congenital CMV
infection are available at the present time. The disease is probably
transmitted by intimate contact. Handwashing and gown technique
are recommended when working with patients who are actively ex-
creting the virus. The duration of communicability is likely quite
prolonged since viral excretion has persisted following congenital
infection for as long as eight years.

Although initial steps toward development of a live virus vaccine
have been taken, considerably more information concerning this
disease must be acquired before a vaccine can ever be utilized.
The use of gamma globulin or interferon holds little promise.

The possible use of drugs, such as cytosine arabinoside (ara-C),
5-iodo-2-deoxy-uridine (IDUR) and adenine arabinoside (ara-A),
for the treatment of infants with severe infection are being evaluated. Incomplete information at this time suggests that viruria diminishes temporarily in treated infants, but striking clinical improvement are not observed. Until the safety and efficacy of these
drugs are established, their indiscriminate use in children with
congenitally or naturally acquired infection is not indicated.

::

7.2: HERPES SIMPLEX VIRUS

GENERAL CHARACTERISTICS: Herpes simplex virus (HSV, Herpesvirus hominis) chiefly produces subclinical infection, but it may
cause a variety of clinical responses involving localized tissues
(e.g. mucous membranes, skin, eye and central nervous system)
and/or generalized systemic infection (Table 7-6). Localized infections occur primarily in normal host, in contrast, disseminated
infections usually occur in newborn infants and in patients with compromised host responses.

TABLE 7-6: CLINICAL FEATURES OF HSV INFECTION	
SITE OF PRIMARY INFECTION	LESIONS
1. Mouth	Gingivostomatitis
2. Genital	Genital herpes
3. Eye	Keratoconjunctivitis
4. Skin	Traumatic herpes Eczema herpeticum
5. Central Nervous System	Encephalitis Meningitis Myelitis
6. Viscera	Disseminated disease

Symptomatic disease caused by HSV may appear in two forms: primary or recurrent infection. Following the primary infection, HSV
often becomes latent and the disease tends to be reactivated at irregular intervals by various provocations such as fever, trauma,

emotional upsets, gastrointestinal disorders, etc. Other characteristic features of HSV infection include: (1) production of vesicular
lesions, (2) production of intranuclear inclusions, (3) easy isolation
of virus in cell cultures, and (4) circulating antibodies do not prevent recurrence of the disease.

EPIDEMIOLOGY: HSV infection is one of the most common viral
diseases seen in children and adults. The majority of primary infections occur between one and five years of age. The prevalence
of HSV antibodies varies with different populations; among the lower
socio-economic group, HSV infections are prevalent and tend to occur at an earlier age. In the United States, the sera of most adults
(over 80%) contain antibodies.

As in cytomegalovirus infections, herpes infection in women is more
common during pregnancy and the risk of infection increases as gestation progresses. The incidence of HSV infection in mothers during pregnancy is variable, ranging from 0.02% to 1% (Ng. et al.,
1970; Nahmias et al., 1971). Hanshaw (1973) estimated that with an
annual birth rate of about 3.2 million per year in the U.S., there
would be 160 cases of neonatal herpes annually if infection occurred
at the rate of 1/20,000 deliveries.

1. ETIOLOGY AND PATHOGENESIS

1.1: The Agent: Recent studies indicate that HSV has two types
(1 and 2) with minor biologic, immunologic, biochemical and epidemiological differences between them. In general, type 1 virus (oral
type) infects the mouth, eyes, skin, and central nervous system,
whereas type 2 virus (genital type) causes genital as well as neonatal infections. However, type 1 infection can also involve the areas
mentioned for type 2 and vice versa. After neonatal period, primary infection in infancy and early childhood is usually due to type
1 virus. In contrast, type 2 infections are generally acquired at
puberty or later in life. Antibodies to types 1 and 2 can be differentiated by various methods, but there is a great deal of cross reaction between the two types. There also appears to be cross immunity between type 1 and type 2 infection, but the protection is
incomplete.

Recent epidemiological surveys also suggest that there may be a relationship between cervical cancer and type 2 HSV.

1.2: Mode of Transmission: During acute infections, either primary
or recurrent, the virus may be transmitted to susceptible individuals, presumably by direct contact. The virus can be isolated from
the herpetic lesions intermittently for several weeks. The route of
infection is presumably through oral mucosa, traumatized skin or
mucous membrane, and possibly through sexual contact. It is also
known that carriers (latent infection) may excrete virus without the
presence of an active lesion.

1.3: Pathogenesis and Latency: After the initial infection, occurring through a break in the mucous membranes (mouth, throat, eye, genital) or skin, the virus multiplies locally and produces local lesions. From this site the infection spreads to the regional lymph nodes where the virus multiplies further. The acute phase generally lasts 5 to 10 days and is self-limited. In rare cases, such as in the newborn or in the immunologically compromised host, the virus may spread into the blood and to distant organs resulting in disseminated infection.

Following the primary infection, antibodies develop and persist for a prolonged period. Antibodies alone do not seem to limit the spread of infection. Cell-mediated immunity seems to be more important in limiting the spread of the disease. Recent observations suggest that antibodies may interact with other host immune factor in controlling the infection.

When the primary infection subsides, HSV is not eradicated from the host, the infection becomes latent and the virus presumably remains in the ganglia for years or even for life, with recrudescence of activity at irregular intervals. Recurrent herpes tends to occur at the same site of the primary infection (skin, eye or oral mucosa, etc.). The lesions are usually small and are localized. Recurrent infection usually does not have associated systemic symptoms and has a shorter period of virus excretion from the lesions.

Circulating antibodies and hypersensitivity reaction are generally present during latency or reactivation stages. Antibodies do not affect the intracellular virus and do not limit cell-to-cell spread of the virus or prevent reactivation of the disease.

2. CLINICAL MANIFESTATIONS

2.1: Neonatal Herpes: Neonatal herpes is usually acquired during passage through the infected birth canal and the majority (90%) of infants develop symptoms 3 to 7 days after birth. Infection may also be acquired via intrauterine or transplacental routes, since approximately 10% of infants show clinical disease at birth. HSV infection in neonates may be generalized or localized. The frequency of each type of infection and its outcome are shown in Table 7-7.

The presenting symptoms of neonatal herpes are variable and often cannot be differentiated from neonatal sepsis produced by other infecting agents (Chapter 8). The general symptoms include lethargy, poor feeding, vesicular rash, respiratory distress, vomiting, diarrhea, jaundice, fever or hypothermia, hepatosplenomegaly, seizures, keratoconjunctivitis, and bleeding. The two most characteristic features are the presence of vesicular skin lesions and keratitis. Skin lesions occur in approximately 50% of patients and are most useful in differentiating herpes from other congenital infections. The

TABLE 7-7: CLINICAL SPECTRUM AND OUTCOME OF 298 CASES OF NEONATAL HERPETIC INFECTION				
		OUTCOME (%)		
CLINICAL SPECTRUM	CASES (No.)	Died	Survived with Sequelae	Survived without Sequelae
1. Disseminated:				
With CNS involvement	33	92	1	7
Without CNS involvement	32	70	16	14
2. Localized:				
CNS	17	37	47	16
Skin	11	3	24	73
Eye	5	0	40	60
Oral Cavity	1	0	0	100
3. Asymptomatic:	1	0	0	100
Total Number and (%)	298	176 (60%)	54 (18%)	66 (22%)

Modified from Nahmias et al. 1975. (see Krugman & Gershon, 1975)

vesicular lesions often appear in clusters (Fig. 7.3), and may appear anywhere on the skin. In disseminated infection, systemic symptoms may develop within a few days after the appearance of the vesicles. The skin lesions resemble neonatal impetigo, and usually resolve spontaneously within days, but some infants have recurrent crops of skin lesions for weeks or months without other systemic symptoms.

Involvement of the central nervous system occurs in about 50% of infected newborn infants and is usually manifested by irritability and seizures. The CSF usually shows a moderate pleocytosis (50 to 200 WBC's/mm^3) and a marked elevation of protein.

Mortality rates of neonatal herpes depend upon the extent of involvement. CNS involvement or disseminated infection carry a poor prognosis. Localized infection (except CNS) generally has a better prognosis. The prognosis for survivors with CNS involvement is poor, and severe growth and psychomotor retardation occur in about 75% of patients. Blindness may occur as the result of corneal scarring, chorioretinitis, cataracts, or optic atrophy. Prognosis for infants with isolated skin lesions is generally good, although some infants

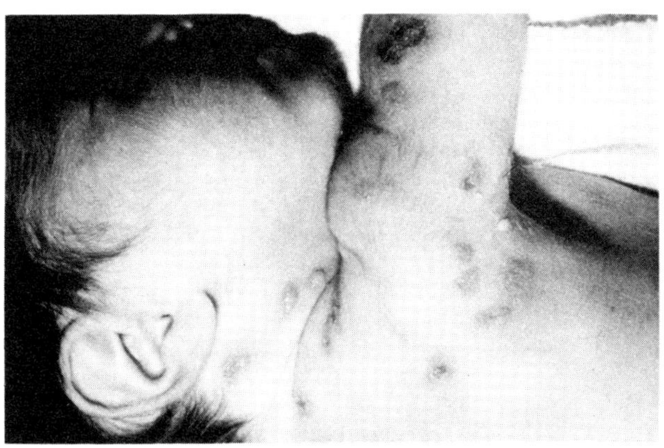

FIG. 7.3: A 4-day-old infant with vesicular lesions due to
herpes simplex virus (type 2) infection.

have developed severe psychomotor retardation and ocular sequelae
in late infancy or early childhood. Subclinical infection due to HSV
have been reported in a few infants, but the frequency of this occurrence is not known. Congenital malformations associated with HSV
infection have also been described in a limited number of cases; they
are manifested by microcephaly, intracranial calcification, microph-
thalmus, and retinal dysplasia.

2.2: HSV Infections Beyond the Newborn Period: The primary HSV
infection in older infants and children is subclinical in the majority
(90%) of patients and probably less than 10% may express clinical
involvement such as gingivostomatitis, mucocutaneous lesions,
traumatic herpes, eczema herpeticum, genital herpes, meningoencephalitis, or rarely, disseminated herpes.

Primary herpetic infection of the skin, mouth, or eye usually occurs
between one and five years of age and is often associated with constitutional symptoms such as fever, malaise, chills and regional
lymphadenopathy. The lesions consist of crops of thin walled vesicles on an erythematous base. They generally progress from macular to papular lesions, then vesicles, pustules, and crusts in 7 to
10 days (up to 2 weeks) without leaving a scar. The lesions may
regress at the papular or vesicular stage without forming pustules
or crusts. Traumatized skin can be readily infected by direct contamination from the infected sites (traumatic herpes); lesions may
appear 2-3 days after trauma. Secondary bacterial infection of these
lesions is not uncommon.

3. DIAGNOSIS

Diagnosis of neonatal herpes is not difficult if the infant develops
typical vesicular lesions during the first week of life. About 50%
of infants with disseminated infection have herpetic lesions of the
skin, mouth, or eyes (Nahmias et al., 1970). A history of maternal genital herpes is often helpful. Similarly, clinical diagnosis of
primary or recurrent herpes involving the skin, mucous membrane,
or eyes is relatively simple in older infants and children. However, when infection involves the central nervous system or other
internal organs in the absence of external lesions, diagnosis may be
quite difficult. The following tests are generally used to confirm
the clinical diagnosis of HSV infection:

1) Virus Isolation: Isolation of HSV in cell cultures is the most
   reliable method for diagnosis. Swabs from the infected lesions
   (i.e. skin, mouth or eyes) or tissues (i.e. brain biopsy) generally show characteristic cytopathic effects in most cell cultures
   within 1 to 3 days. Other specimens (such as urine, stool, and
   CSF) should be submitted for viral isolation in order to determine the extent of involvement. A cervical swab specimen from
   the mother may help to trace the source of infection.

2) Cytologic Examination: Smears from the infected lesions or
   tissue sections may be stained with hematoxylin-eosin, Giemsa
   or Papanicolaou (cervical smears). Demonstration of characteristic multinucleated giant cells containing intranuclear eosinophilic inclusions is suggestive of HSV infection. This finding
   should be supported by viral isolation.

3) HSV Antigen: Infected cells (smears or tissue sections) containing HSV antigens can be detected rapidly within one to two hours
   by the use of fluorescent antibody staining technique (Fig. 7.4).

4) Antibody Studies: As in other congenital infections, determination of herpes IgG in infant's serum is not easy to interpret because of the presence of maternally transferred antibodies. Persistent elevation of these antibodies for several months may
   suggest fetal or neonatal infection. Specific herpes IgM can be
   determined in a specialized laboratory. Documentation of a rise
   in herpes antibody (IgG) in primary infections in older infants
   and children is useful and this may be accomplished by various
   methods, such as neutralization, complement fixation, indirect
   fluorescent antibody, indirect hemagglutination inhibition, etc.

4. MANAGEMENT AND PROGNOSIS

4.1: Prevention: Active immunization against HSV infection is not
available and it is doubtful that it will become feasible in the near
future. Unlike other congenital infections (e.g. rubella and toxoplasmosis), therapeutic abortion is not indicated in HSV infections.

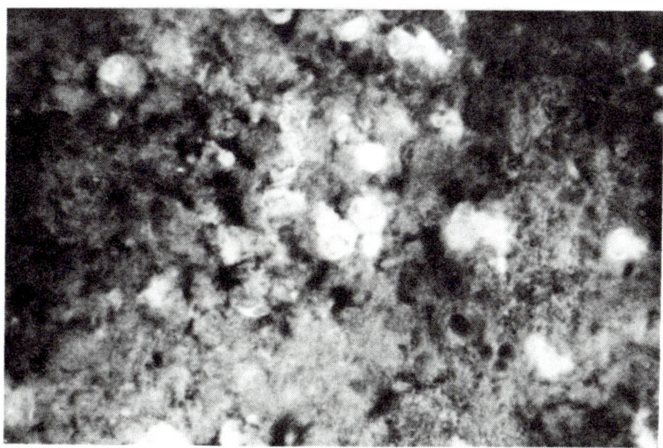

FIG. 7.4: Herpes simplex virus (HSV) encephalitis in
a 10-day-old infant. Neurons containing
antigens, as shown by immunofluorescent
staining, are present in brain biopsy
specimens.

Although congenital HSV infection may occur in early pregnancy,
the majority of neonatal herpes is acquired at the time of delivery
through the contaminated birth canal.

Prevention in neonatal herpes is difficult because inapparent or
minor recurrent infections in the mother are common. Currently
recommended methods for prevention of neonatal herpes include
delivery of mother by cesarean section and avoidance of contact of
infants with personnel who have active herpetic lesions.

A) Cesarean Section: It is believed that the major source of neonatal HSV infection is exposure to the virus during passage through
the infected birth canal. It is, therefore, suggested that delivery by
cesarean section be performed if cervical herpes is diagnosed close
to the time of delivery (Nahmias et al., 1967). The data, though
not extensive, to support such a recommendation is shown in Table
7-8. The findings suggest that the risk of neonatal infection is increased if the baby is delivered vaginally or if there is a rupture of
membranes for more than four hours prior to delivery.

If the mother has a history of recurrent cervical herpes or if the
father has herpectic penile lesions, cervical cultures should be performed in the last month of gestation. It should be pointed out that
HSV infection also occurs not infrequently in neonates born to mothers
who deny genital lesions.

TABLE 7-8: RISK OF NEONATAL HERPETIC INFECTION FROM MOTHER WITH GENITAL HERPES AT DELIVERY	
TYPE OF DELIVERY	NO. OF INFANTS INFECTED/ NO. OF CASES (%)
Vaginal	14/26 (54%)
Cesarean Section:	
After membrane rupture more than 4 hours	18/19 (94%)
Before or within 4 hours of membrane rupture	2/28 (7%)
Nahmias et al. (1975) (see Krugman & Gershon, 1975)	

B)   Isolation: Newborns should be protected from exposure to nursery personnel or family members with observable active infection, either primary or recurrent. Such precautions should also be applied to patients with open skin lesions (i.e. eczema, burns) and patients with compromised cellular immunity.

C)   Immune Globulin: Commercial preparations of immune serum globulin generally contain high titers of antibodies against HSV. However, the efficacy of immune globulin administration in prevention or treatment of neonatal herpes has not been established in humans. Animal studies have shown that early administration of antisera (or human immune globulins) retards and, in some cases, arrests the progress of herpetic infection; late administration (48 to 72 hours after infection) usually results in no protection (Cho et al., 1976). Nahmias et al. (1970) recommended that large doses of immune serum globulin be given to the infant at birth because it might prevent dissemination of the virus. At the present time, data to support such a recommendation are not yet available. It is likely that high titers of antibodies in the circulation will modulate the infection in the early course of the disease, but once dissemination has occurred the effect of antibodies is limited.

4.2: Treatment: Specific antiviral agent for neonatal herpes is not available at this time. Iododeoxyuridine (IDUR), cytosine arabinoside (ara-C) and adenine arabinoside (ara-A) have been tested. The drug concentrations of IDUR or ara-C that are required to inhibit the virus are too toxic and immunosuppressive to be used systemically. Ara-A appears to be less toxic and may be a more promising agent. A controlled interhospital study on the effect of ara-A in severe HSV infection is still underway (Alford C. et al., University of Alabama).

Topical therapy of herpes keratoconjunctivitis with IDUR or ara-A
has been shown to be effective; preparations for topical therapy are
available.

The efficacy of other therapeutic approaches to HSV infection including interferon, humoral antibodies, transfer factor, hyperthermia, BCG, and photoinactivation, has not been established clinically
and needs further evaluation.

4.3: Prognosis: The majority of primary HSV infection beyond the
newborn period is self-limited and the prognosis is generally good.
Fatality may occur in newborns and in patients with meningoencephalitis, severe eczema herpeticum, or severe malnutrition. Neurologic sequelae are common among those recovering from meningoencephalitis. Recurrent attack of gingivostomatitis may be frequent
and cause temporary pain and inconvenience. Recurrent keratitis
may result in scarring of the cornea and blindness.

:::

7.3: TOXOPLASMOSIS

INTRODUCTION: Congenital toxoplasmosis, caused by Toxoplasma
gondii, is the result of primary infection occurring in a pregnant
woman. The incidence of congenital infection varies with geographi-
cal location, cooking habits and hygiene. In Paris, the risk of maternal infections is 6.3 per 100 pregnancies per year (Desmonts et
al., 1974), whereas in the U.S. the risk is 0.15 to 0.6 per 100 pregnancies per year (Kimball, 1971). The high incidence in Paris is
related to high risk of exposure in the endemic area to their habit of
eating raw or undercooked meat.

Toxoplasmosis in the pregnant mother is usually asymptomatic. Involvement of the fetus may lead to abortion, prematurity, stillbirth,
asymptomatic or symptomatic infection in the newly born infant.
Asymptomatic infection is the most common form; some of these infants may develop symptoms months or even years later with clinical presentation of central nervous system involvement or chorioretinitis. Symptomatic infection occurs in approximately 10 to 20%
of infants born with congenital toxoplasmosis, and a wide spectrum
of clinical syndromes may accompany this disease. The classic
triad of chorioretinitis, hydrocephalus, and intracranial calcification
occurs only in small numbers of the most severely affected infants.
Chorioretinitis is common but easily overlooked in newborn infants.

Natural infection with toxoplasma is worldwide and involves many
vertebrate species. Recent studies indicate that only cats excrete
oocysts and serve as the complete host (Frenkel, 1973; Jacobs, 1974).
In the cat, ingestion of the organism (trophozoites, tissue cysts or
oocysts) results in intestinal replication with development of oocysts

(mature sexual forms). The oocysts are excreted in feces, and may retain infectivity in the soil for a prolonged period. If these oocysts are ingested by other animals (intermediate host), trophozoites are formed and multiply intracellularly during acute infection and can cross the placenta resulting in congenital infection. Trophozoites also can disseminate to many other tissues. Subsequently trophozoites form tissue cysts which persist during chronic infection and are important in transmission of the disease by carnivorism.

1. ETIOLOGY AND PATHOGENESIS

Toxoplasma gondii is an ubiquitous obligate intracellular protozoan. Three forms exist in nature: trophozoites, tissue cysts and oocysts. Man is infected by: 1) the tissue cysts from the meat of infected animals, 2) the oocyst that is present in soil contaminated by cat feces, or 3) with trophozoites by the transplacental route.

Congenital toxoplasmosis is the result of an acute infection in a pregnant woman. The risk of fetal involvement by toxoplasma organisms depends upon the time of maternal infection in relation to the gestational age. Primary infections acquired prior to conception do not result in fetal involvement. Approximately 40% of maternal infections spread to the fetus (Table 7-9). The majority of fetal

TABLE 7-9: OUTCOME OF 180 PREGNANCIES WITH ACQUIRED MATERNAL TOXOPLASMOSIS	
Uninfected infant	61%
Neonatal death	3%
Congenital toxoplasmosis:	36%
severe	(3.9)%
mild	(6.1)%
subclinical	(26.0)%
	36.0%
Total	100%

Modified from Desmonts, G. and Couvreur, J. (1975) (see Krugman & Gershon, 1975).

infection (66%) occurs during the third trimester; maternal infection during the first and second trimester results in fetal infection in 17% and 27% of cases respectively. Infection acquired during the first and second trimesters is associated with a more severe disease, whereas infection acquired during the third trimester often results in asymptomatic toxoplasmosis.

Toxoplasma gondii multiplies at the site of entry and enters the blood stream. Parasitemia is a part of primary infection; the organism is disseminated to organs and tissues such as placenta, lung, heart,

brain, bone marrow, lymph node, liver, spleen, eye and muscles.
Variable degrees of inflammatory reactions may be seen in different tissues. In pregnant women the placenta is an intermediate stop
and necrotic lesions are formed there. From the placenta, toxoplasma organisms enter the fetal circulation resulting in infection of
the fetus. The pathologic lesions are more severe in the fetus and
newborns than those seen in the adult, and infection remains active
longer. Brain involvement in the congenitally infected fetus and
newborn is manifested by severe meningoencephalitis with necrosis,
calcification and cyst formation. Single or multiple foci of inflammatory lesions may occur in the retina of the eyes. Cellular infiltrates and focal necrosis may involve heart, lung, liver, spleen,
muscles and other tissues. The pathologic lesions may result from:
1) destruction of parasitized cells, 2) tissue necrosis following rupture of cysts, 3) infarction necrosis due to vascular involvement,
and 4) periaqueductal and periventricular necrosis (Frenkel, 1974).

Infection of <u>Toxoplasma gondii</u> is followed by development of antibodies and delayed hypersensitivity reaction. Antibodies can be detected by various methods. The dye test (Sabin and Feldman) is the
most commonly used method for measuring the neutralizing antibody.
This test is based on the principle that the presence of antibodies in
serum diminish toxoplasma's staining affinity for methylene blue.

Presence of antibodies in maternal serum is associated with immunity to fetal infection. Occurrence of infection in successive pregnancies has been reported but it is an exceptional event (Garcia,
1968).

2. CLINICAL MANIFESTATIONS

The majority of infants with congenital toxoplasmosis are asymptomatic. It has been estimated that perhaps only 10% of the infected
infants show signs of clinical disease by routine examination, however, this figure may increase to 30% if careful eye examinations
are performed (Desmonts et al., 1974; Alford et al., 1974). Symptomatic newborns have chorioretinitis, hepatosplenomegaly, lymphadenopathy, jaundice, anemia, hydromicrocephaly, convulsions,
cerebral calcification, and CSF pleocytosis occurring in different
combinations. Other symptoms such as fever, hypothermia, vomiting, diarrhea, pneumonia, skin rash, and hemorrhage may also
occur.

Some infants born with subclinical infection may develop signs of infection months or even years later and present with chorioretinitis,
strabismus, blindness, deafness, seizures, hydro- or microcephaly,
psychomotor and mental retardation.

Acquired toxoplasmosis is also asymptomatic in the majority of patients. Clinically the disease may be expressed by a variety of signs

and symptoms including fever, malaise, lymphadenopathy, hepatomegaly, splenomegaly, maculopapular rash, pneumonia, myocarditis, myalgia, arthralgia, meningoencephalitis, and chorioretinitis.
Disseminated infections are more often seen in immunosuppressed
patients, particularly those with Hodgkin's disease, lymphosarcoma
and leukemia.

3. DIAGNOSIS

Laboratory methods for confirmation of congenital toxoplasmosis
include: 1) isolation of toxoplasma in susceptible animals (mice,
hamsters, or rabbits), 2) demonstration of the organism in tissue
sections or smears, 3) serological testing and 4) levels of IgM in
cord serum. Serological testing and IgM levels in cord serum are
most commonly used.

1) Isolation of toxoplasma by inoculation of blood or other tissues
   (placenta) into susceptible mice (or other animals) and then determine the development of antibody in infected animals by serological testing. Desmonts et al. (1975) reported that toxoplasma
   can be frequently isolated from the placenta (95%) and from the
   blood (43%) of congenitally infected neonates.

2) Toxoplasma may be identified with Giemsa or PAS staining of
   smears and tissue sections (placenta). Morphological identification is only suggestive and requires further confirmation.

3) Serological diagnosis by Sabin-Feldman dye test or other methods
   is useful but may be difficult during the first few weeks or even
   months of life, because maternal IgG is transferred to the fetus.
   Two methods are available to differentiate between maternal antibodies and antibodies synthesized by the infant: (a) demonstration of the presence of specific IgM antibodies by indirect fluorescent antibody (IgM-IFA) method, and (b) quantitation of the
   amount of antibodies persisting in the infant's serum in the early
   months of life. Follow-up serological testing is the only method
   for diagnosis in infants who show negative IFA-IgM or negative
   toxoplasma isolation.

4. PREVENTION AND TREATMENT

4.1: Prevention: Neither active nor passive immunization against
toxoplasmosis is available at the present time. Susceptible pregnant
women should avoid exposure to T. gondii. This can be accomplished
by the following measures: (1) avoiding ingestion of raw or undercooked meats and careful hand washing after handling raw meat;
(2) keep the household cat from hunting and feed it only dried, canned
or cooked meat; (3) delegate maintenance of the cat to someone else
and change litterboxes daily and disinfect them with boiling water;
(4) use gloves when working in soil contaminated with cat feces;

(5) cover children's sandboxes when not in use; (6) control flies and
cockroaches; and (7) wash hands before meals and before touching
the face (Frenkel, 1974).

A satisfactory means for preventing or controlling of fetal infection
following the diagnosis of primary infection in the pregnant mother
is not available. European workers have used spiramycin with
some success (Desmonts et al., 1974). The use of sulfadiazine and
pyrimethamine is probably too teratogenic, and therefore is not
recommended during the first trimester. The safety of these drugs
in the second and third trimester is not known. If the infection occurs during the first trimester, therapeutic abortion may be
recommended.

<u>4.2: Treatment</u>: For all congenital infections, either symptomatic
or asymptomatic, combined use of sulfadiazine (150 mg/kg/day in
4 divided doses) and pryimethamine (1 mg/kg/day in two divided
doses) is recommended. Both drugs are given orally and the duration of therapy is approximately 4 weeks or longer. Folinic acid
(1 to 2 mg per day in single dose) is given to reduce the anti-folate
effect of pyrimethamine. The side effect of sulfadiazine-pyrimetha-
mine is bone marrow depression and is dose-related. Blood counts
(WBC, platelet, reticulocyte) should be twice weekly to monitor the
side effects of drug therapy.

Spiramycin has been used in Europe for the treatment of toxoplasmosis but it has not been licensed for use in the United States.

REFERENCES

GENERAL

Alford, C.A.: The immunologic status of the newborn. Hosp. Prac.
June, 1970, p. 88.

Alford, C.A., Jr., Stagno, S., and Reynolds, D.W.: Diagnosis of
chronic perinatal infections. Am. J Dis. Child. 129:455, 1975.

Altemeier, W.A. and Smith, R.T.: Immunologic aspects of resistance in early life. Pediatr. Clin. N.A. Vol. 12, No. 3, August
1965.

Blattner, R.J.: The role of viruses in congenital defects. Am. J.
Dis. Child. 128:781, 1974.

Catalano, L.W., Jr., and Sever, J.L.: The role of viruses as
causes of congenital defects. Ann. Rev. Microbiol. 25:255, 1971.

Eichenwald, H.F., McCracken, G.H., Jr., and Kindberg, S.J.:
Virus infections of the newborn. Progr. Med. Virol. 9:35, 1967.

Horstmann, D.M.: Viral infections in pregnancy. Yale J. Biol. Med. 42:99, 1969.

Krugman, S., Gershon, A.A. eds.: Symposium on infection of the fetus and the newborn infant. Alan R. Liss, Inc., New York, 1975.

McCracken, G.H., Jr., Hardy, J.B., Chen, T.C., Hoffman, L.S., Gilkeson, M.R., and Sever, J.L.: Serum immunoglobulin levels in newborn infants. II. Survey of cord and follow-up sera from 123 infants with congenital rubella. J. Pediatr. 74:383, 1969.

Medearis, D.N , Jr.: Comparative aspects of reproductive failure induced in mammals by viruses. In, Comparative aspects of reproductive failure, Benirschke, K., editor, Springer-Verlag, New York, 1967, p. 333.

Mims, C A.: Pathogenesis of viral infections of the fetus. Progr. Med. Virol. 10:194, 1968.

Monif, G.R.G.: Viral infections of the human fetus. The Macmillan Co., Collier-Macmillan Ltd., London, 1969.

Nahmias, A.J.: The TORCH complex. Hosp. Pract., May 1974, p. 65.

Overall, J.C. and Glasgow, L.A.: Virus infections of the fetus and newborn infant. J. Pediatr. 77:315, 1970.

Remington, J.S. and Klein, J.O., eds.: Infectious diseases of the fetus and newborn infant. W.B. Saunders Co., Philadelphia, 1976.

Sever, J.L.: Viral teratogens: A status report. Hosp. Pract. April, 1970, p. 75.

CYTOMEGALOVIRUS

Baron, J., Youngblood, L., Siewer, C.M.F., and Medearis, D.N. Jr.: The incidence of cytomegalovirus, herpes simplex, rubella, and toxoplasma antibodies in microcephalic, mentally retarded, and normocephalic children. Pediatrics 44:932, 1969.

Birnbaum, G., Lynch, J.I., Margileth, A.M., Lonergan, W.M., and Sever, J.L.: Cytomegalovirus infections in newborn infants. J. Pediatr. 75:789, 1969.

Diosi, P., Moldovan, E., and Tomescu, N.: Latent cytomegalovirus infection in blood donors. Br. Med. J. 4:660, 1969.

Hanshaw,J.B., Steinfield,H.J., and White, C.J.: Fluorescent antibody tests for cytomegalovirus macroglobulin. NEJM 279:566, 1968.

Hanshaw, J.B.: Congenital cytomegalovirus infection: Laboratory methods of detection. J. Pediatr. 75:1179, 1969.

Hanshaw, J.B.: Congenital cytomegalovirus infection: A fifteen-year perspective. J. Infect. Dis. 123:555, 1971.

Hanshaw, J B., Scheiner, A.P., Moxley, A.W., et al.: School failure and deafness after "silent" congenital cytomegalovirus infection. NEJM 295:468, 1976.

Henle, W., Henle, G., Scriba, M., et al.: Antibody responses to the Epstein-Barr virus and cytomegalovirus after open-heart and other surgery. NEJM 282:1068, 1970.

Klemola, K. and Kaariainen, L.: Cytomegalovirus as a possible cause of a disease resembling infectious mononucleosis. Br. Med. J. 2:1099, 1965.

Kumar, M.L., Nankervis, G.A., and Gold, E.: Inapparent congenital cytomegalovirus infection: A follow-up study. NEJM 288: 1370, 1973.

McCracken, G H., Jr., Shinefield, H.R., Cobb, K., Railsen, A.R., Dische, R., and Eichenwald, H.F.: Congenital cytomegalic inclusion disease: A longitudinal study of 20 patients. Am. J. Dis. Child. 117:522, 1969.

Medearis, D.N., Jr.: Observations concerning human cytomegalovirus infection and disease. Bull. Hopkins Hosp. 114:181, 1964.

Neiman, P., Wasserman, P.B., Wentworth, B.B., et al.: Interstitial pneumonia and cytomegalovirus infection as complications of human marrow transplantation. Transplantation 15:478, 1973.

Prince, A.M., Szmuness, W., Millian, S.J., et al.: A serologic study of cytomegalovirus infections associated with blood transfusions. NEJM 284:1125, 1971.

Reynolds, D.W., Stagno, S., Hosty, T.S., Tiller, M., and Alford, C.A., Jr.: Maternal cytomegalovirus excretion and perinatal infection. NEJM 289:1, 1973.

Smith, S.D., Cho, C.T., Brahmacupta, N., and Lenahan, M.F.: Pulmonary involvement with cytomegalovirus infections in children. Arch. Dis. Child. 52:441, 1977.

Starr, J.G. and Gold, E.: Screening of newborn infants for cytomegalovirus infection. J. Pediatr. 73:820, 1968.

Stagno, S., Reynolds, D.W., Tsiantos, A., et al.: Comparative serial virologic and serologic studies of symptomatic and subclinical congenitally and naturally acquired cytomegalovirus infections. J. Infect. Dis. 132:568, 1975.

Weller, T.H.: The cytomegaloviruses: Ubiquitous agents with protean clinical manifestations. NEJM 285:203, 267, 1971.

Weller, T.H. and Hanshaw, J.B.: Virologic and clinical observations on cytomegalic inclusion disease. NEJM 266:1233, 1962.

HERPES SIMPLEX VIRUS

Altshuler, G.: Pathogenesis of congenital herpesvirus infection: Case report including a description of the placenta. Am. J. Dis. Child. 127:427, 1974.

Ch'ien, L.T., Whitley, R.J., Nahmias, A.J., Lewin, E.B., Linnemann, C.C., Frenkel, L.D., Bellanti, J.A., Buchanan, R.A., and Alford, C.A.: Antiviral chemotherapy and neonatal herpes simplex virus infection: A pilot study experience with adenine arabinoside (Ara-A). Pediatrics 55:678, 1975.

Cho, C.T., Feng, K.K., Brahmacupta, N.: Synergistic antiviral effects of adenine arabinoside and humoral antibodies in experimental encephalitis due to Herpesvirus hominis. J. Infect. Dis. 133:157, 1976.

Florman, A.L., Gershon, A.A., Blackett, P.R., and Nahmias, A.J.: Intrauterine infection with herpes simplex virus. JAMA 225: 129, 1973.

Hanshaw, J.B.: Herpesvirus hominis infections in the fetus and the newborn. Am. J. Dis. Child. 126:546, 1973.

Nahmias, A J., Josey, W.E., and Naib, Z.M.: Neonatal herpes simplex infection: Role of genital infection in mother as the source of virus in the newborn. JAMA 199:164, 1967.

Nahmias, A.J., Dowdle, W., Josey, W., Naib, Z., Painter, L., and Luce, C.: Newborn infection with herpesvirus hominis types 1 and 2. J. Pediatr. 75:1194, 1969.

Nahmias, A J., Alford, C.A., and Korones, S.B.: Infection of the newborn with herpesvirus hominis. Adv. Pediatr. 17:185, 1970.

Nahmias, A.J., Josey, W., Naib, Z., Freeman, M., Fernandex, R., and Wheeler, J.: Perinatal risk associated with maternal genital herpes simplex virus infection. Am. J. Obstet. Gynec. 110: 825, 1971.

Nahmias, A J., and Roizman, B.: Herpes simplex viruses. NEJM 289:667, 719, 781, 1973.

Ng, A B., Regan, J.W., and Yen, S.S.: Herpes genitalis. Clinical and cytopathologic experience with 256 patients. Obstet. Gyn. 36:645, 1970.

Rawls, W.E., Garden, J.L., Flanders, R.W., Lowry, S.P., Kaufman, R.H., and Melnick, J.L.: Genital herpes in two social groups. Am. J. Obstet. Gynec. 110:682, 1971.

Sieber, O.F., Fulginiti, V.A., Bragie, J., and Umlauf, H.J., Jr.: In utero infection of the fetus by herpes simplex virus. J. Pediatr. 69:30, 1966.

Smith, I.W., Peuthere, J.F., and MacCallum, F.O.: The incidence of Herpes-virus hominis antibody in the population. J. Hyg. 65:395, 1967.

South, M A., Tompkins, W.A.F., Morris, R., and Rawls, W.E.: Congenital malformation of the central nervous system associated with genital type (type 2) herpes virus. J. Pediatr. 75:13, 1969.

St. Geme, J.W., Jr., Gailey, S.R., Koopman, J.S., Oh, W., Hobel, C.J., and Imagawa, D.T.: Neonatal risk following late gestational genital Herpesvirus hominis infection. Am. J. Dis. Child. 129:342, 1975.

Torphy, D.E., Ray, C.G., McAlister, R., and Du, J.N.H.: Herpes simplex virus infection in infants: A spectrum of disease. J. Pediatr. 76:405, 1970.

TOXOPLASMOSIS

Alford, C.A., Stagno, S., and Reynolds, D.W.: Congenital toxoplasmosis: Clinical, laboratory and therapeutic considerations, with special reference to subclinical disease. Bull. N.Y. Acad. Med. 50:160, 1974.

Desmonts, G. and Couvreur, J.: Congenital toxoplasmosis: A prospective study of 378 pregnancies. NEJM 290:1110, 1974.

Eichenwald, H.F.: A study of congenital toxoplasmosis with particular emphasis on clinical manifestations, sequelae, and therapy. In, Human Toxoplasmosis, Slim, J.C., editor, Munksgaard, Copenhagen, 1959.

Feldman, H.A.: Toxoplasma and toxoplasmosis. Hosp. Pract. March, 1969, p. 64.

Feldman, H.A.: Toxoplasmosis: An overview. Bull. N.Y. Acad. Med. 50:110, 1974.

Frenkel, J.K.: Toxoplasma in and around us. BioScience 23:343, 1973.

Frenkel, J.K.: Pathology and pathogenesis of congenital toxoplasmosis. Bull. N.Y. Acad. Med. 50:182, 1974.

Garcia, A.G.P.: Congenital toxoplasmosis in two successive sibs. Arch. Dis. Child. 43:705, 1968.

Jacobs, L.: Toxoplasma gondii: Parasitology and transmission. Bull. N.Y. Acad. Med. 50:128, 1974.

Kimball, A C., Kean, B.H., and Frech, F.: Congenital toxoplasmosis: A prospective study of 4,048 obstetric patients. Am. J. Obstet. Gynec. 3:211, 1971.

Remington, J.S., and Desmonts, G.: Congenital toxoplasmosis: Variability in the IgM fluorescent antibody response and some pitfalls in diagnosis. J. Pediatr. 83:27, 1973.

CHAPTER 8. NEONATAL INFECTIONS

8.1: NEONATAL SEPSIS

INTRODUCTION: Neonatal sepsis is an acute systemic disease associated with the invasion of bloodstream and various tissues by microorganisms and their toxic products. In the past, the term neonatal sepsis meant bacterial sepsis or septicemia, but it is becoming clearer that other infecting agents such as viruses, fungi, or protozoa can also produce a clinical response similar to that of bacterial sepsis. The tissues most frequently involved in neonatal sepsis include the brain, meninges, lungs, liver, spleen, peritoneum, kidneys, heart, skin, middle ear, bones and joints.

The incidence of neonatal sepsis is difficult to determine because it is not a reportable disease. The incidence varies in different nursery populations, ranging from 1 to 5 per 1000 live births. The incidence also fluctuates with the season of the year and with outbreaks in the nurseries. The case fatality rate for neonatal sepsis is about 30 to 50%. Neurological sequelae occur in a significant number among those who survive.

The high morbidity and mortality of neonatal sepsis is partly related to difficulties in diagnosis. The difficulties are three-fold: (1) when the onset is insidious, the signs and symptoms are nonspecific and the physician may unwisely elect to adopt a "wait and see" policy before taking specific action; (2) when the onset is sudden and dramatic, with death occurring within hours, the physician has little time in which to act; and (3) bacterial sepsis is complicated by a high incidence (12 to 40%) of meningoencephalitis in newborn infants, which in itself is difficult to diagnose except by examining spinal fluid.

Thus, neonatal sepsis is a relatively common and severe illness. Early recognition of its onset, appropriate microbiological diagnostic studies, and management with specific antibiotics and supportive care are required if the infant is to survive and be free of sequelae. For practical purposes, all babies with clinical features of neonatal sepsis should be managed as if they have bacterial infection, until proven otherwise.

1. ETIOLOGY AND PATHOGENESIS

1.1: Etiologic Agents: The etiologic agents usually responsible for neonatal sepsis are shown in Table 8-1. Bacteria are the major causes of neonatal sepsis. Viruses and other agents play a less important role. Reports of neonatal bacterial sepsis in the United States between the 1920's and 1970's demonstrated an important shift

TABLE 8-1: ETIOLOGIC AGENTS OF NEONATAL SEPSIS		
AGENTS	COMMON	LESS COMMON
Bacteria	E. coli Streptococci, group B Klebsiella Staphylococci	Listeria, Proteus, Pseudomonas Enterococci, Salmonella Pneumococci, Meningococci Paracolon, Anaerobes*
Viruses	-	Coxsackie, Echo, RSV, Adeno CMV, Rubella, Herpes simplex Hepatitis**

* Other less common bacteria include Achromobacter, Aerobacter, Alcaligenes fecalis, Brucella abortus, Clostridium welchii, Corynebacterium diphtheriae, Edwardsiella tarda, Flavobacterium, Hemophilus influenzae, Mimae, Mycobacterium, Neisseria gonorrhoea, Pasteurella multocida, Serratia, Shigella, Streptococcus viridans, Vibrio fetus. (Modified from Davis, P.A., Arch. Dis. Child. 46:1, 1971).

** Other less common viruses: See Table 8-2. RSV = respiratory syncytial virus, CMV = cytomegalovirus.

in etiologic agents from gram-positive to gram-negative organisms, and also an increased incidence of group B streptococcal infections in recent years. During the past several years, E. coli and group B streptococci have been the two major organisms responsible for the majority of cases of neonatal sepsis. Less frequently encountered bacteria include klebsiella, staphylococci, pseudomonas, proteus, listeria, salmonella, pneumonocci, meningococci, and anaerobic bacteria. Some low virulent and nonpathogenic bacteria can also produce disease in newborn infants, particularly in premature and debilitated infants.

Septic-like clinical findings in infants can be caused by viruses such as cytomegalovirus, rubella, coxsackie, echo, respiratory syncytial virus, adenovirus, herpes simplex, varicella, hepatitis B, etc. Nonspecific viral infections are not uncommon during pregnancy, but only a small number of maternal infections lead to infection in the fetus and newborns. The consequences of these maternal viral infections are listed in Table 8-2. Diseases caused by cytomegalovirus, rubella, and herpes simplex are discussed elsewhere (see Chapter 7).

TABLE 8-2: VIRAL INFECTIONS AFFECTING THE FETUS OR NEWBORN	
MATERNAL INFECTION	EFFECTS ON FETUS OR NEWBORN
1. Influenza	Abortion, malformation (?)
2. Measles	Abortion, stillbirth, congenital measles
3. Mumps	Fetal death, endocardial fibro-elastosis (?)
4. Herpes simplex	Generalized herpes, encephalitis, death, malformation (?)
5. Chickenpox-"shingles"	Congenital chickenpox or "shingles," abortion, stillbirth
6. Hepatitis (serum)	Neonatal hepatitis
7. Smallpox	Congenital smallpox, abortion, stillbirths
8. Vaccinia	Congenital generalized vaccinia, abortion
9. Poliomyelitis	Congenital spinal or bulbar polio-myelitis, abortion
10. ECHO	Subclinical-mild-severe infections, diarrhea
11. Coxsackie	Myocarditis, subclinical-mild-severe infections
12. Equine encephalitis	Congenital encephalitis

Cytomegalovirus and rubella are not included in this Table (see Chapter 7).

<u>1.2: Source of Infection:</u> **There are three major sources of neo-**natal infections: (1) in utero via the placenta, (2) through the infected amniotic fluid and contaminated birth canal, or (3) from the environment after birth, either by contact with human carrier or from contaminated equipment. The common types of infecting organisms from these sources are listed in Table 8-3.

TABLE 8-3: MAJOR SOURCES OF NEONATAL INFECTIONS		
SOURCE	MECHANISMS OF TRANSMISSION	EXAMPLES OF KIND OF INFECTION
1. Ante-natal	Transplacental (maternal to fetal blood)	<u>Congenital infections</u> (e.g. rubella, cytomegalovirus, toxoplasma, syphilis, listeria, hepatitis, mycobacteria)
2. Peri-natal	a. Ascending infection (vagina to uterus)	<u>Early onset neonatal sepsis</u> (e.g. E. coli, group B streptococci, gram-negative enteric, gonococci) <u>Late onset disease</u> (e.g. Candida albicans, Herpes simplex, Cytomegalovirus, chlamydia, group B streptococci)
3. Post-natal	Environmental Contamination (nursery, equipments, hospital personnel, family members)	<u>Late onset neonatal sepsis</u> (e.g. staphylococci, pseudomonas, enteropathogenic E. coli) <u>Late onset viral infections</u> (e.g. Coxsackie, Echo, Adeno, respiratory syncytial)

Most of the intrauterine infections occurring prior to rupture of fetal membranes are by transplacental route resulting from maternal bloodstream infections. These infections produce variable effects on fetuses, resulting in premature delivery, growth retardation, developmental delay, congenital anomalies, abortion, fetal death and even resulting in apparently normal infants. Infections acquired through the infected amniotic fluid or contaminated birth canal are common and usually associated with early onset of illness. For example, recent observations indicate that there are two forms of group B streptococcal infection in neonates. The early-onset disease occurs in the first 10 days of life, whereas the late-onset disease occurs from 11 days to 3 months of life. The female genitourinary tract is

the major reservoir for this organism. It is likely that infants
with early-onset disease acquired the organism either in utero or
during passage through the birth canal, whereas those with late-
onset acquire the organisms post-natally.

Infections acquired from the environment after birth are important
causes of neonatal sepsis and often can be prevented (see Prevention of Neonatal Infection). Premature and sick infants are particularly susceptible. Staphylococcus aureus, enteropathogenic
E. coli, and Pseudomonas are of great concern. The rates of colonization of staphylococci vary greatly in different nurseries. Some
of these infants, although small in number, may develop serious
infections weeks or months after going home.

1.3: Portal of Entry: The portal of entry of bacteria and viruses
is usually undetermined. Because of the immaturity of inflammatory responses, newborns may fail to localize the infection with a
vigorous local inflammatory reaction; therefore, the site of infection may not be clinically apparent. Theoretically, all the obvious
portals such as mucous membranes, skin, gastrointestinal tract,
and genitourinary tract should be considered. Special attention
should be given to the umbilicus because it is frequently contaminated and infected. The area of circumcision is not frequently mentioned as a possible portal of entry, but it would be difficult to think
of an area with greater potential.

1.4: Predisposing Factors: Predisposing factors in neonatal sepsis are numerous. The most important factors are: (1) maternal
infection, (2) prolonged and difficult delivery, (3) premature rupture of the membranes, and (4) prematurity.

Focal and generalized infections in the mothers contribute significantly to sepsis in their infants. Infections in the mother may be
silent or clinically apparent, such as urinary tract infection, cellulitis, mastitis, pelvic peritonitis, herpetic lesions, and nonspecific
viral illness. In addition, many of the common pathogenic or non-
pathogenic organisms inhabiting the genital or intestinal tract of the
mother may produce disease in infants. Obstetrical complications
are important contributing factors to neonatal infection. In one
study of neonatal meningitis, obstetrical complications were present
in approximately 50% of the mothers (Overall, 1970). It is apparent
that many of the common non-pathogenic inhabitants of the genital
tract may become pathogenic in the presence of traumatized tissues
and blood clots.

The fetus is protected from exposure to microbial agents. Rupture
of the fetal membranes before the onset or at the time of labor provides an opportunity for exposure to infecting agents. The risk of
fetal infection increases with the interval between rupture of membranes and delivery. Neonatal sepsis may develop at any time with

more than half of the cases occurring in the first week after birth. Illness developing within the first 2 days of life is closely associated with perinatal complications, such as premature rupture of membranes, maternal bleeding, toxemia, infection, cesarean section, and precipitous delivery.

Premature infants are more susceptible to neonatal sepsis. There is also a higher mortality associated with the disease in premature infants. Overall (1970) found that the incidence of bacterial meningitis in premature infants was about 3 to 4 times higher than in full term infants.

In regard to sex of the infant, there is a highly significant preponderance of male infants with sepsis. Washburn et al. (1965) reviewed 438 cases of neonatal sepsis and found a ratio of male to female of 2:1.

1.5: Host Defense Mechanisms: A special predisposing factor in septicemia in newborn infants is the inadequate maturation of naturally inherent defense mechanisms. There is a passive transfer of maternal IgG to the fetus, and the level of circulating IgG in the infants' blood at birth is equal to or higher than that of the mothers. However, IgM and IgA are not transferred passively from mother to fetus; consequently, levels in babies' blood are very low. It is likely that such deficiencies may lead to an increased susceptibility to infection. In addition, newborn infants have a lower level of serum complement, and phagocytic activities appear to be less effective, particularly during stress situations. Cell-mediated immunity in premature and newborn infants is also believed to be less well developed. Premature infants have fewer capillaries in all their tissues than full term infants and, consequently, mobilization of natural defenses may be poorer in premature infants. Inflammatory responses in immature hosts are also deficient. For example, Fruend (1931) showed that young and adult rabbits have different capacities to develop and to localize inflammation at the site of injection of pneumococci. In adult rabbits, a very extensive local inflammation develops and bacteremia occurs only in a relatively few number of rabbits. In contrast, young rabbits fail to develop extensive inflammation and consequently die with bacteremia. Local reactions in these young rabbits were variable (51% had no reaction, 36% had local redness only, and 13% had redness and swelling). Such findings are probably similar to those observed in human newborns.

2. CLINICAL MANIFESTATIONS

The signs and symptoms of neonatal sepsis are nonspecific and often of insidious onset. They are in sharp contrast to the toxic manifestations of sepsis observed in older children and adults. The relative immaturity of the inflammatory responses and of the host defensive factors may be responsible for such a variation.

Presenting signs and symptoms of sepsis are variable and may involve multiple organs or systems. Fever, although not a common symptom of sepsis, may be present in full term infants. Subnormal temperatures and irregular fluctuations are often seen in infected premature infants. "Not doing well" is the common feature of sepsis. Gastrointestinal signs include poor feeding and sucking, vomiting, diarrhea and abdominal distension. Respiratory signs may include dyspnea, irregular breathing, apnea and cyanosis. Symptoms referable to the central nervous system are irritability, lethargy, feeding difficulty, apnea, convulsion, and fever. Meningeal irritation signs, such as stiff neck and Kernig's, are not often seen in newborns with proven meningitis. Skin manifestations may include jaundice, cellulitis, impetigo, omphalitis, abscess, sclerema, petechiae, and skin lesions (Fig. 8.1).

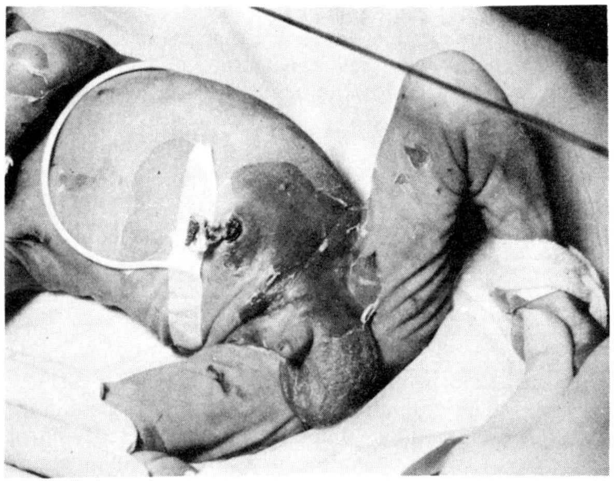

FIG. 8.1: Cutaneous manifestations of toxic epidermolysis due to Staphylococcus aureus (Staphylococcal scalded skin syndrome) in an infant.

Dramatic and sudden onset of sepsis may appear at birth, or hours, days or even weeks later. Neonatal sepsis can be confused with the respiratory distress syndrome that manifests itself at birth or a few hours after birth. The septic infant at birth may have pneumonia, which on roentgen examination can be confused with aspiration of amniotic fluid, blood, meconium or gastric contents, or with the "wet-lung" syndrome, atelectasis, or even with hyalin membrane disease.

The infant with a sudden and dramatic onset may show signs of circulatory collapse, such as ashen gray color in skin, rapid feeble pulse, gallop rhythm on auscultation of the heart, cool extremities, hypotonia, lethargy, stupor, and oliguria. Signs of disseminated intravascular coagulation may be present. Renal failure may develop in rare cases.

3. DIAGNOSIS

The signs and symptoms of neonatal sepsis are nonspecific. Many newborns exhibit the same clinical manifestations for reasons other than sepsis. The physician must explore all possible causes. Sepsis should be suspected in all sick infants, particularly in the presence of predisposing factors. Laboratory work-up of neonatal sepsis includes: (1) cultures for bacteria (blood, urine, stool and/or swabs from umbilicus, throat, and ear canal), (2) examination of the cerebro-spinal fluid for cells, sugar, protein, and for gram stain and culture, (3) roentgenograms of the chest, (4) serum bilirubin, complete blood count including platelets, urinalysis, blood sugar, blood urea nitrogen and creatinine, and serum electrolytes, and (5) gastric aspirates for the presence of increased number of polymorphonuclear leukocytes. The value of other tests, such as the Limulus test for endotoxin, are less well defined. The general approaches to diagnosis of neonatal sepsis are shown in Fig. 8.2. Other studies for viral or fungal causes of neonatal sepsis can be performed when suspected. Diagnosis of congenital infections is discussed in Chapter 7.

4. MANAGEMENT

4.1: <u>Antibiotic Treatment</u>: Specific treatment of neonatal sepsis with antibiotics is under constant change because of: (1) the increasing resistance of certain bacterial strains to some antibiotics, (2) new antibiotics continue to appear, and (3) rapidly changing physiologic processes of the neonate which affect the pharmacokinetic properties of antimicrobial agents. Failure to take these factors into consideration when giving antibiotics to neonates may result in therapeutic failure or toxic drug reactions.

Prevalence of bacterial resistance to antibiotics may reflect the patterns of antibiotic usage in a particular nursery or community. For example, the level of resistance (i.e. <u>E. coli</u> to kanamycin, Pseudomonas to carbenicillin) differs in varying communities and at varying times in the same community. Thus, there is a need for continuing surveillance of hospital and nursery strains of bacteria for their susceptibility to the commonly used antimicrobials.

A number of enzyme systems (e.g. those in the liver) and physiologic processes (e.g. excretion of drug by the kidneys) are deficient or immature in early life and may result in an altered drug metabolism and excretion. Toxic effects of antimicrobial agents occur frequently in premature infants in whom enzyme systems and physiologic

<table>
<tr><td colspan="2" align="center">HISTORY

1. "Not doing well" - insidious or dramatic

2. Predisposing factors:
Maternal infection
Prolonged labor
Premature rupture of membranes
Premature birth</td></tr>
<tr><td valign="top">PHYSICAL EXAMINATION

1. G-I signs (poor feeding and sucking, vomiting, diarrhea, distension)

2. Respiratory signs (dyspnea, tachypnea, apnea, cyanosis)

3. CNS signs (lethargy, irritability, convulsions, hypothermia, fever)

4. Skin signs (petechiae, rash, jaundice, cellulitis)</td><td valign="top">LABORATORY EXAMINATION

1. Bacterial cultures

2. CSF examinations and cultures

3. Chest roentgenograms

4. Gastric aspirates

5. Others (e.g. CBC, urinalysis, blood sugar, electrolytes, BUN, creatinine, etc.)</td></tr>
</table>

FIG. 8.2: Approach to Diagnosis of Neonatal Sepsis

processes are most immature (Table 8-4). Excessive doses of chloramphenicol may result in cardiovascular collapse and death (gray syndrome) Sulfonamides may interfere with bilirubin binding to albumin, thus allowing free bilirubin to circulate in the central nervous system and lead to kernicterus in infants with hyperbilirubinemia. Tetracyclines concentrate in newly formed calcium complexes, leading to dental staining and depression of bone growth.

Because of the inherent risk associated with the use of antibiotics in neonates, it is important to be familiar with the use of penicillin, ampicillin, kanamycin and gentamicin, which have been commonly used in neonatal sepsis. These antibiotics have been proven to be safe and effective for treating neonatal sepsis if appropriate dosages are given and if resistance is not a factor. Because renal clearance of drug is slower in premature infants, the half-life of these antibiotics in serum correlates with the age of the infants. The daily dosage for premature infants is less than for full term infants.

Newborn infants suspected of having sepsis should be treated with combinations of antibiotics, covering both gram positive and gram negative bacteria, after bacteriological studies have been obtained.

TABLE 8-4: COMPLICATIONS INDUCED BY ANTIMICROBIAL AGENTS IN PREMATURE AND NEWBORN INFANTS		
DRUG	COMPLICATIONS	MECHANISMS
1. Chloramphenicol	Gray syndrome	Immaturity of hepatic glucuronyl transferase
2. Sulfonamide	Kernicterus	Compete with bilirubin for binding to albumin
3. Tetracycline	Dental staining and depression of bone growth	Drug concentrates in the newly formed calcium complexes
4. Novobiocin	Hyperbilirubinemia	Drug inhibit hepatic glucuronyl transferase
5. Sulfonamide Nitrofurantoin	Hemolysis	In infants with red cells G-6-P-D deficiency

Because of the immaturity of host defense mechanisms in the neonates, bactericidal rather than bacteriostatic agents are chosen. These include either ampicillin (or penicillin) in combination with kanamycin (or gentamicin). The dosage and route of administration are shown in Table 8-5. Penicillin or ampicillin are effective against streptococci, pneumococci and susceptible staphylococci. Some clinicians believe ampicillin has an advantage over penicillin when combined with kanamycin or gentamicin because of its broader spectrum of antimicrobial activity, particularly against enterococci and E. coli. When clinical or epidemiologic features suggest the possibility of a staphylococcal infection, a semi-synthetic penicillin resistant to penicillinase (such as nafcillin, methicillin) should substitute for penicillin or ampicillin. Patients with skin lesions suggestive of a pseudomonas infection should be given gentamicin instead of kanamycin. Wide variations in peak serum levels may be observed in infants receiving kanamycin and gentamicin. Serum levels of antibiotics should be monitored whenever possible.

Once the organism has been identified and the sensitivity patterns are known, an appropriate single antibiotic may be used. The duration of antibiotic therapy will depend on the nature of the infection, the infecting agent, and the clinical course of the infant. In general, the antibiotic treatment of neonatal sepsis should continue for a minimum of ten days.

The value of intrathecal or intraventricular administration of antibiotics for neonatal meningitis has not been well defined. Recent observations indicated that intrathecal administration of gentamicin did not significantly improve the morbidity or mortality of gram-negative neonatal meningitis (McCraken, 1975).

TABLE 8-5: ANTIMICROBIAL AGENTS FOR NEWBORN INFANTS	
Notes: 1. The median of the dosage ranges is generally used. 2. The lower doses and lesser frequency in the ranges should be used in premature infants. 3. The larger doses and greater frequency are reserved for full-term infants one to four weeks of age with serious infection.	
AGENT	**DOSAGE/KG OF BODY WEIGHT/ 24 HRS.**
Penicillin, G. crystalline	50,000 to 200,000 units in 2 to 3 doses, IV, IM
Methicillin, sodium	75 to 200 mg in 2 to 3 doses, IV, IM
Oxacillin, sodium	50 to 100 mg in 2 to 3 doses, IV, IM
Nafcillin, sodium	50 to 100 mg in 2 to 3 doses, IV, IM
Ampicillin	100 to 200 mg in 2 to 3 doses, IV, IM
Carbenicillin, disodium	200 to 400 mg in 2 to 3 doses
Kanamycin	15 mg in 2 doses, IM
Gentamicin	5 to 7.5 mg in 2 to 3 doses, IM, IV
Polymyxin B	2.5 mg in 4 doses, IM
Colistin sulfate	10-15 mg in 4 doses, PO
Neomycin sulfate	100 mg in 3-4 doses, PO
Chloramphenicol*	25 to 50 mg in 2 to 3 doses
Nystatin	200,000 to 400,000 units in 4 doses PO
* Rarely indicated.	

4.2: Supportive Therapy: Supportive therapy for infants with neonatal sepsis is essential. Correction of dehydration, shock and
acidosis is often life-saving (also see Chapter 22). Treatment of
recurrent apnea, dyspnea, and cyanosis may require not only adequate administration of extra oxygen, but assisted ventilation as
well. Maintaining proper blood levels of glucose, calcium, sodium
and potassium is obviously important. Treatment and prevention
of convulsions, increased intracranial pressure, and excessive irritability may be necessary. Disseminated intravascular coagulopathy and renal failure associated with neonatal sepsis present spe-
ial problems in management.

One special type of supportive therapy is the administration of whole
blood or its components to the septic newborn infants. Red blood
cells may be needed to correct rapidly developing anemia. Whole
blood or plasma is beneficial for expanding blood volume in hypovolemia related to dehydration and circulatory collapse. Platelet
transfusions or granulocyte transfusions are indicated in severe
thrombocytopenia or granulocytopenia observed in some infants with
sepsis. Whole blood transfusions, or exchange transfusions of
whole blood, have been used by some clinicians on the grounds that
there are incompletely defined humoral and cellular components in
the blood that may appear to have a beneficial effect on the course
of disease.

::

8.2: LOCALIZED INFECTIONS

1. THRUSH (MONILIASIS)

Thrush, a common oral lesion caused by <u>Candida albicans</u>, is usually acquired at birth from the mother's birth canal. The disease
may also be acquired from other infected infants, or from contaminated hands or feeding facilities. The lesions usually appear within
a few days after birth and appear as small white flakes or patches
on the gums, palate, buccal mucosa, or tongue. Diagnosis can
easily be made clinically. Oral thrush is easily distinguished from
milk curds by using a swab; milk curds are easily wiped off, whereas
thrush is not. Confirmation of the diagnosis is made by smears
stained with methylene blue, and by routine bacterial or fungal
culture.

Oral thrush is generally a mild and self-limited disease leaving no
scars. Often the moniliasis may involve other organs, such as skin
of perineal or perianal region, fingernails, and gastrointestinal
tract. Persistence or recurrence of thrush with protracted skin lesions may suggest underlying immunodeficiency disease, malignancy,
malnutrition, prolonged antibiotic therapy or endocrine dysfunction.
Debilitated infants, particularly those receiving prolonged total parental nutrition, may develop candida septicemia with involvement of
kidney, lung, brain, esophagus or stomach.

Treatment of oral thrush includes swabbing the mouth four times
daily with an oral suspension of nystatin (Mycostatin) 100,000 units
(1 ml.), until the lesions have cleared, and for a few days afterward. Aqueous gentian violet (1%) is also useful; it can be applied
directly to the lesions four times a day by using a moistened cotton
swab. Nystatin or gentian violet may also be applied to the skin
infection. Disseminated candidiasis may be treated with amphotericin B (see Chapter 15).

2. CONJUNCTIVITIS (OPHTHALMIA NEONATORIUM)

Two major causes of acute inflammation of the conjunctiva in newborn infants are chemical irritation and infection. Chemical conjunctivitis usually occurs following the application of silver nitrate
for prophylaxis of gonococcal eye infection. It generally subsides
within one or two days and the bacteriological studies are negative.
The microbial agents encountered in conjunctivitis in this age group
include gonococci, staphylococci, streptococci, pneumococci, pseudomonas, and chlamydia oculogenitalis (inclusion conjunctivitis).
Most of these infections are acquired from an infected birth canal
during parturition. Most bacterial conjunctivitis are staphylococcal
in origin. The time of onset of the conjunctivitis varies, e.g.,
chemical conjunctivitis occurs within 24 hours after birth, bacterial
conjunctivitis within 2 to 5 days, and inclusion conjunctivitis 5 to 10
days.

Gonococcal conjunctivitis, once the most common cause of blindness
in infants and children, is rare. This is attributed to the routine
prophylactic use of 1% silver nitrate solution or other antibiotics to
the eye immediately after birth. Gonococcal conjunctivitis is a serious disease manifested by a marked edema, fiery red conjunctivae
with a copious creamy discharge, and a high risk of corneal ulceration and permanent scarring, leading to blindness. Diagnosis can
be confirmed by Gram stains and by cultures of the exudates. Treatment includes: (1) systemic penicillin G, 30,000 units/kg, I.M.
every 12 hours; (2) topical penicillin G, (2,500 units/ml) every one
to two hours; (3) frequent irrigation of conjunctivae with isotonic
saline solution; and (4) atropine drops (0.25%) twice daily if cornea
is threatened. Consultation with an ophthalmologist is desirable.

Conjunctivitis is further discussed in Chapter 2.

The edema, redness, and discharges caused by other bacteria (e.g.
staphylococci) are generally less severe and with fewer complications. Gram stain and cultures of the exudate are usually positive
for the bacterial agent. Initial treatment generally consists of local
antibiotics, such as ophthalmic bacitracin or neomycin every 4 to 6
hours. The choice of antibiotic depends upon the nature of the pathogen. Infection of the conjunctiva associated with panophthalmitis
with rapid progress of orbital cellulitis indicates a serious infection

and requires systemic antibiotic therapy. Staphylococcus aureus,
group A streptococci, pneumonococci, and H. influenzae type B are
the common agents responsible for such infections.

Inclusion conjunctivitis (inclusion blenorrhea) in the newborn is acquired from the infected birth canal in the mother. The infected
conjunctiva is characterized by hyperemia, follicular hypertrophy,
and mucopurulent exudate, and may be associated with rhinitis. The
chlamydia infects mainly the superficial epithelial cells, and the infection heals spontaneously over a period of weeks or months, usually leaving little scarring. Diagnosis can be made by examining
the smears or scrapings by Giemsa or immunofluorescent staining;
cultures for chlamydia in embryonated eggs or in tissue cultures
can also be accomplished. Giemsa stain shows bluish granular
cytoplasmic inclusions in the epithelial cells. Treatment consists
of local application of sulfonamide ophthalmic drops. Systemic
therapy may be required in some cases. Recently Beem et al.
(1977) described a distinctive pneumonia associated with Chlamydia
infection in infants; conjunctivitis was also present in these patients.

3. OMPHALITIS

Infection of the skin and soft tissues around the umbilicus (omphalitis) ranges from mild erythema with scanty purulent discharge to a
severe cellulitis with redness and edema of the surrounding tissue.

Local infection of the umbilical stump is most often due to staphylococcus aureus. It is largely preventable with adequate cord and
skin care. Mild infection can be treated simply with topical alcohol, or with a neomycin-bacitracin preparation and an occlusive
dressing. In chronic or neglected cases, a granuloma may develop
in the umbilical stump; cauterization with a silver nitrate stick is
generally adequate in treating the granuloma. Daily application of
table salt for 2-3 days is also effective in treating umbilical
granulomas.

In severe cases of omphalitis, the infection may spread along the
falciform ligament to the liver where abscesses and septicemia develop, or the infection may spread via the umbilical vein resulting
in portal vein thrombosis. Systemic antibiotic therapy, as outlined
for neonatal sepsis, is needed for some severe cases of cellulitis.
Local measure may be applied and include a moist, warm compress
or a lamp providing heat.

In rare cases, local maceration and cellulitis around the umbilical
stump may be secondary to the structural anomalies, such as patent
urachus or enteric fistula.

8.3: PREVENTION OF NEONATAL INFECTION

1. GENERAL PROPHYLACTIC MEASURES

Since environmental factors play an important role in infection, particularly in premature and debilitated infants, every effort should be made to reduce the infection rates and to abolish epidemics. "The first requirement of a hospital is that it should do the sick no harm" (Florence Nightingale). This famous dictum clearly illustrates the importance of infection control in the hospital, particularly in the newborn nurseries. The general preventive measures in newborn nurseries are listed in Table 8-6 (also see Chapter 24).

TABLE 8-6: GENERAL PROPHYLACTIC MEASURES FOR INFECTIONS IN NEWBORN NURSERIES

1. Thorough hand washing before <u>and</u> after handling any infants.

2. Avoid overcrowding of the babies and the staff.

3. Exclude personnel with active infections (such as skin and wound infections) in the nursery.

4. A small isolation unit (an incubator may be considered as an isolation unit) for infected infants or infant born to infected mother.

5. Regular surveillance of the rates of bacterial colonization (such as <u>Staphylococcus aureus</u>) in the babies.

<u>Staphylococcus aureus</u> is of great concern during the neonatal period. It may present in three forms: (1) asymptomatic colonization, (2) localized infections (such as pustules, omphalitis, conjunctivitis, and paronychia), and (3) outbreak of severe sepsis in newborn nurseries. Epidemics of staphylococcal disease are usually caused by certain phage types (such as 80/81). The infection is primarily transmitted from one baby to the next by the hands of personnel. Therefore, vigorous hand washing is critical in controlling the spread of infection.

In addition, premature and sick infants requiring intensive care should be housed in specially designed nurseries. Special nursing techniques and adequate nursing staff are needed in nurseries. Incubators and equipment must be cleaned after use. Floor and walls of the nurseries should be washed regularly.

2. PREVENTION OF SPECIFIC INFECTIONS

Many of the neonatal infections can be prevented by early recognition and early treatment of the maternal infections, such as urinary tract infection, gonococcal infection, etc. Reduction of obstetrical complications will also reduce the risk of neonatal infection. Recently, fetal infection by rubella virus has been reduced by appropriate vaccination against rubella in susceptible women who reach the child-bearing age. Infection of the fetus by the spirochete of syphilis can be eliminated by appropriate serological testing and antibiotic therapy in the mother during pregnancy. The mother with an active genital herpes simplex virus infection is a potential threat to the fetus born by the vaginal route; therefore, delivery by cesarean section should be considered. The recent rise in neonatal sepsis and meningitis caused by group B streptococci has been well documented. Carrier rates of 10-25% in some institutions are reported. Some investigators have suggested treating carriers of group B streptococci during pregnancy with penicillin, but such recommendations have not been generally accepted at the present time. Routine vaginal cultures of pregnant women would at least alert the physician responsible for the newborn infant to the potential threat of infection by group B streptococci.

REFERENCES

Ablow, R.C., et al.: A comparison of early-onset group B streptococcal neonatal infection and the respiratory-distress syndrome of the newborn. NEJM 294:65, 1976.

Baker, C.J., Barrett, F.F., Gordon, R.C., and Yow, M.D.: Suppurative meningitis due to streptococci of Lancefield group B: A study of 33 infants. J. Pediatr. 82:724, 1973.

Balagtas, R.C., Bell, C.E., Edwards, L.D., and Levin, S.: Risk of local and systemic infections associated with umbilical vein catheterization: A prospective study in 86 newborn patients. Pediatrics 48:359, 1971.

Benirschke, K.: Routes and types of infection in the fetus and the newborn. Am. J. Dis. Child. 99:714, 1960.

Bland, R.D.: Otitis media in the first six weeks of life: Diagnosis, bacteriology, and management. Pediatrics 49:187, 1972.

Blane, W.A.: Pathways of fetal and early neonatal infection: Viral placentitis, bacterial and fungal chorioamnionitis. J. Pediatr. 59: 473, 1961.

Buetow, K.C., Klein, S.W., and Lane, R.B.: Septicemia in premature infants. Am. J. Dis. Child. 110:29, 1965.

Chow, A.W., Leake, R.D., Yamauchi, T., Anthony, B.F., and Guze, L.B.: The significance of anaerobes in neonatal bacteremia: Analysis of 23 cases and review of the literature. Pediatrics 54: 736, 1974.

Davies, P.A.: Bacterial infection in the fetus and newborn. Arch. Dis. Child. 46:1, 1971.

Eichenwald, E.F., McCracken, G.H., Jr., and Kindberg, S.J.: Virus infections of the newborn. Progr. Med. Virol. 9:35, 1967.

Eickhoff, T.C., Klein, J.O., Daly, A.K., Ingall, D., and Finland, M.: Neonatal sepsis and other infections due to Group B beta-hemolytic streptococci. NEJM 271:1221, 1964.

Francios, R.A., Knostman, J.D., and Zimmerman, R.A.: Group B streptococcal neonatal and infant infections. J. Pediatr. 82:707, 1973.

Freund, J.: Reaction of young and adult rabbits to pneumococci injected into the skin. J. Exp. Med. 54:171, 1931.

Gluck, L., Wood, H.F., and Fousek, M.D.: Septicemia of the newborn. Pediatr. Clin. N.A. 13:1131, 1966.

Gotoff, S.P., and Behrman, R.E.: Neonatal septicemia. J. Pediatr. 76:142, 1970.

Hosmer, M.E. and Sprunt, K.: Screening method for identification of infected infant following premature rupture of maternal membranes. Pediatr. 49:283, 1972.

Johnson, R.B. and Sell, S.H.: Septicemia in infants and children. Pediatrics 34:473, 1964.

Kaslow, R.A., Taylor, A., Dweck, H.S., Bobo, R.A., Steele, C.D., and Cassady, G.: Enteropathogenic Escherichia coli infection in a newborn nursery. Am. J. Dis. Child. 128:797, 1974.

McCracken, G.H., et al.: Relation between Escherichia coli Kl capsular polysaccharide antigen and clinical outcome in neonatal meningitis. Lancet 2:246, 1974.

McCracken, G.H., Jr.: Pharmacological basis for antimicrobial therapy in newborn infants. Am. J. Dis. Child. 128:407, 1974.

McCracken, G.H., Jr., Eichenwald, H.F.: Leucocyte function and the development of opsonic and complement activity in the neonate. Am. J. Dis. Child. 121:120, 1971.

McCracken, G.H., Jr., and Shinefield, H.R.: Changes in the pattern of neonatal septicemia and meningitis. Am. J. Dis. Child. 112:33, 1966.

Mims, L.C., Medawar, M.S., Perkins, J.R., and Grubb, W.R.: Predicting neonatal infections by evaluation of the gastric aspirate: A study in two hundred and seven patients. Am. J. Obstet. Gynecol. 114:232, 1972.

Najem, G R., Riley, H.D., Ordway, N.K., and Yoshioka, H.: Clinical and microbiologic surveillance of neonatal staphylococcal disease. Am. J. Dis. Child. 129:297, 1975.

Overall, J.C., Jr.: Neonatal bacterial meningitis. J. Pediatr. 76:499, 1970.

Overall, J.C., Jr., and Glasgow, L.A.: Virus infections of the fetus and newborn infant. J. Pediatr. 77:315, 1970.

Ray, C.G. and Wedgewood, R.J.: Neonatal listeriosis. Six case reports and a review of the literature. Pediatrics 34:378, 1964.

Sarff, L.D., Platt, L.H., and McCracken, G.H.: Cerebrospinal fluid evaluation in neonates: Comparison of high-risk infants with and without meningitis. J. Pediatr. 88:473, 1976.

Shurin, P.A., Pelton, S.I., and Klein, J.O.: Otitis media in the newborn infants. Ann. Otology, Laryngology, Rhinology, Suppl. #2, p. 216, 1976.

Tyler, C.W. and Albers, W.H.: Obstetric factors related to bacteremia in the newborn infant. Am. J. Obstet. Gynecol. 94:970, 1966.

Wilson, M.G., Armstrong, D.H., Nelson, R.C., and Boak, R.A.: Prolonged rupture of fetal membranes. Effect on newborn infant. Am. J. Dis. Child. 107:138, 1964.

CHAPTER 9. GASTROINTESTINAL INFECTIONS

INTRODUCTION: The major symptoms of acute infection involving
the gastrointestinal tract are diarrhea and/or vomiting. Acute
gastroenteritis is a common pediatric problem and may result in
a high morbidity and mortality in infants and children, particularly
in the very young and the malnourished. The incidence and severity
of infectious diarrhea vary with factors such as age, climate, season, nutrition, sanitation, etc. Diarrhea during the first month of
life presents a special problem and raises the possibility of neonatal sepsis (see Chapter 8). Both incidence and severity of acute
gastrointestinal infections decline progressively after two or three
years of age.

High rates of infant mortality have been attributed to acute diarrhea
in many parts of the world, particularly in areas in which poverty,
poor hygiene and malnutrition exist. The relationship between malnutrition and diarrhea is discussed in Chapter 21.

In most studies of acute diarrheal disease in infants and children,
isolation of pathogenic bacteria or viruses is accomplished in only
20 to 40% of the cases and the rest have no known causes. The major known pathogens of infantile diarrhea include enteropathogenic
Escherichia coli (EPEC), Salmonella and Shigella species. Recent
epidemiologic and laboratory studies suggest that viral agents (i.e.
rotaviruses) and E. coli, other than the classical enteropathogenic
serotypes (i.e. enterotoxigenic strains), play an important role in
acute gastroenteritis in infants and children. The actual incidence
and clinical spectrum produced by these newly recognized agents
are being evaluated. It is possible that other unrecognized agents
have yet to be discovered. The known bacterial and viral pathogens
responsible for acute gastroenteritis in infants and children are
listed in Table 9-1. Gastrointestinal infections caused by protozoa
(e.g. amebiasis, giardiasis) and other parasitic diseases are discussed separately in Chapter 16. Food poisoning, that is, the ingestion of foods contaminated with Staphylococcus aureus, Clostridium perfringens, Bacillus cereus or Vibrio parahaemolyticus, must
also be included in the differential diagnosis of acute diarrhea.

9.1: ESCHERICHIA COLI

INTRODUCTION: Escherichia coli is a normal inhabitant of the intestinal tract of man and animals and is widely distributed in nature.
Infantile diarrhea remains a major problem in the U.S., despite advances in nutrition and improved sanitation. These infections begin
as sporadic, isolated events in the nursery but soon spread by fecal

TABLE 9-1: ETIOLOGIC AGENTS OF ACUTE BACTERIAL AND VIRAL GASTROENTERITIS	
COMMON	**LESS COMMON**
1. Rotaviruses	1. Viruses (Entero, Adeno, Norwalk, Hawaii)

2. E. coli:
  a. Enteropathic
  b. Enterotoxic
	2. Clostridium perfringens, Cl. botulinum

3. Salmonella	3. Bacillus cereus
4. Shigella	4. Staphylococcus aureus
	5. Vibrio parahaemolyticus, V. fetus
	6. Yersinia enterocoliticus

contamination of the environment or through contact with the contaminated hands or clothing of nursery personnel. The situation abruptly develops into an epidemic involving the majority of infants within the contaminated area. The outbreak may be quite prolonged and may result in a high number of infantile deaths. The majority of reported epidemics of gastroenteritis in newborn infants are caused by enteropathogenic E. coli (EPEC). Infants are usually not asymptomatic carriers. Recent reports indicate that enterotoxigenic strains of E. coli are an important cause of acute diarrhea of childhood in some areas. The relationship of various strains of E. coli to diarrhea is not well defined at the present time and requires further study.

1. ETIOLOGY AND PATHOGENESIS

E. coli infantile diarrhea can be the result of the action of an enterotoxin or the result of invasion of the distal intestinal mucosa. Capabilities to produce enterotoxin and to invade the epithelial cells are not exclusive and may co-exist in the same E. coli strain. The release of enterotoxin depends on outward diffusion or transport through the bacterial cell wall and not on cell lysis. The unique property of the enterotoxin is that it acts on the mucosa of the small intestine causing intracellular increase in cyclic AMP which, in turn, leads to increased electrolyte and fluid secretion. There is no damage to the epithelium, and recovery is dependent upon supportive therapy to counteract acidosis and dehydration.

In some recent epidemics, 10 to 30 percent of the illnesses have been caused by invasive E. coli. These organisms proliferate in the lamina propria where PMN leukocytes accumulate. Occasionally there is lymphatic involvement with spread to the mesenteric lymph nodes. Production of inflammatory exudate is manifested by the presence of PMN leukocytes in the stool.

Numerous specific antibodies including hemagglutinins for E. coli have been found in the secretory IgA fraction of colostrum. Resistance of breast-fed babies to attacks of diarrhea suggest that colostral antibodies against E. coli are protective. Secretory IgA, which resists digestion and does not fix complement, has a tendency to adhere to the mucosal surface without being absorbed by the mucosa. Although plasma cells in the lamina propria produce IgA following antigenic stimulation, the wide variety of serotypes of organisms combined with age of these patients preclude the use of oral vaccines for infants. The best measures remain preventive, that is, minimizing fecal contamination of the environment, monitoring personal habits and whenever possible, isolating infants who acquire the illness.

Transfer of the toxin producing capability to other strains of E. coli involves a plasmid, that is, the transfer of an extra chromosomal genetic determinant located in the cytoplasm. The mechanism for such a transfer is conjugation, the same mechanism responsible for unit transfer of multiple antibiotic resistance.

2. CLINICAL MANIFESTATIONS

Following ingestion and passage through the stomach, E. coli organisms colonize and multiply in the upper gastrointestinal tract. Manifestations of this host-parasite interaction are usually evident after 2 to 6 days, but the incubation time can be as short as 18 hours. In toxigenic diarrhea, the enterotoxin is adsorbed to the mucosa in the small intestine and results in the production of a watery stool which is yellow-green in color and foul smelling. There may be a low grade fever or no fever, vomiting and some abdominal cramps. Sigmoidoscopic examination will be normal. In severe cases, acidosis and dehydration may lead to rapid circulatory collapse.

The invasive strains of E. coli multiply in the lumen and spread to the distal intestine, where invasion of the epithelium proceeds, producing colitis associated with positive findings on sigmoidoscopy. Fever abdominal cramps and leukocytosis are common. In the watery stools, PMN leukocytes are abundant, along with mucus strands and occasionally blood.

A complication of invasive E. coli enteritis is the development of bacteremia.

3. DIAGNOSIS

The presence of PMN leukocytes in the stool is a basis for differentiating invasion disease from toxigenic disease. However, the specific etiology as shown in Table 9-2 cannot be determined on this

TABLE 9-2: ORGANISMS MOST FREQUENTLY IMPLICATED IN BACTERIAL DIARRHEA IN CHILDREN AND INFANTS

Organism	Mode of Transmission	Incubation Time	Toxin	Mucosal Invasion	Leukocytes	Fever	Vomiting	Blood in Stools
E. coli (Enterotoxic)	Food, water, fecal contamination	8–14 hrs.	+	–	–	$\pm$	+	–
E. coli (Enteropathic)	Food, water, fecal contamination	8–24 hrs.	–	$\pm$	PMNs	+++	–	++
Shigellosis	Man to man	1–5 days	–	+	PMNs	+++	$\pm$	++
Salmonellosis (except typhoid)	Food, water	8–48 hrs.	–	++	PMNs	++	++	+

basis alone, or simply on the basis of signs and symptoms. The
stool specimen should be microscopically examined for the presence
of WBCs. The sample, which consists of a small amount of feces
taken from the edge and not the middle of the fresh specimen, is
emulsified in a small drop of saline on a clean glass slide and then
mixed with 2 drops of Loeffler's methylene blue. The mixture is
covered with a glass coverslip and after 2 to 3 minutes examined
microscopically. PMNs are present in invasive E. coli infection
but absent in a strictly toxigenic disease. PMNs are not seen in
EPEC stool specimens obtained from healthy people.

Laboratory identification of the specific etiologic agent is readily
achieved through culture procedures or by using the fluorescent
antibody technique for presumptive diagnosis. Cultures can be obtained by rectal swabs or from fresh fecal specimens. Laboratory
differentiation of bacterial pathogens is summarized in Table 9.3.

Serologic typing of E. coli is useful for monitoring an epidemic or
for determining whether recurrence of disease is due to relapse or
reinfection. The antigens which make up the complete serotype include: (1) the O or somatic lipopolysaccharide - protein cell wall
(endotoxin), (2) the H or flagellar protein antigen, and (3) the K or
envelope polysaccharide antigens which are further subclassified
into L A and B types. Less than 10% of the 150 O types are associated with gastroenteritis. Serologic typing, that is, identification of
O group, may be partially carried out by the hospital diagnostic laboratory. It is necessary to use a reference laboratory for more specific serotype identification in differentiating the 150 O, 50 H and
80 K antigens.

Laboratory determinations for enterotoxin production are not routinely carried out at the present time. A simple biochemical assay
is not yet available. Three different assays which are available include: (1) induction of fluid secretion in the ligated ileal loop of
adult rabbit intestine, (2) fluid accumulation in the intestine of infant
rabbits following orogastric inoculation of broth culture as measured
by increased weight, and (3) a most recently developed tissue culture
assay using Chinese hamster ovary cells in which morphological
changes result after exposure to toxin.

4. MANAGEMENT

Management of gastroenteritis caused by E. coli consists primarily
of administering oral or parenteral fluids and electrolytes to correct
dehydration and acidosis resulting from diarrhea. Use of drugs
which decrease bowel motility are not indicated because such therapy
may enhance the invasive disease by promoting further in vivo proliferation of the bacteria. Further, these drugs are potentially harmful in infants and children. The use of antibiotics for treatment is
controversial. Antibiotic treatment of invasive infections has been

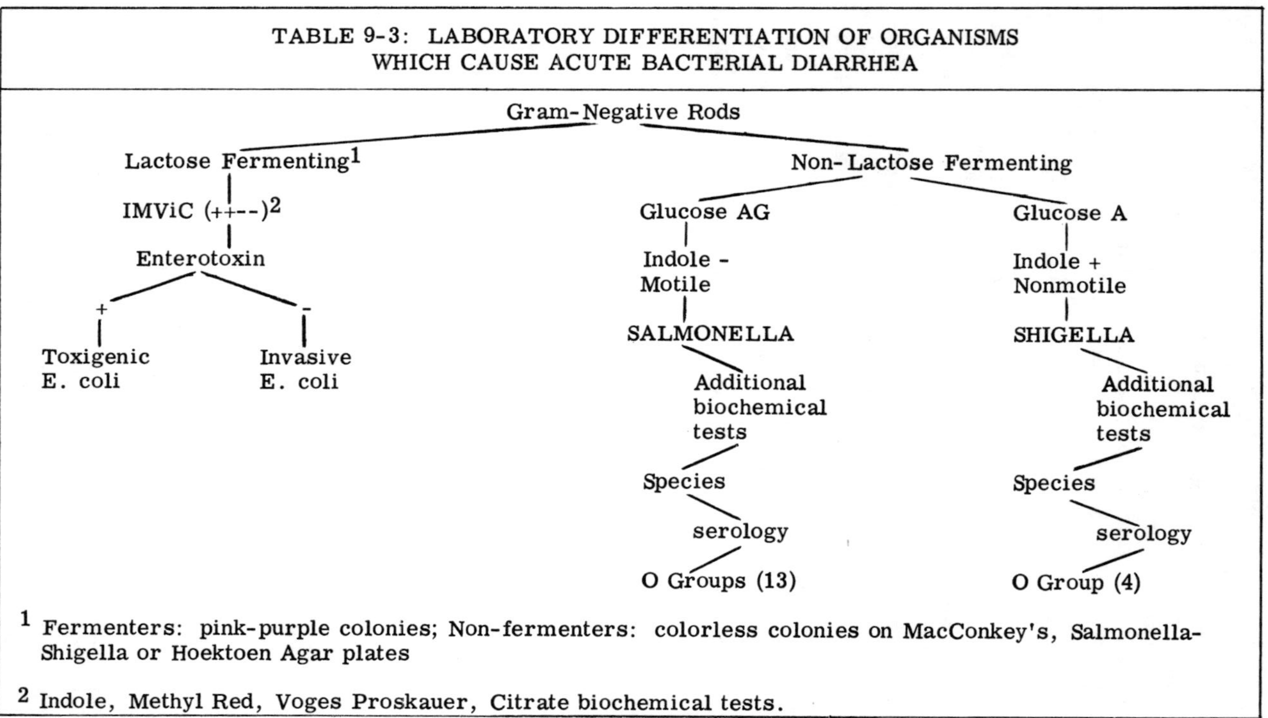

[1] Fermenters: pink-purple colonies; Non-fermenters: colorless colonies on MacConkey's, Salmonella-Shigella or Hoektoen Agar plates

[2] Indole, Methyl Red, Voges Proskauer, Citrate biochemical tests.

shown to decrease the manifestations of systemic clinical illness
and to decrease the number of organisms excreted in the stool. A
nonabsorbable bacterial antibiotic such as neomycin or colistin may
be used for 3 to 5 days.

Chemoprophylaxis should be limited to use for control of nursery
epidemics, since illness usually develops in all infants in the contaminated area. The antibiotic of choice for exposed infants is
neomycin.

::

9.2: SALMONELLOSIS

INTRODUCTION: Nontyphoidal salmonellosis accounts for approximately 5% of infectious diarrheas during infancy. Sporadic outbreaks, which account for 55 percent of isolates, occur most frequently in children under 5 years of age. In infants, the overall
mortality rate for salmonellosis is 6 percent but varies depending
on the species of salmonella responsible for the epidemic. This
compares to an overall mortality in the U.S. of 1 to 2% in 2,000,000
adult cases of salmonellosis during 1975. In man, the source of infection is food or water contaminated with any of over 1400 serotypes of Salmonella. The vast natural reservoir for these organisms
is lower animals, which includes pets such as turtles, birds, dogs,
mice, rats and horses. Food sources include chickens, turkeys,
ducks and other animal meats which are cooked insufficiently. Even
after proper cooking, foods can be recontaminated with dirty uten-
sils, or prepared foods may be contaminated following handling by a
convalescent patient or human chronic carrier. In addition, hospital supplies such as carmine dye, used in gastroenterologic examinations, thyroid tablets, liver extracts and lactalbumin have been
found to be contaminated with Salmonella and responsible for hospital acquired infections. In 1965, an epidemic in Riverside, California, involving over 16,000 people, was traced to inadequate chlorination of the drinking water. The organism responsible for this
epidemic was S. typhimurium.

Neonatal exposure to organisms can occur during the process of
delivery or contamination following delivery, for example through
maternal exposure, by nursery personnel or environmental contamination. Gastroenteritis which persists can lead to bacteremia.

1. ETIOLOGY AND PATHOGENESIS

Non-typhoidal salmonellosis includes over 1400 different serotypes
of Salmonella. These organisms have no particular host preference
and readily multiply in the gastrointestinal tract of the invaded host.
In the U.S., the 10 species which account for 70% of human salmonellosis are typhimurium (responsible for 20 percent of cases), en-
teritidis, newport, heidelberg, infantis, st. paul, thompson, blockley,

derby and typhi. The incubation time is a function of dose of organisms contained in the ingested food or water. Gastroenteritis in young children usually develops in 8 to 48 hours but can begin as early as 6 hours after ingestion or require several days before becoming manifest. The ingested bacteria multiply in the lumen of the small intestine and colon and then invade the epithelial lining with minimal destruction of the mucosa. Within the lamina propria, PMN leukocytes accumulate in the cases of non-typhoidal salmonellosis, whereas in S. typhi infection, monocytes predominate. If the inflammatory response is not contained, infection spreads via the lymphatics to the Peyer's patches or mesenteric lymph nodes (enteric fever) from which point invasion of the bloodstream proceeds. Ulceration, hemorrhage and perforation in the intestine is very seldom seen in children. Serum agglutinins develop in response to both lymphatic and bloodstream involvement.

Some predisposing conditions are known to promote salmonellosis. These include reduced gastric acidity, alteration of normal flora after antibiotic treatment, hemolytic anemias and disorders of immunity, such as immunosuppressive therapy, leukemia or lymphoma.

2. CLINICAL MANIFESTATIONS

Gastroenteritis due to infection by Salmonella has an abrupt onset characterized by fever, myalgia, headache and malaise. Within hours, cramps, nausea, vomiting and diarrhea are manifested, along with a more pronounced fever. Additional physical findings are scant. The stools are watery and numerous. Microscopic examination of the fecal material may show pus, blood and mucus. Usually the fever will drop within 1 to 2 days, while the diarrhea persists for 2 to 4 days, followed by complete recovery. Excretion of organisms in the stool continues for 2 to 4 weeks or longer. In the more severe form of Salmonella gastroenteritis, dehydration may lead to cyanosis, hypothermia and circulatory collapse. Sepsis, meningitis, pneumonia, and osteomyelitis may be present.

3. DIAGNOSIS

Gastroenteritis due to Salmonella cannot be differentially diagnosed on the basis of signs and symptoms. It is therefore necessary to isolate and identify the organisms recovered from a fresh stool specimen or a rectal swab specimen. The fecal material is emulsified in sterile saline or broth and inoculated on Desoxycholate citrate, Salmonella-Shigella or MacConkey's agar plates, and into Selenite F or Tetrathionate enrichment broths. On these selective agar plates colorless colonies (non-lactose fermenting organisms) grow out in 24 hours and are then subcultured into the appropriate differential media for identification of species. Salmonella are gram negative, non-spore forming, non-lactose fermenting rods and are motile.

The Kaufmann-White scheme defines the serologic types in immunologic terms by antigenic formulas, identifying the somatic (O), the
flagella (H), and the polysaccharide envelope (Vi) antigens for each
isolate. Using monospecific O antisera, the Salmonella are grouped
into 13 O types. In the U.S., 98 percent of organisms causing gastroenteritis fall into eight O groups, A through E3. Within an O
group the nomenclature used for identifying species usually reflects
the geographic location in which the isolate was identified as the
etiologic agent in the outbreak. For monitoring epidemics, the
more reliable method for identification of organisms is phage typing.
The phage groups are A through T, with arabic numbering of strains
within a group. For example, there are 80 phage types of S. typhimurium. These combined methods have produced the current classification scheme for over 1400 serotypes.

4. MANAGEMENT

Gastroenteritis caused by Salmonella is characterized by numerous
watery stools. Prolonged diarrhea can lead to dehydration and acidosis for which supportive measures, such as fluid and electrolyte
replacement, may be necessary. In children, peristaltic function is
more effective in cleansing the intestines than antibiotics. It has
been shown that antibiotic treatment does not shorten the clinical
course, but it prolongs fecal excretion of organisms and increases
the problem of transfer of multiple drug resistance to any organism
within the family Enterobacteriaceae. Antibiotics are not indicated
for uncomplicated enteritis except in neonates, in seriously ill patients, or in patients with immunologic deficiencies. Kanamycin,
ampicillin, or chloramphenicol have been effective in treating these
patients; however, because of the multiple drug resistance problem,
continued treatment should be governed by the results of the antibiotic susceptibility tests.

9.3: TYPHOID FEVER

INTRODUCTION: Typhoid fever, a multisystem disease with a wide
spectrum of clinical manifestations, is caused by S. typhi, whereas
the clinical syndrome, enteric fever, can be caused by S. typhi,
S. paratyphi A or S. paratyphi B. During 1975 there were 375 cases
of typhoid fever in the U.S. In a recent study reported from Scotland, the incidence of typhoid fever among children for the period
1967-1974 was 194 cases, with the lowest incidence (15.5%) being
among children less than 5 years of age and the highest incidence
being in the 15-24 year age group. There appears to be some seasonal variation coincident with vacation travel to areas where endemic infections are recognized.

1. ETIOLOGY AND PATHOGENESIS

The etiologic agents of enteric fever are <u>S. typhi</u>, <u>S. paratyphi A</u> and <u>S. paratyphi B</u>.

The portal of entry is by way of the mouth, following ingestion of food such as eggs or canned meat, or following the drinking of contaminated water. The ingested organisms multiply in the gastrointestinal tract and invade the mucosa with continued multiplication in the submucosa. The bacteria are phagocytized by macrophages but remain viable within these cells and, therefore, are disseminated systemically as facultative intracellular parasites. After prolonged fever, bacteremia and relocation of infection in the submucosal lymphoic tissue of the small intestine, gastrointestinal symptoms are manifested. Constipation or diarrhea may result. In the terminal ileum, the lymph follicles become hyperplastic with buttonlike protrusions into the lumen. Within the bowel, the Peyer's patches become enlarged, raised and sharply delineated. Necrosis may develop and lead to ulceration of the mucosa, without involvement of the muscularis, followed by complete healing without any scarring. Although secondary spread of infection frequently occurs in adults, it is not usually seen in children.

2. CLINICAL MANIFESTATIONS

In children, the gastrointestinal manifestations of typhoid fever vary considerably. These include vomiting, constipation and diarrhea. Bloody stools and abdominal distension may occur.

Typhoid fever in infants differs significantly from the disease seen in older children and adults. The diagnosis is often made by the chance isolation of <u>S. typhi</u> from stool cultures. Clinical manifestations may be minimum or resemble bacillary dysentery. Rose spots are less common than in adults and leukocytosis is the rule, with white blood counts frequently above 20,000 cells/mm^3. The course of the disease is usually abbreviated, rarely lasting more than 2 weeks.

In children, severe complications of typhoid fever include bowel perforation. These complications are associated with high mortality rates. Other complications include meningitis, pneumonia, cholecystitis, arthritis, nephritis and osteomyelitis. A rare but usually fatal complication of typhoid fever is acute disseminated encephalomyelitis.

3. DIAGNOSIS

In 90 percent of the typhoid fever cases, <u>S. typhi</u> may be recovered from the blood, urine or stool. Injudicious use of antibiotics may result in failure to recover organisms from these specimens and, in such cases, one should examine the bone marrow for facultative

intracellular parasites residing in the macrophages. The Widal
test, an assay for elevation of humoral antibody response to the O
and Vi antigens, is based on a 4-fold or greater increase in titer
over a 2-3 week interval. This test, while useful, is frequently
inaccurate, and therefore only suggestive for the diagnosis of typhoid fever. Another useful diagnostic test is to X-ray the bowel
and look for uniform dilatation of the ileum, but not the jejunum.

S. paratyphi A or B are more routinely recovered from cultures of
stool specimens rather than from blood or urine specimens.

4. MANAGEMENT

Patients with typhoid fever should be placed in strict isolation in the
hospital. The antibiotics of choice for treating this infectious disease are chloramphenicol, ampicillin, amoxicillin or trimethoprim-
sulfamethoxazole (see page 571). Although clinical improvement is
evident within 48 to 72 hours, treatment should be continued for two
to three weeks. The complications of chloramphenicol treatment
include granulocytopenia and aplastic anemia. Antibiotic susceptibility tests should be made for every isolate, and should be the basis for selecting the appropriate antibiotic.

Hydration and electrolyte balance must be monitored carefully during the primary phase of this illness. No laxatives or enemas should
be given because of the danger of intestinal perforation and hemorrhage. In children, the latter complication has been surgically managed with a simple suture or resection of the intestine.

Following an episode of typhoid fever, the patient may excrete the
organisms for months. Therefore, stool cultures should be taken
every 2 weeks to survey for carrier state. If the specimens are
persistently positive for up to 3 months, the patient is classified a
carrier. Those individuals should be given an X-ray of the biliary
tract to check for the presence of stones in the gall bladder for which
cholecystectomy is the treatment of choice. In lieu of gall bladder
stone formation, antibiotic treatment for an additional 4-6 weeks is
usually needed.

Three consecutive negative specimens are consistent with successful
eradication of the infection. The latter response is generally observed in children.

9.4: SHIGELLOSIS

INTRODUCTION: Shigella are naturally found in man and monkeys.
Man-to-man transmission of disease may result from ingestion of
fewer than 200 organisms transmitted via contaminated fingers, food,

flies or feces. Epidemic shigellosis is seen in military camps, institutions for the mentally retarded and on Indian reservations in the United States. The species most frequently isolated in the U.S. are S. sonnei (72%) and S. flexneri (24%). The highest incidence of dysentery for species other than S. dysenteriae is among children 1 to 4 years of age. Overall, shigellosis accounts for 1.5 percent of infectious diarrheas in infancy. Although infections can occur during any season, they are more prevalent during the warm months of the year.

1. ETIOLOGY AND PATHOGENESIS

The Shigella are classified into 4 groups: A, B, C and D, which are synonymous with the species names: dysenteriae, flexneri, boydii and sonnei. Within each of these species there are several different serologic types.

The small number of ingested organisms invade the epithelial cells lining the mucosa of the distal colon, sigmoid colon and rectum. The incubation period is usually less than 4 days but ranges from 1 to 7 days. The bacteria multiply in the lamina propria, evoking an intense PMN leukocyte inflammatory response. The mucosa becomes diffusely swollen, with engorged vessels and punctate hemorrhages. There is increased secretion of mucus. Thrombosis of arterioles results in necrosis followed by formation of a yellow membrane over the surface of a shallow irregular ulceration that usually stops at the submucosa. The ulcer seldom perforates, rather it heals with formation of granulation tissue containing both PMN and monocytic leukocytes. New epithelium grows from the margins of the mucosa covering the ulcer. Shigella also produce an enterotoxin which may contribute to the production of the watery diarrhea by promoting fluid and electrolyte loss. The mode of action of this enterotoxin is at present unknown. It does not cause an increase in cyclic AMP levels in the cells and therefore is not similar to the enterotoxins of E. coli or Vibrio cholerae.

2. CLINICAL MANIFESTATIONS

In children, shigellosis is manifested by high fever, headaches, delirium, lethargy and convulsions. Diarrhea is explosive, with watery stools during the initial phase which, in time, decrease in quantity, even though the number of movements remains high. Tenesmus is a common problem. The stools contain many PMN leukocytes, mucus and blood. The acute symptoms may persist for 7 to 10 days. Convalescence may be prolonged, and is characterized as a time in which the patient may have as many as 7 to 12 movements per day. Dehydration becomes apparent, in that the eyes are sunken, the skin and mucus membranes are dry and, in infants, the anterior fontanelle is sunken. Severe acidosis develops because of electrolyte losses. These combined effects lead to prostration, peripheral

vascular collapse and death within 1 to 2 days. The mortality rate
varies inversely with the socioeconomic level and is highest for
children under 2 years of age.

3. DIAGNOSIS

Shigellosis is an invasive gastroenteritis which, on the basis of
signs and symptoms, cannot be differentially diagnosed from salmonellosis or invasive E. coli disease. Because overgrowth by
other organisms in the fecal specimen is a practical consideration,
specimens for culture must be processed promptly. Culture procedures are similar to those for Salmonella. Shigella can easily be
differentiated from Salmonella (see Table 9-3). The Shigella also
produce a heat labile and low molecular weight enterotoxin.

As with any invasive enteritis, microscopic examination of a methylene blue preparation of the stool specimen will reveal many fecal
leukocytes, blood and mucus. Excretion of leukocytes persists for
up to 8 days after symptoms have subsided. Sigmoidoscopic examination reveals intense inflammation of the mucosa with a fibrinous
membrane or localized ulceration of the mucosa surrounded by a
gray area of necrosis.

4. MANAGEMENT

Supportive measures are generally needed in severe cases. These
include administration of electrolytes and fluids to control acidosis
and dehydration, and blood or plasma transfusions to manage circulatory collapse. Following reinstitution of oral alimentation with
fluid, the patients should then be maintained on a low residue, high
protein diet for several days.

Antibiotic treatment has been shown to reduce the period of morbidity
and the duration of excretion of bacteria in the stool. However, the
effectiveness of treatment may be limited by rapid selection of antibiotic resistant organisms. Multiple resistance factors, plasmids,
are rapidly transferred by conjugation to other organisms within the
family Enterobacteriaceae. Ampicillin, chloramphenicol, colistin,
kanamycin, or neomycin have been used in the past. Final selection
should be based on results of the laboratory antibiotic susceptibility
tests. Recently, trimethoprim-sulfamethoxazole (page 571) has been
used with good results.

The best methods for control and prevention of shigellosis include
improved sanitation, purification and protection of water supplies,
pasteurization of milk, care in food preparation, and fly control.
Handwashing and hygiene are very important considerations.

An oral vaccine has been developed using attenuated organisms.
When tested in human volunteers this vaccine has not provided long
lasting protection. Repeated oral vaccination may be useful in institutional settings or in hyperendemic regions.

::

9.5: FOOD POISONING

INTRODUCTION: Food poisoning can be classified as an infection
or an intoxication resulting from the ingestion of food or water contaminated at some point during production, processing or storage.
The outcome of exposure to contaminated food will be determined
by the number of organisms present and the method of food preparation. An outbreak is defined as an incident in which 2 or more persons experience a similar illness after ingesting a common food.
The incidence of confirmed bacterial food poisoning in the United
States is listed in Table 9-4. The incidence of food poisoning is
steady throughout the year with only salmonellosis showing any seasonal trend, that is, occurring more frequently in the months from
April through November. Improper food handling is responsible for
more than half of these outbreaks.

1. ETIOLOGY AND PATHOGENESIS

Among the bacteria which have been implicated as etiologic agents of
food poisoning are C. perfringens, Staph. aureus, Salmonella species, hemolytic Streptococci, Escherichia coli, Vibrio parahaemolyticus and Bacillus cereus. Food poisoning is less frequently caused
by Brucella species and C. botulinum (see Table 9-4). Pathogens
which are suspected, but not confirmed, to be etiologic agents in
foodborne disease include group D Streptococcus, Yersinia entero-
coliticus, Citrobacter, Enterobacter, Klebsiella, Pseudomonas,
and presumably viral agents.

The foods involved include cereal, custards, pudding, meat loaf,
sauces and gravy, stews, cooked meats, dairy products, vegetables,
rice, lettuce and home prepared foods and preserves. In food poisoning classified as infections, the organisms are present in the food,
survive passage in the stomach, and multiply in the intestine and
other parts of the alimentary tract resulting in acute diarrhea and
vomiting. The intoxication form of food poisoning may result following ingestion of food containing preformed enterotoxin, i.e., Staph.
aureus or C. botulinum, or following proliferation of the toxin-pro-
ducing bacteria in the intestine, i.e., enteropathogenic E. coli or
C. perfringens. In the former type of food poisoning, the outcome of
exposure will be influenced by the heat stability or heat lability of the
toxin and, therefore, by the method of food preparation. Whereas
the enterotoxin of Staph aureus is heat stable, that of C. botulinum is
heat labile (Table 9-5).

TABLE 9-4: CONFIRMED BACTERIAL FOODBORNE DISEASE IN THE UNITED STATES, 1973-1974		
	NO. OF OUTBREAKS (NO. OF CASES)	
BACTERIA	1973	1974
B. cereus	1 (2)	1 (11)
Brucella	1 (4)	0 (0)
C. botulinum	10 (31)	21 (32)
C. perfringens	9 (1,424)	15 (863)
Salmonella	33 (2,462)	35 (5,499)
Shigella	8 (1,388)	3 (212)
Staphylococcus	20 (1,272)	43 (1,565)
Group A Streptococcus	1 (250)	1 (325)
V. cholerae	0 (0)	1 (6)
V. parahaemolyticus	1 (2)	0 (0)
Suspect Group D Streptococci	0 (0)	2 (38)
Total	84 (6,835)	122 (8,551)

From "Foodborne and waterborne diseases outbreak," Center for Disease Control, DHEW Publication No. (CDC) 76-8185, January 1976.

2. CLINICAL MANIFESTATIONS

Because the food poisoning syndrome is caused by a variety of bacteria and/or preformed toxins, there is considerable variability in the time of incubation and in the clinical manifestations of the illness. In general, the incubation time is short, varying between 1 and 24 hours. The duration of symptoms is also relatively short, ranging from 1 to 2 days, except for salmonellosis, for which the mean duration time is 5 to 6 days. In general, the manifestations include abdominal cramps, diarrhea, and nausea or vomiting. Fever is relatively uncommon, except for food poisoning caused by Salmonella. For the majority of patients, complete recovery is evident after 48 hours.

TABLE 9-5: PROPERTIES OF ENTEROTOXINS CONTRIBUTING TO GASTROINTESTINAL INFECTIONS

ENTEROTOXINS		CHARACTERISTIC OF TOXIN	
Organism	Disease	Heat Lability	Mode of Action
E. coli	Neonatal diarrhea	+	Elevation of cyclic AMP -->electrolyte and fluid loss via intestinal lumen.
Vibrio cholerae	Cholera	+	Elevation of cyclic AMP -- >electrolyte and fluid loss via intestinal lumen.
Shigella dysenteriae	Dysentery	+	Unknown.
Staph. aureus	Food poisoning	-	Absorbed; acts on CNS
Clos. perfringens	Food poisoning	+	Causes fluid accumulation in lumen of intestine.
B. cereus	Food poisoning	+	Unknown
Clos. botulinum	Food poisoning	+	Blocks neural transmission at neuromuscular junction of skeletal muscle.
Ps. aeruginosa	Enteritis necroticans	+	Unknown

Botulism, however, is an exception, in that the effects of the toxin are systemic and progressive. The toxin which acts by blocking neural transmission at the neuromuscular junction of skeletal muscles causes a paralysis of the muscles of the larynx, pharynx and eyes. This intoxication also paralyzes the muscles of the respiratory tract, thereby interfering with respiratory function, and causes a general weakness of the muscles in the extremities.

Recently, infant botulism has been described (Pickett, et al., 1976; Midura, et al., 1976). Clinical features of infant botulism include constipation, poor feeding, weak cry, hypotonia, and muscle weakness with loss of head control. Cranial nerve abnormalities are common (e.g. ptosis, ophthalmoplegia, flaccid facial expression, pooled oral secretions, dysphagia, and a weak gag reflex). Respiratory arrests develop in a significant number of patients. The incidence and clinical spectrum of this newly recognized disease have yet to be defined.

Staph aureus, a common cause of food poisoning, can produce a severe prostrating illness resulting from the ingestion of preformed enterotoxin in the food. The illness has an explosive onset, usually within 7 hours after ingesting the food, but rapid recovery without complications is the rule.

3. DIAGNOSIS

For the diagnosis of food poisoning, a complete patient history must be taken and should include history of exposure to contaminated food, as well as a check for similar symptoms among other people who may have eaten the suspected food. The most useful specimens include samples of the gastric contents, feces and suspected food. A gram stain of a smear of the specimens and both aerobic and anaerobic cultures are necessary for laboratory confirmation of bacterial food poisoning. Admission to the hospital is recommended only for patients in which dehydration is severe, or for patients who have some underlying illness.

4. MANAGEMENT

Most cases of food poisoning associated with Staph aureus and C. perfringens are mild and self-limited. The usual treatment consists of bed rest, no food intake for 12 to 24 hours if vomiting is severe, and replacement of fluid and electrolyte losses through oral administration of an electrolyte-glucose-water solution. If dehydration is severe, the hospitalized patient should be given the electrolyte and glucose solution parenterally. Administration of antibiotics is usually not recommended except for outbreaks of streptococcal food-borne infections and for botulism.

Botulism is a very serious intoxication, the systemic manifestations of which must be carefully monitored in order to make available the appropriate life supporting equipment. A primary consideration is the removal of any unabsorbed toxin. This is done by inducing vomiting, performing gastric lavage and giving an enema after oral administration of magnesium citrate. Serum, gastric contents and food specimens should be analyzed for toxin. The patient should be skin tested for hypersensitivity to horse serum before administration of the trivalent (ABE) antitoxin. If hypersensitivity to horse serum is present, human antitoxin is available from the Center for Disease Control in Atlanta, Georgia. If the patient is not hypersensitive, antitoxin is administered intravenously and intramuscularly every two hours as needed. To eradicate any viable organisms present in the intestinal contents phenoxymethyl penicillin should be given for 2 days. The role of botulinum antitoxin and antibiotics in the treatment of infant botulism has not been evaluated.

If commercial products are involved in food poisoning, prompt notification of local health authorities is necessary to avoid additional cases. The suspected food should be saved for laboratory confirmation.

The best control measure for preventing food poisoning is education. Although individuals involved in food preparation and who practice poor hygiene or have active skin lesions, may contaminate foods at any point in the processing, everyone may participate at all times in preventing food poisoning through the proper handling, storage and preparation of all foods destined for human consumption.

::

9.6: VIRAL GASTROENTERITIS

INTRODUCTION AND EPIDEMIOLOGY: Recently, morphologically identical viruses have been detected in fecal extracts in many parts of the world. Because these viruses have not been fully characterized, different investigators have applied a variety of names, e.g. rotaviruses, orbiviruses, reo-like viruses, duoviruses, infantile gastroenteritis virus, etc. (Bishop, R.F. et al., 1973; Flewett, T.H. et al., 1974-a; Kapikian, A.Z. et al., 1974). Before the official name is given to these viruses, we shall temporarily refer to this group of agents as rotaviruses.

Available evidence suggests rotaviruses are the major cause of acute diarrheal disease in infants and young children throughout the world. As many as 50 to 80% of infants and children hospitalized with gastroenteritis may have infections caused by this virus, which are particularly prevalent during the colder months of the year. Most of the infections occur in infants and children between 6 months and 3 years of age. Rotaviruses are rarely seen in adults and in children older than 6 years of age, or in children who have experienced previous gastroenteritis. Infection is associated with a rise in antibody titer and apparent induction of long-lasting immunity.

Transmission of infection probably occurs by the fecal-oral route. Disease may be transmitted by close contact and is highly contagious among hospitalized infants.

Two antigenically distinct agents, Norwalk and Hawaii, isolated from an outbreak of diarrhea, may also induce a self-limited disease characterized by vomiting and/or diarrhea in adults and children (Kapikian, A.Z. et al., 1972; Wyatt, R.G. et al., 1974-a). Although enteroviruses and adenoviruses have been associated with localized outbreaks of acute gastroenteritis in humans, they will probably be less prevalent than the rotaviruses.

The clinical features and histopathological lesions produced by these newly identified viruses are very similar to the general features of viral gastroenteritis and are not diagnostic of disease caused by a specific agent. This chapter will discuss primarily what is known about rotaviruses.

1. ETIOLOGY AND PATHOGENESIS

The role of bacteria in infectious diarrhea is well established. On the other hand, the etiologic role of viruses in gastroenteritis, with the exception of rotaviruses, is less well defined. As mentioned above, several agents produce acute viral gastroenteritis, a common illness in infants and children characterized predominantly by vomiting and diarrhea. Among those agents, the newly recognized rotaviruses are probably the most important cause of acute infantile diarrhea (Davidson et al., 1975) (Table 9-6). Other viral agents involved in acute diarrheal diseases in humans and animals are listed in Table 9-7.

1.1: Rotaviruses: The evidence that suggests human rotaviruses are an important etiologic agent of infantile diarrhea includes: (1) the virus is seen in large numbers in feces, upper intestinal juice and epithelium of duodenal mucosa in acute cases, but not in normal controls or in convalescent cases, (2) seroconversion is demonstrated in most infected children, and (3) oral transmission of infection has been successful with one adult volunteer (Middleton et al., 1974).

The human rotavirus has not been well characterized. The rotavirus is a 60-65 nm RNA virus belonging to the family Reoviruidae. Although morphologically similar to reoviruses and orbiviruses, it differs in its fine structure and serological response (Kapikian, A.Z. et al., 1974; Flewett, T.H. et al., 1974-b). The virus consists of a core (38 nm) surrounded by a characteristic double-shelled capsid with the inner layer of capsids radiating outward in a wheel-like (or rotary fashion "rota"). Antigenically, by complement-fixation and immunofluorescent testing, the human rotaviruses are related to the epidemic diarrhea of infant mice virus and Nebraska calf diarrhea virus. However, the human virus and the animal viruses are probably not identical.

TABLE 9-6: ENTERIC PATHOGENS IN FECES FROM 378 CHILDREN WITH ACUTE ENTERITIS AND 116 CONTROL GROUP (MELBOURNE, AUSTRALIA)

AGENTS	PATIENT (%)	CONTROL (%)
"Rotaviruses"	52	0
Salmonella spp.	11	1
Adenoviruses	7	8
Enteroviruses	2	8
"Enteropathogenic" E. coli	2	3
Shigella spp.	1	0

(Modified from Davidson, G.P. et al. Lancet 1:242, 1975)

TABLE 9-7: VIRAL AGENTS INVOLVED IN DIARRHEA IN HUMANS AND ANIMALS

HUMANS	ANIMALS
1. Rotaviruses*	1. Neonatal calf (pig) diarrhea virus
2. Norwalk	2. Epidemic diarrhea of mice
3. Hawaii	3. SA 11 virus (sheep)
4. Enteroviruses (?)	4. O agent (cattle)
5. Adenoviruses (?)	

* Rotaviruses are antigenically related to neonatal calf (pig) diarrhea virus and epidemic diarrhea of mice.

The excretion of rotaviruses is greatest during the 3rd and 4th day
of illness and is usually not detectable after one week. Viral particles are seen in the epithelial cells of duodenal mucosa during the
acute stage of illness when associated histological abnormalities
and depressed dissacharidase levels in duodenal mucosa are also
present (Bishop et al., 1974). In some patients, severe morphological changes with flattening of villi and derangement of surface
epithelium occur (Bishop et al., 1973; Middleton et al., 1974). But
in others no lesions are found. Histopathological changes of duodenal mucosa usually return to normal in 4 to 6 weeks.

1.2: Norwalk Agent: During an outbreak of gastroenteritis in Norwalk, Ohio, a small (27 nm), RNA relatively heat-stable virus was
detected in stools. Transmissability of infection due to this virus
has been demonstrated in volunteers. This virus induces symptoms
consisting of vomiting, diarrhea, often accompanied by low-grade
fever, abdominal cramps, and malaise. Both viral particles and
antibody responses are detected in naturally and experimentally infected individuals (Kapikian et al., 1972; Wyatt, et al., 1974-a).

Histopathological changes occur primarily in the jejunal mucosa and
consist of blunted villi with infiltration of predominantly mononuclear, and some polymorphonuclear, leukocytes in the lamina propria. This cellular infiltration occurs with the onset of clinical illness (48 hours) and resolves during convalescence (Agus et al.,
1973; Dolin et al., 1972; Schreiber et al., 1973). Transient lymphopenia occurs within 48 hours of the infection when symptoms of
acute clinical illness are present (Dolin et al., 1976). The depletion
of circulating lymphocytes temporally coincides with the onset of
clinical illness and parallels the accumulation of lymphocytes in the
jejunal mucosa. Thus, the lymphopenia is likely due to redistribu-
tion of circulating lymphocytes to the site of viral infection in the
gut.

1.3: Hawaii Agent: This agent was isolated from an outbreak of
gastroenteritis that occurred in Hawaii. Hawaii agent has also produced disease in volunteers. The clinical, epidemiological, and
histopathological features of infection are similar to Norwalk agent.
Cross-challenge studies in volunteers suggest that Hawaii and Norwalk agents may be immunologically distinct (Wyatt, 1974-a).

2. CLINICAL MANIFESTATIONS

The incubation period is brief, usually 48 hours. Vomiting, the first
symptom, occurs in 90 to 100% of patients, which is twice as common as that seen in bacterial infections. Fever is also a prominent
component of thise disease. Following the vomiting, a watery diarrhea containing no blood or excess fat occurs. The diarrhea may be
aggravated by feeding and relieved by fasting. The vomiting and
fever last for 1 to 2 days, while the diarrhea usually subsides within
4 days. Isotonic dehydration is not uncommon, although 15 or 20% of

patients may develop hypernatremic dehydration. Associated symptoms of upper respiratory infections may be present. Recovery is usually rapid and complete in 5 to 7 days. However, fulminating disease with rapid progression to dehydration, collapse, and death may occur.

3. DIAGNOSIS

The viral particles can be seen by electron microscopy in fecal extracts taken during the acute phase of the disease. The use of immune electron microscopy may facilitate the identification of the viral particles. This technique involves the use of convalescent serum which serves as the source of antibody, enabling the recognition of the viral agent.

Antibodies can be detected by complement-fixation (CF), immunofluorescense (IF), and immune electron microscopy (IEM). Stool extracts rich in viral particles or a cross-reacting virus (e.g. Nebraska calf diarrhea virus) may be used for antigens in CF test. Virus-infected intestinal organ cultures (Wyatt, R.G. et al., 1974-b) may be used for titrating antibodies by IF.

Propagation of human rotaviruses in tissue cultures has not been achieved. This will be a step toward routine diagnosis in the virus laboratory, and preparation of a vaccine.

Examination of the stools usually show no blood or excess fat. Stools, when examined for presence of cells, show predominantly lymphocytes in the majority of patients. In contrast to the prevailing belief that pus cells are not seen in viral gastroenteritis, an excess number of polymorphonuclear cells have been observed in 16% of those infected; therefore, this parameter is not specific in diagnosis (Rodriques et al., 1976).

4. MANAGEMENT AND PROGNOSIS

The majority of human infections due to rotaviruses are self-limited. Specific therapy is not available. Dietary restriction during the acute diarrhea phase may be helpful. Serum electrolytes and hydration status of the patient should be monitored. Supportive care and appropriate fluids and electrolytes should be used for correction of dehydration and electrolyte imbalance.

Recovery is generally rapid and complete but transient recurrence of diarrhea may occur. Some patients have died of rapid progression of dehydration and collapse. Since the virus can easily be transmitted to other infants and young children, particularly in hospitalized infants, special precautions with isolation of patients and appropriate cleansing of hands and all objects contaminated by the infected child are recommended.

The ultimate means for control of this disease must be prevention.
The protective effect of mother's milk has not been objectively assessed. An attenuated, orally administered, calf diarrhea virus
vaccine has been shown to reduce the incidence of diarrhea in calves.
Active immunization against human rotaviruses may become a re-
alistic possibility.

REFERENCES

GASTROINTESTINAL INFECTIONS

Ager, E.A. and Top, F.H.: Salmonellosis. In, Communicable
and Infectious Diseases, edited by Top, F.H., Sr. and Wehrle,
P.F. C.V. Mosby Co., St. Louis, pp. 567-580, 1972.

Banwell, J.G. and Sherr H.: Effect of bacterial enterotoxins on
the gastrointestinal tract. Gastroenterology 65:467, 1973.

Bishop, R.F., et al.: An epidemic of diarrhea in human neonates
involving reovirus-like agents and enteropathogenic serotypes of
Escherichia coli. J. Clin, Path. 29:46, 1976.

Boyer, K.M., et al.: An outbreak of gastroenteritis due to E. coli
1042 in a neonatal nursery. J. Pediatr. 86:919, 1975.

Cramblatt, H.G., et al.: The etiology of infectious diarrhea in infancy, with special reference to enteropathogenic E. coli. Ann.
N.Y. Acad. Sci. 176:80, 1971.

DuPont, H.L., et al.: The response of man to virulent Shigella
flexneri 2 a. J. Infect. Dis. 119:296, 1969.

DuPont, H.L.: Diagnosis and treatment of infectious diseases.
Infect. Dis. Rev. 2:201, 1973.

Dupont, H.L.: Recent developments in immunizations against diarrheal diseases. South. Med. J. 68:1027, 1975.

Gall, D.G. and Hamilson, J.K.: Chronic diarrhea in childhood: A
new look at an old problem. Pediatr. Clin. N.A. 21:1001, 1974.

Giannella, R.A.: Acute bacterial diarrhea. J. Kentucky Med. Asso.
72:667, 1974.

Gorbach, S.L. and Khurana, C.M.: Toxigenic Escherichia coli: A
cause of infantile diarrhea in Chicago. NEJM 287:791, 1972.

Gordon, J.E.: Diarrheal disease of early childhood: Worldwide
scope of the problem. Ann. N.Y. Acad. Sci. 176:9, 1971.

Guerrant, R.L., et al.: Role of toxigenic and invasive bacteria in acute diarrhea of childhood. NEJM 293:567, 1975

Harris, J.C., et al.: Fecal leukocytes in diarrheal illness. Ann. Int. Med. 76:697, 1972.

Lewis, N.N. and Gangarosa, E.J.: Shigellosis. In, Communicable and Infectious Diseases, edited by Top, F.H., Sr. and Wehrle, P.F. C.V. Mosby Co., St. Louis, pp. 585-591, 1972.

Riley, H.D.: Antibiotic therapy in neonatal enteric disease. Ann. N.Y. Acad. Sci. 176:360, 1971.

Rosenstein, B.J.: Salmonellosis in infants and children. J. Pediatr. 70:1, 1967.

Rudoy, R.C. and Nelson, J.D.: Enteroinvasive and enterotoxigenic Escherichia coli. Occurrence in acute diarrhea of infants and children. Am. J. Dis. Child. 129:668, 1975.

Sack, R.B., et al.: Enterotoxigenic Escherichia coli associated diarrheal disease in Apache children. NEJM 292:1041, 1975.

Sanders, D.Y., et al.: Chronic salmonellosis in infancy. Clin. Pediatr. 13:640, 1974.

Schroeder, S.A., et al.: Epidemic salmonellosis in hospitals and institutions. NEJM 279:674, 1968.

Watanabe, T.: Transferable antibiotic resistance in Enterobacteriaceae. Relationship to the problems of treatment and control of coliform enteritis. Ann. N.Y. Acad. Sci. 176:371, 1971.

Wheeler, W.E.: Diarrhea, infantile, caused by Enteropathogenic E. coli. In, Communicable and Infectious Diseases, edited by Top, F.H., Sr. and Wehrle, P.F. C.V. Mosby Co., St. Louis, pp. 182-189, 1972.

Winter, S.T.: The age factor in acute diarrhea during childhood. Clin. Pediatr. 13:17, 1974.

ENTERIC FEVER

Calderon, E.: Amoxicillin in the treatment of typhoid fever due to chloramphenicol resistant Salmonella typhi. J. Infect. Dis. 129: S219, 1974.

Farid, Z., et al.: Trimethoprim - sulfamethoxazole in enteric fevers. Brit. Med. J. 3:323, 1970.

Farid, Z., et al.: Treatment of chronic enteric fever with amoxicillin. J. Infect. Dis. 132:698, 1975.

Geddes, A.M.: Trimethoprim-sulfamethoxazole in the treatment of gastrointestinal infections including enteric fever and typhoid carriers. Can. Med. Asso. U. 112:355, 1975.

Kabakian, H.A., et al.: Roentgenographic findings in typhoid fever. Am. J. Roentgenology, Rad. Thera. and Nuclear Medicine 125:198, 1975.

Kaul, B.K.: Operative management of typhoid perforation in children. Internatl. Surg. 60:407, 1975.

Lampe, R.M., et al.: Glucose-6-phosphate dehydrogenase deficiency in Thai children with typhoid fever. J. Pediatr. 87:576, 1975.

Levin, D.M., et al.: Vi antigen from Salmonella typhosa and immunity against typhoid fever. Infect. Immunity 12:1290, 1975.

Ramachandran, S., et al.: Acute disseminated encephalomyelitis in typhoid fever. Brit. Med. J. 1:494, 1975.

Robertson, R.P., et al.: Evaluation of chloramphenicol and ampicillin in Salmonella fever. NEJM 278:171, 1968.

Sharp, J.C.M. and Heymann, C.S.: Enteric fever in Scotland. J. Hygiene 76:83, 1976.

Vaierub, S.: Tracking down Salmonella typhi. JAMA 233:1196, 1975.

Vargas, M. and Pena, A.: Perforated viscera in typhoid fever: A better prognosis for children. J. Pediatr. Surg. 10:531, 1975.

FOOD POISONING

Barker, W.H., Jr., et al.: Foodborne disease surveillance. Am. J. Public Health 64:854, 1974.

Cimino, J.A., et al.: A Salmonellosis outbreak in New York City attributed to a catering establishment. Public Health Reports 89: 468, 1974.

Dakin, W.P.H., et al.: Gastroenteritis due to non-agglutinable (non-cholera) vibrios. Med. J. Australia 2:487, 1974.

Eckman, M.R.: Brucellosis linked to Mexican cheese. JAMA 232: 636, 1975.

Editorial: Epidemiology: Staphylococcal infections. II. Food poisoning. Brit. Med. J. 4:291, 1975.

Fantasia, L.D., et al.: Detection and growth of enteropathogenic Escherichia coli in soft ripened cheese. App. Microbiol. 29:179, 1975.

Hauschild, A.H.W.: Criteria and procedures for implicating Clostridium perfringens in foodborne outbreaks. Can. J. Public Health 66:388, 1975.

Hughes, J.M., et al.: Foodborne disease outbreaks in the United States, 1973. J. Infect. Dis. 132:224, 1975.

Midura, T.F. and Arnon, S.S.: Infant botulism. Lancet 2:934, 1976.

Pickett, J., Berg, B., Chaplin, E., and Brunstetter-Shafer, M.: Syndrome of botulism is infancy. NEJM 295:770, 1976.

Taylor, A.J. and Gilbert, R.J.: Bacillus cereus food poisoning: A provisional serotyping scheme. J. Med. Microbiol. 8:543, 1975.

Todd, E., et al.: Two outbreaks of Bacillus cereus food poisoning in Canada. Can. J. Public Health 65:109, 1974.

Todd, E. and Pivnick, H.: The significance of food poisoning in Canada. Can. J. Public Health 65:89, 1974.

VIRAL GASTROENTERITIS

Agus, S.G., Dolin, R., Wyatt, R.G., Tousimis, A.J., and Northrup, R.S.: Acute infectious nonbacterial gastroenteritis: Intestinal histopathology. Histologic and enzymatic alterations during illness produced by the Norwalk agent in man. Ann. Intern. Med. 79:18, 1973.

Bishop, R.F., Davidson, G.P., Holmes, I.H., and Ruck, B.J.: Virus particles in epithelial cells of duodenal mucosa from children with acute nonbacterial gastroenteritis. Lancet 2:1281, 1973.

Bishop, R.F., Davidson, G.P., Holmes, I.H., and Ruck, B.J.: Detection of a new virus by electron microscopy of faecal extracts from children with acute gastroenteritis. Lancet 1:149, 1974.

Davidson, G.P., Bishop, R.F., Townley, R.W., Holmes, I.H., and Ruck, B.J.: Importance of a new virus in acute sporadic enteritis in children. Lancet 1:242, 1975.

Dolin, R., Blacklow, N.R., DuPont, H., Formal, S., Buscho, R.F., Kasel, J.A., Chames, R.P., Hornick, R., and Chanock, R.M.: Transmission of acute infectious nonbacterial gastroenteritis to volunteers by oral administration of stool filtrates. J. Infect. Dis. 123:307, 1971.

Dolin, R., Reichman, R.C., and Fanci, A.S.: Lymphocyte populations in acute viral gastroenteritis. Infect. Immun. 14:422, 1976.

Eichenwald, H.F., Ababio, A., Arky, A.M., and Hartman, A.P.: Epidemic diarrhea in premature and older infants caused by Echo virus type 18. JAMA 166:1563, 1958.

Flewett, T.H., Bryden, A.S., and Davies, H.: Virus particles in gastroenteritis. Lancet 2:1497, 1974.

Flewett, T.H., Davies, H., Bryden, A.S., and Robertson, M.J.: Diagnostic electron microscopy of faeces. II. Acute gastroenteritis associated with reovirus-like particles. J. Clin. Pathol. 27: 608, 1974.

Kapikian, A.Z., Wyatt, R.G., Dolin, R., Thornhill, T.S., Kalica, A.R., and Chanock, R.M.: Visualization by immune electron microscopy of a 27-nm particle associated with acute infectious nonbacterial gastroenteritis. J. Virol. 10:1075, 1972.

Kapikian, A.Z., Kim, H.W., Wyatt, R.G., Rodriques, W.J., Ross, S., Cline, W.L., Parrott, R H., and Chanock, R.M.: Reoviruslike agent in stools: Association with infantile diarrhea and development of serologic tests. Science 185:1049, 1974.

Middleton, P.J., Szymanski, M T., Abbott, G.D., Bortolussi, R., and Hamilton, J.R.: Orbivirus acute gastroenteritis of infancy. Lancet 1:1241, 1974.

Ramos-Alvarez, M., and Olarte, J.: Diarrheal disease of children. Am. J. Hyg. 77:283, 1963.

Rodriques, W.J., Kim, H.W., Brandt, C.D., Chanock, R.M., Kapikian, A.Z., Wyatt, R., and Parrott, R.H.: Clinical features of human reovirus-like agent gastroenteritis in infants and children. Pediatr. Res. 10:402, 1976.

Schreiber, D.S., Blacklow, N.R., and Trier, J.S.: The mucosal lesion of the proximal small intestine in acute infectious nonbacterial gastroenteritis. NEJM 288:1318, 1973.

Wyatt, R.G., Dolin, R., Blacklow, N.R., DuPont, H.L., Buscho, R.F., Thornhill, T.S., Kapikian, A.Z., and Chanock, R.M.: Comparison of three agents of acute infectious nonbacterial gastroenteritis by cross-challenge in volunteers. J. Infect. Dis. 129:709, 1974.

Wyatt, R.G., Kapikian, A.Z., Thornhill, T.S., Sereno, M.M., Kim, H.W., Chanock, R.M.: In vitro cultivation in human fetal intestinal organ culture of a reovirus-like agent associated with non-bacterial gastroenteritis in infants and children. J. Infect. Dis. 130:523, 1974.

CHAPTER 10. INTRA-ABDOMINAL INFECTIONS

GENERAL CONSIDERATIONS: In the normal abdominal cavity, bacteria are confined to the gut lumen. It is only in pathologic situations that bacteria are found beyond the lamina propria of the gut wall. Disturbance of this barrier by disease, trauma or surgical operation may permit the escape of gut organisms capable of causing intra-abdominal infections. These infections may take the form of peritonitis, intra-peritoneal abscesses, retro-peritoneal abscesses or visceral abscesses (Table 10-1). Since most of the agents causing these infections are indigenous to the gut, an understanding of the normal gastrointestinal flora is required.

TABLE 10-1: CLASSIFICATION OF INTRA-ABDOMINAL PEDIATRIC INFECTIONS

I.   Peritonitis
 	
     A. Primary
     B. Secondary
 	
II.   Intra-peritoneal abscess
 	
III. Retro-peritoneal abscess
 	
IV. Visceral abscesses

Adapted from Altemeier et al., Advances in Surgery, Vol. 5, 1971.

The intestine of the newborn is rapidly colonized with lactobacilli and other bacteria largely dependent on diet (nursing vs. bottle feeding). Gastric acidity and rapid peristaltic action maintain relatively low bacterial counts in the stomach and proximal small intestine. When pathologic states such as pyloric stenosis or achlorhydria interfere with these processes, excessive bacterial proliferation may result.

After weaning, lactobacilli continue to be present in the stomach. Most of the bacteria derived from saliva or food are destroyed by gastric acid in the stomach. Those surviving organisms are generally acid resistant lactobacilli, streptococci (enterococci) and fungi. In the presence of normal gut motility, they colonize the upper regions of the small intestine in relatively low concentrations of 10^3 to 10^4 organisms per ml. of intestinal fluid. The sites of absorption in the duodenum and jejunum are thus relatively free of microorganisms which can interfere with fat and vitamin absorption. Perforation of

the upper small bowel carries a relatively low risk of bacterial contamination into the abdominal cavity.

In the lower ileum, the bacterial flora increase in number and
type. Gram negative organisms such as aerobic coliforms and anaerobic bacteroides, as well as bifidobacterium (anaerobic lactobacilli), may be present in concentrations of 10^5 to 10^8 per ml.
Tremendous bacterial overgrowth in the ileum results from disorders that impair intestinal motility, such as Crohn's disease, adhesions, or diabetic neuropathy.

In the large intestine, anaerobes comprise 95 to 99 percent of the
normal flora. A wide variety of anaerobic species have been isolated, but two large groups predominate: Bacteroides and bifidobacterium. These anaerobes outnumber aerobic and facultative
organisms by 1000 to 10,000 times (Gorbach, 1971). The most prevalent anaerobe is invariably Bacteroides fragilis, present in concentrations of 10^{10} to 10^{11} per gram of wet feces. Bifidobacterium is
found in over two-thirds of fecal samples in concentration of 10^9 per
gram. The coliforms, mainly Escherichia coli, are the most prevalent aerobic bacteria at levels of 10^6 to 10^7 per gram, accounting
for less than .1% of the total bacterial population (Finegold, 1971).
Additional aerobic or facultative forms present include lactobacillus,
enterococcus, and Streptococcus viridans. Other anerobes frequently found in normal fecal flora are Clostridium spp., Fusobacterium, Eubacterium, Propionibacterium, Veillonella and other anaerobic cocci. The important point is that in the normal host, the
intestinal flora is primarily anaerobic and E. coli may account for
only a small percentage of bacteria present.

Both the frequency and species of anaerobes present in the feces may
be determined by the diet or state of nutrition. When compared to
Americans, subjects consuming a Japanese diet have higher counts
of E. coli and lower counts of certain bacteroides species. Fusobacterium nucleatum is frequently absent in Japanese, whereas other
fusobacteria are found more frequently in Japanese than in Americans (Attebery et al., 1974). Mata and Urrutia (1971) studied the
influence of malnutrition on the development of indigenous bacterial
flora in breast-fed children of low socioeconomic status in Guatemala. E. coli established itself early in these infants, presumably
due to primitive sanitary conditions present at birth. However, by
the first week of breast-feeding, bifidobacteria were the predominant
intestinal flora and E. coli counts were relatively low. With food
supplementation and eventual weaning, bacteroides, streptococci and
veillonellae became more frequent. As the weaning process prog-
ressed, all children were colonized with E. coli.

Altered host defenses occurring in such states as malnutrition, prematurity, and primary immune deficiency may result in the addition
of pathogens to the endogenous flora, or possibly even the breakdown
of the mucosal barrier itself, resulting in clinical disease (Walker,

1976). In the United States, the appearance of non-indigenous pathogens is more commonly correlated with overzealous use of broad
spectrum antibiotics. These antibiotics prevent the competitive interaction of normal gut bacteria from acting as a deterent to the
overgrowth of fungal and bacterial pathogens. Other important gastrointestinal defenses include peristalsis, gastric acidity and the
ability of the liver to inactivate a variety of noxious substances which
gain access to the portal circulation from the gut. Walker (1976)
discusses the importance of these factors, as well as immunologic
defenses in the gastrointestinal tract supplied by secretory IgA and
other immunoglobulins.

BACTERIOLOGY OF INTRA-ABDOMINAL INFECTIONS: Since intra-
abdominal infections are mainly derived from gastrointestinal tract
contamination, their bacteriology is remarkably similar. Characteristically, multiple organisms are cultured from a given site usually consisting of a mixture of anaerobes and facultative aerobes that
normally colonize the gut. Lorber and Swenson (1975) prospectively
studied 76 cases of intra-abdominal infection using recent techniques
for collection, isolation and identification of anaerobic bacteria, as
well as facultative and aerobic organisms. Anaerobic bacteria predominated regardless of anatomic location (Table 10-2). Anaerobes

TABLE 10-2: FREQUENCY OF ANAEROBIC BACTERIA CULTURED FROM INTRA-ABDOMINAL INFECTIONS, 1969-1974			
		ANAEROBIC BACTERIA	
INFECTION	NO. OF CASES	PRESENT	MULTIPLE SPECIES
Peritonitis	30	28	24
Intraperitoneal Abscess	16	14	10
Retroperitoneal Abscess	5	3	3
Visceral Abscess	15	11	7
Adapted from Lorber and Swenson, Surgical Clinics of North America, Vol. 55, No. 6, Dec. 1975.			

were isolated in 84% of the 76 cases, and multiple anaerobic bacteria were present in 66%. In 39% (30 cases), anaerobes were the
only organisms isolated. It is important to note that no patients had
"sterile pus" or cryptogenic abscesses, a finding that was commonplace prior to modern techniques for isolating anaerobes. In the
entire series, there was an average of 3.9 organisms per infection
(2.6 anaerobes: 1.3 aerobes). The principle anaerobic pathogens
were Bacteroides fragilis (36% of all anerobes) and anaerobic gram
positive cocci. E. coli was the most frequent facultative aerobe
isolated (Table 10-3). Bacteremia was a common event, Bacteroides
fragilis being the most frequently isolated organism from the blood.

Similar bacteriology has been reported by other recent studies of
intra-abdominal infections. Gorbach (1971) found three types of
anaerobes were the most frequent virulent pathogens in intra-
abdominal infections, i.e. Bacteroides fragilis, Clostridia spp. and anaerobic cocci (esp. the peptostreptococcus). There was an average
of five bacterial species per intra-abdominal infection with a ratio
of 3 anaerobes to 2 aerobes. The recovery of multiple bacteria
from infected sites questions the relative importance of each organism to the pathogenesis of intra-abdominal infection. This is a
practical question as well, concerning which organisms, aerobic,
anaerobic or both, require specific antibiotic therapy.

Weinstein et al. (1974) developed an animal model to study the evolution of intra-abdominal abscesses. A gelatin capsule containing
large bowel contents was implanted in the abdominal cavities of rats,
followed by quantitative bacteriologic analysis of the infected sites.
Three stages of the disease were seen: peritonitis, bacteremia and
abscess formation. Initially, there was an acute generalized peritonitis during which E. coli and enterococci were the major bacterial
isolates. During this acute stage, there was a 43% mortality and
blood cultures were frequently positive for E. coli. All animals that
survived the acute peritonitis went on to develop discrete intra-
abdominal abscess by the seventh postoperative day. The major
isolates in the abscess cavities were anaerobes, Bacteroides
fragilis, and fusobacteria. Bacteremia was seldom detected during
the abscess stage of infection. Whereas aerobic bacteria played a
prominent role in producing the acute peritonitis, anaerobes were the
dominant isolates concurrent with abscess formation (Onderdonk et
al., 1974).

In another set of experiments using this same animal model, selected
antibiotics were targeted against either aerobic or anaerobic bacteria
during various stages of intra-abdominal infection. During acute
peritonitis, animals treated only with clindamycin (effective against
bacteroides and most anaerobic bacteria) had no significant improvement in mortality rate (35%) over the untreated controls (37%),
whereas use of gentamicin (effective against coliforms and other
aerobic bacteria), used either alone or in combination with clindamycin, lead to 90% survival. The early mortality during acute

TABLE 10-3: BACTERIOLOGY OF 76 INTRA-ABDOMINAL INFECTIONS	
ORGANISM	**NUMBER OF ISOLATES**
ANAEROBIC BACTERIA:	
Gram-negative nonsporulating rods	
Bacteroides	116
(B. fragilis: 71)	
(B. melaninegenicus: 30)	
Fusobacterium spp.	15
Cocci	
Peptostreptococcus spp.	22
Peptococcus spp.	21
Gram-positive nonsporulating rods	
Eubacterium spp.	8
Clostridium perfringens	7
Others	9
Total	198
AEROBIC AND FACULTATIVE BACTERIA:	
Gram-negative rods	
Escherichia coli	43
Proteus spp.	8
Klebsiella spp.	6
Pseudomonas spp.	2
Gram-positive cocci	
Streptococcus sp.	37
Others	4
Total	100

Adapted from Lorber and Swenson, Surgical Clinics of North America, Vol. 55, No. 6, Dec. 1975.

peritonitis appeared to be due to gentamicin sensitive coliform bacteria. Interestingly, 100% of the animals left untreated and 98% of those given gentamicin alone went on to develop discrete intra-abdominal abscesses. In contrast, only 5 to 6 percent of those receiving clindamycin alone or in combination with gentamicin went on to develop these abscesses. This response to clindamycin suggests the importance of anaerobes in abscess formation as a late complication of peritonitis (Finegold et al., 1975).

10.1: PERITONITIS

Peritonitis is a nonspecific inflammation of the serous lining of the abdominal and pelvic cavity. The peritoneum is composed of a single layer of mesothelial cells overlying connective tissue, blood vessels and lymphatics. The peritoneum is reflected over abdominal viscera as their outer covering and lines both the abdominal and pelvic cavities. This forms a potential space which is closed from outside contamination, except for the fimbriated ends of the fallopian tubes in the female. The surface area of the peritoneum has been calculated to be approximately 22,000 sq. cm. in an adult, roughly equivalent to 50% of the surface area of the skin. The importance of this tremendous surface area is due to the ability of the peritoneum to act as a semi-permeable membrane, allowing rapid bidirectional transfer of substances across its surface. Serous fluid normally secreted by the peritoneum, moistens surfaces thereby permitting intestinal peristalsis and other movements of the abdominal viscera. When chemical irritants and/or infective agents injure the peritoneum, a characteristic inflammatory response occurs resulting in the clinical signs and symptoms of peritonitis.

Aseptic peritonitis may result when chemical irritants such as blood, gastric juice, bile, urine, pancreatic secretions or meconium are introduced into the peritoneal cavity, following intra-abdominal disease, trauma or surgery. If bacterial contamination occurs, septic peritonitis may result. Septic peritonitis is termed secondary when the infection is disseminated by rupture of gut lumen or extension from an intra-abdominal viscus or abscess. Primary peritonis results when the focus of infection is outside the abdominal cavity and reaches the peritoneum via hematogenous or lymphatic routes.

1. PRIMARY PERITONITIS

1.1: ETIOLOGY: Although primary bacterial peritonitis is usually found in children, it is a rare form of diffuse peritonitis occurring most often in children with nephrosis or post-necrotic cirrhosis. Unlike secondary peritonitis, the peritoneum is invaded by a single bacterial species and preceding intra-abdominal injury or disease is not necessary. The infecting organism presumably reaches the peritoneum via the blood stream, lymphatics or by ascending the female genital tract. Prior to the 1950's the pneumococcus was

responsible for most of the cases of primary peritonitis. Since
this time, several studies have reported a decreasing frequency of
the pneumococcus, with a corresponding increase in the frequency
of the hemolytic streptococcus and gram-negative organisms as the
cause of primary peritonitis. Whereas 50 of 72 cases of primary
peritonitis between 1925 and 1955 were due to the pneumococcus,
only 6 of 33 cases were due to the pneumococcus between 1956 and
1970 (Fowler, 1971). Gram-negative organisms were responsible
for 69% (17 of 26 cases) of primary peritonitis occurring during the
past decade in a study by McDougal et al., (1975). E. coli accounted
for 42% (11 cases) of these infections. In high risk children, with the
nephrotic syndrome, there has also been a shift toward gram-negative
organisms as a cause of primary peritonitis (Speck et al., 1974).

The incidence of primary peritonitis does not appear to be decreasing. A review of 84,352 pediatric admissions to two large metropolitan hospitals over the past 10 years revealed 26 patients with
primary peritonitis and 157 patients with diffuse peritoneal sepsis
of other etiologies (McDougal et al., 1975) (Table 10-4). These
patients with primary peritonitis accounted for 2.1 percent of all
pediatric abdominal emergency admissions. When only the cases of
diffuse peritonitis are considered, primary peritonitis accounted for
17.6 percent of the cases in infancy and 13.4 percent of the diffuse
peritonitis seen in children ages 2 to 16. Clearly, it would be helpful to distinguish primary peritonitis from diffuse secondary peritoneal sepsis that requires immediate surgical intervention.

1.2: CLINICAL MANIFESTATIONS: The distinguishing characteristics of primary peritonitis in infants and children are outlined in
Table 10-5. Primary peritonitis is less common than secondary
peritonitis, but the age distribution is similar. Females tend to
predominate in primary peritonitis except when the nephrotic syndrome is present, whereupon the increased frequency in males reflects the sex distribution of nephrosis. The presence of associated
disease may give some clue as to whether primary or secondary
peritonitis is present. McDougal et al., (1975) found that 15 patients
or 58 percent of those with primary peritonitis had urinary tract disease. Ten of these patients had urinary tract infections, four had
the nephrotic syndrome and one had hydronephrosis. Post necrotic
cirrhosis was present in three patients. Among 22 children with well
documented nephrotic syndrome (proteinuria, hypercholesterolemia,
and edema), 39 episodes of primary peritonitis occurred (Speck et
al., 1974).

The onset of primary peritonitis in infants is usually insidious over
1 to 2 days and is manifested by lethargy, abdominal distension and
a fall in temperature. A preceding infection, such as pneumonia,
is a frequent finding. Abdominal x-ray reveals a nonspecific pattern
without evidence of free air. Infants who present with secondary
peritonitis tended to have a sudden onset, developing the signs of

TABLE 10-4: ETIOLOGY OF 183 CASES OF PERITONITIS ADMITTED TO TWO METROPOLITAN HOSPITALS* (1964 - 1974)		
DISEASE	**INFANTS** (<2 yrs)	**CHILDREN** (2-14 yrs)
PRIMARY PERITONITIS:		
Nephrotic Syndrome		4
Post-necrotic Cirrhosis		3
Hydronephrosis		1
Urinary Tract Infection		10
Hyaline Membrane Disease	1	
Cystic Fibrosis		1
Adrenogenital Syndrome		1
Preceding Pneumonia	3	
No Associated Disease	2	
Total	6	20
SECONDARY PERITONITIS:		
Spontaneous Enteric Perforation		
Stomach	10	
Duodenum (ulcer)		1
Jejunum	3	
Ileum	7	
Sigmoid	2	
Meconium Peritonitis	1	
Pancreatitis with Ruptured Pseudocyst	1	
Subhepatic Abscess	1	
Infected Omphalomesenteric Cyst	1	
Pelvic Inflammatory Disease with Diffuse Peritonitis		4
Ruptured Appendix	2	123
Total	28	128

* Adapted from McDougal, Izant and Zollinger, Annals of Surgery 181, No. 3, 311, 1975.

TABLE 10-5: DISTINGUISHING CHARACTERISTICS OF PRIMARY AND SECONDARY PERITONITIS IN INFANTS AND CHILDREN		
	Primary Peritonitis	Secondary Peritonitis
Etiology:	Hematogenous, lymphatic or genital route No intra-abdominal source	Extension of intra-abdominal source
Pathogens	Single species: gram-negative; bacillary (E. coli) streptococcus; pneumococus	Intestinal flora: Multiple species of aerobes and anaerobes
Frequency:	Rare, less than 2% of abdominal emergencies	Common
Age:	Infants: less than 2 months Children: 5-9 years	Common
Sex:	Females predominate (except when Nephrosis present)	No sex difference
Associated Disease:	Nephrotic Syndrome Post-necrotic cirrhosis Urinary Tract Infection	Appendicitis Ruptured abdominal viscus Post-surgery
Clinical Manifestation:	Infants: insidious onset preceding pneumonia frequent; Abdominal x-ray: non specific pattern, no free air	Infants: sudden onset no evidence of prior infection; Abdominal x-ray: free air evident
	Childhood: onset less than 24 hours; Abdominal x-ray: non-specific pattern occasional air-filled loop of small intestine	Childhood: usually over several days; Abdominal x-ray: indistinguishable from 1° peritonitis in most cases (may see appendicolith or free air)

peritonitis over a period of hours. Although the clinical signs, symptoms and laboratory findings are similar to patients with primary peritonitis, they have no evidence of prior infection and free air is evident on abdominal x-ray in the majority of cases (McDougal et al., 1975).

Among children over the age of 2 years with primary peritonitis, the time from the onset of symptoms to the presentation of abdominal findings is usually less than 24 hours, although the development of primary peritonitis may be more insidious in children with underlying cirrhosis or nephrosis. The time from onset of symptoms to the presentation of abdominal findings in children with secondary peritonitis is significantly longer. Fever, nausea, vomiting, diffuse abdominal tenderness, rebound tenderness, abdominal rigidity and spasm of the rectus muscle occurs with equal frequency in patients with primary and secondary peritonitis; neither is there any difference in the temperature or white blood cell count. Abdominal x-rays are similar for both infants and children with primary peritonitis, showing a nonspecific pattern with an occasional air-filled loop of small bowel. Whereas abdominal x-rays are helpful in identifying infants with enteric perforations, free air is seen in only one of the 123 children who presented with ruptured appendix. The majority of children with diffuse secondary peritonitis have abdominal x-rays that are indistinguishable from children with primary peritonitis.

1.3: DIAGNOSIS: Although it is possible to have a strong suspicion of primary peritonitis in a child who has nephrotic syndrome and presents with diffuse abdominal pain and fever, the diagnosis is usually difficult to make on clinical or laboratory grounds alone prior to exploratory laparotomy. Diagnostic paracentesis with gram staining of aspirated fluid may be preferable to diagnostic exploration in high risk patients, such as neonates or nephrotics. A gram stain showing a single gram-positive organism excludes an enteric source of infection, and exploratory surgery may be avoided. If gram-negative organisms are present, primary peritonitis cannot be excluded and the diagnosis should be established at laparotomy.

1.4: MANAGEMENT: Before antibiotics are administered to a patient presenting with diffuse peritonitis, sputum, urine, and blood cultures should be obtained and microscopic examination of stained urine and sputum specimens should be performed. In addition to complete blood count and serum amylase, a urinalysis may give evidence of active renal disease as manifest by significant proteinuria. Plain film of the abdomen is always helpful since pneumonitis is common in children and may be confused with the abdominal pain seen in peritonitis. A diagnostic peritoneal tap can further improve the accuracy of the diagnosis and may be particularly helpful in seriously ill patients who are poor surgical risks. If, at this point, primary peritonitis is suspected, antibiotics should be targeted against the pneumococcus, streptococcus and gram-negative organisms. A rational antibiotic choice would consist of the combination of a penicillin effective against the streptococcus and pneumococcus and an aminoglycoside effective against gram-negative rods. A combination of ampicillin with kanamycin or gentamicin would meet this criteria. The initial antibiotics should be changed only if antibiotic sensitivity testing suggests a more efficacious antimicrobial agent. If the diagnosis of primary peritonitis is not strongly suspected, or if after 48 hours of appropriate parenteral antibiotic therapy, the child's clinical condition fails to improve, or physical findings show localization, then surgical exploration is indicated.

2. SECONDARY PERITONITIS

2.1: ETIOLOGY: Peritonitis secondary to abdominal disease or injury is a common infection. In children, this type of peritonitis usually results from perforation of an inflamed appendix or other abdominal viscus. Less frequently, peritonitis may be secondary to intussusception, volvulus, incarcerated hernia, rupture of a Meckel's diverticulum or perforation of the intestine or abdominal viscera following blunt trauma or introduction of foreign body. Peritonitis may develop during the neonatal period following perforation of the intestine in meconium ileus or following spontaneous rupture of the stomach, intestine or appendix. Peritonitis may also result from umbilical infection.

The bacteriology of secondary peritonitis in children is characterized by the multiple species of both anaerobes and aerobes that make up the normal flora of the gastrointestinal tract. In some cases, other organisms may be introduced from outside the gut in the course of trauma, surgery, or invasive procedures, such as during peritoneal dialysis. Table 10-6 illustrates the wide variety of anaerobes cultured from the peritoneal fluid of 22 children with appendicitis or perforated viscus. _Bacteroides fragilis_ was the anaerobic microorganism isolated most frequently. More than one anaerobe was recovered from 16 of 22 patients, including a maximum of 6 organisms from one patient. Aerobic organisms, predominantly _Escherichia coli_, were recovered from 19 of the 22 children.

2.2: PATHOGENESIS: Bacterial contamination of the peritoneum does not automatically result in diffuse peritonitis. It is surprisingly difficult to produce fatal peritonitis in experimental animals with pure cultures of intestinal flora, unless either massive doses of the culture are used, or the defenses of the peritoneum are devitalized or injured by chemical irritants, intestinal enzymes, foreign bodies or other trauma (Altemeier et al., 1971). In order for bacterial contamination to result in diffuse peritonitis, there must be a continued source of bacteria within the peritoneal cavity and a foreign material such as bile, feces or necrotic tissue that protects bacteria from the aggressive defense of the peritoneum. The majority of transient bacterial contaminants are overcome by the presence of leukocytes and fibrin deposits resulting in a localization process that ends in resolution.

**TABLE 10-6: MICROORGANISMS CULTURED FROM
22 CHILDREN WITH CLINICALLY SIGNIFICANT
SECONDARY PERITONITIS***

ANAEROBES	NUMBER
Gram-negative nonsporulating rods	29
Bacteroides (B. fragilis: 24)	
Fusobacterium	3
Cocci	
Peptostreptococcus	1
Peptococcus	6
Veillonella	1
Microaerophilic streptococcus	1
Gram-positive nonsporulating rods	
Eubacterium	2
Propionibacterium	1
Bifidobacterium	1
Clostridia	11
AEROBES	
Gram-negative rods	19
(pred. E. coli)	

* Peritoneal fluid obtained from children with appendicitis or
a perforated viscus.

Adapted from Dunkle, Brotherton and Feigin, Pediatrics, Vol.
57 No. 3, March, 1976.

Injury to the peritoneum results in an inflammatory response characterized by vascular dilatation and increased capillary permeability.
The inflamed peritoneum pours out plasma-like fluid rich in leukocytes capable of phagocytosis of bacteria and foreign material. Exudate accumulates and fibrin deposits on the peritoneal surface localize or wall off the infection by plastering omentum and bowel loops
to the inflamed areas. This process may end in resolution of the
inflammation or it may prevent diffuse disease, only to give rise to
abscesses. If localization fails, spreading diffuse peritonitis results. Extensive or diffuse inflammation of the peritoneum may lead
to enormous extracellular fluid loss into the peritoneal cavity and
adjacent tissues, resulting in hypovolemia and shock. Hypovolemia
is further potentiated by vomiting, gastrointestinal suction, or by
the presence of adynamic ileus during which the intestine becomes
distended with air and fluid. This dilatation increases fluid within
the intestine and impairs the absorption of water and salt from the
lumen of the bowel. In addition, bacteria and toxins may be absorbed

by the peritoneum resulting in bacteremia and septicemia. Mechanical effects of abdominal distension, severe shifts in body fluids,
and toxic effects of septicemia combine to produce profound changes
in the cardiorespiratory system that may lead to hypoxia, metabolic
and respiratory acidosis, and death.

2.3: CLINICAL MANIFESTATIONS: The precipitating abdominal
disease or injury determines the early symptoms of secondary peritonitis, which may be sudden after traumatic perforation of the gut
or insidious after a ruptured appendix. Steady aching or burning
abdominal pain usually dominates the clinical picture. Depending
on the extent of peritoneal inflammation the pain may be localized or
generalized, but is always aggravated by movement. Other typical
symptoms are anorexia, nausea, vomiting, fever and chills. Excessive thirst and decreased urination result as dehydration develops.

Physical signs include abdominal tenderness over a widening area,
rebound tenderness and tenderness on rectal examination. Decreased
or absent abdominal respiration due to intensified abdominal pain
on inspiration result in rapid, shallow respiratory movements. Increasing toxemia may be evident by fever, tachycardia, increased
irritability and signs of dehydration. As ileus develops, the abdomen becomes distended, bowel sounds diminish and vomiting is more
frequent. Exceptions to this clinical picture are frequent. For example, abdominal pain and other signs of peritonitis may be decep-
tively absent in infants or children on corticosteroid therapy. In
early infancy, the temperature may be normal or even subnormal.

Acute appendicitis with perforation is the most common cause of
secondary peritonitis. During the first two months of life, however,
appendicitis is extremely rare. Presenting findings are failure to
feed, vomiting and abdominal distension. Early perforation results
in a high mortality rate (Parsons et al., 1970). From infancy through
childhood there is a steady increase in the frequency of appendicitis,
but perforation and mortality are more common in younger children
and infants. In one series of 837 cases of appendicitis, 83% of children under the age of 4 years had perforation at the time of diagnosis. In the preschool age group, perforation occurred in 67%, compared to an overall frequency in children of 30% (Fig. 10.1, Boles
et al., 1954).

Since the typical history of periumbilical pain shifting to the right lower
quadrant, followed by vomiting and fever, is frequently not obtained
in children under 6 years of age, delay from onset of symptoms to
hospitalization frequently occurs. The delay averaged 67 hours in
the series represented in Fig. 10.1 (Boles et al., 1954). Pain may
not be apparent in infants and preschool children. Rather, appendicitis may be manifest by changes in behavior such as irritability,
restlessness and refusal to sleep or feed. Vomiting is often the first
real indication that the child is ill, and alterations in bowel habits,

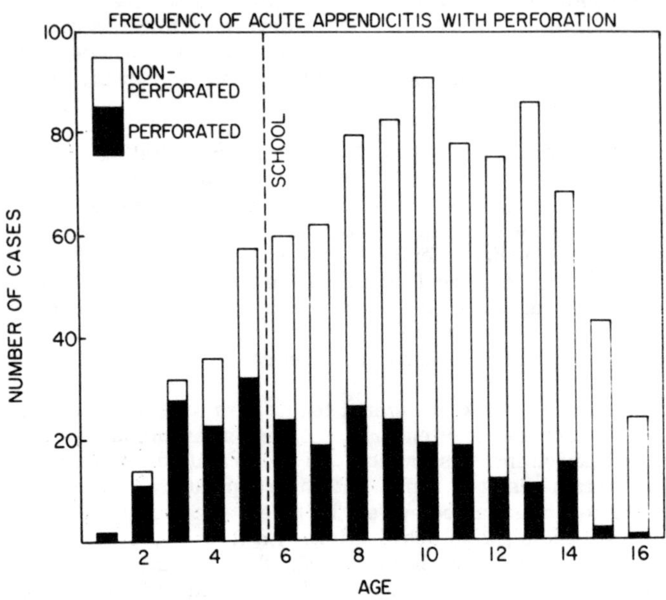

FIG. 10.1: Frequency of Acute Appendicitis with Perforation.
(Boles et al., Arch. Surg. 79:447, 1954.)

such as constipation or diarrhea frequently occur. In general, the
symptoms of appendicitis with perforation are not significantly different from appendicitis without perforation. Duration of symptoms,
however, is frequently longer in the presence of perforation. In one
series of 100 children with acute appendicitis and perforation, 53%
had periumbilical pain which localized to the right lower quadrant,
40% diffuse abdominal pain which followed no particular pattern, and
5% did not complain of any pain (Holgerson et al., 1971). Cessation
of pain, however, may be coincidental with perforation of the appendix.

High fever and leukocytosis occurring late in the illness suggests
perforation. Marked guarding and abdominal tenderness over the
right lower quadrant are present in both perforated and nonperforated
cases of acute appendicitis, although diffuse or generalized abdominal
tenderness is more prominent as peritonitis spreads. Rectal examination is not particularly helpful in determining the presence of perforation, but occasionally localized tenderness can be found only by
this examination. Clinical dehydration, abdominal distension and decreased or absent bowel sounds are more frequently found in children
with perforation (Blair et al., 1969).

2.4: DIAGNOSIS: Prompt diagnosis is important in reducing morbidity and mortality from secondary peritonitis. Early recognition is

difficult when history is unobtainable, or typical physical signs are absent, as in infants and very young children, or the presence of mental retardation, shock, stupor, or coma. Symptoms and signs also may be modified by steroid therapy, prior antibiotics or previous debilitating disease, such as diabetes, leukemia, or malabsorption syndromes.

Of the variable clinical manifestations of peritonitis described in the foregoing discussion, constant abdominal pain and tenderness are the most frequent findings. If the diagnosis is uncertain, frequent re-examination of the abdomen is imperative. The blood leukocyte count is usually higher than 13,000 cells per mm^3. Serial determinations revealing increasing leukocytosis suggests perforation of the appendix or spreading peritonitis. Boles et al. (1954) found a white blood cell count of 20,000 or more in 38% of perforated cases, compared to 9% of nonperforated cases of appendicitis. Leukopenia may occur in infants and very young children, or in the presence of overwhelming infection. The blood smear usually shows a shift to immature polymorphonuclear forms. Blood chemistry documents the degree of dehydration and acidosis present, and serum amylase and glucose determination help to exclude pancreatitis and diabetes. Some increase in serum amylase is commonly associated with secondary peritonitis of most any cause. Urinalysis is helpful in excluding urinary tract disease, although mild pyuria and acetone are frequently present in children with peritonitis.

Plain films of the abdomen (supine, upright or left lateral decubitus) may reveal the roentgenographic picture of diffuse ileus with distension of small bowel loops and colon, and obliteration of psoas shadows. Free air may be visualized if a ruptured viscus has occurred, although this is a rare finding following a perforated appendix. Plain films of the abdomen in appendicitis, with or without perforation, are usually nonspecific. A "sentinel loop" ileus is occasionally seen in the right lower quadrant. The presence of a appendicolith or fecolith (an oval density 5 to 28 mm in diameter) in the right lower quadrant is diagnostic of appendicitis and is an especially valuable finding in a child with a perplexing clinical picture.

In the presence of diffuse peritonitis where either the patient is a poor surgical risk or the diagnosis is not clearcut, diagnostic needle aspiration of the peritoneal cavity may be helpful. Aspirated fluid is examined for blood, bile and amylase, and gram stained for evidence of gram-negative flora or other microorganisms. The fluid should be cultured for both anaerobic and aerobic bacteria. A dry or negative tap is of no diagnostic value.

In addition to peritonitis following trauma or surgery, the differential diagnosis includes a long list of medical conditions that are capable of either causing peritonitis or mimicking acute abdominal inflammation. Table 10-7 lists some of these conditions that led to the finding

TABLE 10-7: CONDITIONS MIMICKING ACUTE APPENDICITIS
IN CHILDREN AND ADULTS AT OPERATION

Acute Mesenteric Lymphadenitis	26
Gynecological Disease	21
Fibrotic Appendix	12
Sigmoid Diverticulitis	4
Urinary-tract Infection	3
Small-bowel Obstruction	3
Acute Regional Ileitis (Crohn's Disease)	3
Tuberculous Ileitis	1
Cholecystitis	1
Meckel's Diverticulitis	1
No Cause Found	24
TOTAL	98

Adapted from Gilmore et al., Lancet, Vol. II, No. 7932:422,
September 6, 1975.

of a normal uninflamed appendix in 98 of 444 patients who underwent
acute appendectomy, a diagnostic error of 22% (Gilmore et al., 1975).
In this study, 12% of children under 11 years of age had acute mesenteric lymphadenitis. This diagnosis is frequently made when the
only abnormality found at operation is enlargement of the mesenteric
lymph nodes. Since symptoms include fever, abdominal pain, nausea
and vomiting, a presumptive diagnosis of appendicitis frequently results. This syndrome may follow an upper respiratory infection, although cultures of the mesenteric nodes are often negative. Pathogens
recovered from the mesenteric nodes include strains of staphylococcus, the beta-hemolytic streptococcus, pasteurella (Yersinia) species and adenoviruses. A few cases of coxsackie A virus enteritis
have been associated with mesenteric lymphadenitis (Blattner, 1969).

Although the gynecologic disorders listed in Table 10-7 simulated
acute appendicitis more frequently in women over 30, of 106 females
age 11 to 20 years of age, nine were discovered to have either ruptured, twisted, or bleeding ovarian cysts, and two had salpingitis.
Diverticulitis and cholecystitis are found almost exclusively in adults,
whereas regional ileitis and urinary tract infections are well-known
mimickers of appendicitis in children. Other relatively common conditions not mentioned in Table 10-7 that simulate either appendicitis
or other causes of abdominal pain in children include epidemic pleurodynia, pneumonia, gastroenteritis, and multiple non-infectious causes
such as intussusception and incarcerated hernia. As previously discussed, primary peritonitis is an important consideration in children
with nephrosis. Although hepatitis is usually sub-clinical in children,
moderately severe abdominal pain may occur. Acute pancreatitis is
a relatively common cause of peritoneal inflammation in adults, but
this is a rare syndrome in children.

2.5: MANAGEMENT: Following a presumptive diagnosis of uncomplicated acute appendicitis, early surgery is clearly the treatment of choice. Procrastination with antibiotics or prolonged observation only increases the risk of perforation (Table 10-8). In

TABLE 10-8: COMPLICATIONS FOLLOWING APPENDICITIS WITH PERFORATION IN 100 INFANTS AND CHILDREN	
Wound Abscess	24
Pelvic Abscess	17
Intraperitoneal Abscess	2
Intestinal Obstruction	5
Fecal Fistula	3
Rectal Bleeding	2
Gram-negative Sepsis	2
Acute Orchitis	1

Adapted from Holgersen, L.O. and Stanley-Brown, E.G., Am. J. Dis. Child, 122:292, 1971.

the more complex patient with progressive secondary peritonitis, as might occur following a ruptured viscus, vigorous effort may be required to improve the patient's condition prior to surgery. Impending shock, hyperthermia, and dehydration are corrected during the preparation period prior to operation. Since large losses of protein containing fluid occur as a consequence of peritonitis, fluid replacement should begin immediately. With central venous pressure or pulmonary wedge pressure as a guide, hypovolemia, dehydration and metabolic acidosis may be corrected with plasma, or albumin and appropriate electrolyte solutions. A urinary catheter is inserted so that urine output can be monitored hourly, along with vital signs and hematocrit. Decompression of adynamic ileus is achieved by use of a nasogastric or long intestinal tube. After appropriate cultures, systemic antibiotic therapy is targeted against the predictable mixture of aerobes and anerobes. A rational choice would be a combination of an aminoglycoside, effective against gram-negative pathogens such as E. coli, and parenteral clindamycin or chloramphenicol, effective against Bacteroides fragilis and other anaerobes. In addition to antibiotics, cooling measures are used to prevent seizures and excessive hyperthermia.

Subtle respiratory decompensation may occur during the course of peritonitis. It may only be detectable by a decreased arterial PCO_2 from hyperventilation in an attempt to maintain adequate oxygenation, or by a rapid pulse that persists, despite restoration of blood volume. Blood gas studies detect and monitor decompensation both before and after oxygen therapy has been instituted (Storer, 1974). In most cases, surgery is performed to remove the source of infection at the earliest possible time the patient is medically stable. Repeated

examinations of the abdomen to determine the course of the disease
and the appearance of any localizing signs is an important part of
the continued management of the patient.

::

10.2 INTRA-PERITONEAL ABSCESSES

1. ETIOLOGY

Intra-peritoneal abscesses follow diffuse peritonitis when the infection is localized or walled off by omentum or bowel loops plastered
to the inflamed peritoneal surface. Polymorphonuclear leukocytes,
bacteria and cellular debris accumulate within this space, and tissue necrosis continues until the purulent exudate and necrotic tissue
are removed by surgical excision or spontaneous rupture of the abscess cavity. Resolution also occurs when proteolytic enzymes convert the cellular debris to sterile fluid, creating a cyst. An abscess
may also follow a localized focus of peritonitis in which the peritoneal
defense has time to prevent spreading or diffuse peritonitis. The
periappendiceal abscess is an example. These are termed secondary
abscesses because an intra-abdominal lesion due to disease or trauma
is evident prior to abscess formation. Primary abscess formation
also occurs in which no apparent cause is found within the abdominal
cavity. Presumably, the infecting organism reaches the peritoneal
cavity by hematogenous or lymphatic spread. These abscesses are
rare in children who have normal host defense mechanisms. Finally,
abscesses form following postoperative procedures, especially surgical invasion of the gastrointestinal tract or biliary tree. Fluids
leaking from the operative site are localized and infection supervenes.

The bacteriology of intra-abdominal abscesses is discussed in the
earlier section (Bacteriology of Intra-abdominal Infections). Anaerobic bacteria predominate and multiple species are usually present
(Table 10-2 and Table 10-3). Studies in humans and in experimental
animals indicate that anaerobes are the dominant organisms responsible for abscess formation (Onderdonk et al., 1974). When modern
techniques of isolating anaerobes are utilized, there is a marked decrease in the number of sterile abscesses. Altemeier et al. (1973)
isolated anaerobes in 70% of 501 cases of intra-abdominal abscesses.

Intra-peritoneal abscesses are also classified anatomically, forming
the basis for surgical treatment. The spaces which accumulate peritoneal fluid are the usual sites of abscess formation. These are the
subphrenic, which includes the left and right subphrenic or suprahepatic spaces, the right subhepatic space, the lesser sac, the right
and left paracolic gutters and the pelvis (most commonly the cul-de-
sac of Douglas) (Storer, 1974). Abscesses may be present in more
than one area, or may form adjacent to diseased viscera. Subphrenic
abscesses commonly follow appendicitis and other diseases of the

stomach, duodenum, liver, biliary tract, or pelvis. Abdominal surgery is one of the most common causes of subphrenic abscesses, as are automobile accidents resulting in laceration of the liver or bowel. The left-sided lesser sac abscesses are less common and primarily occur after gastrointestinal surgery or diseases of the stomach, pancreas, or duodenum. Paracolic abscesses occur more frequently, especially on the right following appendicitis or regional enteritis. Pelvic abscesses also follow appendicitis with perforation or any form of diffuse peritonitis, but more often are related to pelvic inflammatory disease.

2. CLINICAL MANIFESTATIONS

The clinical signs and symptoms of intra-peritoneal abscesses are usually nonspecific and highly varied. The onset may be acute, especially following a perforated peptic ulcer or ruptured appendix, but often the process is insidious with vague symptoms showing no evidence of localization. The patient may present with only intermittent fever, malaise, and weight loss. Even in the postoperative patient, symptoms and signs are frequently not diagnostic. Abdominal pain and tenderness, fever, tachycardia, and leukocytosis are common postoperative findings. The administration of antibiotics further clouds the symptom complex, allowing the intra-abdominal process to continue for weeks or months before becoming manifest.

The clinical manifestations of 82 children and adults with documented subphrenic abscess are presented in Table 10-9 (Magilligan et al., 1968). Pain, in the upper abdomen or lower chest, and fever were constant findings. It is important to note the frequency of chest pain, shoulder pain and dyspnea, all symptoms causing the clinician to suspect a respiratory or intrathoracic condition. The presence of rales or dullness over the lung bases, and abnormalities on chest x-rays, further point toward a respiratory problem. Actual rupture of the abscess through the diaphragm to the lung with the production of foul smelling sputum was rare, occurring in only four percent. Direct evidence of an intra-abdominal condition, as manifest by nausea and vomiting, occurred in only nine percent of patients, although abdominal tenderness along the costal margin was a frequent finding.

Abdominal findings are more prominent in other types of intra-peritoneal abscesses. An enlarging, tender, poorly defined mass along the right upper quadrant is suggestive of a right subhepatic abscess. In addition to deep, lower abdominal pain and fever, pelvic abscess is frequently associated with diarrhea. If the abscess compresses the bladder, urinary frequency, urgency, and dysuria may also occur. The pelvic abscess is usually not detected by abdominal palpation, but rectal examination reveals a tender mass bulging against the anterior rectal wall.

TABLE 10-9: CLINICAL MANIFESTATIONS OF SUBPHRENIC ABSCESS IN 82 CHILDREN AND ADULTS

SYMPTOMS	PERCENTAGE
Chest pain	59
Abdominal pain	94
Shoulder pain	37
Weight loss	59
Dyspnea	24
Nausea and vomiting	9
Production of foul sputum	4
SIGNS	
Fever	97
Abdominal tenderness	80
Dullness or rales	72
LABORATORY DATA	
Leukocytosis > 15,000	66
ROENTGENOGRAPHIC FINDINGS	
Pleural effusion	73
Elevated diaphragm	69
Immobile diaphragm	34
Ileus	18
Lower lobe atelectasis or infiltrate	18

Adapted from Magilligan, D.J., Arch. Surg. 96:14-19, 1968.

3. DIAGNOSIS

The lack of specific clinical findings during abscess formation requires the clinician to be alert to clinical settings in which intraperitoneal abscesses arise. An important clue is relapse following recovery from surgical procedures, trauma, or peritonitis. The patient who initially appears to improve following peritonitis or abdominal operation, only to develop prolonged malaise, anorexia, weakness or vomiting, should be suspect for an intra-peritoneal abscess. Recurrence of fever or rise in white blood cell count after initial improvement during the postoperative course further suggests the possibility of abscess formation. In some cases, antibiotics suppress symptoms and signs of infection, thereby delaying the diagnosis and resulting in a prolonged postoperative course. In this situation, briefly stopping the antibiotics permits the definitive diagnosis to be made.

Subphrenic abscesses are difficult to diagnose by evaluation of clinical signs and symptoms alone. The white blood cell count is frequently elevated, but there is no specific laboratory test. A leukocytosis of >15,000 in 66% and >25,000 in 23% of cases is reported by Magilligan et al., 1971 (see Table 10-9). Roentgenographic examination is the most helpful diagnostic aide. Pleural effusion is an early and frequent sign of subphrenic abscess occurring in 73% of cases (Table 10-9). Elevated diaphragm is also a common finding, and either during fluoroscopy or by comparing inspiratory and expiratory films, decreased motion of the diaphragm is established. Atelectasis, pneumonitis and evidence of adynamic ileus are also frequent findings. Clearly, subphrenic abscesses must be differentiated from pneumonia, pulmonary embolism or infarction and postoperative atelectasis, as well as from other types of intra-abdominal abscesses.

Radiologic signs permitting location of other types of intra-abdominal abscesses are visualization of soft tissue densities, localized extraluminal gas, and displacement or obliteration of normally visualized structures. Abscesses of the lesser sac displace the stomach anteriorly and the colon downward. Pelvic abscesses distort the dome of the urinary bladder (Aeriel and Kazarian, 1971). Combined liver-lung or spleen-lung radioisotope scan also helps to localize a subphrenic abscess. Other techniques to localize intra-abdominal abscesses have been employed with varying success. These include ultrasonography (Goldberg et al., 1975), computerized tomography and the gallium scan.

4. MANAGEMENT

Early surgical drainage reduces the morbidity and mortality from intra-peritoneal abscesses. Roberts et al. (1974) demonstrated a mortality of 16% with aggressive surgical drainage of subphrenic abscesses, compared to a 43% mortality in patients treated with antibiotics alone. Complications resulting from delay in surgery include empyema, pneumonia, mediastinal abscesses, bronchopleural fistula, and rupture of the intra-peritoneal abscess into the abdomen or through the diaphragm.

As with diffuse peritonitis, preoperative preparation, including correcting dehydration, is important. Intravenous antibiotics help to abort cellulitis and control sepsis, thereby preventing further suppurative complications. In general, surgery should not be delayed to institute a trial of antibiotic therapy. During surgery, both anaerobic and aerobic culture are obtained from the abscess, allowing specific antibiotic therapy during the postoperative period.

10.3: RETRO-PERITONEAL ABSCESSES

The differential diagnosis of intra-peritoneal abscesses includes
localized areas of infection arising within the retro-peritoneum.
Retro-peritoneal abscesses occur in the space between the peritoneum and the transversalis fascia lining the posterior abdominal
wall (Altemeier, 1973). This space extends from the diaphragm to
the pelvic brim, and is divided into anterior-posterior planes by
renal fascia containing the kidneys. Retroperitoneal abscesses are
mainly secondary to infection, trauma or malignancy of the genito-
urinary tract. The perinephric space is the most frequent site of
abscess formation, and pyelonephritis is the most common etiology.
During the neonatal period, the majority of intra-abdominal masses
are retroperitoneal, but these usually represent multicystic kidney,
hydronephrosis, neuroblastoma, and nephroblastoma (Wilms' tumor), rather than abscess formation (Blakenship et al., 1975). The
bacteriology of retroperitoneal abscesses reflects the etiology of
the infection. Monomicrobic infection due to gram negative rods,
such as E. coli or Klebsiella species, is likely when the urinary
tract is the primary source. Both Lorber and Swenson (1975)
(Table 10-2), and Altemeier et al. (1973) reported a high frequency
of anaerobic infection.

The clinical manifestations of retroperitoneal abscesses are similar to those of intra-peritoneal infection. Malaise, fever, weight
loss, leukocytosis and pain predominate. Localized tenderness
may be felt over the kidneys, costovertebral angle or spine, and a
tender mass may be occasionally palpated in the area of the abscess.
Pyuria, hematuria or difficulty with urination suggests urinary tract
involvement.

Diagnosis is achieved by use of urinary tract studies, particularly
intravenous or retrograde pyelography and renal arteriography.
The intravenous pyelogram frequently reveals displacement of the
ureter, bladder, or kidney by an external mass. Plain films of the
abdomen will show a soft tissue mass, obliteration of psoas shadow
or loss of normal renal outline. Elevation of the diaphragm can
also be present. Even though retroperitoneal abscess is strongly
suspected, the diagnosis may only be made at laparotomy.

Adequate surgical drainage is the primary treatment. Reconstruc-
tion of the urinary tract is often delayed until after the abscess is
drained and the infection has subsided. Appropriate antibiotic therapy is started either empirically or on the basis of urine culture
results prior to surgery, but survival without surgical drainage is
rare.

10.4: VISCERAL ABSCESSES

Abscesses in the liver, pancreas, spleen and kidneys are difficult to diagnose and treat, resulting in a high mortality. Fortunately, they are extremely rare in children. Between 1917 and 1967, the frequency of pyogenic liver abscess based on autopsy study of children under 15 years of age was 0.35% (27 in 7,697 autopsies) (Dehner and Kissane, 1969). These children were mainly under five years of age and were compromised by leukemia, immunosuppressive therapy, previous surgery or sepsis. Only two of the 27 liver abscesses were diagnosed prior to autopsy. Eighty percent of the liver abscesses were multiple and 60% were associated with extrahepatic abscesses of the spleen, kidney or lungs.

1. ETIOLOGY OF LIVER ABSCESSES

Prior to antibiotics, liver abscesses mainly followed unmanageable infections in otherwise normal children. Since the 1940's, most of the reported cases are in children with leukemia or chronic granulomatous disease, or in children who are immunosuppressed. In a review of 92 patients with chronic granulomatous disease, 41 patients were noted to have hepatic or parahepatic abscesses (Johnston, 1971). In these children, systemic bacteremia resulting in hematogenous spread to the liver is the main mechanism of liver abscess development. Liver abscess also results from invasion by contiguous structures, or from direct inoculation during recent abdominal surgery or trauma. Liver abscesses in adults are usually secondary to pylephlebitis (septic thrombosis of the portal vein), or are associated with suppurative cholangitis.

The gastrointestinal flora frequently isolated from liver abscesses are E. coli, Klebsiella, Pseudomonas and Enterococcus (Streptococcus species). Staphylococcus aureus is the most frequent pathogen isolated from liver abscesses in children with chronic granulomatous disease (Johnston, 1971) and has been reported recently as a cause of liver abscess in normal children (Kaplan, 1976). Many studies report a high percentage of sterile liver abscesses varying from 11% (Dehner and Kissane, 1969) to 40% (Ochsner et al., 1938). In studies utilizing modern techniques for the isolation of anaerobes, sterile abscesses are rare. Sabbaj et al., (1972) report anaerobes in pure or mixed culture in 45% of liver abscesses in adults. Blood cultures were also positive for anaerobes in 54% of these patients. In another report, including both children and adults, Altemeier (1974) recovered anaerobes from all twelve liver abscesses cultured between 1970-1972. Anaerobes were the only isolates in eight of these twelve and included Bacteroides, Fusobacterium and Peptostreptococcus species.

2. CLINICAL MANIFESTATIONS AND DIAGNOSIS OF LIVER ABSCESS

Since the diagnosis is usually made at autopsy, there is very little information in the literature summarizing the clinical and laboratory features of pyogenic liver abscess in living children. Recently, Kaplan and Feigin (1976) described two previously healthy children in which liver abscesses were successfully diagnosed and treated. Both children presented with abdominal pain and met the criteria for fever of unknown origin. Autopsy studies reveal the signs and symptoms to be nonspecific and often related to underlying primary disease (Dehner and Kissane, 1969). The diagnosis should be suspected in any patient with chronic granulomatous disease who presents with fever and abdominal pain. Fever, malaise, abdominal pain and tenderness in the right upper quadrant are the most frequent findings. Leukocytosis ranging from 12,000 to 41,000 cells per mm^3 is the most common laboratory finding (Dehner and Kissane, 1919). Mild hyperbilirubinemia, low serum albumin and elevated alkaline phosphatase are nonspecific laboratory findings (Silverman, 1971). Liver function tests, however, may be entirely normal (Kaplan and Feigin, 1976).

Liver abscess is difficult to distinguish from subphrenic abscess on the basis of roentgenographic findings alone. Pleural effusion, alteration of the right hemi-diaphragm, and limited diaphragmatic excursion are common to both conditions. Enlargement of the liver, and evidence of air in the liver abscess cavity are helpful findings. The most useful diagnostic aid is the radioisotope (technetium 99m) liver scan. In contrast to normal liver parenchyma, the abscess cavity does not accumulate the radioisotope, allowing the localization of abscesses two centimeters or greater. Once a space-occupying mass has been located, arteriography and ultrasound can further distinguish between solid tumor and a fluid-filled abscess cavity.

Pyogenic liver abscess is differentiated from amoebic abscesses by history of travel, previous dysentery, or the finding of amoebae on stool examination. High antibody titer by indirect hemagglutination test is a sensitive indicator of amoebiasis. These antibodies are present in over 90% of the patients with amoebic liver abscesses (Jessee et al., 1975). The differential diagnosis is aided by use of the gallium 67 scan which highlights pyogenic liver abscesses as "hot" areas, but amoebic abscesses as "cold" areas (Meyer and Finegold, 1976).

3. MANAGEMENT OF LIVER ABSCESSES

Like other intra-abdominal abscesses, the treatment for liver abscess is primarily surgical. Antibiotics are instituted to prevent sepsis and suppurative complications. Prior to culture results, antibiotics effective against Bacteroides, such as clindamycin or chloramphenicol, should be utilized in conjunction with antibiotics effective against gram-negative organisms (i.e. Gentamicin). Gentamicin is also effective against Staphylococcus aureus, a pathogen frequently isolated from liver abscesses. In a patient with chronic granulomatous disease, a specific anti-staphylococcal drug would be an appropriate choice. Anaerobic and aerobic cultures at the time of surgery permit specific antibiotic therapy, which should be continued for at least two months, and perhaps four months in patients with multiple liver abscesses (Meyer and Finegold, 1976).

REFERENCES

Altemeier, W.A.: Liver Abscess: The Etiologic Role of Anaerobic Bacteria, In Anaerobic Bacteria: Role in Disease. Balows, A. et al., ed. Charles C Thomas, Springfield, 1974, pp. 387-398.

Altemeier, W.A. and Alexander, J.W.: Retroperitoneal abscess. Arch Surg 83:44-56, 1961.

Altemeier, W.A., Culbertson, W.R and Fuller, W.D.: Intra-abdominal sepsis. Advances in Surg 5:281-333, 1971.

Altemeier, W.A., Culbertson, W.R., Fuller, W.D., and Shock, D.C.: Intra-abdominal abscess. Am. J. Surg. 125:70-79, 1973.

Ariel, I.M. and Kazarian, K.K.: Diagnosis and Treatment of Abdominal Abscesses. Williams and Wilkins Co., Baltimore, 1971.

Attebery, H.R., Sutter, V.L. and Finegold, S.M.: Normal Human Intestinal Flora, In Anaerobic Bacteria: Role in Disease. Balows, A., et al., ed., Charles C Thomas, Springfield, 1974, pp. 81-97.

Barbour, G.L. and Juniper, K., Jr.: A clinical comparison of amebic and pyogenic abscesses of the liver in sixty-six patients. Am. J. Med. 53:323-334, 1972.

Blair, G. L. and Gaisford, W.D.: Acute appendicitis in children under six years. J. Pediat. Surg. 4:445-451, 1969.

Blankenship, W J., Bogren, H., Stadalnik, R.C., and Vitale, D.E.: Suprarenal abscesses in the neonate: A case report and review of diagnosis and management. Pediatrics 55:239-243, 1975.

Blattner, R.J.: Acute mesenteric lymphadenitis. J. Pediat. Vol. 74, No. 3, 479-481, 1969.

Boles, E.T., Jr., Ireton, R.J. and Clatworthy, H.W., Jr.: Acute appendicitis in children. Arch Surg 79:447-454, 1954.

Carter, R., Brewer, L.A. III: Subphrenic abscesses: A thoracoabdominal clinical complex: The changing picture with antibiotics. J. Surg. 180:165-174, 1964.

Dehner, L.P. and Kissane, J.M.: Pyogenic hepatic abscesses in infancy and childhood. J. Pediat. 74:763-773, 1969.

de la Mazu, L.M., Faramarz, N. and Berman, L.D.: The changing etiology of liver abscess. JAMA 227:161-163, 1974.

Donaldson, R.M.: Normal bacteriologic populations of the intestine and their relation to intestinal function. NEJM 270:938,944,1050, 1964.

Douglas, B. and Vesey, B.: Bacteroides: A cause of residual abscess? J. Pediat. Surg. 10:215-220, 1975.

Dunkle, L.M., Brotherton, M.S., and Feigin, R.D.: Anaerobic infections in children: A prospective study. Pediatrics 57:311-320, 1976.

Finegold, S.M.: The significance of the intestinal microflora. Infect. Dis. Rev. I:67-72, 1971.

Finegold, S.M.: Pylephlebitis and liver abscess, in Infectious Diseases, Heoprich, P.D., ed., Harper & Row, New York, 1972, pp. 699-702.

Finegold, S.M. and Dineen, P.: Subphrenic and Other Intra-Abdominal Abscesses, in Infectious Diseases, Hoeprich, P.D., ed., Harper & Row, New York, 1972, pp. 703-708.

Finegold, S.M., Bartlett, J.G., Chow, A.W., Flora, D.J., Gorbach, S.L., Harder, E.J., and Tally, F.P.: Management of anaerobic infections. Ann. Int. Med. 88:375-389, 1975.

Fowler, R. Jr.: Primary peritonitis: Changing aspects, 1956-1970, Australian Pediat. J. 7:73, 1971.

Fraga, J.R., Javate, B.A., and Venkatessan, S.: Liver abscesses and sepsis due to klebsiella pneumoniae in a newborn, A complication of umbilical vein catheterization. Clin. Pediat. 13:1081-1082, 1974.

Gilmore, O.J.A., et al.: Appendicitis and mimicking conditions: A prospective study. Lancet Vol. II, No. 7932, 421-424, Sept. 6, 1975.

Goldberg, B.R., Pollack, H.M., Capitanio, M.A., and Kirkpatrick, J.A.: Ultransonography: An aid in the diagnosis of masses in pediatric patients. Pediatrics 56:421-428, 1975.

Gorbach, S.L.: Intestinal microflora. Gastroenterology 60:1110-1129, 1971.

Gorbach, S.L., Thadepalli, H., Norsen, J.: Anaerobic Microorganisms in Intra-Abdominal Infection, in Anaerobic Bacteria: Role in Disease, Balows, A., et al., eds., Charles C Thomas, Springfield, 1974, pp. 399-407.

Gwinn, J.L., Lee, F.A., and Baker, C.J., et al.: Pyogenic liver abscess. Am. J. Dis. Child. 123:49, 1972.

Haller, J.A., Shaker, I.J., Donahoo, J.S., Schnauffer, L., White, J.J.: Peritoneal drainage versus non-drainage for generalized peritonitis from ruptured appendicitis in children. Ann. Surg. 177:595-599, 1973.

Holgersen, L.O. and Stanley-Brown, E.G.: Acute appendicitis with perforation. Am. J. Dis. Child. 122:288-293, 1971.

Holliday, R.L.: Peritonitis - Old and new thoughts. Heart and Lung 4:456-460, 1975.

Jensen, F. and Pedersen, J.F.: The value of ultrasonic scanning in the diagnosis of intra-abdominal abscesses and hematoma. Surg. Gyn. Obstet. 139:326-328, 1974.

Jessee, W.F., Ryan, J.M., Fitzgerald, J.F., Grosfeld, J.L.: Amebic liver abscess in childhood. Clin. Pediat. 14:134-145, 1975.

Johnston, R B. and Baehner, R.L.: Chronic granulomatous disease: correlation between pathogenesis and clinical findings. Pediatrics 48:730-739, 1971.

Kaplan, S.L. and Feigin, R.D.: Pyogenic liver abscess in normal children with fever of unknown origin. Pediatrics 58:614-616, 1976.

Konvolinka, C.W. and Olearczyk, A.: Subphrenic Abscess, in Current Problems in Surgery, Year Book Medical Publishers, Inc., Chicago, January, 1972.

Lorber, Bennett and Swenson, R.M.: The bacteriology of intra-abdominal infections. Surg. Clin. N.A. 55:1349-1354, 1975.

Magilligan, D.J.: Suprahepatic abscess. Arch. Surg. 96:14-19, 1968.

Marchildon, M.B. and Dudgeon, D.L.: Perforated appendicitis: Current experience in a children's hospital. Ann. Surg. 185:84-87, 1977.

Martin, L.W., Altemeier, W.A., and Reyes, P.M.: Infections in pediatric surgery. Pediat. Clin. N.A. 16:735-766, 1969.

Mata, L.J. and Urrutia, J.J.: Intestinal colonization of breast-fed children in a rural area of low socioeconomic level. Ann. N.Y. Acad. Sci. 176:93-109, 1971.

McDougal, W.S., Izant, R.J., Zollinger, R.M.: Primary peritonitis in infancy and childhood. Ann. Surg. 181:310-313, 1975.

Meyer, R.D. and Finegold, S.M.: Anaerobic infections: Diagnosis and treatment. South. Med. J. 69:1178-1195, 1976.

Middleton, H.M., Patton, D.D., Hoyumpa, A.M., and Shenker, S.: Liver-lung scan in the diagnosis of right subphrenic abscess. Am. J. Diges. Dis. 21:215-222,

Moore, W.E.C., Cata, E.P., and Holdeman, L.V.: Anaerobic bacteria of the gastrointestinal flora and their occurrence in clinical infections. J. Infect. Dis. 119:641-649, 1969.

Ochsner, A., DeBakey, M.E., Murray, S.: Pyogenic abscesses of the liver: An analysis of 47 cases with review of the literature. Am. J. Surg. 40:292-319, 1938.

Onderdonk, A.B., Weinstein, W.M., Sullivan, N.M., et al.: Experimental intra-abdominal abscesses in rats: Quantitative bacteriology of infected animals. Infect. Immun. 10:1256-1259, 1974.

Parsons, J.M., Miscall, B.G., McSherry, C.K.: Appendicitis in the newborn infant. Surgery 67:841-843, 1970.

Redfern, W.T., Close, A.S., and Ellison, E.H.: Intra-abdominal abscesses, A review of 100 consecutive patients. Arch. Surgery 85:278-284, 1962.

Roberts, E.A.B., and Nealon, T.F.: Subphrenic abscess, comparison between operative and antibiotic management. Ann. Surg. 180:209, 212, 1974.

Sabbaj, J., Sutter, V.L., and Finegold, S.M.: Anaerobic pyogenic liver abscess. Ann Int. Med. 77:629-638, 1972.

Shandling, B., Sigmund, E.H., Simpson, J.S., Stephens, C.A. and Bandi, S.K.: Perforating appendicitis and antibiotics. J. Pediat. Surg. 9:79-83, 1974.

Sherman, N.J., Davis, J.R., Jesseph, J.E.: Subphrenic abscess, a continuing hazard. Am. J. Surg. 117:117-123, 1969.

Silverman, A., Roy, C.C., Cozzeho, F.J., eds.: Pediatric Clinical Gastroenterology. C.V. Mosby Co., St. Louis, 1971, pp. 351-353.

Speck, W.T., Dresdale, S.S., McMillan, R.W.: Primary peritonitis and the nephrotic syndrome. Am. J. Surg. 127:267-269, 1974.

Stone, H.H.: Bacterial flora of appendicitis in children. J. Ped. Surg. 11:37-42, 1976.

Stone, H.H., Sanders, S.L., Martin, J.D., Jr.: Perforated appendicitis in children. Surgery 69:673-679, 1971.

Storer, E.H.: Peritonitis and intra-abdominal abscesses, in Principles of Surgery, 2nd Ed., McGraw-Hill, New York, 1974, pp. 1297-1311.

Tally, F.P. and Gorbach, S.L.: Antibiotics in surgery. Advances in Surgery 9:41-95, 1975.

Thadepalli, H., Gorbach, S.L., Broido, P.W., Norsen, J., Nyhus, L.: Abdominal trauma, anaerobes and antibiotics. Surgery 137:270-276, 1973.

Walker, A.W.: Host defense mechanisms in the gastrointestinal tract. Pediatrics 57:901-916, 1976.

Weinstein, W.M., Onderdonk, A.B., Bartlett, J.G., et al.: Experimental intra-abdominal abscesses in rats: Development of an experimental model. Infect. Immun. 10:1250-1255, 1974.

Williams, J.W., et al.: Liver abscesses in newborn. Am. J. Dis. Child. 125:111, 1973.

CHAPTER 11. URINARY TRACT INFECTIONS

INTRODUCTION: The urinary tract is second only to the respiratory tract as the most common site of bacterial infection in children. Certainly, urinary tract infections (UTI) represent the most
prevalent and most remedial genito-urinary tract disease during
childhood. Because of the frequency of recurrences and the potential for loss of renal function, the diagnosis of a urinary tract infection in a pediatric patient requires a subsequent commitment by
the physician and the patient's family for evaluation and long-term
surveillance. For these reasons, the diagnosis of a UTI should
never be made casually, and a thorough understanding of the natural
history of UTI is mandatory for all physicians caring for children.

Due to the nonspecificity, and even absence of symptoms in children,
the true incidence of UTI is unknown. In the neonatal period, prospective studies have detected significant bacteriuria in 0.7 percent
to 1.5 percent of neonates. A marked preponderance of males with
bacteriuria (4:1) exists in the neonatal period. From one month to
one year, however, UTI occur equally in male and female infants
with an overall incidence of approximately 1.0 percent. After one
year of age, UTI predominately occur in females.

Prospective studies in school children by Kunin (1962) found persistent bacteriuria in 1.2 percent of girls and 0.04 percent in boys.
These infections were often asymptomatic. Long-term surveillance
of these girls revealed a high rate of recurrence (65% in white girls)
and a conversion of 0.3-0.4% from negative to positive each year.
Thus, five percent of a population of girls will acquire a urinary
tract infection during elementary and high school. The peak incidence of UTI in children, however, occurs between the ages of two
and six years. Both Cohen (1972) and DeLuca (1963) found the peak
incidence of initial UTI to be three years of age. Following the first
UTI, 30-65% of children have recurrent UTI. It is disquieting to
note that 50% of recurrent infections are asymptomatic and are detectable only with routine urine cultures.

1. ETIOLOGY AND PATHOGENESIS

The principle pathogens of the urinary tract of children are the gram-
negative bacteria. Of these bacilli, Escherichia coli account for as
many as 75% of acute infections. Often, the serotype of E. coli
identified in the urine is also isolated from the patient's vaginal and
intestinal flora. Klebsiella and Proteus mirabilis are the next most
frequently encountered agents in uncomplicated infections. Other
gram negative organisms occasionally encountered include Pseudomonas aeruginosa, Enterobacter species, Serratia marcesens, and

rarely, Hemophilus influenzae. Recently, an increasing awareness of the pathogenicity of gram positive organisms in UTI has developed. Staphylococcus epidermidis has been identified as a significant pathogen, particularly in boys. Other gram positive agents include Enterococcus and Staphylococcus aureus. When UTI occur following instrumentation, or in the presence of functional or anatomical abnormalities, a much greater prevalence of "non-coliform" bacterial agents occurs. Bergstrom (1972) also noted fewer E. coli infections in boys with a much greater frequency of Proteus mirabilis.

Because of the frequency with which E. coli infects the urinary tract, a great deal of investigative work has attempted to elucidate the pathogenic nature of this bacteria. Studies have shown that E. coli serotypes 01, 02, 04, 06, 07, 011, 015, 062, and 075 account for as many as 60% of UTI in children. All of these serotypes have been identified in non-urinary infections, however, and are the most commonly isolated gastrointestinal serotypes. At present, it is not possible to predict upper versus lower tract infection on the basis of the O-antigen alone. Hanson et al. (1975) have noticed that the above O-serotypes are isolated more often from the urine of patients with symptomatic UTI. Asymptomatic UTI on the other hand, were more often associated with the spontaneously agglutinating rough strains of E. coli which seldom caused symptomatic infection. These rough strains were much more sensitive to antibiotic therapy than the E. coli encountered with symptomatic infection. This data suggest that modification of the bacterial cell envelope may reduce the virulence of the agent in asymptomatic infections. The K capsular antigen may also be important for the virulence of E. coli in the human urinary tract, although experimental work has not substantiated this hypothesis.

The causative role of L-forms (cell-wall defective organisms) in UTI remains controversial. When diligently sought, L-forms have been identified in 20% of adult patients with chronic pyelonephritis. Whether the presence of these L-forms is significant in the pathogenesis of recurrent infections is speculative.

Viruses do not appear to be an important etiology of UTI in children. Virus isolation from the urine usually occurs in the course of a systemic infection. Acute hemorrhagic cystitis associated with dysuria, frequency and urgency, however, may result from infection with adenovirus types 11 and 21.

Mycobacterium tuberculosis, fungi and protozoa causing UTI in children are extremely rare and will not be discussed in this chapter.

Pathogenic organisms enter the urinary tract either from the bloodstream or by ascending through the urethra. There is no present evidence to implicate lymphatic spread of bacteria into the human kidney. Experimental and clinical findings suggest that the hematogenous route is not the principal method of bacterial entry into the kidney. In the experimental model, the inoculation of bacteria into the bloodstream produces pyelonephritis only when obstruction is present. Furthermore, in children, most UTI occur in the lower urinary tract, are not accompanied or preceded by septicemia, and do not have associated structural abnormalities. The neonatal period is somewhat unique since males are infected more often than females, structural abnormalities are frequent and associated sepsis is seen. For these reasons, the hematogenous route of infection is likely in the neonatal period.

Most UTI originate through the ascending transurethral passage of bacteria. This concept readily explains the marked female preponderance, the greater incidence of lower tract infections and the infection with the patient's bowel flora. The ascending route is particularly common in young children in whom perineal contamination is unavoidable. The capability of bacteria to travel across the short female urethra is suggested since bacteria have been shown to inhabit the male urethra as far as 6 cm proximal to the meatus. Inoculation of bacteria into the bladder, however, will not produce a UTI in a normal urinary tract. UTI routinely result from such bacterial inoculation if there is ureteral reflux or obstruction.

Since contamination of the urinary tract may be a universal phenomenon in the young female, host factors must also influence the development of UTI in children. As seen in experimental data and from clinical experience, UTI are associated with major anatomic abnormalities. Obstructive lesions such as complete ureteropelvic or vesicourethral obstruction frequently present as a UTI. Such congenital obstructive lesions are seen more frequently in boys with UTI. Functional obstruction to urine flow caused by a neurogenic bladder or by bladder distortion secondary to fecal impaction may also result in UTI. Although rare in children, obstruction from urolithiasis may also lead to infection.

Vesicoureteral reflux is another urologic abnormality associated with urinary tract infection. A brief summary of this very complex topic is necessary in any discussion of UTI in children. Reflux is defined as the retrograde flow of urine into the ureter and kidney. It is caused by the incompetence of the normal valvular action of the ureterovesical junction caused by congenital anatomical defects, distortion from disease or from distal obstruction. Reflux is classified by Smellie (1975) according to severity by the following system: Grade 1, reflux into the ureter with voiding; Grade 2 and 3, reflux into the renal pelvis with reflux, only upon micturition in Grade 2; and Grade 4, reflux associated with dilatation of the ureter and renal pelvis. Vesicoureteral reflux may be found in up to 30-50% of children with UTI and is by far the most common abnormality identified in these children. It is best diagnosed with voiding cystography.

Since reflux provides a means for bacteria to reach the kidney and for residual bladder urine in which bacteria may multiply, children with reflux would empirically appear to be at greater risk for developing infections and renal scarring. The role of reflux alone, reflux plus infection, or infection without reflux in progressive renal scarring remains unanswered. Smellie (1975) found a high incidence of renal scarring with Grade 4 reflux, particularly in young boys. Rolleston (1975) also noted that renal scarring occurred in patients with severe reflux in the first year of life. Recent data implicate intrarenal reflux (reflux demonstrated into the renal parenchyma) as being necessary for renal scarring. Hodson (1975) has found that renal scarring in the pig will occur with intrarenal reflux without concomitant infection.

It is also known that reflux becomes less common with advancing age and that reflux is seen much less frequently with UTI in adults. Smellie et al. (1975) demonstrated that chronic reflux disappeared in 50% of 126 refluxing ureters during continuous antibiotic therapy. In their population, loss of reflux occurred even in children with Grade 4 reflux and despite renal scarring. Most children with Grade 1 and Grade 2 reflux reverted to normal. In the absence of UTI, progression of reflux did not result in a renal scar. Kunin (1969) has shown that reflux will disappear with short-term antibiotic therapy for each infection. Decreasing reflux with age may either be a result of controlling urinary infections, or maturational development of the vesicourethral valve. Surgical correction of reflux in cases of recurrent infections refractory to medical management may be effective in controlling reinfection. In summary, it appears that renal scarring may occur from severe reflux, usually when accompanied by infection. In addition, it appears that renal scarring usually occurs with reflux at an early age and that reflux tends to improve over time without surgery.

Host immunity may also be important in the pathogenesis of UTI. However, since patients with immune deficiency states are not particularly subject to UTI, the role of systemic immunity is questionable. Children with pyelonephritis often, but not always, develop a circulating antibody response to the infective organisms. The finding of an elevated serum antibody titer in a patient with a UTI has been advocated as a means of identifying renal parenchymal infections. It has now been shown that antibody titers may also be elevated in patients with both cystitis and asymptomatic bacteriuria. Although experimental evidence suggests that an antibody response may be protective against reinfection of the urinary tract in rabbits, such protection has not been demonstrated in humans.

On the other hand, antibodies produced locally in the urinary tract may be of more significance. Urine from uninfected humans may contain IgG, IgA and IgE. At least part of the urinary IgA represents secretory IgA. Both IgG and IgA are produced within the urinary tract and both may be present in high levels in the urine of children with UTI. The significance of these antibodies in patients with recurrent or asymptomatic infections remains to be clarified. The association of antibody-coated bacteria in the urine of patients with pyelonephritis may be of clinical importance and will be discussed later.

Local factors appear to be important in the pathogenesis of UTI. The hypertonic renal medulla, for example, provides a favorable environment for bacterial multiplication and for the development of bacterial L-forms. In addition, granulocytic mobilization is markedly inhibited in such hypertonic media. The presence of ammonia in the renal interstitium inhibits chemotaxis by inactivating the fourth component of complement. Antibacterial activity, in contrast, has been demonstrated in prostatic secretions and in the bladder mucosa. Clearly, many factors contribute to the prevention and genesis of an infection following the introduction of bacteria into the urinary tract. The question of how each of these factors influence the problem of UTI in children remains unanswered.

2. CLINICAL MANIFESTATIONS

The clinical diagnosis of UTI in children is not an easy task for the physician. Not only are the symptoms nonspecific, but they also vary with the age of the child. This difficulty in diagnosis was emphasized by DeLuca (1963), who found an average delay of 18 months from the onset of symptoms to the diagnosis of UTI in children less than three years of age.

Table 11-1 illustrates the changing pattern of symptoms with UTI according to the age of the patient. During the first months of life, most symptoms are associated with the gastrointestinal tract. Failure to thrive, feeding problems, diarrhea, vomiting, jaundice and abdominal distension may occur. In the neonate, a UTI may be a presentation of bacterial sepsis and may be accompanied by the symptoms of irritability, hypotonis, respiratory symptoms and even convulsions.

After 2 years of age, fever is the most common symptom. As seen in Table 11-1, symptoms referable to the urinary tract, such as frequency, dysuria, abdominal pain, flank pain and hematuria, become more prevalent with advancing age. The common symptoms of dysuria and frequency in children should not be accepted as a priori evidence of a UTI since trauma, perineal irritation, masturbation and many other etiologies may produce this same symptom complex. All patients with these symptoms should have culture documentation to make the diagnosis of UTI. The recurrence of enuresis after successful toilet-training certainly suggests the possibility of a UTI. When UTI are associated with obstructive uropathy, which is more commonly seen in young infants and in boys, symptoms such as dribbling of urine, straining with urination, or a decrease in the force or size of the urinary stream may bring the patient to the physician.

TABLE 11-1: PRESENTING SYMPTOMS OF 200 INFANTS AND CHILDREN WITH URINARY TRACT INFECTIONS

	Birth-1 Month	1 Month-2 Years	2-5 Years	5-12 Years	
	45 Patients	45 Patients	44 Patients	66 Patients	Total
Failure to thrive, feeding problems	24	16	3	–	45
Screaming attacks, irritability	–	6	2	–	8
Offensive or cloudy urine	–	4	6	–	10
Diarrhea	8	7	–	–	15
Vomiting	11	13	7	2	33
Fever	5	17	25	33	80
Convulsions	1	3	4	3	11
Hematuria	–	3	7	4	14
Frequency or dysuria	–	2	15	27	44
Enuresis	–	–	12	19	31
Abdominal pain	–	–	10	29	39
Loin pain	–	–	–	8	8

From Riley, H.: Pyelonephritis in Children: The Long-Term Problem, Hospital Practice 7:141, 1972 by permission of the author and publisher.

As shown by Kunin (1971) and Cohen (1972), it is not uncommon for
the older child with documented bacteriuria to be totally asymptomatic with the first infection. Recurrent infections, however, present the greatest challenge in diagnosis. Over 50% of children with
recurrent UTI are asymptomatic, regardless of whether symptoms
were present with the first infection.

Following the initial UTI, a child has a 40-65% risk for recurrence
even without a predisposing urologic abnormality. Over 50% of
these recurrences occur within six months of the initial infection,
and 70% occur within one year. The asymptomatic nature of these
recurrences must be emphasized.

Complications may result from both acute and chronic UTI. In most
instances, an acute UTI is an uncomfortable nuisance; however, in
cases of acute pyelonephritis, septicemia may occur with life-
threatening consequences, particularly in the neonate and infant.
Since vomiting and diarrhea often accompany a UTI in young children, dehydration may intervene, requiring hospitalization. On the
other hand, an acute UTI may itself represent a complication of an
underlying congenital urological disorder whose correction may be
necessary to preserve renal function. The value of radiographic
investigations to diagnose such problems will be discussed in a subsequent section.

The effects of chronic pyelonephritis may be devastating to the afflicted child. In a review of 1279 hospitalized children with UTI,
De Luca (1963) found 35% ultimately developed severe renal damage
and that 20% died. In less select populations, the frequency with
which recurrent pyelonephritis leads to end-stage renal disease and
hypertension in the absence of anatomical abnormalities remains unanswered. Certainly, cases of progressive renal impairment from
recurrent pyelonephritis without urologic complications have been
reported. It is clear, however, that the child with chronic pyelonephritis associated with severe ureteral reflux or obstructive uropathy
is at greatest risk for developing the growth failure, anemia, hypertension and metabolic aberrations of chronic renal failure. The data
of Kunin (1971) and Winberg et al. (1975) suggest that early detection and appropriate antibiotic therapy of UTI are effective in preventing progressive renal scarring.

3. DIAGNOSIS

Urinary tract infections are generally defined as the presence of
greater than 10^5 bacteria per milliliter of properly collected midstream voided urine. To apply this definition to all children, one
must assume that bacterial excretion, method of collection, state of
hydration, bladder incubation time and the time between the sample
collection and culture plating are uniform. Since these variables
obviously cannot always be controlled in children, a more practical
definition seems in order. A UTI has been defined by Kunin (1971)

as the bacterial colonization of any part of the urinary tract, with
the number of organisms appearing in the urine being greater than
can be accounted for by the system of collection. This definition
serves two purposes. First, it emphasizes that the diagnosis of a
urinary tract infection is based on the identification of bacteria in a
urine culture. Second, it stresses that physicians understand the
techniques and limitations of urine collection in children.

Before discussing the methods of collecting urine samples, it is important to discuss some of the factors affecting bacterial growth in
the urine. Usually, urine provides an excellent medium for bacterial
multiplication. Therefore, in order to obtain an accurate reflection
of the number of organisms in a urine sample, the length of time between obtaining a urine sample and plating a culture should be minimal (less than one hour). When it is impossible to plate a urine sample in such a short time, refrigeration may inhibit bacterial growth
until culturing is possible. In addition, several circumstances may
decrease the bacterial count in a urine sample. These include: low
urine pH and specific gravity; previous antibiotic therapy; polyuria
which decreases bladder incubation time; and collecting a sample in
late afternoon when bacterial excretion tends to decline.

The most widely employed method of collecting urine samples for
culture is the midstream clean-voided urine. This method requires
a cooperative toilet-trained patient which makes it impractical for
young children. With this technique, after the labia majora are
spread or the foreskin retracted, the external genitalia are thoroughly cleansed with hexachlorophene and rinsed with sterile water.
A midstream sample of urine is then collected in a sterile container.
Growth of greater than 10^5 colonies of a single organism per ml of
urine on two consecutive specimens is diagnostic of a UTI. Colony
counts of a single organism between 10,000 and 100,000 per ml are
suspicious of a UTI and require confirmation with either repeated
midstream clean-catch samples, suprapubic bladder aspiration or
catheterized urine culture. Less than 10,000 colonies per ml in a
clean-voided urine is considered negative. Making the diagnosis of
a UTI on the basis of a specimen collected in a sterile urine collection bag, regardless of the colony count, is hazardous. Before concluding that a UTI exists in this situation, the positive culture should
be reconfirmed with a suprapubic bladder aspiration or catheterization.

In young children and in cases with indeterminate bacterial counts
from clean voided specimens, percutaneous suprapubic bladder aspiration has proven to be a safe and reliable means of accurately
diagnosing a UTI. Aspiration is performed with the patient supine
and the lower extremities held in a "frog-leg" position. After cleansing the suprapubic area with iodine and alcohol, a needle is inserted
in the midline 1.5 cm above the symphysis pubis and angled 30⁰ toward the bladder. In small children, a 21 gauge 1.5 cm needle is
adequate. In older children, a 5 cm spinal needle is occasionally
necessary. To avoid failure, a period of time should have elapsed

since the patient last voided or wet the diaper. Transient hematuria may rarely complicate this procedure. Bladder aspiration should be avoided in cases of abdominal distension to avoid perforation of the gastrointestinal tract. The presence of any gram-negative bacterial growth on a single bladder aspiration is sufficient for diagnosis of a urinary tract infection. Small numbers of gram positive organisms might represent contamination from the skin and should be confirmed with repeated aspiration.

The introduction of office bacteriologic screening techniques has provided an accurate, inexpensive and simple means of screening children for urinary tract infections. One of these methods is the filter strip culture method which uses miniature trypticase soy agar trays. This technique has been found to be 98% accurate when compared to standard cultures, and is the least expensive of the bacteriologic methods (as little as $0.10 per culture). It has the slight disadvantage of not differentiating gram-negative or gram-positive organisms. The dip-slide or dip-strip techniques, which use discriminating agars, allow differentiation of gram negative and gram positive bacteria. When a positive culture is found on either the filter-strip, dip-slide or dip-strip culture, the organism can then be identified definitely and antimicrobial sensitivities performed. These methods can be used efficiently for screening for UTI in an out-patient population; however, they do not replace traditional culture techniques in the complicated case where decreased numbers of bacteria might be expected.

Pyuria of greater than five white blood cells per cubic millimeter in an uncentrifuged urine sample has been shown to be unreliable for screening for urinary tract infections in children. Riley (1972) found pyuria to be absent in up to 60% of children with documented UTI. The presence of pyuria, however, does not necessarily indicate the presence of infection. Table 11-2 lists some etiologies of pyuria without bacteriuria. Hence, the diagnosis of UTI should never

TABLE 11-2: SOURCES OF PYURIA WITHOUT BACTERIURIA	
Dehydration	Trauma
Irritants	Calculi
Renal tuberculosis	Acute glomerulonephritis
Vaccinations	Viral gastroenteritis
Renal tubular acidosis	Systemic lupus erythematosus
Viral cystitis	Interstitial nephritis

be made on the basis of pyuria alone. A gram stain of an uncentrifuged urine sediment collected under sterile conditions is more helpful in screening for UTI. The identification of one organism per high power field in a gram stain of uncentrifuged urine has a 90% correlation with 10^5 organisms per ml of urine. A gram stain, while not a substitution for culture, may support a tentative diagnosis of UTI when symptoms require therapy before the results of cultures are known.

Chemical screening tests for detecting UTI, such as the Greiss nitrate-nitrite test, the tetrazolium reduction test, urinary glucose determination and the presence of catalase in the urine, have not been widely accepted in pediatrics. These tests require patient co-operation and an overnight bladder incubation time, making them impractical for infants and young children. All of these tests require subsequent confirmation by appropriate urine cultures before the diagnosis of UTI can be made with certainty. The availability of the inexpensive bacteriologic screening techniques would seem to limit the usefulness of these less sensitive and less specific chemical tests.

The laboratory may be helpful in localizing the site of infection within the urinary tract. Since the patients with bacteriuria of renal origin are thought to be at greatest risk for renal scarring and loss of renal function, this information is of major importance. Some of the laboratory tests that have been used to identify pyelone-phritis include elevated erythrocyte sedimentation rate, elevated C - reactive protein, loss of renal concentrating capacity, elevated serum antibody titers and the presence and pattern of lactic dehy-drogenase isoenzymes in the urine. The most direct methods are cultures of urethral urine or renal biopsy specimens. These methods, however, lack practicality because of their associated risks. In addition, because of the focal nature of pyelonephritis, renal biopsy cultures have not been reliable in documenting upper tract infection. The bladder wash-out technique has been advocated to differentiate upper and lower tract infection. This method requires bladder cath-eterization and irrigation with an antibiotic solution. After allowing the antibiotic solution to remain in the bladder for 30 minutes, the bladder is washed four times with sterile saline. The urine is cul-tured after the saline washings and after three consecutive 20-minute collecting periods. Upper tract infection is diagnosed by greater than 10^3 bacteria per ml in any of the final three collections, if this growth represents a five-fold increase above the sample obtained immedi-ately following the saline washings. Intermittent excretion of bac-teria from the renal parenchyma could cause the washout test to be negative in the presence of upper-tract disease, while ureteric re-flux may lead to a false positive washout test if infected bladder urine is retained in the ureters and emptied into the bladder after the saline washings.

An interesting noninvasive method of differentiating upper-tract and lower-tract infection was reported by Jones et al. (1974), Thomas et al., (1974), and Forsum et al., (1976) who detected antibody-coated bacteria in the urine of adult patients with pyelonephritis. Using florescein-conjugated antihuman globulin, these authors found antibodies (primarily IgG) coating bacteria in patients with renal in-fection. IgA and IgM coated bacteria were also occasionally identi-fied. An elevated serum antibody titer was not a prerequisite to developing the antibody-coating. Although this method has not yet been reported in children, it is extremely appealing because of its ease and safety. False positives have been reported in patients with prostatitis.

4. MANAGEMENT

The goals of management in urinary tract infections in children are to eradicate infection, to recognize and correct anatomical abnormalities, to preserve renal function and to prevent recurrences. To attain these goals requires patient compliance in completing antimicrobial therapy, radiographic evaluation of the urinary tract, careful screening for recurrent infections with repeated urine cultures and correction of any predisposing hygienic inadequacies. Because of the time, effort and expense of these endeavors, it is imperative to first accurately diagnose a UTI and to allow time for informing parents of the significance of the diagnosis and management program.

Antimicrobial therapy should be instituted once the diagnosis is confirmed and antimicrobial sensitivities obtained. If symptoms require immediate therapy prior to culture reports, every effort should be made to obtain a urine culture by suprapubic aspiration or catheterization, since once antibiotics have been started it is impossible to reconfirm a questionable culture result. As mentioned earlier, a gram stain of an unspun sterile urine collection may be of great assistance in deciding whether to immediately start antibiotics after obtaining a diagnostic culture.

McCracken and Eichenwald (1974) have recently outlined an initial approach for the antimicrobial treatment of UTI in children. Since E. coli are responsible for most initial infections, oral sulfisoxazole 120-150 mg/kg/day is the first choice if therapy is begun prior to culture results. Ampicillin, 50-100 mg/kg/day in four oral doses or amoxicillin, 20-40 mg/kg/day in three doses are acceptable alternatives. After antimicrobial sensitivities are known, an adjustment in therapy may be required. The best index of the efficacy of therapy, however, is a repeat culture after 48-72 hours of treatment. If the repeat culture is still positive, antibiotics should be changed regardless of in vitro sensitivities. When pyelonephritis is suspected, or when signs of sepsis are present, hospitalization with parenteral antibiotic therapy is indicated. Neonatal UTI should be considered a manifestation of neonatal sepsis, and parenteral therapy should be started after urine and blood cultures are obtained.

Considerable controversy exists concerning whether to treat an acute infection with two weeks of antibiotic therapy or for longer periods. Although UTI were traditionally treated for six weeks, data from Cohen (1972) and Bergstrom et al. (1968) showed that two weeks of antibiotic therapy is equally effective in eradicating infection. Furthermore, recurrent infections were as common following six weeks of therapy as with two weeks of antibiotics.

Recurrent infections should be treated in an identical manner to acute infections. However, in some patients with unexplained and frequent recurrences, or in patients with structural defects which can't be corrected, prolonged therapy with bacteriostatic drugs may be required after eradication of infection with a bactericidal agent. Nitrofurantoin (1-2 mg/kg/day) is the preferred drug in young children. The length of chronic therapy depends on the clinical situation. Patients with structural abnormalities may require suppressive therapy for many years. Children who are receiving chronic suppressive therapy should have urine cultures examined at regular intervals for intercurrent UTI. A new drug combination, trimethoprim-sulfamethoxazole, has been recently approved for the treatment of UTI in children. This combination (2 mg trimethoprim/10 mg sulfamethoxazole/kg/day) may also be quite helpful as suppressive therapy.

In addition to antibiotic therapy, several general measures may be of benefit in hastening eradication of the acute infection and in preventing recurrences. A generous fluid intake should be encouraged to replace increased insensible water losses from fever and the increased urinary fluid losses that result from the impaired concentrating ability produced by pyelonephritis. In addition, children are encouraged to void frequently since the retention of urine in the bladder may serve to maintain an infection. Multiple voidings before bedtime may be suggested. Proper perineal hygiene should be emphasized since enteric organisms usually are the source of UTI. Wiping from anterior to posterior following defecation is recommended. Prolonged tub baths, particularly with bath perfumes or bubble bath preparations, should be avoided. Constipation has also been associated with UTI in children by Neumann et al. (1973). It is thought that chronic constipation produces distension of the rectum, which in turn distorts the bladder. Elevation of the posterior bladder thereby makes it difficult to initiate voiding. Neumann found that correcting the constipation in his patients with laxatives, dietary measures and stool softeners greatly reduced the incidence of recurrent UTI.

The success in eradicating an infection should be assessed with a urine culture 4-7 days following the completion of two weeks of antibiotic therapy. Because of the frequent and early recurrence of urinary infections, a program for regular urine cultures is proposed in Table 11-3. The asymptomatic nature of recurrent infections requires that such a program be instituted even in an apparently healthy child. The inexpensive microculture techniques are particularly suited for such a program.

Radiologic investigation of the urinary tract for structural abnormalities is also an important part of the management of UTI in children. A high incidence of urologic lesions has been found in children presenting with UTI in the first months of life. Although radiographic abnormalities are more common in boys at all ages, Tsingoglou (1972) reported a series in which 35 cases of lower urinary tract obstructions occurred in girls less than 1 year old. In addition, Smellie

<table>
<tr><td colspan="1">TABLE 11-3: FOLLOWING AN INITIAL URINARY TRACT INFECTION, URINE CULTURES SHOULD BE PERFORMED:</td></tr>
<tr><td>
1. 4-7 days following completion of antibiotic therapy
2. At 6 weeks
3. At 3-month intervals for 1 year
4. At 6-month intervals for 5 years thereafter
</td></tr>
</table>

(1975) reports that renal scarring from severe reflux occurs very early in life. For these reasons, an intravenous pyelogram and voiding cystourethrogram should be performed following the initial infection in all children less than two years old and in boys of all ages. Because transient reflux may occur during an acute infection, it is advisable to wait 2-4 weeks after completion of therapy to obtain the voiding cystourethrogram. There is much debate about when radiologic studies should be obtained in girls over two years of age. Because of the high recurrence rate and the asymptomatic nature of these recurrences, it seems reasonable to perform an intravenous pyelogram (IVP) following the first infection in girls over two years of age. If the IVP is normal, there seems to be little benefit from proceeding with the voiding cystourethrogram. However, if significant abnormalities are found on the IVP, or if the girl develops numerous recurrences, a voiding cystourethrogram should also be obtained. Cystoscopy is not a part of the routine evaluation of a child with a UTI. Cystoscopy is considered if the IVP or voiding cystourethrogram is abnormal, or if repeated infections occur while receiving good medical management.

The role of surgery in the management of UTI is primarily to correct obstructive lesions and to correct severe reflux in young children. Ureteral reimplantation may be required in older children to control repeated infections which occur despite good medical management. The importance of uretheral obstruction in the development of UTI in girls has been recently questioned by urologists, radiologists and pediatricians. Forbes (1969) found in a controlled study that meatotomy had no beneficial effect in preventing recurrent infections in girls with the radiologic diagnosis of meatal stenosis. Walker and Richard (1973), in a review of urethral obstruction in girls, state that little evidence supports the assumption that urethral obstruction plays an important role in UTI in girls. Therefore, indiscriminant meatotomy or urethrotomy appears to be unwarranted in the treatment of UTI in girls.

REFERENCES

Abbott, G.D.: Neonatal bacteriuria: A prospective study in 1,460 infants. B. Med. J. 1:267, 1972.

Allen, T.D.: Pathogenesis of urinary tract infection in children. NEJM 273:1421-1425, 1965.

Amar, A. and Chabra, L.: The practical management of urinary tract infections in children. Clin. Pediatr. 13:532, 1974.

Bergstrom, T.: Sex differences in childhood urinary tract infection. Arch. Dis. Child. 47:227, 1972.

Bergstrom, T. et al.: Studies of urinary tract infections in infancy and childhood. XII: Eighty consecutive patients with neonatal infection. J. Pediatr. 80:858, 1972.

Bergstrom, T. et al.: Studies of urinary tract infections in infancy and childhood. X: Short or long-term treatment in girls with first or second-time urinary tract infections uncomplicated by obstructive urological abnormalities. Acta Paediatr. 57:186, 1968.

Brumfitt, W. et al.: Antibiotic-resistant Escherichia coli causing urinary tract infection in general practice: Relation to faecal flora. Lancet 1:315, 1971.

Brun, C., Raaschou, F. and Eriksen, K.: Simultaneous bacteriologic studies of renal biopsies and urine. In, Progress in Pyelonephritis, Kass, E.H., ed., F.A. Davis Co., Philadelphia, 1964, p. 461.

Cohen, M.: Urinary tract infections in children. I. Females age 2 through 14, first two infections. Pediatrics 50:271, 1972.

DeLuca, F.G., Fisher, J.H. and Swenson, O.: Review of recurrent urinary tract infections in infancy and early childhood. NEJM 268: 75, 1963.

Dodge, W. et al.: Detection of bacteriuria in children. J. Pediatrics 74:107, 1969.

Edlemann, C.M. et al.: The prevalence of bacteriuria in full-term and premature newborn infants. J. Pediatr. 82:125, 1973.

Forbes, P., Drummond, K. and Nogrady, M.: Initial urinary tract infections: Observations in children without major radiologic abnormalities. J. Pediatr. 75:187, 1969.

Forbes, P., Drummond, K. and Nogrady, M.: Meatotomy in girls with meatal stenosis and urinary tract infection. J. Pediatr. 75: 937, 1969.

Forsum, U., Hjelm, E., Jonsell, G.: Antibody-coated bacteria in the urine of children with urinary tract infections. Acta. Paediatr. 65 639, 1976.

Gillenwater, J.V. et al.: Home culture by the Dip-Strip method. Pediatrics 58:508, 1976.

Gruneberg, R.N.: Relationship of infecting urinary organism to the faecal flora in patients with symptomatic urinary infection. Lancet 2:766, 1969.

Gutman, L., Schaller, J. and Wedgewood, R.: Bacterial L-forms in relapsing urinary tract infection. Lancet 2:11, 1967.

Hanson, L.A. et al.: The host parasite relationship in urinary tract infections. Kidney Int. Supplement 8:S-28, 1975.

Harding, G. and Ronald, A.: A controlled study of antimicrobial prophylaxis of recurrent urinary infection in women. NEJM 291: 597, 1974.

Harkness, J., Anderson, F. and Dalta, N.: R-factors in urinary tract infection. Kidney Int. Supplement 8:S-122, 1975.

Hermansson, G. et al.: Coagulase negative staphylococci as a cause of symptomatic urinary infections in children. J. Pediatr. 84:807, 1974.

Hodson, J. et al.: Reflux nephropathy. Kidney Int. Supplement 8: S-50, 1975.

Jodal, U., Lindberg, U. and Lincoln, K.: Level diagnosis of symptomatic urinary tract infections in childhood. Acta Paediatr. 64: 201, 1975.

Jones, S., Smith, J. and Sanford, J.: Localization of urinary tract infections by detection of antibody coated bacteria in urine sediment. NEJM 290:591, 1974.

Kaye, P.: Urinary Tract Infection and Its Management. C.V. Mosby Co., St. Louis, 1972.

Kunin, C.M.: Epidemiology and natural history of urinary tract infection in school age children. Pediatr. Clin. N.A. 18:245, 1971.

Kunin, C.M.: Tendency of vesico-ureteric reflux to disappear coincident with specific chemotherapy. In, Renal Infection and Renal Scarring, Kincaid-Smith, P. and Fairley, K.F., eds., Mercedes Publishing Services, Melbourne, 1970, p. 287.

Kunin, C.M.: Detection, Prevention and Management of Urinary Tract Infections. Lea and Febiger, Philadelphia, 1972.

Kunin, C.M., Zurha, E. and Paguin, A.J.: Urinary tract infections in school children. I. Prevalence of bacteriuria and associated urologic findings. NEJM 206:1287, 1962.

Lincoln, K. and Winberg, J.: Studies of urinary tract infections in infancy and childhood. II. Quantitative estimation of bacteriuria in unselected neonates with special reference to occurrence of asymptomatic infections. Acta Paediatr. 53:307, 1964.

McCracken, G. and Eichenwald, H.: Antimicrobial therapy: Therapeutic recommendations and a review of the newer drugs. J. Pediatr. 85:292-312, 451-456, 1974.

Mufson, M.A. et al.: Adenovirus infection in acute hemorrhagic cystitis. Am. J. Dis. Child. 121:281, 1971.

Neter, E.: The microbiologic aspects of urinary tract infection. In, Pediatric Nephrology, Rubin, M.I. and Barrat, T.M., eds., Williams and Wilkins Co., Baltimore, 1975.

Neter, E. et al.: I. Patterns of antibody response of children with infections of the urinary tract. Pediatr. Res. 4:500, 1970.

Neumann, P., deDomenico, I. and Nogrady, M.: Constipation and urinary tract infection. Pediatrics 52:241, 1973.

Pryles, C. and Eliot, C.: Pyuria and bacteriuria in infants - the value of pyuria as a diagnostic criterion of urinary tract infections. Am. J. Dis. Child. 110:628, 1965.

Pryles, C. and Lustik, B.: Laboratory diagnosis of urinary tract infections. Pediatr. Clin. N.A. 18:233, 1971.

Retik, A.: Urinary reflux in children: An approach to management. Hospital Practice 11:125, 1974.

Riley, H.: Pyelonephritis in children. Hospital Practice 7:141, 1972.

Rolleston, G., Shannon, F. and Utley, W.: Follow-up of vesico-ureteric reflux in the newborn. Kidney Int. Supplement 8:S-59, 1975.

Scott, J.: The role of surgery in the management of vesico-ureteric reflux. Kidney Int. Supplement 8:S-73, 1975.

Shopfner, C.E.: Modern concepts of lower urinary tract infection and obstruction in pediatric patients. Pediatrics 45:194, 1970.

Smellie, J. et al.: Vesico-ureteric reflux and renal scarring. Kidney Int. Supplement 8:S-65, 1975.

Steihm, R. and Uchling, D.: Secretory IgA in urinary tract infections. Pediatrics 47:40, 1971.

Tsingoglou, S., Dickson, J.: Lower urinary obstruction in infancy. Arch. Dis. Child. 47:215, 1972.

Walker, D. and Richard, G.: A critical evaluation of urethral obstruction in female children. Pediatrics 51:272, 1973.

Winberg, J., Bergstrom, T. and Jacobsson, B.: Morbidity, age and sex distribution, recurrences and renal scarring in symptomatic urinary tract infection in childhood. Kidney Int. Supplement 8:S-101, 1975.

CHAPTER 12. VENEREAL DISEASES

12.1: GONORRHEA

INTRODUCTION: It is well known that venereal diseases in general
and gonorrhea specifically are reaching epidemic proportions. In
the United States, nearly one million cases were reported in 1975
and the number of unreported cases is estimated to be at least 2-3
times that number.

Gonorrhea is currently the most common reportable and commonly
reported communicable disease in the U.S. Two-thirds of the cases
are in individuals 25 years-old and younger, and one-fourth of the
cases occur in the 10 to 19-year-old age group. Reasons for the increase in gonorrhea include a short incubation period, asymptomatic
carriage, absence of immunity following infection, lack of serological test, high communicability, increased resistance of the organism
to antibiotic therapy, changing sexual mores, and contraception. The
pediatric population reflects this increase also, especially in young
adolescents and young children. The mode of transmission in young
adolescents is probably voluntary sexual contact, while in young children it is more likely to be sexual abuse or nonvenereal transmission.
The pediatrician and family physician, through their unfamiliarity
with the high incidence and atypical presentations of gonorrhea in
children, probably fail many times to recognize this disease in their
young patients.

1. ETIOLOGY AND PATHOGENESIS

The causative organism of gonorrhea is Neisseria gonorrheae, an
aerobic, gram negative diplococci. There are four types (1, 2, 3
and 4) of gonococcus. Only types 1 and 2 have pili and cause disease
in man. The organism adheres to the surface with pili, penetrates
the epithelium, and multiplies submucosally. An inflammatory reaction takes place at the point of entry with submucosal capillary
dilatation, mobilization of polymorphonuclear leukocytes, and epithelial desquamation. In the male, this is manifest by a penile discharge. In the female, infection and abscess formation in the para-
urethral and vaginal glands occurs. After approximately one to two
weeks, fibrous tissue results. The chance of dissemination is more
likely if the victim is inoculated by the anorectal or pharyngeal
routes, especially in the male. Although measureable immunological
responses occur, both local and systemic, and cellular and humoral,
infection does not confer protective immunity against subsequent
infections.

2. CLINICAL MANIFESTATIONS

The manifestations of gonococcal infection best known to the pediatrician is ophthalmia neonatorum. The baby is usually exposed to the organism upon passage through the birth canal, although babies born by Cesarean section have been infected, presumably by the ascension of gonococcal organisms after rupture of membranes. Newborns may also be infected from the hands of contaminated handlers. The incubation period is one to three days and the disease begins as a conjunctivitis followed by a watery discharge which rapidly becomes purulent. The eyes become hyperemic and the lids swollen. Ophthalmia neonatorum must be recognized and treated early as it attacks the cornea, causing ulceration and perforation, resulting in blindness. With the advent of silver nitrate prophylaxis, the incidence of this form of gonococcal infection has decreased, but prophylaxis is not 100% effective (see Chapter - Conjunctivitis).

The prepubescent female shows a propensity to infection with gonococci because of a thin vaginal epithelium which has an alkaline pH. There is also a lack of pubic hair, and the child has gaping labia. The disease presents as a vulvovaginitis with a profuse, thick, creamy discharge, often accompanied by secondary urethritis and proctitis. Primary gonococcal infection in the adolescent female is usually a cervicitis which, when symptomatic, presents with a purulent discharge, dysuria and, on occasion, dyspareunia. The cervix is usually hyperemic and tender. The incidence of asymptomatic infections in adolescent girls has been estimated to be 10-20%.

In the male, symptomatic infection of the urethra presents with dysuria, discharge and erythema. In young males, pyuria may be the only sign of gonococcal infection (Dawar and Hellerstein, 1972). Asymptomatic infections do occur in young males and, although their exact incidence is unknown, in older males the incidence is reported in the range of 10%.

In complicated infections, the organism may spread along the mucous membranes from the site of entry and ascend in the female, causing endometritis and more. If it reaches the tubes, it may cause acute salpingitis, manifested by fever and chills in an acutely ill-appearing patient. There is bilateral low abdominal pain, and the patient may complain of diarrhea, nausea, vomiting, constipation, or dyspareunia. Blood samples will show an increased white blood cell count with a left shift and an elevated sedimentation rate. On the other hand, acute salpingitis may follow a prolonged subacute course with only a sensation of a dull ache or pressure in the lower abdomen, with a tendency for this to be unilateral. The white blood cell count in this case will be normal and the sedimentation rate will not be elevated. If the salpingitis is allowed to become chronic, there may be damage to the tubes, resulting in pyosalpinx, hydrosalpinx, adhesions, or a cystic ovary which diminishes fertility and may lead to an ectopic pregnancy. Clinically, the patient with chronic salpingitis will be afebrile with a normal count and sedimentation rate, but have symptoms of a unilateral adnexal mass which is tender to palpation.

In rare cases, gonococci may spread from the pelvis over the peritoneal surface of the liver, causing perihepatitis. The symptoms consist of right upper quadrant pain which may be pleuritic and often referred to the shoulder. The patient also displays tenderness, guarding, and a friction rub over the liver. Complicated gonorrhea in the male may result from direct extension to the prostate accompanied by enlargement and urinary obstruction or, if a mass is present in the scrotum which is tender, erythematous, and warm, gonococcal epididymitis must be considered.

When hematogenous extension occurs, skin lesions, arthritis, tenosynovitis, meningitis, and rarely, endocarditis may result. The skin lesions are described as tender papules 1 to 2 mm. in diameter with an erythematous or hemorrhagic base and a central pinpoint-size vesicular or pustular area. More lesions are seen on the extremities than the trunk. Arthritis occurs twice as frequently in females as males. It begins with fever and occasionally chills with arthralgia, followed by arthritis of one or more joints. The wrists, knees, and ankles are most commonly affected.

Oral and anal gonorrhea should be considered in sexually active adolescents. The former, most likely resulting from oral intercourse, manifests as cryptic tonsillitis and pharyngitis with or without an exudate, erythema, and swelling of the palate. Anal gonorrhea is becoming more common as homosexuality becomes more accepted. Anal gonococcal infections may be asymptomatic or may cause tenesmus and a bloody mucoid discharge.

Finally, gonorrhea in the young child may not present with the more typical clinical manifestations noted above. Low et al. (1976) reviewed 11 cases of gonococcal infections in children under 10 years of age. Five female children presented with evidence of vulvovaginitis. However, of the remaining six children, two had asymptomatic infections (one pharyngeal, one rectal), one presented with a sore throat, one with an infected thumb (a $1\frac{1}{2}$year old), one with recurrent hematuria, and one with a history of child abuse and a positive vaginal culture but no vulvovaginitis. All of these children were from lower socio-economic families and in 10 of 11 cases the source of infection could be traced to an adult in the household who was infected.

3. DIAGNOSIS

The diagnosis of gonorrhea depends solely upon the isolation of the gonococcus, although a presumptive clinical diagnosis may be supported by gram stain of exudate in the urethra of the male and the finding of gram negative cocci. Similar findings in the female are misleading because of organisms of similar morphology and staining characteristics which may inhabit the vagina. Fluorescent staining, although another adjunct to diagnosis, is not conclusive, as the fluorescent antibody may cross-react with other species of neisseria or other organisms. Obviously, serologic diagnosis of this infection would greatly augment case finding efforts and, although this is currently being investigated, serologic tests are not routinely available for use at present.

Careful culture technique is essential in order to assure optimal results. The gonococcus is a fastidious organism and the chances of isolation will be greatly increased if the specimen is collected properly, placed on a selective media (such as Thayer-Martin) and grown under optimal conditions (2-10% CO_2 at 35-37°C.). The swabs used for specimen collection should be cotton and certified free of fatty acids, for these will inhibit organism growth. The cervix is the preferred cite of culture for the female and lubricants should not be used prior to obtaining the specimens as they are often bactericidal.

4. MANAGEMENT

The drug of choice in the treatment of any form of gonorrhea is penicillin. For those patients with known penicillin sensitivity, spectinomycin is used. The dosage and duration of drug therapy depends upon the clinical form of the disease.

In the newborn with ophthalmia neonatorum, systemic therapy should consist of at least 50,000 units/kg/day of penicillin G parenterally for five days, along with topical applications of tetracycline or chloramphenicol. All newborns should receive prophylaxis with silver nitrate 1% solution immediately after delivery.

In cases of cervicitis, vaginitis, or urethritis, whether the patient is male or female, therapy consists of 4.8 million units of aqueous penicillin G IM preceded by one gram of probenecid. If the patient is allergic to penicillin, two grams of spectinomycin intra-muscularly are administered. All patients should be followed up and recultured to assure that the gonorrhea has been eradicated.

Any form of gonorrhea which has spread, such as pelvic inflammatory disease of disseminated gonorrhea, is treated with intravenous penicillin for seven to ten days. The dose is six to ten million units in an adult or adolescent and 100,000-200,000 units/kg/day in children.

In addition to treatment of the gonococcal infection, complete management should include treatment of the adolescent's sexual partner, evaluation of the patient for co-existent venereal diseases by obtaining a VDRL or fluorescent treponema antibody test, and emotional support. Whenever infection is diagnosed in the young child, the potential for child abuse must be assessed and efforts made to identify the source of infection in the child's family or household.

:::

12.2: SYPHILIS

INTRODUCTION: Syphilis is the second most prevalent venereal disease in the United States, but unlike gonorrhea, the incidence has remained relatively constant for the past 10 years. Syphilis is usually classified into congenital and acquired forms. It is of interest that despite the relative constancy of reported cases of the acquired form (25,000 cases per year of primary and secondary syphilis, over the past 10 years), the incidence of congenital syphilis has dropped markedly from 2,052 cases reported in 1971 to 916 cases in 1975.

Although the majority of cases of the acquired form occur in young adults, the disease can occur in any age group, and in 1975 there were nearly 4,000 cases reported in children and adolescents 19 years of age and under. As is the case with gonorrhea, it is estimated that the actual number of cases exceeds by 4-5 times the number of reported cases.

1. CONGENITAL SYPHILIS

The spirochete, Treponema pallidum, which is the infectious agent, invades the placenta sometime during the course of pregnancy and from that vantage point infects the fetus. Although it has been widely held that spirochetes could not penetrate the placenta until the latter stages of pregnancy following atrophy of Langhan's cell layer, this has recently been disputed (Benirschke, K., 1974), and the precise pathogenesis of congenital syphilis is still poorly understood. However when the placenta is or has been infected, it will be large, edematous and pale at birth, and this should always alert the clinician to the possibility of congenital syphilis. A careful microscopic examination of the placenta and appropriate diagnostic studies on the mother and infant should then be mandated.

Congenital syphilis occurs in two forms - early and late. In the early form, manifesting within the first few weeks of life, bone lesions (osteitis) are the most frequent finding (Grossman and Drutz, 1974). Roentgenograms may show areas of destruction and growth disturbances in the metaphysis, primarily in long bones. Erosion of the medial proximal metaphysis of the tibia (Wimberger's sign) is sometimes present.

The earliest manifestation of early untreated congenital syphilis may be nothing more than a benign appearing rhinitis or a red, maculopapular rash. The rhinitis, which can occur in the first few days of life, is a clear discharge that when secondarily infected by bacteria, may become purulent and bloody. The skin lesions, which typically involve the palms and soles, may at first be maculopapular, progressing later to bullous or vesicular lesions. Pseudoparalysis, although "classic," is uncommon. Involvement of the Central Nervous System is common, although the infant is usually asymptomatic. The cerebrospinal fluid cell count and protein are elevated. Other manifestations of untreated early congenital syphilis include jaundice, hemolytic anemia, hepatosplenomegaly, lymphadenopathy, pneumonitis and/or the nephrotic syndrome.

The late form of congenital syphilis is manifested by a symptom complex called Hutchinson's triad, consisting of Hutchinson's teeth, interstitial keratitis and 8th nerve deafness. Other associated findings are "mulberry molars," Clutton's joints and the saddle nose. Of greater importance are the manifestations of CNS involvement which range from an elevated CSF cell count and protein in an otherwise asymptomatic person, to juvenile paresis. These sequelae may not be totally prevented by treatment of the infant after birth, and their prevention thus lies in the early identification and treatment of the infected mother during gestation.

In the newborn infant suspected of having congenital syphilis, the diagnosis is confirmed by finding a positive IgM-fluorescent treponemal antibody absorption test in the infant's serum (Kauffman, R.E. et al., 1974). Since IgM antibodies from the mother do not cross the placenta, their presence in the infant signifies an intrauterine treponemal infection. The VDRL (reagin) test which is routinely performed on cord blood in many institutions simply indicates the presence of reagin which: 1) may be due to active infection in the infant; 2) may have been passively transferred from the mother who had (has) an infection which may or may not have been treated; or 3) may be caused by a biologically false positive reaction. Thus, the VDRL while useful as a screening test, does not confirm the diagnosis of congenital syphilis.

The treatment of congenital syphilis has recently been critically reviewed by McCraken and Kaplan (1974). Acknowledging the lack of data regarding proper dosage and choice of penicillin preparations for treating this disease, they recommend that infants with active congenital syphilis without CNS involvement be treated either with procaine penicillin G, 10,000 u/Kg, administered once daily IM for 10 days, or benzathine penicillin G, 50,000 u/Kg, administered in one injection. For infants with congenital neurosyphilis, larger amounts of penicillin are required to assure adequate spirocheticidal levels in the cerebrospinal fluid, and procaine penicillin G in dosage of 50,000 u/Kg is given in one daily dose for 10-14 days.

2. ACQUIRED SYPHILIS

Acquired syphilis is heralded by the appearance of a chancre on the glans penis, labia, vagina, cervix, anus, rectum, or mouth about three to six weeks after exposure. It may be accompanied by regional, nontender lymphadenopathy. With or without treatment, the primary lesion will eventually disappear, but the serology will usually become positive within one week after the lesion appears. The infected individual then enters the second stage of syphilis. This consists of a generalized, painless, nonpruritic rash which may be macular, papular, or pustular, and it usually involves the palms and the soles. Condylomas in the anogenital region, mucous membrane patches in the mouth, lymphadenopathy, and general malaise are other clinical manifestations of the second stage. After approximately six weeks, these symptoms too will disappear, and the patient enters the latent stage. It is important to remember that the disease is very contagious in the second stage and non-venereal transmission of the infection is known to occur.

The adolescent or adult with primary or secondary acquired syphilis (including pregnant women) should be treated either with 2.4 million units of benzathine penicillin G intramuscularly (usually given in two 1.2 million unit doses at the same time) or 600,000 units of procaine penicillin administered daily for 10 days. Tetracycline is considered the second drug of choice but should be used only in the penicillin-allergic patient. The treatment of patients with neurosyphilis requires larger doses of penicillin, usually in a total dose range of 6-9 million units. As in the patient with gonorrhea, other aspects of management include treatment of the sexual partner, protecting the confidentiality of the minor, excluding the possibility of coexistent venereal disease of other causes and providing emotional support.

12.3: LYMPHOGRANULOMA VENEREUM (LGV), CHANCROID AND GRANULOMA INGUINALE

These venereal diseases are uncommon in the United States and very rare in the pediatric age group. LGV is caused by a large virus in the psittacosis-lymphogranuloma-trachoma (P-L-T) group and is common in the tropics. The infection presents as a transient penile vesicle followed by inguinal lymphadenopathy, malaise and low grade fever. Anorectal involvement may result in stricture formation. The diagnosis is substantiated by a positive Frei test and treatment consists of tetracycline administered orally for 3 weeks.

Chancroid is caused by <u>Hemophilus ducreyi</u>, a gram negative coccobacilliary rod which characteristically causes a soft chancre or multiple ulcerations on the glans penis, accompanied by tender regional lymphadenopathy. Preferred therapy is tetracycline but sulfasoxazole is also effective.

Granuloma inguinale is caused by an intracellular organism, calymmatobacterium granulomatis. The infection manifests as a vesicle, papule or nodule on the genitalia which ulcerates. The ulcer is painful, accompanied by regional lymphadenopathy and a destructive granulomatous process. The diagnosis is confirmed by the presence of Donovan bodies in tissue scrapings. Tetracycline is effective in treating this infection.

In all three of the above infections, it is important to exclude the coexistence of other venereal diseases by appropriate laboratory tests.

REFERENCES

Benirschke, K.: Syphilis - The placenta and the fetus. Am. J. Dis. Child. 128:142-143, 1974.

Dawar, S. and Hellerstein, S.: Gonorrhea as a cause of asymptomatic pyuria in adolescent boys. J. Pediatr. 82:357-258, 1972.

Grossman, M. and Drutz, D.: Venereal disease in children, In Advances in Pediatrics, Vol. 21, Schulman, J., ed., Yearbook Medical Publishers, Chicago, 1974, pp. 97-137.

Kauffman, R.E., Olansky, D.C. and Weisner, P.J.: J. Am. Venereal Disease Assoc. 1:79-84, 1974.

Litt, I.F., Edberg, S.C. and Finberg, L.: Gonorrhea in children and adolescents: A current review. J. Pediatr. 85:595-607, 1974.

Low, R.C., Cho, C.T. and Dudding, B.A.: Social, familial and clinical aspects of gonococcal infections in young children. Clin. Pediatr. 16:623-626, 1977.

McCraken, G. and Kaplan, M.: Penicillin treatment for congenital syphilis-A critical reappraisal. JAMA 228-855, 1974.

CHAPTER 13. CARDIOVASCULAR INFECTIONS

13.1: PERICARDITIS

INTRODUCTION: Pericarditis occurs infrequently in children, and
when present is most commonly due to acute rheumatic fever or one
of the systemic collagen diseases, such as rheumatoid arthritis.
Epicarditis is almost always coexistent. However, infectious agents
may cause pericarditis, which will be the primary thrust of this discussion. Approximately one in a thousand hospitalized children has
primary pericarditis.

1. ETIOLOGY

In older children, acute rheumatic fever and rheumatoid arthritis
are the most common causes of pericarditis. However, in tertiary
care centers, myopericarditis as a complication of oncologic disease or its therapy is noted with increasing frequency. Postpericardiotomy syndrome following open-heart surgery may be due to
viral etiology or a nonspecific hypersensitivity reaction. Most certainly in infants under one year of age, viral etiology of pericarditis
predominates.

The viral agents are similar to those listed in the myocarditis discussion. It is common not to be able to establish or confirm a viral
etiology by culture and/or serologic studies even when the presentation and clinical course highly suggest probably viral cause. Purulent pericarditis is also uncommon but requires urgent diagnosis and
specific management.

2. CLINICAL MANIFESTATIONS AND DIAGNOSIS

Precordial pain, which usually lessens upon sitting, occurs in about
half of the older children but is less frequent than in adults. Antecedent infections, particularly of the upper respiratory tract, may
be present. The child is frequently febrile. When systemic symptoms and signs coexist, the pericarditis is likely to be an inflammatory manifestation of a disease involving multiple organ systems such
as acute rheumatic fever, rheumatoid arthritis or systemic lupus
erythematosus. The vast majority of children with rheumatic pericarditis also have mitral and/or aortic valvulitis with regurgitation
of those respective valves.

A pericardial friction rub is the cardinal physical sign. Auscultation
at frequent intervals, particularly early in the course of the pericarditis, may establish the diagnosis. Usually small amounts of pericardial effusion develop which may cause the rub to disappear. This

fluid accumulation usually does not produce symptoms. However, when present in large amounts, or rapidly accumulating, evidence of cardiac tamponade becomes apparent. This includes distant heart sounds, tachycardia, pulsus paradoxus, low cardiac output, hypotension, peripheral vasoconstriction and venous congestion with liver enlargement.

The electrocardiogram usually shows one or more of the following: low voltage, current of injury pattern with ST segment elevation, prolonged QT, abnormal T vector with a wide QRS-T angle in the frontal plane, and electrical alternans. The sedimentation rate may be moderately elevated with viral pericarditis, and markedly elevated with bacterial disease. The chest roentgenogram may show a normal cardiac size if the effusion is small. However, serial studies usually show progressive increase of the cardiac silhouette size and, in the upright position, the heart shadow may have a pear or water-bottle shape with bulging of the inferior borders. The pulmonary venous markings are normal unless cardiac tamponade is present. Echocardiography is an excellent noninvasive diagnostic tool which usually demonstrates an echo-free space between the two pericardial surfaces when appreciable effusion is present (Fig. 13.1). Pericardiocentesis is always indicated when cardiac tamponade exists and is frequently helpful in diagnosis of infectious etiologies.

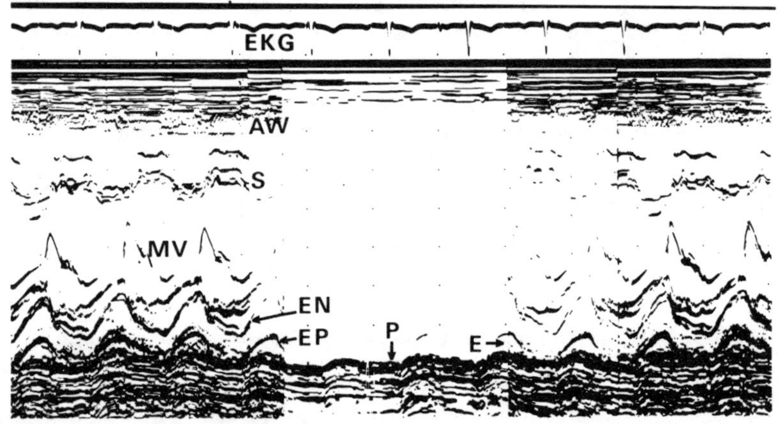

FIG. 13.1: Echocardiogram demonstrating pericardial effusion.
EKG: electrocardiogram; AW: anterior wall; S: septum; MV: mitral valve; EN: endocardium; EP: epicardium; P: parietal pericardium; E: pericardial effusion.

The salient features in diagnosis of pericarditis are the presence
of a pericardial friction rub, the progressive increase of the cardiac size over a short interval of days or weeks in the absence of a
heart murmur, the electrocardiographic and echocardiographic
changes, and the confirmation of fluid by pericardial tap.

3. MANAGEMENT AND PROGNOSIS

Therapy of pericarditis secondary to, or associated with, a systemic
disease should be aimed primarily at the basic disease itself. The
precordial pain of pericarditis may respond to salicylates. Corticosteroid therapy is usually indicated in children with progressive
pericardial effusion caused by acute rheumatic fever or rheumatoid
arthritis, and occasionally in the postpericardiotomy syndrome.
Since myocarditis frequently coexists, therapy should be for the congestive heart failure. Aspiration of fluid by pericardial tap not only
may be lifesaving in the presence of cardiac tamponade but cultures
for bacteria and viruses are mandatory. Occasionally, malignant
cells can be identified which may require the use of antimitotic
agents. However, clear fluid in the pericardial aspirate usually indicates viral etiology or so-called acute benign pericarditis. When
purulent pericarditis is detected, the prognosis is grave unless tube
drainage is established immediately, the causative organism identified and its sensitivity to antimicrobials determined, and appropriate
intravenous antibiotics utilized in large dosages for 4-6 weeks. Fortunately, tuberculous pericarditis is rare in children in the United
States since even with antituberculous therapy results are poor.

Prognosis of pericarditis is usually favorable when due to acute rheumatic fever, rheumatoid arthritis and viral infectious agents. However, there may be exceptions to the latter when significant epicarditis or myocarditis coexists. Occasionally, myocardial cell
destruction may be significant and followed by fibrosis with variable
degrees of reduction of myocardial performance. With purulent pericarditis, the outlook has improved with drainage tube insertion and
antimicrobial therapy, but the mortality rate remains close to fifty
percent. Constrictive pericarditis, as a late complication of acute
pericarditis, is rare in children, but the prognosis is favorable with
pericardiectomy.

13.2: MYOCARDITIS

INTRODUCTION: Inflammation of the muscle walls of the heart, or
myocarditis, may be caused by a wide variety of infectious agents, as
well as other etiologies. Although new biochemical and immunologic
techniques have advanced our knowledge on the noninfectious causes of
myocarditis, such as the collagen or connective tissue diseases, emphasis will be on the myocarditis caused by infectious agents.

1. ETIOLOGY

Acute rheumatic fever with myocarditis and valvulitis remains as a significant cause of inflammation of the myocardium in children. There seems little question that all initial, as well as recurrent episodes of rheumatic fever are preceded by a Group A beta-hemolytic streptococcal infection. Since the diagnosis and management of streptococcal infections will be dealt with in another chapter, rheumatic myocarditis will be limited to discussion under differential diagnosis. Viruses, bacteria, rickettsia, fungi, spirochaeta and parasites have been reported as causes of myocarditis. The frequency with which nonviral infectious agents cause myocarditis in children in the United States is rare. Furthermore, systemic manifestations of the infectious process either predominate or coexist.

Viral infections may involve the myocardium to a minor or major degree. The more common etiologic agents include coxsackie A and B, rubella, vaccinia, varicella, cytomegalovirus, herpesvirus, enterovirus, arbovirus, adenovirus, influenza, rubeola, hepatitis, mumps and infectious mononucleosis. Rarely lymphocytic choriomeningitis, poliomyelitis, psittacosis and rabies may be associated with myocarditis. With systemic viral infections, the myocardial involvement is initially that of an acute infective myocarditis. Some days later a primary autoimmune myocardiopathy may develop. For the primary infective myocarditities, various terminologies have been used, such as acute aseptic myocarditis, isolated myocarditis, acute interstitial myocarditis, acute nonspecific myocarditis and idiopathic myocarditis. For a number of years, it was suspected that viruses could cause myocarditis, but it was not until 1956 that coxsackie viruses were proven capable of producing myocarditis in humans. This particular group of viruses seems to have a high degree of cardiotropism, and more than 100 fatal cases of myocarditis in infants and children have been reported, due to any one of the various antigenic types of coxsackie (B1 to B5). Newborn and young infants seem particularly prone to serious and sometimes fatal coxsackie myocarditis. This corroborates experimental data in that the newborn mouse is significantly more susceptible to coxsackie myocarditis than the adult mouse. Perhaps some of the poorly understood myocardiopathies, such as endocardial fibroelastosis, may be sequelae to acute or chronic myocarditis.

The myocarditic heart is usually somewhat increased in weight, is soft, flabby and moderately pale with some areas of streaked pallor due to scarring. Three stages of lesions are seen microscopically. Acute myocarditis shows diffuse or patchy infiltration by plasma cells, nests of mononuclear leukocytes and some eosinophils, and varying degrees of muscle cell necrosis. In the subacute form, inflammation may still be present but fibrosis begins to predominate; the muscle fibers are swollen with decay of the cross bands. Later, giant cell infiltrations with fibrosis of some muscle cells and hypertrophy of surviving muscle fibers predominate.

2. CLINICAL MANIFESTATIONS AND DIAGNOSIS

Newborns with myocarditis usually present with anorexia, vomiting, and lethargy, but occasionally severe pallor, with peripheral circulatory collapse and shock, may suddenly become manifest. Most of such infants have hypo or hyperthermia, respiratory distress, especially tachypnea, and cyanosis. A gallop rhythm with poor heart tones and tachycardia almost always exist. A soft systolic regurgitant murmur of tricuspid insufficiency and hepatomegaly may be evident. Cardiomegaly on chest roentgenogram (Fig. 13.2) and low voltage QRS complexes with ST segment and T wave changes on the electrocardiogram are characteristic.

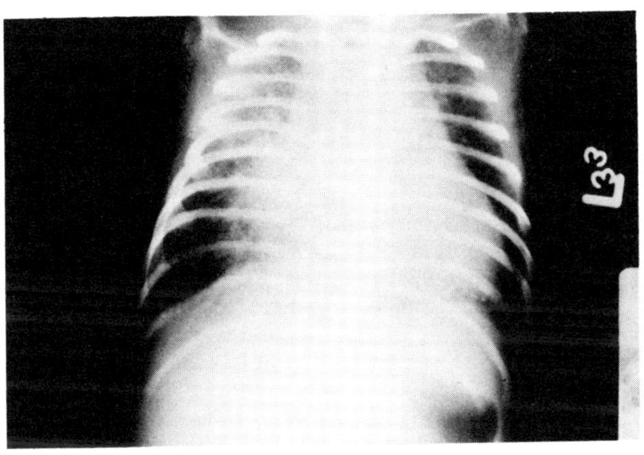

FIG. 13.2: An infant with acute myocarditis due to coxsackie B-3 virus.

In older children, the onset may be more subtle with a history of a preceding upper respiratory infection, low grade fever, listlessness and occasionally chest pain. Irregular rhythms on auscultation may be shown to be due to supraventricular or ventricular ectopic beats. The erythrocyte sedimentation rate is usually moderately elevated, as is the serum glutamic oxaloacetic acid.

Any infant or child who presents with symptoms and signs of congestive heart failure in the absence of congenital heart disease, paroxysmal supraventricular tachycardia, or manifestations of acute rheumatic fever should be considered to have an infectious myocardiopathy. Complete virus isolation studies with acute and convalescent serum samples for serologic assay are always indicated. The diagnosis can absolutely be confirmed only by isolation of the virus from the heart, cerebrospinal fluid or blood, or from the stool or oropharynx coupled with an appropriate serologic titer rise. However, since in many instances viral etiology cannot be established, the clinical course may be helpful in differentiating a primary myocardial disease, such as endocardial fibroelastosis, from the myocardiopathy secondary to a viral agent. Whenever infectious myocarditis other than of viral etiology is being considered, appropriate additional laboratory studies to include blood, stool, and urine cultures for bacterial, protozoan and parasitic agents should be obtained as well as a tuberculosis skin test.

The recent introduction of the noninvasive procedure of echocardiography to identify chamber size, muscle wall thickness and movement, as well as the presence or absence of pericardial fluid, has been an asset to our diagnostic armamentarium. However, in those children in whom cardiomegaly, with or without congestive heart failure, persists, cardiac catheterization should be done to assess myocardial performance, as well as to determine ventricular chamber size ratio to muscle wall thickness by selective angiocardiography and to exclude silent, uncommon congenital diseases, such as anomalous origin of the coronary artery from the pulmonary artery, Ebstein's abnormality of the tricuspid valve, Uhl's disease, and right atrial aneurysm.

A friction rub is frequently present in pericarditis. When effusion is present, the rub may disappear. Differentiation of pericarditis from inflammatory myocarditis may be difficult. However, it may not be too important since not only do pericarditis and myocarditis frequently coexist, but their differentiation usually is not of clinical importance unless cardiac tamponade due to effusion is present.

Toxic myocarditis is a poorly used term to designate some type of biochemical abnormality of the myocardium secondary to some other systemic process, such as drug ingestion, altered electrolytes or blood gases, and other toxic or anoxic agents. These must be considered by appropriate laboratory studies. The myocardium is particularly susceptible to reduced function by hypothermia, hypocalcemia and acidemia.

3. MANAGEMENT AND PROGNOSIS

In those children with heart failure due to myocarditis, decongestive measures should be instituted. When decompensation is marked, the parenteral use of a rapidly acting diuretic such as ethacrynic acid or furosemide, 1 mg/kg of body weight, is indicated. Fowler's position and oxygen for dyspnea and orthopnea are helpful measures. If the myocardial performance is markedly reduced with very low cardiac output, Isoproterenol may have a significant inotropic effect, thereby improving peripheral and coronary perfusion. Sodium bicarbonate may be needed to combat acidosis.

Cautious digitalization usually results in significant improvement, but patients with myocarditis may be exquisitely sensitive to this drug. The dosage of digitalis should be smaller than the usual recommended dose and careful electrocardiographic monitoring is necessary. Long-term oral diuretics should be used when cardiomegaly and congestive heart failure persist. Although isolated reports of significant clinical improvement with corticosteroids have appeared in the literature, their role is unclear in the management of infectious myocarditis.

Milder forms of myocarditis usually have an excellent prognosis. Bed rest followed by gradual ambulation over several weeks as the heart size, electrocardiogram and sedimentation rate return to normal is necessary. However, about half of the children with marked cardiomegaly and heart failure require continued use of decongestive measures because of irreversible myocardial damage. Late death may rarely occur due to uncontrolled heart failure or fatal arrhythmias. However, the fatality rate of acute myocarditis in the newborn due to the coxsackie group of viruses may be as high as fifty percent. In those that survive, recovery is usually complete. Recurrent acute myocarditis is very rare.

::

13.3: INFECTIVE ENDOCARDITIS

There are two forms of infective endocarditis, both rare in infants and children. The first is subacute bacterial endocarditis which usually occurs in children who have underlying cardiovascular abnormalities. The second, even more rare, is acute bacterial endocarditis which may develop (on endocardial surfaces) during the course of septicemia in the absence of underlying structural defects.

1. SUBACUTE BACTERIAL ENDOCARDITIS

INTRODUCTION: Patients of all ages are encountered, although it is very rare in children under two years of age. Incidence of endocarditis in children accounts for about 0.5 per 1,000 hospital admissions, excluding postoperative bacterial endocarditis.

1.1: PATHOGENESIS AND ETIOLOGY

Prerequisites for the initiation and localization of the subacute bacterial endocarditis are bacteremia (even transient) and a cardiac anomaly in which there is usually a significant pressure gradient across a defect or superimposed on a deformed valve. A Venturi effect is produced when blood is driven from a high-pressure area through an orifice to a lower-pressure blood vessel or chamber, and a deposition of bacteria appears in the low-pressure side. A jet effect establishes the other site of potential involvement. The frequent site(s) of vegetation in various cardiac anomalies are explained by this mechanism (Table 13-1).

<table>
<tr><td colspan="2">TABLE 13-1: SITE OF VEGETATION IN VARIOUS CARDIAC ANOMALIES</td></tr>
<tr><td>LESIONS</td><td>LOCATION OF VEGETATION</td></tr>
<tr><td>Ventricular Septal Defect</td><td>Right ventricular rim of the defect, on the opposing septal leaflet of tricuspid valve</td></tr>
<tr><td>Patent Ductus Arteriosus Systemic-to-Pulmonary Shunts</td><td>Pulmonary artery</td></tr>
<tr><td>Aortic Stenosis
Pulmonary Stenosis</td><td>On the superior surface of the valve
At the site of a jet stream lesion</td></tr>
<tr><td>Aortic Insufficiency
Pulmonary Insufficiency</td><td>Ventricular surface of semilunar valve</td></tr>
<tr><td>Mitral Insufficiency
Tricuspid Insufficiency</td><td>Atrial surface of the atrioventricular valve</td></tr>
<tr><td>Coarctation of Aorta</td><td>Distal to the coarctation (Superior surface of associated bicuspid aortic valve)</td></tr>
<tr><td>Tetralogy of Fallot</td><td>In the outflow tract of right ventricle
Pulmonary valve
Pulmonary side of systemic-to-pulmonary shunt</td></tr>
</table>

The streptococcus (S. viridans, enterococcus) and staphylococcus (S. aureus, S. albus) are the organisms responsible for 90-95% of the cases. Less commonly encountered bacteria include pneumococcus, pseudomonas, E. coli, aerobacter, proteus, Hemophilus influenzae and Listeria. Endocarditis due to fungi (Candida species being the most common) may occur in patients receiving long-term antibiotics or steroid therapy, and in narcotic addicts. The most common organism encountered in postoperative endocarditis is the staphylococcus.

Practically every form of congenital cardiac defect predisposes to endocarditis, but the most commonly encountered congenital cardiac lesions are tetralogy of Fallot with or without palliative systemic-to-pulmonary shunt, small ventricular septal defects and aortic stenoses. The secundum type atrial septal defect is least likely to develop the infection. Mitral insufficiency is the most frequent rheumatic lesion to have superimposed bacterial endocarditis.

1.2: CLINICAL MANIFESTATIONS

HISTORY:

a) Almost all patients have heart disease

b) A history of recent infection or a surgical procedure (dental extraction, tonsillectomy) is occasionally present.

c) Insidious onset with fatigue, loss of appetite and pallor are common.

SIGNS:

a) Heart murmur (100%). The change in the intensity of a heart murmur or the development of a new murmur are of diagnostic importance. Congestive heart failure may be the first sign of this disease.

b) Fever (80-90%) may range between 38.5° and 39.5° with considerable daily fluctuation.

c) Splenomegaly (70%).

d) Skin manifestations (50%) are probably due to microemboli.

    (1) Petechiae are the most frequent skin lesions, although not pathognomonic, and are seen on the skin, mucous membranes or conjunctivae.

    (2) Osler's node is usually not seen in children.

    (3) Janeway lesions, small painless hemorrhagic areas on the palms or the soles, are also rare.

    (4) Splinter hemorrhages are linear hemorrhagic streaks beneath the nails and, when present, are highly suspect of the diagnosis.

e) Embolic phenomena (50%).

    (1) Pulmonary emboli are rare but may occur in patients with either ventricular septal defect or tetralogy of Fallot.

    (2) Central nervous system complications (20%) occur more frequently in patients with cyanotic heart diseases or leftsided valvular lesions (aortic and mitral valves). Seizures and hemiparesis may be neurological manifestations.

(3) Renal: Hematuria is common. Renal failure may follow chronic endocarditis.

f) Clubbing in the absence of cyanosis is rare (2%).

LABORATORY FINDINGS:

a) Anemia is frequently present (80%) with hemoglobin levels below 12 gm%.

b) Leukocytosis with increased polymorphonuclear cells and increased sedimentation rate are usually present.

c) Microscopic hematuria is seen in 30%.

d) Hypergammaglobulinemia with inversion of albumin/globulin ratio is a late finding, and a positive rheumatoid factor may be present.

1.3: DIAGNOSIS

In a patient with a known underlying heart lesion (either congenital or rheumatic) and fever of unknown origin of one week's duration or longer, infective endocarditis should be highly suspect. If any of the above mentioned signs or laboratory changes are present in such patients, subacute bacterial endocarditis should be considered as the diagnosis until proven otherwise. Definitive diagnosis is made by positive blood culture.

1.4: MANAGEMENT, PROGNOSIS AND PREVENTION

When clinical findings suggest infective endocarditis, six blood cultures drawn in rapid succession over 24-48 hours are recommended. Blood cultures are positive in 75-80% of the cases. If a positive blood culture is obtained and the organism identified, specific treatment as indicated by sensitivity testing should be started immediately. After obtaining the blood cultures, treatment with penicillin in combination with streptomycin should be initiated, since Streptococcus viridans and enterococcus are the most common etiologic agents.

When Streptococcus viridans is the causative agent, intravenous penicillin is recommended in doses of 100,000 units/kg/day (maximun 4-6 million units/day), administered for a total of four weeks. Streptomycin, administered intramuscularly, in doses of 20 mg/kg/day (in two doses), is also added. Enterococcal endocarditis requires larger doses of intravenous penicillin (usually 250,000 units/kg/day - minimum 20 million units daily) combined with intramuscular streptomycin for four weeks.

The drug of choice for staphylococcal endocarditis is methicillin (200-300 mg/kg/day) intravenously in 4-6 doses. Alternative drugs include nafcillin, oxacillin, dicloxacillin, cloxacillin and cephalothin. The therapy should be continued for at least six weeks. Amphotericin B may be effective against Candida. In case of postoperative endocarditis, reoperation and removal of the infected prosthetic material, in conjunction with aggressive antibiotic therapy, is recommended.

With currently available potent antibiotics, overall recovery rate is 80-85% (90% or better for Streptococcus viridans and enterococcus and 50% for staphylococcus). Prognosis is better in patients in whom the disease is recognized and treated early (90% recovery when recognized within one month after onset and 50% recovery when recognized three months after onset) and in whom blood culture is positive and the organism is sensitive to the commonly used antibiotics. Presence of congestive heart failure or embolic phenomena indicate a poor prognosis.

Almost as important as treatment of infective endocarditis is its prevention. All patients with congenital or rheumatic heart disease who undergo certain dental or surgical procedures or instrumentation of the upper respiratory tract, genito-urinary or gastrointestinal tract, and those who undergo cardiac surgery, must receive antibiotic prophylaxis in therapeutic dosages (Table 13-2). In choosing antibiotics for prophylaxis, one should consider the organisms that are most likely to cause bacterial endocarditis from any given procedure and appropriate antibiotic(s) should be chosen accordingly.

2. ACUTE BACTERIAL ENDOCARDITIS

The pathoanatomic mechanisms involved in the development of acute endocarditis are quite different, and previously normal valves may be involved. The organisms responsible for the acute bacterial endocarditis are highly invasive and it is usually a complication of a bacterial sepsis. It may also occur in a child under two years of age. The most common infecting agent is Staphylococcus aureus, Less commonly encountered are gram-negative bacilli, enterococci, pneumococci and fungi.

Cardiac findings may be overshadowed by the signs of severe sepsis; high fever, prostration or shock.

Since the mortality rate is very high (approximately 50%), three blood cultures should be drawn in rapid succession within 1-2 hours and treatment should be started immediately with large intravenous doses of methicillin. When the offending organism is isolated from blood culture, modification of the antibiotic therapy should be adjusted consistent with the organism's sensitivity.

TABLE 13-2: PREVENTION OF BACTERIAL ENDOCARDITIS

INDICATIONS	ORGANISM MOST LIKELY ENCOUNTERED	SUGGESTED ANTIBIOTICS
Dental Extraction Periodontal Procedures Oral Surgery Tonsillectomy and Adenoidectomy Bronchoscopy	S. viridans	Penicillin*

Surgery or Instrumen-
  tation of Genitourinary
  or Gastrointestinal
  (colon, rectum, gall
  bladder) tract
Complicated Deliveries
	Enterococcus
	(e.g. S. fecalis)
		Penicillin* or
		Ampicillin**
		+
		Streptomycin †

Cardiac Surgery	S. aureus (coag +) S. epidermidis or albus (coag -)	

Status After Cardiac
  Surgery
	Same as outlined
	  above for the un-
	  operated patients	

Other Indications:
  Surgery of infected tissue
    (incision & drainage of abscess)
  Extensive burn
  Indwelling vascular catheter

*Penicillin (IM)   Procaine pen. G. 600,000 U +
                    Crystalline pen. G 200,000 U,
                        1 Hr. prior to procedure (PTP) and
                        once daily for 2 days

                            OR

        (Oral) Pen. V 500 mg 1H PTP and then
                    250 mg q 6H for 2 days, or
                Pen. G 1.2 million U 1H PTP and then
                    0.6 million U q 6H for 2 days

IF SENSITIVE TO PENICILLIN: Erythromycin (Oral) 20 mg/
kg 2 H PTP and 10 mg/kg q 6H for 3 days

** Ampicillin (Oral, IV) 25-50 mg/kg 1H PTP and 25 mg/kg for
   3 days

 † Streptomycin (IM) 40 mg/kg 1H PTP and once daily for 2 days

REFERENCES

PERICARDITIS

Ingram, D.L., Anderson, P., and Smith, D.H.: Counter-current immuno-electrophoresis in the diagnosis of systemic diseases caused by Hemophilus Influenza type B. J. Pediatr. 81:1156, 1972.

Lenure, F., Tajik, A.J., Giuliani, E.R., Gau, G.T. and Schattenburg, T.T.: Further echocardiographic observations in pericardial effusion. Mayo Clin. Proc. 51:13, 1976.

Navaqui, S. and Kobins, S.A.: Acute meningococcal pericarditis without meningitis. Arch. Intern. Med. 135:314, 1975.

Roberts, K.B. and Neff, J.M.: Meningococcal pericarditis without meningitis in a child. Am. J. Dis. Child. 124:440, 1972.

Rooney, J.J. Crocco, J.A. et al.: Tuberculous pericarditis. Ann. Int. Med. 72:73, 1970.

Rubin, R.H., and Moellering, R.C., Jr.: Clinical microbiologic and therapeutic aspects of purulent pericarditis. Am. J. Med. 59: 68, 1975. (Review Article)

Schlossberg, D., Zacarias, F. and Shulman, J.A.: Primary pneumococcal pericarditis. JAMA 234:853, 1975.

Simon, H.B., Tarr, P.I., Hutter, A.M., Jr., and Erdmaun, J., III: Primary meningococcal pericarditis. JAMA 235:278, 1976.

Smith, E.W.P. and Ingram, D.L.: Counter-immunoelectrophoresis in Hemophilus Influenza type B epiglottitis and pericarditis. J. Pediatr. 86:571, 1975.

MYOCARDITIS

Burch, G.E., De Pasquale, N.P., Hale, A.R., Mogabgab, W.J., and Sun, S.C.: Experimental viral myocarditis. Circulation Suppl. II to 31, 32:61, 1965.

Burch, G.E., Sun, S.C., Cololough, H.L., Sobol, R.S. and De Pasquale, N.P.: Coxsackie B viral myocarditis and valvulitis identified in routine autopsy specimens by immunofluorescent techniques. Am. Heart J. 74:12, 1967.

Cheetham, H.D., Hart, J., et al.: Rabies with myocarditis: Two cases in England. Lancet 1:921, 1970.

Flexner, G.E. and Pullen, R.L.: Mumps myocarditis: Review of literature and report of a case. Am. Heart J. 31:238, 1946.

Gore, I. and Saphir, O.: Myocarditis. A classification of 1,402 cases. Am. Heart J. 34:827, 1947. (Review Article)

Grist, N.R. and Bell, E.J.: Coxsackie group B fatal neonatal myocarditis associated with cardiomegaly. J. Clin. Path. 19:325, 1966.

Hardman, J.M. and Earle, K.M.: Myocarditis in 200 fatal meningococcic infections. Arch. Pathl. 87:318, 1969.

Jennings, R.C.: Coxsackie group B fatal neonatal myocarditis associated with cardiomegaly. J. Clin. Path. 19:325, 1966.

Lang, D.J. and Hanshaw, J.B.: Cytomegalovirus infection and the postperfusion syndrome. NEJM 280:1145, 1972.

Sanyal, S.K., Mahdoug, M., Gabrielson, M.O., Vidone, R.A. and Browne, M.J.: Fatal myocarditis in an adolescent caused by coxsackie virus, group B, type 4. Pediatrics 35:36, 1965.

Saphir, O. and Cohen, N.A.: Myocarditis in infancy. Arch. Pathl. 64:446, 1957.

Schieken, R.M. and Myers, M.G.: Complete heart block in viral myocarditis. J. Pediatr. 37:831, 1975.

Weinstein, S.B.: Acute benign pericarditis associated with coxsackie virus, group B., type 5. NEJM 257:265, 1957.

Whitehead, R.: Isolated myocarditis. Brit. Heart J. 27:230, 1965.

INFECTIVE ENDOCARDITIS

Blumenthal, S.: Infective endocarditis. In, Heart Disease in Infants, Children and Adolescents, Moss, A.J. and Adams, F.H., eds., Williams and Wilkins Co., Baltimore, 1968, Chapter 38.

Caldwell, R.L., Hurwitz, R.A. and Girod, D.A.: Subacute bacterial endocarditis in children: Current status. Am. J. Dis. Child. 122:312, 1971.

Committee on Prevention of Bacterial Endocarditis by the Rheumatic Fever Committee and the Committee on Congenital Cardiac Defects of the American Heart Association: Prevention of Bacterial Endocarditis. Circulation 46:3, 1972.

Felner, J.M. and Dowell, V.R.: Antimicrobic bacterial endocarditis. NEJM 283:1188, 1970.

Johnson, D.H. Rosenthal, A. and Nadas, A.S.: A forty-year review of bacterial endocarditis in infancy and childhood. Circulation 51:581, 1975.

Kislak, J.W.: The treatment of endocarditis. Am. Heart J. 79: 713, May, 1970.

McCraken, G.H. Jr. and Eichenwald, H.F.: Antimicrobial therapy: Therapeutic recommendations and a review of newer drugs. J. Pediatr. 85:297-312, 1974.

Peterson, L.J. and Peacock, R.: The incidence of bacteremia in pediatric patients following tooth extraction. Circulation 53:676, 1976.

Shafer, R.B. and Hall, W.H.: Bacterial endocarditis following surgery. Am. J. Card. 25:602, 1970.

Scott, R.M.: Bacterial endocarditis due to Neisseria flava. J. Pediatr. 78:673, 1971.

Weinstein, L. and Schlesinger, J.: Pathoanatomic, pathophysiologic and clinical correlations in endocarditis. NEJM 291:832, 1974 and 291:112, 1974.

CHAPTER 14. RICKETTSIAL DISEASES

INTRODUCTION: Four diseases caused by Rickettsiae are known
to occur in the United States: Rocky Mountain Spotted Fever
(RMSF), Endemic Typhus, Q fever and Rickettsialpox. Of these
diseases, RMSF is the most severe and, since this disease does
respond to appropriate antibiotic therapy, the present mortality of
7-8 per cent is primarily the result of incorrect diagnosis, delay
in treatment and improper supportive care. Thus this rickettsial
disease will be reviewed in greater detail and the other three infections considered only briefly at the conclusion of the chapter.

14.1: ROCKY MOUNTAIN SPOTTED FEVER

INTRODUCTION: Rocky Mountain Spotted Fever (RMSF) is a severe, acute, endemic noncontagious infectious vasculitis caused by
a rickettsial organism, Rickettsia rickettsii. RMSF is now a relatively uncommon disease with only 500-600 cases reported each
year, in contrast to the 7000 cases which occurred yearly before
1909.

Although scattered cases have been reported in 48 of the 50 states,
the disease has traditionally been described as endemic in two areas:
the Rocky Mountain states and the south Atlantic states (see Fig.
14.1). Rocky Mountain Spotted Fever is most prevalent in the states
east of the Mississippi River, particularly the south Atlantic states
(50 percent of the reported cases) which include the Piedmont Pla-
teau, as well as in the west south central states of Oklahoma, Texas
and Arkansas. This large geographic area accounted for more than
90 percent of the reported cases in 1975, while less than 5 percent
of the cases were in the Rocky Mountain states.

The peak incidence of Rocky Mountain Spotted Fever in the United
States occurs in the summer months - June, July and August -
coinciding with maximum tick activity. In the northeast as far south
as Virginia, the maximum number of cases are reported from late
June to early August, concurrent with the activity of the adult dog
tick. The southern tier of states have shown a recent increase in
cases from early May to June which Rothenberg and Sonnenshine
(1970) have hypothesized may be circumstantial evidence of the lone
star tick as a vector. However, the possibility exists that this may
be a function of solar activity on the dog tick. In the Mountain states,
the wood tick is the major vector and cases are seen from late March
through June.

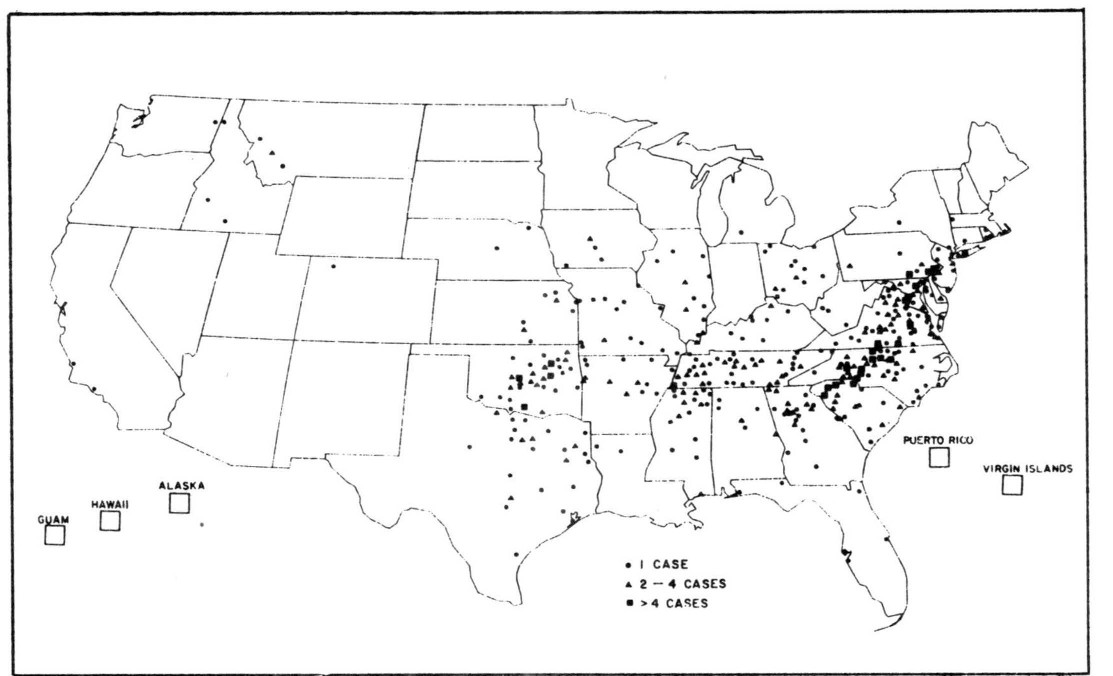

FIG. 14.1: Rocky Mountain Spotted Fever (Tick-borne Typhus) - Reported cases by County, United States, 1975. MMWR Annual Supplement, 1975 (in MMWR, August, 1976, Vol.24, No.54).

The distribution of Rocky Mountain Spotted Fever cases by age and sex has changes significantly since Ricketts' initial description, when the disease was primarily an occupational hazard of farmers, lumbermen, sheepherders and trappers who were middle-aged males. With the decline of the number of cases in the west and the preponderance of cases in the east due to the bite of the dog tick, the distribution has shifted toward the pediatric age group. Today, 30-40 percent of the cases occur in children from 0-9, and from 60-90 percent in people less than 20 years old. The distribution is a function of increased exposure to the domestic dog, delay in the removal of attached ticks, and increased exposure to immature and unattached adult ticks in the field. In the adult population, the majority of cases of Rocky Mountain Spotted Fever are occupational or recreational. Recreational exposure is particularly challenging to the physician, because of travelers' movement from endemic to non-endemic areas during the incubation period of the disease. In contrast to the preponderance of cases in males in the 1900's, the ratio of males to females is 1:1.

Rocky Mountain Spotted Fever has a great propensity to occur in Caucasians, which is a puzzling fact noted by several authors, and the etiology remains obscure. In the literature, less than 10 percent of the published cases of Rocky Mountain Spotted Fever occurred in Blacks (Peters, A., 1971).

1. ETIOLOGY, TRANSMISSION AND PATHOPHYSIOLOGY

1.1: Etiology: Rickettsiae are the approximate size of bacteria (1 micron x 0.3 micra), divide by binary fission and contain both RNA and DNA. Although very porous and largely nonselective, the rickettsiae seem to have a cell wall. In addition, it has been suggested that rickettsiae have toxin-like properties in vivo which are quite distinct from bacterial endotoxins. In guinea pigs and rats, pure isolates of rickettsiae produce vasoconstriction and shock too rapidly to be explained by a vasculitis. Although RMSF is caused primarily by Rickettsia rickettsii, it is possible that another rickettsial species, R. canada, may cause a clinical picture indistinguishable from RMSF (Bozeman et al., 1970).

1.2: Transmission: Infection is transmitted to man at the time of engorgement during tick infection by R. rickettsii. The most important tick vector of RMSF is the American dog tick Dermacentor variabilis. However the lone star tick (Ambloyomma americanus, the Rocky Mountain wood tick, Dermacentor andersoni, and the rabbit tick, Haemaphysalis leporispalustris) are also of importance in the distribution, maintenance and transmission of RMSF in the United States.

The perpetuation of R. rickettsii depends upon a complicated interrelationship between the ticks, vectors, and the animal hosts. The relationship between the tick and the rickettsia is probably a commensal one and the tick is exceedingly well suited for its role as vector and reservoir. Ticks are very hardy, able to survive long periods without feeding and have few natural enemies (James and Harwood, 1969). They have a wide host range, are persistently slow feeders and difficult to dislodge, which gives adequate time for reactivation and transmission of the rickettsiae. Transmission of RMSF is impossible if the rickettsiae are not "reactivated" which occurs late in the course of the first blood meal, or after extended incubation in the warm sun. The necessity for reactivation explains the paucity of cases of RMSF in the early spring and emphasizes the importance of the prompt removal of ticks in prevention of RMSF.

1.3: Pathophysiology: During the engorgement of an infected tick, the "activated" rickettsiae enter the endothelial cells of the host's capillaries and small arteries. It has been suggested that the endothelial cells are invaded because of the relatively high oxygen tension. As the intranuclear rickettsiae multiply, a notable change in intracellular morphology takes place with mitochondrial condensation and the loss of free RNA along the endoplasmic reticulum. Because immunofluorescent studies fail to show the presence of gamma globulin, fibrinogen or complement, it has been suggested that the intracellular changes are a reflection of toxin activity (Brito, J., 1973). The cellular response - endothelial proliferation and mononuclear infiltration - gives the microscopic appearance of an infectious vasculitis.

The second phase of cell injury is mediated through antigen-antibody complexes which actively fix complement, thus releasing chemotactic factors which attract PMN's. Either the direct effect of complement or the release of lysozymal enzymes from the PMN's give rise to a necrotizing or immediate type hypersensitivity arteritis. This concept is supported by immunofluorescent studies, which have demonstrated a large amount of gamma globulin and complement in a linear pattern at the luminal side of the small vessels (Brito, T., 1973). The loss of function of endothelial cells allows small intravascular proteins to leak into the extravascular space (Brito, T., et al., 1968), which is confirmed by the presence of fibrinogen, a small plasma protein, in the vessel walls and in the adventitia. Petechiae and ecchymoses appear when large defects in the endothelium allow red blood cells to pass into the tissue. The diffuse vascular involvement gives rise to the diverse clinical features.

2. CLINICAL MANIFESTATIONS

The incubation of Rocky Mountain Spotted Fever is from 3-12 days, averaging seven days and ranging from 1-21 days. A short incubation usually signals a more severe infection. Tick bite or tick exposure can be elicited in the history of 70-90 percent of the patients. The prodrome is characterized by vague symptoms of malaise, low back pain, anorexia, dizziness, lethargy, irritability, occipital headaches resistant to salicylate therapy, and gastrointestinal disturbances of constipation, nausea and vomiting. The onset of fever is abrupt, usually in the afternoon, accompanied by prostration, severe myalgias and "bad shaking" chills. The temperature rises quickly to 39-40° C and is characteristically followed by dramatic morning remissions of 1-3°C (3-5°F) rarely returning to normal. In the second week, both hyperthermia 41-42°C (106-108°F) and hypothermia of 36°C (95°F) may be present and represent very grave signs (Baker, G., 1951). The fever resolves by lysis in 14-21 days (range 10-42 days). The use of antibiotics, especially in combination with steroids, will cause a rapid defervescence in 1-3 days. After the temperature has returned to normal for 24 hours, any exacerbation of fever is frequently a sign of a secondary pyogenic infection, which is most commonly pneumonia.

The sine qua non of Rocky Mountain Spotted Fever is the characteristic rash, which usually appears on the second to fourth febrile day (Fig. 14.2). It is light pink or red, macular, non-fixed, blanches

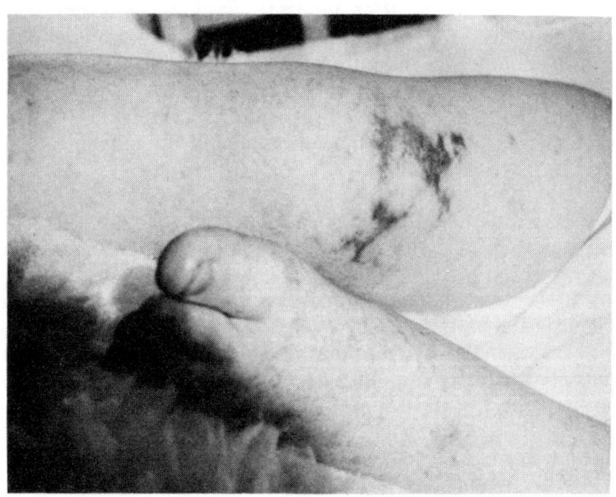

FIG. 14.2: Typical petechial eruption of Rocky
Mountain Spotted Fever.

with pressure and is accentuated by local application of heat or with the increase of fever. The rash begins on the flexor surfaces of the wrist and ankles, spreading rapidly to involve the entire extremity. Most striking is the presence of the rash on the palms of the hands and soles of the feet. In 24 hours the rash becomes very diffuse and maculopapular which can be appreciated by light palpation. An extensive rash usually indicates a more severe disease. In time, the rash becomes petechial and may even become ecchymotic and mottled. Ecchymoses represent severe vascular compromise, which may result in ischemic necrosis of the tonsils, fingers, toes, ears, nose, scrotum, vulva and buttocks. During the recovery period, the copper brown lesions slowly subside and undergo brawny desquamation. A visible residua of the rash may be demonstrated by exposure to heat or cold for months following the illness.

Other findings typical of RMSF are dehydration with soft doughy skin and dry mucous membranes; dry, sufused conjunctivae; photophobia, venous engorgement of the fundus with retinal edema, cytoid bodies, hemorrhages and vascular occlusion (Presley, G.D., 1969; Raab, E.L., et al., 1969). The spleen is enlarged and firm in more than one-half of the cases, and coincident hepatic enlargement occurs in 50% of patients.

The predominant neurologic manifestations in RMSF are headache, alteration in sensorium, insomnia, convulsions, and paralysis. Occipitofrontal headache, the most consistent symptom, occurring in 80% of the patients, is severe and unremitting. Alterations in sensorium include confusion, restlessness, somnolence, lethargy, irritability, stupor and coma, which has a grave prognosis. Rocky Mountain Spotted Fever can mimic encephalitis, meningitis, and convulsive disorders, with nuchal rigidity, transient EEG abnormalities, ataxia, grand mal or focal seizures, incontinence or deafness, but these usually disappear upon recovery (Harrel, G.T., et al., 1951).

The diffuse peripheral vasculitis and myocarditis have a profound effect on the cardiovascular integrity. The second week is marked by rapid and significant cardiovascular deterioration, which ultimately terminates in vasomotor collapse and death. The severe myalgia secondary to thrombosis and ischemia are early signs of cardiovascular insufficiency. EKG findings, such as S-T segment depression, low voltage, and conduction defects (flat T and prolonged Q-T), imply further cardiac impairment. At this time, the patient may experience exceedingly intense myalgias. Severe abdominal pain, rigidity and rebound tenderness may mimic an appendicitis. The gradual onset of retinal periorbital and peripheral edema, a rapid weak pulse (110-200/min.) out of proportion to the fever, and a decrease in systolic blood pressure (often 90 mm Hg.) signify vascular compromise (Aqilina, J.T. et al., 1952). Renal perfusion and glomerular filtration rate decrease resulting in renal vasoconstriction, medullary shunting, olguria, azotemia, and finally anuria. With renal function severely compromised, fluid imbalance progresses to pulmonary edema, hypoxia and cardiovascular collapse. Reversal of this trend is heralded by a voluminous diuresis, decrease in pulse rate, increase in the blood pressure and gradual disappearance of the edema.

3. DIAGNOSIS

The diagnosis must first be suspected based on clinical grounds alone since the laboratory findings are of little value in early diagnosis of

RMSF, but are nonetheless essential in monitoring the patient's progress. The white blood count (WBC) during the incubation period may be depressed ($2000\text{-}4000/\text{mm}^3$) without alteration in the differential. With the onset of fever, leukopenia, leukocytosis or a normal count may be present, often with a 5-10 percent shift to the left. Toxic granulation of the PMN's, a marked leukocytosis ($13{,}000\text{-}30{,}000/\text{mm}^3$), and a marked shift to the left (90 percent band forms) may be present late in the course of RMSF. The hemoglobin and hemocrit are often low and peripheral smear indicates a normocytic, normochromic anemia. Prolonged prothrombin time secondary to liver damage and thrombocytopenia are frequently encountered. The presence of a disseminated intravascular coagulopathy will result in a prolonged partial thromboplastin time, prolonged clotting time, decreased fibrinogen, increased fibrinolysis, increased quantity of fibrin split products and RBC fragments on peripheral smear (Atkin, M.D., et al., 1965).

The urine volume may be diminished with a high specific gravity. Transient albuminuria and microscopic hematuria, with occasional casts, are often present. Gross hematuria is seen in association with a coagulopathy. Urine osmolality has been shown to be increased, with losses of both sodium and potassium followed by profound sodium retention and potassium loss (Beisel, W.R., et al., 1967). Bilirubininuria may be present secondary to hepatic dysfunction.

Lumbar puncture usually reveals a mild to moderate increase in opening pressure, but the CSF appears grossly normal. Slight pleocytosis with a predominance of mononuclears (up to 300 cells/mm^3) may be seen. Protein and glucose are usually normal in the CSF; however, slight elevation of the protein is not uncommon. Grossly bloody CSF is seen, indicating intracranial bleeding which is an infrequent complication of Rocky Mountain Spotted Fever.

The Weil-Felix Test, which depends on the agglutination of various Proteus antigens by the patient's serum, is helpful in the diagnosis of Rocky Mountain Spotted Fever. A four-fold rise in the OX19 (1:320) or OX2 titers is considered diagnostic of spotted fever (Bergolon and Topping, 1942). The test is sensitive but nonspecific. Therefore, specific diagnosis depends on a four-fold increase in complement fixation titers of R. rickettsii or R. canada. Although the C-F test is very specific, antigens are not commercially available (but are available from the Center for Disease Control) and the test is difficult to interpret by inexperienced personnel (Hershey, D.F. et al., 1957).

4. MANAGEMENT

4.1: Treatment: The antibiotics used in treating RMSF are tetracycline and chloramphenicol. Therapy is most effective when begun early in the course of infection. The dosage used for chloramphenicol is 50-100 mg/K/day to a maximum of 2-3 Gms daily. For

tetracycline, the dose is 20 mgm/K/day (maximum 1-2 Gms daily).
Both drugs are continued for 48 hours after the patient is afebrile.

Although antibiotics are essential in treating RMSF, supportive care
is of equal importance. The vasculitis comprises the normal balance
between intravascular and extravascular fluids, and the most difficult problem is therefore to maintain adequate intravascular (blood)
volume for adequate perfusion of the vital organs (especially the
kidneys) without compromising ventilation. Intravenous therapy is
necessary to correct the hyponatremia, hypoproteinemia, hemorrhage, nutrition deficiency and blood volume. Electrolyte solutions
should be used judiciously (2/3 maintenance), since the solution
passes freely into the tissues which may increase the tissue edema.
Expansion of intravascular volume may be accomplished with albumin. However, use of albumin is limited because it will slowly leak
into the tissues and may increase edema, which in turn compromises
pulmonary, renal and cardiovascular function. Fresh frozen plasma,
which provides large proteins, albumin and some clotting factors,
can be alternated with albumin in maintaining intravascular volume.
Disseminated intravascular coagulopathy is controlled by heparin
(10,000-20,000 units/day in 6-8 divided doses), but it may be necessary to replace specific clotting factors, especially factor VIII and
fibrinogen.

Nutritional support often requires intravenous vitamin supplementation. Therapeutic doses of vitamins A, B complex, C and D should
be provided, as well as vitamin K (2 mgm/day), until the prothrombin time has been corrected. Seizures are well controlled by pheno-
barbital, and hypoxia can be corrected with oxygen by mask.

Nursing care can be invaluable in preventing many annoying complications. The patient should be turned frequently to avoid decubitis
ulcers, which form very rapidly in RMSF, and necrotic and ulcerated skin should be debrided and dry, soft surgical dressings applied.
In the comatose patient, artificial tears should be used regularly to
prevent corneal ulceration. Conscientious mouth care includes routine mouthwash, which prevents oral stagnation and parotitis. Candida overgrowth in the mucous membranes (mouth, vagina) should be
promptly treated with topical Nystatin (200,000 units/ml) applied
locally four times a day.

4.2: Prevention and Control: The methods of prevention of Rocky
Mountain Spotted Fever (vaccination and personal precautionary
measures) and control of the tick have not changed drastically since
1925. The limited effectiveness of the vaccine developed by Cox in
1938 (Cox, H.R., 1937) and the low incidence of the disease restrict
the population eligible for vaccination to laboratory personnel and
those for whom exposure is a significant occupational hazard. The
vaccine cannot be relied upon to prevent Rocky Mountain Spotted
Fever, so thorough knowledge of personal precautionary measures
is still paramount. Limited control of RMSF may be feasible by

using insecticides in regional and local endemic areas, particularly where children are active such as in vacant lots, playgrounds and schools. Other important steps include stray dog control, and thorough deticking of farm animals and pets, for which there are numerous "pour on" formulas available (Bunch, W.L., 1968).

Precautionary measures and personal hygiene are the most practical methods to prevent RMSF and should include frequent inspections for ticks attached in exposed areas, as well as prompt removal of crawling ticks. Children playing in tick-infested areas should be carefully inspected for ticks, with special attention being paid to the area along the hairline and in body folds. If an attached tick is discovered, it should be removed promptly by exerting gentle traction on the body of the tick with a pair of tweezers. It is important not to touch the tick since the feces and juices may be infective. If this is unsuccessful, strong irritants should be avoided, although nail polish may be effective. Another technique that may be tried is insertion of a sterile needle below the mouth parts and dislodging the tick with a quick upward movement (Slotkin, 1975). After a thorough scrubbing with soap and water, antiseptic should be applied liberally.

::

14.2: ENDEMIC (MURINE) TYPHUS

This rickettsial infection is most common in the west south central region of the United States (especially Texas). However, the disease occurs relatively infrequently, with 30-50 cases reported each year in the entire U.S. In contrast to epidemic typhus, which occurs in the winter and spring, endemic typhus is most frequently in the summer and fall.

The disease is caused by Rickettsia mooseri, which causes a primary infection in rats. Man usually becomes infected when bitten by a rat flea (Xenopsylla cheopis) which has fed on an infected rat. Infection can also occur via the respiratory route by inhaling infected excreta of fleas.

R. mooseri produces a mild, influenza-like illness that is seldom fatal. Following a prodrome consisting of headache and myalgia the temperature rises and, between the first and fifth day of fever, the characteristic dull red macular rash appears, first on the trunk and then on the arms and legs. Unlike the rash of RMSF, the rash of endemic typhus rarely involves the face, palms or soles. The disease is usually mild and infection occurs in both children and adults without the typical rash. The diagnosis is confirmed by demonstrating a rise in R. mooseri complement-fixing antibody titers. In Older's study (1970), the rash occurred in only 25% of patients with the disease. Tetracycline or chloramphenicol are effective drugs in treating the infection and the prognosis is excellent.

::

14.3: RICKETTSIALPOX

Rickettsialpox was first reported in 1946 in New York City (Huebner, R.J. et al., 1946). It is endemic in the northeastern region
of the United States. The disease is caused by Rickettsia akari
which is transmitted to man by the mouse mite, Allodermamyssus
sanguineus.

The mite produces an initial lesion, presumably at the site of the
bite, which is a nontender and red papule that becomes a vesicle
and ruptures after several days, leaving a black, crusted eschar
which may persist for several weeks. Regional lymphadenopathy
is common.

Three to seven days after the bite, fever abruptly develops, accompanied by headaches, malaise, chills and sweating. Within 24 to 72
hours after onset of fever, a maculopapular eruption occurs over
the entire body. Gradually, the lesions enlarge and a vesicle appears in the center of the lesions, eventually taking on the appearance of a varicella eruption, except that the crusts are darker.

The duration of illness rarely exceeds 10 days. Early in the disease, leukopenia with a relative lymphocytosis may occur. As in
the case of other rickettsial infections, the diagnosis is confirmed
by a four-fold or greater rise in complement-fixing antibody titers
in paired sera. The tetracyclines or chloramphenicol are effective
drugs in this infection and the prognosis is usually excellent.

14.4: Q FEVER

Unlike other rickettsial infections, Q Fever caused by Rickettsia
burneti, is characterized by an interstitial pneumonitis and not a
rash. Also, unlike other rickettsial diseases, studies of outbreaks
of Q fever have failed to incriminate insect vectors. The disease is
reported throughout the world and in the United States it occurs most
commonly in the far west (Bell, J.A., et al. 1950; Lennette and
Clark, 1951). The infection is transmitted to man by inhalation of
contaminated material from domestic animals (sheep and cattle) or
by direct contact with wool, hides or other materials in the animal's
environment. In some parts of the world, ingestion of raw milk has
also been associated with sporadic cases of Q fever.

Clinical manifestations of Q Fever, which may resemble influenza,
include malaise, fever, frontal headaches and cough. Chest pain
may be associated with an interstitial pneumonitis seen on roentgenographic studies. Resolution of the roentgen findings is usually slow
(3-4 weeks), although the symptoms disappear after 10-14 days. The
diagnosis is confirmed by a rise in complement-fixing antibody titer.

Treatment with tetracyclines is effective in reducing the duration of illness and morbidity. Infections in children are often asymptomatic and the prognosis is excellent.

REFERENCES

Aquilina, J.T., Rosenburg, F., Wuertz, R.L.: Nodal tachycardia in Rocky Mountain Spotted Fever. Am. Heart J. 43:755, 1952.

Atkin, M.D., Strauss, H.S., Fischer, G.: A case report of Cape Cod Rocky Mountain Spotted Fever with multiple coagulation disturbances. Pediatrics 36:627, 1965.

Baker, B.E.: Rocky Mountain Spotted Fever. Med. Clin. N.A., May, 1951.

Beisel, W.R., Sawyer, W.D., Ryll, E.D., Crozier, D.: Metabolic studies in human subjects during intracellular infections. Ann. Int. Med. 67:744, 1967.

Bell, J.A., Beck, M.D., and Huebner, R.J.: Epidemiologic studies of Q Fever in Southern California. JAMA 142:868, 1950.

Bergolon, I.A., Topping, N.H.: Complement fixation in rickettsial disease. Am. J. Pub. Health 32:48, 1942.

Bozeman, F.M., Elisberg, B.L., Humphries, J.W., Runcik, K., Palmer, D.B., Jr.: Serologic evidence of rickettsia canada infection in man. J. Infect. Dis. 121:367, 1970.

Brito, T.A., Godoy, C.V.F., Renna, D.O., Jordao, F.M.: Glomerular response in human and experimental rickettsial diseases: A light and electron microscopic study. Path. Microbiol. (Base) 31:365, 1968.

Brito, T.: The pathogenesis of the vascular lesions in experimental rickettsial disease of the guinea pig: A light, immunofluorescent electron microscopic study. Virchow's Arch. Path. Anat. 358:205, 1973.

Bunch, W.L., Jr.: Rocky Mountain Spotted Fever. J. Arkansas Med. Soc. 64:300, 1968.

Cox, H.R.: Rocky Mountain Spotted Fever: Protective value for guinea pigs of vaccine from rickettsia cultured in embryonic chick tissues. Pub. Health Rep. 54:1070, 1937.

Harrel, G.T., Masland, R.L., Rosenblum, M.: CNS sequelae as shown by post recovery EEG in Rickettsial Spotted Fever. J. Clin. Invest. 30:645, 1951.

Hersey, D.F., Colvin, M.C., Shepard, C.C.: Studies on serologic diagnosis of murine typhus and Rocky Mountain Spotted Fever: Human infections. J. Immunol. 79:409, 1957.

Huebner, R.J., Stamps, P. and Armstrong, D.: Rickettsialpox - a newly recognized rickettsial disease. I. Isolation of the etiologic agent. Pub. Health Rep. 61:1605, 1946.

James, M.T., Marwood, R.F.: Hermes Medical Entomology. Macmillan Corp., London, 1969.

Lennette, E.H. and Clark, W.H.: Observations on the epidemiology of Q Fever in northern California. JAMA 145:306, 1951.

Older, J.J.: The epidemiology of murine typhus in Texas, 1969. JAMA 214:2011, 1970.

Peters, A.H.: Rocky Mountain Spotted Fever: Epidemiologic trends with particular reference to Virginia. JAMA 216:1003, 1971.

Presley, G.D.: Fundus changes in Rocky Mountain Spotted Fever. Am. J. Ophthal. 67:263, 1969.

Raab, E.L., Leopold, I.H., Hodes, H.L.: Retinopathy in Rocky Mountain Spotted Fever. Am. J. Ophthal. 68:42, 1969.

Rothenberg, R. and Sorenshine, D.E.: Rocky Mountain Spotted Fever in Virginia - Clinical and epidemiological features. J. of Med. Ent. 7:663, 1970.

Slotkin, R.E.: Rickettsial Diseases in Pediatric Therapy, Chapter 63, Shirkey, H., ed., C.V. Mosby Co., Philadelphia, 1975, p. 453.

GENERAL CONSIDERATIONS: The characteristics of fungal infections include: 1) a tendency to produce a more chronic and milder
disease than bacterial infections, 2) usually do not cause epidemics
and are not contagious except for superficial fungal infections, and
3) in tissues they grow slowly, produce granulomatous reactions
and cause a delayed hypersensitivity type of immune response.

A wide variety of fungi are known to cause infection in man and they
tend to limit their infection to specific anatomic areas, namely systemic (or deep), subcutaneous, cutaneous, or superficial. The disease, etiologic agent, and clinical manifestations of each type of
mycoses are summarized in Tables 15-1, 15-2 and 15-3. The mode
of transmission, source of infection, and pathologic characteristics
of each type of infection are shown in Table 15-4.

Fungal infections in infants and children are common, the majority
involve cutaneous or superficial tissues such as mucous membrane,
skin and its appendages, hair, and nails. Systemic or deep tissue
infections are less common except in infants and children with altered host resistance. A group of fungi (Table 15-5), common saprophytes in nature, generally do not cause serious infection in normal
infants and children but may produce localized or disseminated infection in the compromised host, particularly in persons with severe
diabetes mellitus, malignancy of lymphoid tissues, or in those receiving immunosuppressive therapy and/or a broad spectrum antibiotic. The opportunistic behavior of these fungi (opportunistic infection) is not an all-or-none phenomenon.

15.1: SUPERFICIAL FUNGAL INFECTIONS

The dermatophytoses (dermatomycosis, tinea, or ringworm) include
a diverse group of fungi (dermatophytes) characterized by their ability to cause clinical disease affecting the keratinized tissues. Children generally exhibit infection by these organisms more commonly
than adults. Sex and race are not as important as personal hygiene
in the epidemiology of these infections.

1. TINEA CAPITIS

Tinea capitis refers to fungal invasion of the scalp. Microsporum
audouinii is the most common cause of this disorder in the United
States. Organisms causing this clinical disease also include Trichophyton violaceum, T. schoenlenii, and T. tonsurans. Transmission

TABLE 15-1: CUTANEOUS AND SUPERFICIAL MYCOSES

DISEASE	CAUSATIVE AGENT	CLINICAL MANIFESTATION
Dermatomy- coses	Microsporum audouini Microsporum gypseum Microsporum canis	Invasion of hair and skin Ex. - Tinea capitis
	Epidermophyton floccosum	Invasion of skin and nails Ex. - Tinea pedis
	Trichophyton menta- grophytes Trichophyton rubrum Trichophyton tonsurans Trichophyton schoenleini Trichophyton violaceum Trichophyton concentricum Trichophyton spp.	Invasion of skin, hair and nails Ex. - Tinea corporis, Tinea barbae
	Malassezia furfur	Infection of skin Tinea versicolor
	Pityrosporum ovale	Infection of scalp (?)
Erythrasma	Nocardia minutissima	Infection of skin in axillae and genitocrural regions
Trichomycosis	Nocardia tenuis	Infection axillary or pubic hairs
Geotrichosis	Geotrichim candidum	Infection of skin, mucous mem- branes, or lungs

TABLE 15-2: SUBCUTANEOUS MYCOSES		
DISEASE	CAUSATIVE AGENT	CLINICAL MANIFESTATION
Chromoblasto-mycosis	Hormodendrum pedrosoi Hormodendrum compactum Phialophora verrucosa	Cutaneous involvement, usually of foot and leg
Maduromycosis	Allescheria boydii (Monosporium apio-spermum)	Infection of subcutaneous tissues of foot
Nocardiosis	Nocardia asteroides Nocardia brasiliensis Nocardia spp. Streptomyces madurae	Subcutaneous, suppurative tumefactions or mycetomas; sometimes systemic
Sporotrichosis	Sporotrichum schenckii	Involves skin and sucutaneous tissues

by these fungi is principally person to person and by contaminated fomites, although T. mentagrophytes and M. canis are transmitted by animal vectors.

The hair shafts are characteristically involved. Growth strictly within the hair shaft (or endothrix infection) is caused by T. violaceum, T. schoenleinii and T. tonsurous. Exothrix infection is seen with T. verucosum and T. mentagrophytes, which produce erthrospores on the outside of the hair. The fungi grow downward toward the root of the hair shaft. Since the hair is structurally weakened, it may break off above and below the scalp line.

The infection may invade adjacent areas and/or a state of host hypersensitivity may cause a kerion formation. Kerions are boggy, oozing lesions associated with hair loss. Favus reaction is seen with T. schoenleinii, T. violaceum and M. gypseum and is characterized by thick crusting lesions and permanent alopecia.

The usual clinical picture is that of a nickel to a quarter-sized lesion in the scalp with alopecia marked by broken off hair shafts 1-2 mm above the surface and "black dots" representing hair shafts broken below the surface.

Wood's lamp examination will reveal yellow-green fluorescence with Microsporum species. Trichophytons do not fluoresce. Examination with KOH preparation of the involved hair shafts will show long,

TABLE 15-3: SYSTEMIC (OR DEEP) MYCOSIS		
DISEASE	CAUSATIVE AGENT	CLINICAL MANIFESTATIONS
Aspergillosis	Aspergillus fumigatus Aspergillus spp.	Infection of bronchi, lungs, ears, sinuses, and other sites
Actinomycosis	Actinomyces israelii	Cervicofacial, thoracic, abdominal; multiple abscesses which eventually break down to form draining sinuses
Blastomycosis	Blastomyces dermatitidis	Skin, lung, or systemic manifestations
Candidiasis	Candida albicans	Involvement of skin, oral and vaginal mucosa, and/or lungs and bronchi
Coccidioidomycosis	Coccidioides immitis	Involves cutaneous, subcutaneous, visceral, and osseous tissue
Cryptococcosis	Cryptococcus neoformans	May be generalized infection with meningeal involvement; sometimes cutaneous or pulmonary
Histoplasmosis	Histoplasma capsulatum	Generalized infection involving reticuloendothelial system; also pulmonary or cutaneous
Phycomycosis	Mucor spp. Rhizopus spp.	Generalized involvement; invasion of walls and lumina of blood vessels

TABLE 15-4: CHARACTERISTICS OF VARIOUS TYPES OF MYCOSES

Infection	Transmission	Source	Pathology	Contagiousness
1. Systemic or deep tissue	Inhalation of spores	Saprophytic	Acute or chronic	no
2. Subcutaneous	Direct implantation into wounds by spores or mycelia	Soil, vegetation	Abscess, granuloma, mycetoma	no
3. Cutaneous and Superficial	Direct contact	Soil, mammalian skin	Chronic	yes

TABLE 15-5: OPPORTUNISTIC FUNGAL INFECTION

COMMON	LESS COMMON
Candida	Cryptococcus
Aspergillus	Histoplasma
Rhizopus	Blastomyces
Mucor	

hyphal elements. Culture of the scrapings is definitive. Oral griseofulvin (10-15 mg/kg/day in 4 divided doses) is the most effective treatment and should be continued until the clinical signs and fluorescence are gone (usually about 30 days). A single dose of griseofulvin (3 gm) in combination with Whitefield's ointment has been effective, especially for fluorescent tinea infections.

2. TINEA CORPORIS

Tinea corporis is an infection of the glavorous skin. The common etiologic agents include M. canis, T. mentagrophytes, and T. mentagrophytes, usually from infected cats and dogs. The lesions are characterized by circular or oval advancing borders with scales. The border may be raised and is usually vesicular and erythematous. Infections caused by T. rubrum may not be circular, but display the same reactive, advancing borders.

Diagnosis by Wood's lamp may be attempted. Skin scrapings of the border may be examined with KOH preparation and by culture. Therapy should initially be topical. Whitefield's ointment or tolnaftate (Tinactin) may be applied twice or three times daily. Persistent lesions respond to griseofulvin.

3. TINEA VERSICOLOR

Tinea versicolor is a chronic, superficial infection of the skin caused by Melassezia furfur. The presentation varies from single to confluent areas of fawn-colored macules to hypopigmented lesions. Scratching over the affected area causes skin peeling. The shoulders, back, and neck are frequent sites of involvement. Treatment is topical and many antifungal agents are effective.

4. TINEA PEDIS

Tinea pedis is a very common problem seen in the pediatric age group. T. mentagrophytes, T. rubrum and E. floccusum are important etiologic agents. The transmission may be from person to person contact, with the infected epidermal scales and the wearing of contaminated shoes. The earliest lesions are minute vesicles which extend through epidermal cell layers. The usual site of early infection is the interdigital web of the fourth and fifth toes. Physical findings include fissures and white macerated skin in the interdigital area. Spread to the dorsal and plantar surfaces occurs, and scaling with or without tiny clear vesicles is seen. Allergic or id reactions to these fungi may be seen. The patient experiences pain, burning and itching in the affected areas.

Scrapings of vesicles and scales permits examination with KOH preparation and culture. Long-term (two to ten weeks) therapy with Whitefield's ointment or tolnaftate is usually curative. Griseofulvin therapy should be tried if tolnaftate fails. In the acute vesicular inflammatory stage, potassium permanganate solution (1:4,000) or other soaks should be used to dry the lesion prior to application of tolnaftate.

15.2: CANDIDIASIS

INTRODUCTION: Infections caused by Candida species are commonly encountered in the pediatric age group. These are usually mild and limited to localized infection of the cutaneous surfaces and gastrointestinal tract. It is apparent, however, that severe forms of infection are becoming more frequent, especially in the chronically ill and immunologically compromised host.

Candida species are dimorphic, exhibiting hyphal growth on culture media and with yeast phase and mycelial growth in tissue. These fungi are ubiquitous in the mucosal surfaces of man. Differences in diet, social class and climate influence the frequency of mucosal colonization. Vaginal colonization is present in 10 to 20% of normal females and up to 40% of pregnant women. Lower animals are also colonized by Candida species but animal to man transmission is unknown.

1. ETIOLOGY AND PATHOGENESIS

Candida albicans is the most frequently isolated species from patients with thrush, bronchopulmonary infection and disseminated disease. Other common isolates include C. tropicalis, C. pseudotropicalis and C. parasilosis.

The host immunologic status is perhaps the most important factor associated with the ability of any particular strain to cause human disease. Direct colonization occurs in the newborn with passage through the contaminated birth canal. Superficial invasion and proliferation occur in the gastrointestinal tract. Up to 50% of newborns will exhibit this localized infection known as thrush, characterized by shallow ulcerations of the oral mucosal surface with proliferation of blastospores and hyphal elements.

The prepubescent female rarely exhibits Candida vulvovaginitis. Local changes which occur as a result of puberty (i.e. the change in vaginal pH, and the increase in epithelial glycogen content) create a more favorable environment for the proliferation of Candida species, thus accounting for the increase in this disease in the older, fertile female. The poorly controlled diabetic may develop this form of Candida infection in the prepubescent period.

Chronic infection of the cutaneous surfaces is known as mucocutaneous candidiasis. Immunologic studies have demonstrated a defect in cell mediated immunity which renders the individual unable to respond properly to candida antigens and, therefore, chronic cutaneous invasion continues.

The common clinical cutaneous or intertriginous forms of candidiasis represent superficial invasion of the epidermis and occasionally the dermis by the fungus as a result of local environmental conditions which permit Candida growth. Such conditions are present in the macerated diaper area from the continuous contact with urine. Other such areas involved are the axilla and the skin folds of the neck.

The pulmonary colonization by Candida species may occur as a result of any predisposing disease of the bronchial tree. In the severely immunosuppressed host, actual parenchymal invasion may occur. Histologic examination will reveal microabscess formation with an intense polymorphonuclear response.

Septicemia results in widespread microabscess formation. Commonly, the kidneys, bones, lungs and meninges will be affected.

Septicemia commonly arises as the result of instrumentation, the common source being an indwelling catheter for intravenous infusion. The severity with which this can effect the individual depends upon the type and number of organisms shed into the blood stream. Septicemia may also occur through the ulcerative lesions in the gastrointestinal tract (e.g. patients with leukemia).

The susceptibility of the host to Candida infection is enhanced by the administration of antibiotics, corticosteroids and cytotoxic agents. Patients suffering lymphoreticular disorders are predisposed to developing the more severe forms of the disease.

2. CLINICAL MANIFESTATIONS

Infection by Candida species causes a variety of distinct clinical entities. The more common presentations of candidasis include thrush, cutaneous or intertriginous, vulvovaginal, chronic mucocutaneous, pneumonic, and septicemic. Endocarditis has been described in heroin users.

2.1: Thrush: The newborn develops thrush on the third to fourth day of life. A gray-white pseudomembrane is seen in patchy or confluent distribution involving the oral mucosa. When scraped with a tongue blade, an oozing shallow ulcer will lie beneath the membrane. The infant is usually asymptomatic.

2.2: Vulvovaginitis: Vulvovaginal infection is encountered in the diabetic pubertal and pregnant female. Although this infection may also be asymptomatic, the usual presentation is that of burning and itching of the genital and perineal area associated with a thick white, sometime creamy discharge. Upon examination, excoriation of the cervix and vulva may be seen.

2.3: Cutaneous Infection: Cutaneous candidiasis is usually seen in the moist intertriginous areas. The rash is moist and may be papular, scaling and vesicular with an intense erythema. Discrete satelite lesions are found at the periphery of the lesions. Candidids, or sterile grouped vesicles may occur at some distance from the primary rash and represent a nonspecific response to fungal antigens.

2.4: Chronic Mucocutaneous Candidiasis: This form presents a generalized integumentary infection not confined to the intertriginous areas. The nails and surrounding skin are often heavily involved. Mucous membrane involvement is severe. Particularly heavy colonization of the gastrointestinal tract is common.

2.5: Pneumonia: Symptoms of pulmonary involvement include tachypnea, fever, cyanosis and a thick, often blood-tinged sputum. Auscultation reveals diminished breath sounds and rales over affected areas.

2.6: Septicemia: Candida septicemia should be considered in patient with fever, chills, and candida in the urine, and particularly in patient with lymphoreticular disorder, immunodeficiency disease, in postoperative state, or following prolonged antibiotic therapy. Leukopenia may be present. Additional symptoms will be referrable to the particular organ system if microabscess formation occurs. Diffuse intravascular coagulopathy has been described as a complicating event.

3. DIAGNOSIS

The majority of oral and cutaneous intertriginous lesions caused by Candida species may be diagnosed accurately by inspection. The pseudomembrane of thrush must be differentiated from oral diphtheria infection. Involvement of the skin folds and characteristic satellite lesions differentiates candida diaper dermatitis from the other causes of diaper rash. Scrapings for histology and culture aid in the diagnosis.

In the more severe types of infection, such as septicemia, cultures of the blood, urine, cerebral spinal fluid and biopsy specimens are vital.

In systemic infections, histologic examination of tissue specimens may be necessary. Gram stain will often reveal the characteristic budding yeast and pseudoseptate hyphae of Candida species.

4. TREATMENT

The treatment of thrush is oral nystatin 100,000 units/ml given one ml four fimes daily until lesions have diappeared. In severe gastrointestinal infection, such as esophageal moniliasis with ulceration, nystatin has been given in a dose of 100,000 units hourly for one week followed by a gradual tapering of the dose while monitoring clinical symptoms.

Topical application of nystatin is useful for cutaneous and vulvovaginal moniliasis. Candida diaper dermatitis should be treated with water insoluble nystatin ointment in conjunction with orally administered nystatin. Gentian violet may be successful for stubborn lesions. In chronic mucocutaneous candidiasis, transfer factor has been used successfully (see Chapter 19).

Amphotericin B is the drug of choice in pneumonia and disseminated Candida infections. If the patient has an indwelling catheter that may be responsible for Candida septicemia, then removal of the catheter alone may result in clinical improvement. If no response is seen, then amphotericin B therapy is indicated.

15.3: NOCARDIOSIS

INTRODUCTION: Infections caused by nocardia species are rare
in children. Nocardia species are not fungi, but rather are classified as belonging to the Actinomycetaceae family of bacteria. Nocardia asteroides and N. braziliensis are responsible for most
human infections. These organisms are ubiquitous in nature and
are gram positive, nonmotile aerobic forms. Males are infected
four times as frequently as females.

1. ETIOLOGY AND PATHOGENESIS

Nocardia infections are characterized by pyogenic tissue reaction
with abscess formation. The abscesses are not encapsulated, and
spread of infection may occur by local extension and hematogenous
seeding to peripheral organ systems. In children, infection occurs
most commonly in patients with serious underlying disease. Multiple abscesses occur after hematogenous spread. In children, the
most common sites are the central nervous system and bone.

Traumatic implantation of N. braziliensis into the dermis has been
shown to cause mycetomas in tropical areas. These are exuberant
granulomas and abscesses of the extremities, face and bone with
draining sinus tracts.

2. CLINICAL MANIFESTATIONS

Pulmonary nocardiosis presents as a consolidated pneumonia with
eventual extension to the pleura. Effusion occurs with empyema
and draining chest wall sinus tract formation. Pneumonia is heralded by fever, night sweats, cough and copious, thick, often blood-
tinged sputum. When effusions occur, pleurisy results. The chest
x-ray reveals lobar consolidation and abscess formation. Pleural
fluid is commonly found.

Cerebral abscess may present as the sudden onset of focal seizures,
confusion and localizing neurologic deficits. The mortality rate in
adult patients with pulmonary involvement is 50%. With CNS involvement, the rate is 80%. Early recognition is vital to improving
the prognosis.

3. DIAGNOSIS

The diagnosis of nocardial infection is made by culture. The laboratory should be informed about the possible diagnosis to allow for
the slow growth of this bacteria. Specimens obtained by tracheal aspiration and diagnostic lung puncture are better than sputum. Cerebral involvement can only be documented by biopsy. The cerebral
spinal fluid findings which are not diagnostic include elevated protein,
pleocytosis and low sugar. Organisms are generally not demonstrated by stain and culture of CSF.

Histopathologic examination of tissue requires the Brown and Brenn
modification of the gram stains. Grocott's methanamine silver stain
is also helpful in demonstrating the organism. Culture is done in
glucose-neopeptone agar without antibiotics. The organisms are
demonstrable after aerobic growth after 72 hours. The filamentous,
branching organisms can then be examined and identified. In tissue, the filaments will often fragment, leaving a puzzling variety of
coccoid bacillary rod forms.

4. TREATMENT

Sulfonamides (such as sulfadizine or sulfisoxasole 100 to 150 mg/
kg/day in 4 divided doses) are the drugs of choice. Cycloserine
alone or in combination with a sulfonamide preparation has also been
used. Incision and drainage of abscesses is necessary when these
occur in the course of infection.

::

15.4: SPOROTRICHOSIS

INTRODUCTION: Sporotrichosis refers to the pulmonary, subcutaneous, and rarely generalized infection caused by the fungus
Sporothrix schenchii. The disease is world-wide in distribution but
is endemic in tropical countries and temperate areas of the northern
hemisphere. The fungus grows readily in soil and vegetable matter and is considered an occupational hazard of gardeners, farmers,
etc. It is a disease of all age groups, with 10 to 25% of all cases
arising in children living in tropical countries. In adults, the disease more often occurs in men than in women, but the sex difference
is not as apparent in children.

1. ETIOLOGY AND PATHOGENESIS

Sporothri schenchii is a dimorphic fungus which exhibits growth as
septate branching hyphae (1-2 μ diameter) in culture media. In tissue, it is a budding yeast, often cigar-shaped in appearance, with a
diameter of 10 μ .

Sporotrichosis occurs when the fungus is inoculated into the subcutaneous tissue by splinters, thorns, bites of animals, etc. Host
resistance limits infection to the initial site of inoculation and surrounding lymphatics in the majority of cases.

Once inoculation of the organism into the subcutaneous tissue has
occurred, a small, reddened papule develops which is adherent to
the epidermis. Gradual ulceration develops with formation of a central dark crest. Satellite lesions or nodules are seen along the course
of draining lymphatics.

2. CLINICAL MANIFESTATIONS

There are three recognized forms of sporotrichosis: cutaneous-
lymphatic, pulmonary, and disseminated forms.

2.1: <u>Cutaneous-lymphatic</u>: This is the most common form, arising
from trancutaneous inoculation of the fungus, usually by vegetative
material. Early manifestations include formation of a reddened
papule, with progression to ulceration with occasional fluctuance.
These lesions are nontender. Satellite lesions occur along draining
lymphatics. In adults, this form occurs predominantly on the extremities, but in children, the trunk and face are commonly involved.
The disease is chronic but rarely progresses to other forms
(Fig. 15.1).

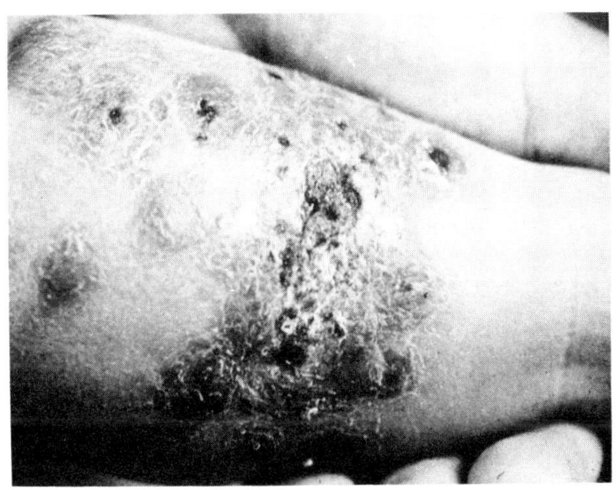

FIG. 15.1: Sporotrichosis involving the lower
extremity.

2.2: <u>Pulmonary Sporotrichosis</u>: This is rare and presents with fever,
cough, and sputum production. No characteristic radiographic presentation has been shown. Fibrosis, fungal ball formation and cavitation are reported.

2.3: <u>Disseminated Sporotrichosis</u>: This occurs in debilitated patients without the usual features of acute sepsis such as fever, chills,
etc. Bone involvement is common. This is a very rare complication.

3. DIAGNOSIS

The clinical presentation is highly suggestive. Aspirates of primary
or satellite lesions should be inoculated onto Sabouraud agar slants.
Typical hyphae with peripheral conidiospores are found when stained

with lactophenol cotton blue. Tissue sections are stained with Gridley stain for the characteristic, but unfortunately rare, cigar-shaped yeasts. Asteroid bodies are suggestive, but not diagnostic of sporotrichosis.

Differential diagnosis of the cutaneous-lymphatic sporotrichosis includes tularemia and blastomycosis. Pulmonary sporotrichosis must be differentiated from tuberculosis, histoplasmosis, sarcoidosis and neoplasia.

4. TREATMENT

Potassium iodide (saturated solution) 0.25 to 1 ml per day divided into 3 doses orally will resolve most cutaneous-lymphatic forms of the disease, and may be helpful in pulmonary sporotrichosis. Therapy should continue for one month after the skin lesions have cleared. Amphotericin B should be used when potassium iodide therapy fails, or in patients with disseminated disease.

::

15.5: ASPERGILLOSIS

INTRODUCTION: Aspergillosis describes any acute or chronic disease caused by any species of Aspergillus. These fungi are ubiquitous in nature with world-wide distribution. They can cause disease in any age group, but the young, old and debilitated are more susceptible to the serious forms of disease. Infections caused by aspergillus are increasing due to the increasing number of people surviving with chronic debilitating diseases.

1. ETIOLOGY AND PATHOGENESIS

Aspergillus fumigatus, A. flavis-oryzae and A. niger are the most important causes of human aspergillosis. Infection follows inhalation of spores into the respiratory tract. Four types of pulmonary infection may occur: 1) allergic aspergillosis due to previous sensitization, 2) local proliferation with pulmonary mycetoma (fungus ball), 3) bronchitis with local proliferation in the bronchial tree, and little or no penetration to the pulmonary parenchyma, and 4) necrotizing pneumonitis and fungal ball formation, which usually occurs in patients with underlying disease.

Hematogenous dissemination from the lungs seeds the fungus to other organs, with the kidneys and brain being involved in greater than 60% of the cases. At autopsy, multiple abscess formation is found in disseminated disease. Endophthalmitis occurs primarily in diabetic patients. Colonization of the paranasal sinuses may lead to spread of the fungus and creates periorbital cellulitis with extension to the central nervous system.

In tissue sections stained with silver methenamine, the fungi are seen as broken fragment of branching hyphae (about 4μ) and the branching characteristically occurs at an angle of about 45°. The organisms have a tendency to invade blood vessels and cause thrombotic angiitis. Acute necrotizing inflammatory changes are found most often in patients dying of disseminated disease. Fungal balls are composed of masses of entangled hyphal elements with little or no inflammatory response in the surrounding tissues. Occasionally, characteristic fruiting conidiophores are found in sections of unobstructed bronchi, when fungal growth takes place in air.

2. CLINICAL MANIFESTATIONS

The clinical features of aspergillosis vary with site of involvement and kind of host response.

2.1: Pulmonary Aspergillosis: As previously stated, pulmonary aspergillosis presents in four ways. Allergic aspergillosis results from inhalation of spores and presents as acute asthma and bronchospasm with expiratory wheezing, cough and tachypnea. Roentgenograms show transient and migratory infiltrates. Marked peripheral eosinophilia may be found and skin tests indicate immediate-type reactivity. Patients with pulmonary mycetoma, bronchitis or necrotizing pneumonitis may have fever, cough, hemoptysis and copious sputum production. On x-ray, an air crescent is seen over a cavitary lesion, suggesting the presence of an aspergillus fungal ball (a pathognomonic sign of mycetoma) (Fig. 15.2).

2.2: Disseminated Aspergillosis: This is an acute, progressive and often fatal infection seen in a compromised host. Symptoms and signs may include fever, headache, seizures, focal neurological signs, embolic skin lesions, azotemia and hematuria. A clinical picture of diffuse or consolidated pneumonia with CNS and renal involvement in a debilitated patient warrants consideration of disseminated aspergillosis.

2.3: Endophthalmitis: Endophthalmitis usually occurs 2 to 3 weeks following eye injury or surgery. It is manifested by periorbital erythema, conjunctional erythema, blurred vision, and pain.

2.4: Primary Cutaneous Aspergillosis: This has been described in debilitated patients. Aspergillus species are often isolated in patients with otitis externa. The etiologic role of these fungi in external ear infection is less well defined.

3. DIAGNOSIS

Laboratory diagnosis of aspergillosis is often difficult. Since Aspergillus species are ubiquitous, they may be present in the laboratory

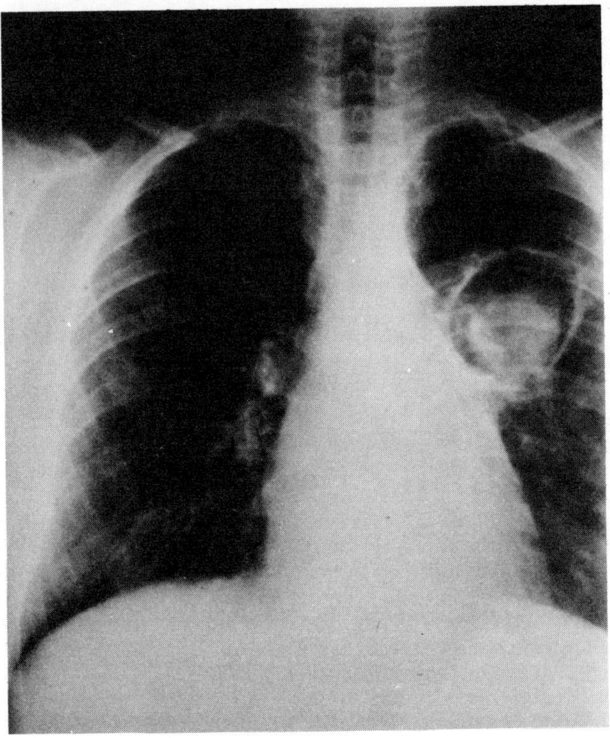

FIG. 15.2: Aspergilloma (fungal ball) in a leukemic child.

environment and may be isolated from sputum, feces, urine, conjunctival and vaginal swabs of uninfected persons. Only isolation of the fungi from deep tissue specimens, together with morphological identification of the fungi from the appropriately stained tissues, are satisfactory. Skin and serologic tests are generally not available, and do not provide consistent results. Eosinophilia and elevation of serum IgE, seen in patients with allergic aspergillosis, must be differentiated from that due to other inhalant allergens and syndromes of pulmonary infiltrates with eosinophilia (e.g. visceral larva migrams). Disseminated aspergillosis closely resembles sepsis due to gram negative bacteria and candida septicemia.

4. TREATMENT

For severe pulmonary involvement endophthalmitis and disseminated disease, intravenous amphotericin B is the drug of choice. Local mycetomas may be removed surgically, but spontaneous resolution may also occur. Enucleation may be necessary in severe endophthalmitis.

15.6: ACTINOMYCOSIS

INTRODUCTION: Actinomycosis is a chronic suppurative disease
caused by the bacteria Actinomyces israelii. This gram positive
anaerobe belongs to the bacterial order Actinomycotales and is part
of the normal flora of the oral cavity. No nonhuman source of this
bacteria has been found. The infection occurs worldwide. In the
United States, males are affected twice as frequently as females.
Person to person colonization is postulated to occur, but person to
person transmission of disease is unknown. Infections are rare in
children.

1. ETIOLOGY AND PATHOGENESIS

Actinomyces israelii is frequently cultured from the tonsillar crypts
and dental surfaces of healthy individuals. Pathogenicity arises
when local conditions render tissue susceptible to invasion and proliferation by this bacteria. Predisposing factors include foreign
body aspiration, prior suppurative dental infections and, most commonly, trauma, such as dental extraction. Local invasion and proliferation initiates a suppurative, granulomatous tissue response.
Cultures often reveal the presence of additional Bacteroides species
and microaerophilic streptococci. Whether these organisms act
synergistically in establishing infection is speculative. Abscesses of
various sizes are formed and these often coalesce. Granulation tissue surround these areas of suppuration. Sulfur granules up to 300μ
in diameter are found in pus and are composed of tangled masses of
growing filamentous actinomyces cemented together by protein and
polysaccharide liberated by the inflammatory response.

Typically the infection spreads following tissue planes. Draining
sinus tracts are frequently observed. Spread to adjacent bone, aspiration to the lung and swallowing infected material may lead to gastrointestinal infections. Hematogenous spread is unusual.

2. CLINICAL MANIFESTATIONS

Three forms of infection are generally seen, namely cervico-facial,
pulmonary and, gastrointestinal actinomycosis. Other unusual forms
include bone, brain, liver, kidney, pelvic organs, and septicemia.

2.1: Cervico-facial Actinomycosis (Lumpy Jaw): This form usually
arises after dental extraction, following previous infections or without apparent cause. The patient experiences the onset of a painful,
firm swelling near the mandible, often at the angle. The overlying
skin becomes purple or reddened, often followed by formation of
draining sinus tracts. Extension to the mandible, maxilla and orbit
with subsequent osteomyelitis may occur.

2.2: Gastrointestinal Actinomycosis: The form of infection arises
when the fungus is swallowed and penetrates mucosal defects, usually

in the ileocecal region. Suppurative inflammation and abscess formation develop in the mesentery and adjacent tissues. Symptoms of appendicitis, liver abscess and pelvic inflammatory disease of a chronic nature are seen. External draining sinuses may occur, and abdominal pain, palpable abdominal mass, jaundice, pyuria, weight loss, and spiking fever typify the constellation of clinical findings. Hematogenous dissemination to the meninges, bone and kidney may occur with this form, and the prognosis is poor.

2.3: Pulmonary Actinomycosis: Thoracic disease occurs with aspiration of the organisms into the lungs, or extension through the esophagus with mediastinal disease. The pulmonary form presents as a low grade pneumonitis which spreads from hilar areas to the pleura. Consolidation and pulmonary abscess are typical. Empyema occurs when the pleural surface is reached and eventual cutaneous fistula formation occurs. Hematogenous spread may occur. Symptoms include early nonproductive cough with progression to chest pain, dyspnea, spiking fever with chills and eventual productive cough with purulent sputum and hemoptysis.

3. DIAGNOSIS

Demonstration of sulfur granules in pus or drainage stained with hematoxylin and eosin should alert the physician to the possibility of Actinomyces israelii. The organisms will be seen as gram positive branching hyphae. Differentiation from Nocardia species should be attempted by partial acid decolorization.

Culture provides the definitive diagnosis. The organism is anaerobic and the laboratory therefore must be alerted to the possibility of actinomycosis. The organism must be grown in agar enriched with brain-heart infusion in 5-10% ambient CO_2. Hyphal elements are demonstrated in 2-5 days. Pure cultures are unusual.

The differential diagnosis of cervico-facial actinomycosis includes nocardial infections, tuberculosis, syphilitic gummas and other pyogenic infections. In the pulmonary form nocardia, other mycoses, tuberculosis and staphylococcal pneumonia must be considered. Gastrointestinal actinomycosis resembles appendicitis, regional enteritis gastrointestinal and pelvic tuberculosis.

4. TREATMENT

Penicillin is the drug of choice. Cervico-facial actinomycosis will respond to parenteral penicillin (30,000-50,000 units/kg/day). Oral phenoxymethyl penicillin 50,000 units/kg/day in four divided doses is continued for three to four weeks after clearing of the lesions.

Intravenous potassium or sodium penicillin 200,000-400,000 units/kg/day in four doses should be used in gastrointestinal and thoracic actinomycosis. Administration should continue 3-4 weeks after clinical symptoms have subsided. Oral penicillin should be instituted for an additional 3-4 weeks after intravenous penicillin has been stopped. Surgical drainage of abscesses is mandatory when they occur during the course of the disease. In patients allergic to penicillin, erythromycin, or tetracycline are usually effective against Actinomyces israelii.

::

15.7: BLASTOMYCOSIS

INTRODUCTION: Blastomycosis, a systemic chronic suppurative disease, is caused by Blastomyces dermatitidis.

Originally, the disease was thought limited to the North American continent, but now cases have been described throughout Africa, South America and Mexico. The fungus is thought to be saprophytic in nature, but successful attempts to isolate Blastomyces from soil have proven inconclusive. Sex distribution of infections in children is approximately equal, and black children are affected more frequently than whites.

1. ETIOLOGY AND PATHOGENESIS

Blastomyces dermatitidis is a dimorphic fungus. At 37°C on Sabouraud's agar, the fungus exhibits growth as thick-walled single budding yeasts. At 30°C it grows as a white mold with spherical conidia arising from conidiophores.

Although no environmental source of Blastomyces is known, the postulated entry site is by inhalation through the respiratory tract. Abortive pulmonary infections may occur but have not been described. From the initial pulmonary site, hematogenous dissemination occurs with suppurative lesions arising at sites of fungal seeding.

Tissue reaction to infection by Blastomyces is characterized by suppuration with predominantly polymorphonuclear leukocytes. Abscess formation occurs and may be of any size. Granuloma formation occurs and giant cells may be found in the periphery of the lesion. Blastomyces dermatitidis may be identified in tissue as 8 to 15 μ budding yeasts. The buds are characteristically broad based, thick-walled with one bud per parent cell. Gomori's silver methenamine and periodic acid Schiff stain will demonstrate the yeast. Blastomyces has several nuclei per cell.

2. CLINICAL MANIFESTATIONS

Blastomycosis usually begins as a mild, lower respiratory infection which progresses to a persistent infiltrate despite antibiotic therapy. The patient experiences a dry cough, chest pain, fever and tachypnea. The roentgenographic appearance is variable, with diffuse involvement of many lobes to lobar consolidation.

When dissemination occurs, the skin, bones and urogenital systems are usually involved. Cutaneous lesions begin as subcutaneous nodules which break through the epidermis and ulcerate. They develop a raised margin sloping sharply outward. Central crusting and pus are present. The lesions are painless and occur on exposed areas of the body such as the scalp and extremities. These are slowly progressive lesions and central healing may be seen. Involvement of the underlying bone is characterized by persistently draining sinus tracts.

Genito-urinary involvement usually affects the internal genitalia and in the male it is manifested by swollen, tender testes, pyuria and hematuria.

Bone infection usually affects the lumbar, sacral and thoracic vertebrae. In children, skull lesions are common and sinus tract formation is a frequent complication. Bony destruction, vertebral collapse and septic joint formation are seen.

The clinical course of untreated cases is one of unrelenting progression and fatal outcome. Spontaneous remissions and cures have been described but are uncommon.

3. DIAGNOSIS

The diagnosis rests upon culture of B. dermatitidis from pus, sputum or tissue. Clinical characteristics give only a presumptive diagnosis. Demonstration of Blastomyces in tissue aids in the diagnosis and may be accomplished with smears of prostatic secretions or pus from skin lesions.

The differential diagnosis of pulmonary blastomycosis includes tuberculotis, other mycoses, bacterial infection and cancer. Skin lesions may represent the presenting complaint and must be differentiated from basal cell carcinoma, the cutaneous-lymphatic variety of sporotrichosis and tuberculosis.

4. TREATMENT

Blastomyces dermatitidis is extremely susceptible to antifungal drugs. Amphotericin B is the drug of choice in pulmonary and disseminated blastomycosis. 2-Hydroxystilbamidine has been used in adult patients with cutaneous blastomycosis. Other drugs, such as saramycetin and hamycin are available only for investigational use.

::

15.8: COCCIDIOIDOMYCOSIS

INTRODUCTION: Coccidioidomycosis (San Joaquim Valley fever) is a fungal infection with a diversity of clinical symptoms and severity, caused by <u>Coccidioides immitis</u>. This disease is endemic within specific geographic areas of the United States, Mexico, Central and South America. In the United States, the disease occurs in southwest areas including southern Arizona, New Mexico, California and southwestern Texas.

Most infections are inapparent, as shown by skin testing. Ten percent of children in endemic areas show positive reactivity to coccidioidin skin test by age one year, and 70% will be positive by ten years of age. Approximately 60% of infections caused by <u>C. immitis</u> are inapparent. Of the remaining 40% who display symptoms, the vast majority will recover completely. Dissemination or severe infection occurs in approximately 1% of infected white males, but disseminated disease is much more frequent among Filipino and black males. Females are much less frequently afflicted with disseminated disease, except during pregnancy when they are exceptionally vulnerable.

1. ETIOLOGY AND PATHOGENESIS

<u>Coccidioides immitis</u> is found in soil. The fungus apparently replicates in areas removed from direct sunlight such as rodent burrows. The capillary action of rainfall in the soil allows the fungus to approach the surface where fungal arthrospores are disseminated with wind currents.

This fungus is dimorphic with free, living mycelial and spherical phases found in infected tissue. Characteristically, the organism appears in culture as mycelia with septate hyphae exhibiting arthrospore and endospore formation after 3-5 days.

Infection usually arises through the inhalation of air-borne arthrospores. This is followed by the conversion of arthrospores to spherules, the parasitic tissue form of the fungus. An intense neutrophilic inflammatory response occurs and is manifested by a pyogenic pneumonitis. Persistent infection incites a variable granulomatous response, with involvement of the draining hilar nodes. Early lesions show integrity of alveolar septa. However, the disease may progress to microabscess formation, consolidation and hyalinization of large areas of the pulmonary parenchyma.

Spherules reproduce by endosporulation. Sporangia are seen when spherules contain endospores and these may be readily identified from tissue, pus and sputum of early lesions. Discharging sporangia and occasional hyphal elements are also reported.

Hematogenous dissemination occurs as a result of compromised host response and/or severe exposure to <u>C. immitis</u>. The central nervous system (CNS), bone, joints, and skin are frequently affected. Intrapulmonary miliary spread is not uncommon. In the CNS, the meninges are frequently the primary site of seeding and granulomatous formation.

Primary cutaneous coccidioidomycosis is rare and results from traumatic implantation of arthrospores through the epidermal barrier. Ulcer formation with induration and regional lymphadenopathy are present.

The primary pulmonary lesions of coccidioidomycosis may heal with sequela or may progress to chronicity with cavity formation, empyema and bronchiectasis.

Some 3-21 days after the initial onset of infection, delay manifestation of hypersensitivity to coccidioidin MM occurs in the form of erythema nodosum, which is commonly seen in adult white females with the disease. Precipitin antibodies are detectable approximately three weeks after exposure and are short-lived. Complement fixation antibodies may not be demonstrable in subclinical infections, but are elevated and remain so in severe and disseminated disease.

2. CLINICAL MANIFESTATIONS

The incubation period is 7-28 days, averaging 14 days. The severity of the infection varies inversely with the duration of incubation. Fever, cough, anorexia, severe headache, night sweats and chest pain are frequent symptoms. The chest pain may be pleuritic and at times very severe. Cough becomes productive with extensive pulmonary involvement. If fever continues and is markedly elevated, dissemination is likely. A morbiliform rash, heaviest in the inguinal area, is sometimes seen in children. With the development of delayed hypersensitivity, erythema nodosum may occur. More than 50% of children with acute symptomatic pulmonary infection display erythema multiforme or nodosum, the latter being characterized by tender, indurated, raised, erythematous nodules, usually over the tibia.

With dissemination, high fever and signs and symptoms of meningitis may arise, which is an ominous finding. Bony lesions resemble osteomyelitis, and draining sinus tracts over bony lesions may occur. Septic arthritis has occurred. Meningitis and miliary hematogenous infection carry an increased mortality rate, while bony joint and cutaneous lesions are marked by periods of exacerbation and remission.

3. DIAGNOSIS

In an endemic area, many cases of coccidioidomycosis go undetected simply because the patient remains asymptomatic or is only mildly ill and does not seek medical attention. In more symptomatic cases, the constellation of fever, chest pain, arthralgia, erythema nodosum and pneumonitis should lead the physician to the possible diagnosis. Skin testing should be done with a 1:1000 dilution of coccidioidin antigen; 0.1 ml is injected subcutaneously and the test is read in 48 hours. Greater than 5 mm induration is a positive test. Patients with erythema nodosum should be tested with a 1:10,000 dilution of antigen.

Complement fixation (CF) antibodies are helpful in the diagnosis.
Cerebral spinal fluid CF antibodies will be detected in 75% of patients with meningitis.

Cultures of C. immitis may be carried out with sputum, pus and
tissue. Specimens should be inoculated on Sabauraud agar slants
and the laboratory must be alerted, as these cultures are extremely
contagious. After a few days, gray fluffy colonies are visible. The
finding of endospores is diagnostic.

Tissue specimens stained with hematoxylin and eosin will readily
demonstrate the large 30-60 μ sporangia with endospores. Special
stains, such as Gridley and silver methenamine, will be helpful.

The differential diagnosis of coccidioidomycosis includes histoplasmosis, sarcoidosis, tuberculosis and pyogenic bacterial pneumonias
with hematogenous dissemination.

4. TREATMENT

Amphotericin B is the drug of choice for patients predisposed to disseminated disease, pregnant women and those with documented disseminated disease. Amphotericin B is given parenterally with attention to the toxic side effects. Intrathecal amphotericin B may be
required for patients with meningitis. Surgical removal of expanding
cavitary lesions and drainage of infected joints and osseous structures is essential. Recent reports suggest chlortrimazole may be
an effective drug, but conclusive studies have yet to be carried out.

15.9: CRYPTOCOCCOSIS

INTRODUCTION: Cryptococcosis (torulosis) is caused by Cryptococcus neoformans and may be manifested by acute or chronic symptoms involving the lungs, central nervous system (CNS) viscera and
skin.

The disease occurs world-wide, and sporadic epidemics with predominantly pulmonary symptoms occur as a result of heavy exposure,
especially in workmen who destroy buildings with pigeon roots, and
in pigeon handlers. Men are affected three times as frequently as
females and infection occurs at all ages. Patients with lymphoreticular disorders, sarcoidosis, diabetes mellities and those receiving
steroid therapy are predisposed to develop the disease.

1. ETIOLOGY AND PATHOGENESIS

Cryptococcus neoformans is a yeast-like fungus which reproduces by
budding. A mucopolysaccharide capsule of variable size surrounds

the fungus. The fungus varies from 4-20 μ in diameter. High concentrations of the fungus are found in areas rich in pigeon excreta.
The pigeons themselves are not infected with the fungus.

Cryptococcosis arises from inhalation of aerosolized fungus. Man-
to-man transmission and direct animal-to-man transmission is rare,
if it occurs at all. An initial pneumonitis results, which may be
transient. Formation of discrete, bordered nodular pulmonary lesions may develop. These lesions consist of solitary intralobar or
subpleural nodules, often with gross myxomatous or gelatinous quality. Early hematogenous dissemination occurs to peripheral organ
systems and, most importantly, to the CNS, bones and skin.

Characteristically, cryptococcal infection incites little tissue reaction. Lesions consist of cystic, mucinous cavities, and contain
numerous fungal cells. Focal lesions develop by physical displacement of surrounding tissue. In some patients, intense cellular reaction occurs and the focal lesions are granulomatous in character.
Histologic examination reveals extra- and intracellular fungal cells.
Single budding forms are demonstrable in early lesions and are rare
in older lesions.

CNS involvement is characterized by small cysts or granulomas involving the pons, basal ganglion and gray matter. The subarachnoid
layer may be found separated from the surface and filled with budding
yeasts, giving it a soap bubble-like appearance. Meningeal involvement characteristically effects the basal and cerebellar areas.

2. CLINICAL MANIFESTATIONS

Often, the initial pulmonary reaction to infection has cleared by the
time the patient seeks medical attention for CNS symptoms. Occasionally a healed subpleural granuloma is found on chest x-ray in
mildly infected patients with nonprogressive disease. Cough, low-
grade fever, scant sputum, dull chest pain and weight loss are complaints of those with pulmonary symptoms. Chest x-ray findings
reveal single or multiple variable sized dense infiltrates with cir-
cumscribed margins. Cavities are rare and are generally thick-
walled.

CNS disease is usually indolent and presents with waxing and waning
symptoms of diplopia, blurred vision, convulsion, headache of increasing severity, focal signs and behavior and personality changes.
Fever is usually low grade. Nuchal rigidity is unusual. Ankle clonus
and exterior plantar responses are seen.

Osseous disease is seen radiographically as a cold abscess with lytic
lesions in approximately 10% of cases. Painless skin lesions of the
scalp, face and extremities are frequently found. Early on they are
pustules or subcutaneous masses which later ulcerate and develop
rolled margins with central granulation tissue. Mucous membrane
ulcerations may occur. Any visceral organ may be involved.

Complications which include permanent neurologic sequelae (e.g.
ataxia, optic atrophy, and obstructive hydrocephalus) have been described following meningitis. Death from involvement of other organ systems has been described following meningitis. In untreated
patients, cryptococcal meningitis is uniformly fatal, while fatality
rates of 25% are seen with antifungal therapy.

3. DIAGNOSIS

The most definitive diagnostic tool is culture. Five to ten ml of
cerebrospinal fluid (CSF) should be collected, centrifuged and the
sediment inoculated onto culture media. Sputum, urine and blood
cultures should be obtained. Biopsy of skin lesions will reveal
organisms.

Approximately 50% of culture positive meningitis cases will have
positive India ink preparation of the CSF. CSF changes seen in
cryptococcal meningitis include elevated protein, pleocytosis with
mostly lymphocytes, and a decreased glucose (in about 50% of cases).

Serologic tests are available and include latex agglutination of complement fixation of cryptococcal antigens. Over 50% of patients with
CNS disease will have positive blood and/or CSF serologic tests.

The differential diagnosis of cryptococcal meningitis includes tuberculous meningitis, neoplastic disease of the meninges and viral
meningoencephalitis. Pulmonary cryptococcosis may appear roent-
genographically as primary or metastatic disease. Skin lesions of
disseminated cryptococcosis resemble lesions of tuberculosis, sarcoid, syphilis and carcinoma.

4. TREATMENT

Amphotericin B given intravenously is the drug of choice. Therapy
should be continued until four to six weeks after the CSF becomes
sterile. If the disease is not controlled by prolonged intravenous
therapy, then intrathecal amphotericin B should be utilized. A subcutaneous reservoir with a valve into the lateral ventricle may be
useful for intrathecal therapy.

Use of antifungal therapy for non-CNS cryptococcal disease is a subject of debate. Surgical excision of pulmonary lesions does not cause
spread of the disease. Observation may be justifiable if cultures of
CSF urine and blood are negative, if the patient does not have any predisposing disease and if all lesions, either cutaneous or pulmonary,
appear stable or are diminishing. Patients with visceral or bony lesions are treated with intravenous amphotericin B.

5-Fluorocytosine, which readily penetrates into the CSF, has been
used with some success in cryptococcal meningitis (Harder and

Hermans, 1975). A combination of amphotericin B and 5-Fluoro-cytosine might act synergistically and reduce the dosage of ampho-tericin B (Utz et al. 1975).

::

15.10: HISTOPLASMOSIS

INTRODUCTION: Histoplasmosis is a disease with a wide clinical spectrum caused by Histoplasma capsulatum. In the mid-1940's, histoplasmin reactivity was demonstrated in nontuberculous cavitary pulmonary disease and the true nature and epidemiology of the disease became known. From skin test reactivity data, the geographic zones within the U.S. in which Histoplasma is endemic were identified. The Ohio and Missouri River Valleys, the eastern coastal states and the southwest are currently endemic areas and account for the largest number of cases.

Histoplasma is recovered from soil samples which are enriched with fecal material of birds and bats. Often the incidence of skin reactivity is higher in rural areas, but patients in urban areas in endemic zones may also display a high incidence of positive skin reactivity.

The milder primary pulmonary form of the disease most often affects adult males, while the severe disseminated form is seen in the young and the old with no sex predilection.

1. ETIOLOGY AND PATHOGENESIS

Histoplasma capsulatum is a dimorphic fungus. Soils enriched by avian excrement serve as the natural reservoir from which aerosol-ized spores are inhaled. Deposition of spores into the lower respira-tory tract causes a discrete focus of infection. Macrophages phago-cytize the invading organisms and, by the process of macrophage migration, the infection crosses the draining hilar nodes. With the onset of delayed hypersensitivity, coagulation necrosis and eventual calcification occur. In the disseminated form of the disease, hema-togenous seeding results from an active primary focus and infection spreads to areas rich in reticuloendothelial cells, such as the liver, bone marrow and spleen. The adrenals and brain may also be involved.

Chronic cavitary disease of the lungs may be seen. When examined histopathologically, histoplasma will be found as an intracellular yeast of approximately 1-5 μ in diameter in fresh lesions, while in old lesions they are found exclusively within the center of coagulation necrosis and have different staining characteristics. Focal periph-eral calcification occurs with healing.

2. CLINICAL MANIFESTATIONS

There are three forms of histoplasmosis seen in the United States:
1) primary pulmonary, 2) disseminated, and 3) chronic cavitary.

2.1: <u>Primary Pulmonary Disease</u>: The most common infection is a
primary pulmonary disease which is asymptomatic or mild. Fever,
cough and chest pain are the presenting symptoms. Physical findings are few and consist of scattered rales and roentgenographic evidence of a local subpleural infiltrate with hilar adenopathy (Fig. 15.3).
Erythema nodosum may be present. With a heavy inoculation of organisms, miliary spread may occur, with x-ray findings much more
striking than clinical symptoms.

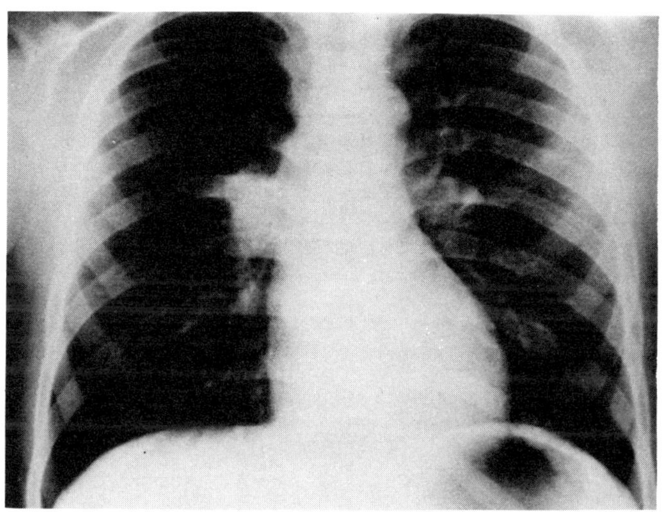

FIG. 15.3: Pulmonary histoplasmosis with hilar adenopathy
in an eight-year-old boy.

2.2: <u>Disseminated Disease</u>: In the young, old and debilitated persons, hematogenous dissemination of H. capsulatum to the liver,
spleen, brain, and bone marrow may occur. Lymphadenopathy,
anemia, and hepatosplenomegaly with anorexia and weight loss are
common. Meningeal involvement is basilar in distribution. Adrenal
seeding can result in adrenal insufficiency. Gastrointestinal involvement characteristically causes ulcerations of the oral mucosa, epiglottis and larynx. Histoplasmosis is a common cause of fever of
unknown origin in children in endemic areas.

2.3: <u>Chronic Cavitary Form</u>: Cavitary histoplasmosis is bilateral in
the majority of cases, often involving the upper lobe. Cough, hemoptysis, fever, anorexia and weight loss are common.

The prognosis of primary infection is good. Progression to disseminated disease is very rare, however, up to 90% of disseminated infections are fatal. Chronic cavitary disease carries a poor prognosis unless therapy is initiated promptly.

3. DIAGNOSIS

The laboratory confirmation of disseminated histoplasmosis depends upon isolating the organisms from cultures of blood, sputum, urine and tissue specimens. Demonstration of fungi in tissue requires experience. In early lesions, histoplasma (intracellular 1-5 μ diameter yeasts) may be seen by staining with hematoxylin and eosin. In granulomas, silver methanamine stains will demonstrate the yeast in the central areas of coagulation necrosis.

Complement fixation antibodies are demonstrable in the sera of the infected patient and a rising titer with a compatible clinical course aids in the diagnosis.

Histoplasmin skin tests may be positive in greater than 80% of people in endemic areas. Skin tests aid in the diagnosis of active infections only when they become positive during clinical infection or when positive in a child less than 1 year of age. The histoplasmin skin test may cause a slight increase in serum antibodies (mycelia phase), and yeast phase antigens must therefore be used to gather information after skin testing.

The differential diagnosis of histoplasmosis includes tuberculosis, viral and other mycotic pneumonia. Disseminated disease closely resembles lymphoma, diffuse viral disease and tuberculosis.

4. TREATMENT

In acute primary infection, observation is all that is necessary in a previously healthy patient. When more severe primary pulmonary involvement occurs, supportive care and oxygen may be required.

Amphotericin B is used in disseminated and chronic cavitary disease. Surgical resection of solitary granulomas and cavities must be considered when medical therapy fails to alter clinical course.

15.11: PHYCOMYCOSIS

INTRODUCTION: Phycomycosis (or mucormycosis) is uncommon in the pediatric age group. The infection is most often seen in the immune compromised host. Patients with poorly controlled diabetes mellitus or patients suffering from lymphoreticular disorders are most susceptible. Age and race do not affect the incidence of this infection.

1. ETIOLOGY AND PATHOGENESIS

Fungi of the class Phycomycetes, including Absildia, Mucor, Rhizopus and Mortierella, are important etiologic agents for phycomycosis. The fungi are ubiquitous in nature, thriving in dung and decaying vegetation, and are common laboratory contaminants.

Phycomycetes are found as broad, nonseptate hyphae with irregular branching. The characteristics of infection produced do not vary among different members of the class.

The organism proliferates in human tissue opportunistically. After establishing an initial invasion site, the fungi characteristically proliferate with the walls of blood vessels. Common sites of infection include the lungs, paranasal sinuses, gastrointestinal tract and epidermis. Patients with acidosis complicating diabetes mellitus are prone to develop infection of the paranasal sinuses.

Tissue reaction seen histologically includes thrombosis and obstruction of blood vessels from fungal proliferation. A pyogenic, principally neutrophilic response is seen, except in subcutaneous tissue where esinophilic granulomas have been described.

2. CLINICAL MANIFESTATIONS

Clinically, three forms of infections caused by Phycomycetes are recognized: rhinocerebral, subcutaneous and pulmonary. Diffuse hematogenous dissemination in patients with the rhinocerebral and pulmonary forms often results in death.

<u>Rhinocerebral phycomycosis</u> begins with infection of the paranasal sinuses, usually in poorly controlled patients with diabetes. A rapidly spreading cellulitis often develops with extension to the orbit. The infection will spread to the meninges and brain if therapy is delayed. Fever, pain and necrosis of the turbinate with bloody nasal discharge are common. Other signs include ptosis and loss of vision.

<u>Subcutaneous phycomycosis</u> has been described in Indonesia and Africa and is characterized by the development of firm, indurated oval-shaped lesions with overlying hyperpigmentation. These lesions are freely mobile and are thought to arise from traumatic implantation via insect bites and contaminated vegetative material.

<u>Pulmonary phycomycosis</u> may arise from hematogenous dissemination and aspiration of necrotic sinus material in a patient with rhinocerebral disease. Pain, fever, effusion and signs of consolidation are seen. The prognosis is poor, even with therapy.

3. DIAGNOSIS

The diagnosis of phycomycosis depends upon histologic findings of infected tissues. Hematoxylin and eosin will demonstrate the broad 10-15 μ nonseptate hyphae with irregular branching. Differentiation from aspergillus species is possible, as aspergillus species display septae in tissues; culture is definitive. Culture may be carried out on glucose neopeptone agar.

The differential diagnosis of the severe forms of phycomycosis includes other opportunistic fungal infections in the compromised host.

4. TREATMENT

Although information concerning the clinical efficacy of amphotericin B is scarce, it is the drug of choice for infections caused by Phycomycetes. In vitro sensitivity tests reveal that these fungi are relatively resistant to amphotericin B. Potassium iodide therapy has been tried but better results have been reported with amphotericin B.

15.12: AMPHOTERICIN B THERAPY

Amphotericin B is efficacious in the treatment of a wide variety of systemic fungal infections. This antibiotic is extremely toxic and must be used with caution in the hospital setting. Immediate toxic effects include headache, chills and fever, nausea and vomiting. Tolerance to these effects occurs rapidly in children, provided the dosage of the drug is increased slowly. Local venous irritation, thrombophlebitis, is a frequent occurrence and necessitates constant vigilance of the intravenous site.

Depression of the bone marrow production of erythrocytes causes an iron resistant anemia in patients receiving the drug. Azotemia and a renal concentrating defect are direct toxic effects which appear to be dose related. Hypokalemia is frequently reported as a hazard to amphotericin B administration.

Intravenous amphotericin B should be given in a dose of 0.1 mg/Kg/ day over a one-week period. Five percent dextrose in water must be used in the infusion as saline will precipitate the drug. The duration of therapy and total dose delivered are governed by the clinical response, provided that toxicity is avoided.

A baseline CBC, liver function tests, blood urea nitrogen and creatinine, serum potassium, urinalysis and creatinine clearance should be carried out before therapy is undertaken. These parameters must be monitored twice weekly during treatment, and monthly examinations should be made for three to four months after amphotericin B has been stopped. When intrathecal therapy is used, the renal toxicity is not as great, since the drug is not absorbed into the vascular space. Intrathecal therapy is recommended to be undertaken twice weekly. Initially, 2 ml of 0.25 mg/ml solution of amphotericin B is diluted 3 to 4 times with 5% dextrose in water. This solution is injected into the lumbar or cisternal space after an equal volume of CSF has been removed. The total dosage given will be 0.50 mg/day. Headache, footdrop, arachnoiditis and radicular neuritis are complications of this therapy.

Alternate day therapy, utilizing twice the daily dosage of amphotericin B, is promising as an effective type of therapy. This method has not undergone extensive investigation.

REFERENCES

Ajello,. L. , et al.: Histoplasmosis. Proceedings of the Second National Conference. Charles C Thomas, Springfield, 1971.

Ballenger, C.W. and Goldring, D.: Nocardiosis in children. J. Pediatr. 50:145, 1957.

Bennett, J.E.: Chemotherapy of systemic mycosis. NEJM 290:30, 290:320, 1974.

Burry, J.N.: Fluorinated corticosteroids and dermatophytosis. Br. Med. J. 3:5974, 1975.

Carlile, J.R., Mullett, R.E., Cho, C.T., et al.: Primary cutaneous aspergillosis in a leukemic child. Arch. Dermatol. 114:78, 1978.

Carrada-Bravo, T.: New observations on the epidemiology and pathogenesis of sporotrichosis. Ann. Trop. Med. and Parasit. 69:267, 1975.

Cawlry, E.P.: Aspergillosis and the aspergilli. Arch. Intern. Med. 80:423, 1947.

Cherry, J.D., et al.: Amphotericin B therapy in children. J. Pediatr. 75:1063, 1969.

Chick, E.W., Balows, A., and Furcolow, M.L. eds.: Opportunistic Fungal Infections. Proceedings of the Second International Conference. Charles C Thomas, Springfield, 1975.

Cho, C.T., Vats, T.S., Lowman, J.T., et al.: Fusariwum solani infection during therapy for leukemia. J. Pediatr. 83:1028, 1973.

Cox, F. and Hughes, W.T.: Contagious and other aspects of nocar-diosis in the compromised host. Pediatrics 55:135, 1975.

Diamond, R.D. and Bennett, J.E.: A subcutaneous reservoir for intrathecal therapy of fungal meningitis. NEJM 288:186, 1973.

Emmons, C., Binford, C., and Utz, J.: Medical Mycology, 2nd ed., Lea and Febiger, Philadelphia, 1970.

Fallo, A.: Candida sepsis and disseminated intravascular coagula-tion in a postoperative infant. Clin. Pediatr. 14:294, 1975.

Feigin, R.D. and Shearer, W.T.: Opportunistic infection in chil-dren. Part III. J. Pediatr. 87:852, 1975.

Fossen, R.B. and Wheeler, W.E.: Short-term treatment of histo-plasmosis. J. Pediatr. 86:32, 1975.

Gaines, J.D. and Remington, J.S.: Diagnosis of deep infection with candida. Arch. Intern. Med. 132:699, 1973.

Goldstein, E and Hoeprich, P.D.: Problems in the diagnosis and treatment of systemic candidiasis. J. Infect. Dis. 125:190, 1972.

Greenburg, R.M. and Kramer, R.: Cryptococcal meningitis. Arch Dis. Child. 45:417, 1970.

Halldorson, T.S.: Actinomycosis in childhood. Clin. Pediatr. 6: 221, 1967.

Harder, E.J. and Hermans, P.E.: Treatment of fungal infections with flucytosine. Arch. Intern. Med. 135:231, 1975.

Harris, J.S.: Mucormycosis. Pediatrics 16:857, 1955.

Hoeprich, P., ed.: Infectious Diseases. Harper and Row, New York, 1972.

Idriss, Z.H., et al.: Nocardiosis in children. Pediatrics 54:479, 1975.

Jones, H.E., et al.: Acquired immunity to dermatophytes. Arch. Dermatol. 109:840, 1974.

Kantrowitz, P.A., et al.: Successful treatment of chronic esophageal moniliasis with a viscous suspension of nystatin. Gastroenterol. 54: 424, 1969.

Krause, W., et al.: Fungaemia and funguria after oral administra-tion of candida albicans. Lancet 1:598, 1969.

Landau, J.W., Newcomer, V.D., and Schultz, J.: Aspergillus-report of two instances in children associated with acute leukemia and review of the pertinent literature. Mycopathol. Myco. Appl. 20:177, 1963.

Lynch, P.J. and Botero, F.: Sporotrichosis in children. Am. J. Dis. Child. 122:325, 1971.

Mann, B. and Pasha, M.: Allergic primary pulmonary aspergillosis and Schonlein-Henoch purpura. Br. Med. J. 1:282, 1959.

Millikan, L.E.: Superficial and cutaneous fungal infections. Postgrad. Med. J. 60:52, 1976.

Orr, R.E. and Riley, H.D.: Sporotrichosis in childhood: Report of 10 cases. J. Pediatr. 78:951, 1971.

Paul, F.M.: Two cases of thoracic actinomycosis in children. Arch. Dis. Child. 37:276, 1963.

Prystowsky, B.V., Vogelstein, B., Ettinger, P.S., et al.: Invasive aspergillosis. NEJM 295:655, 1976.

Schupbach, C.W., Wheeler, C.E., Briggaman, R.A., et al.: Cutaneous manifestations of disseminated cryptococcosis. Arch. Dermatol. 112:1734, 1976.

Tesh, T.B., et al.: Histoplasmosis in children. Pediatrics 33:894, 1964.

Turner, D.J. and Wadlington, W.B.: Blastomycosis in childhood: Treatment with amphotericin B and a review of the literature. J. Pediatr. 75:708, 1969.

Utz, J.P. Garriques, I.L., Sande, M.A., Warner, J.F., Mandell, G.L., MeGehee, R.F., Duma, R.J., and Shadomy, S.: Therapy of cryptococcosis with a combination of flucytosine and amphotericin B. J. Infect. Dis. 132:368, 1975.

CHAPTER 16.   PARASITIC INFECTIONS

INTRODUCTION: Parasitic diseases are the most prevalent world-wide infections of man, however, they are often regarded more as nuisances than as serious health problems.   Jansen (1974) has estimated that one-third of the world population is infected with Ascaris, while hookworm accounts for 800 million affected individuals, and Trichuris and Enterobius another 500 million each.   The World Health Organization (WHO) in 1971, estimated that 480 million people live in areas still endemic for malaria.   Because parasitic infections are more frequent in tropical areas of the world and in the warmer rural areas of the U.S., many physicians in this country are uninformed as to proper diagnosis and treatment.   The increase in foreign travel and the return of soldiers and refugees from Southeast Asia have provided a continuing reservoir for new infections.   This chapter will deal with those infections which are commonly encountered in this country.   Table 16-1 lists these infections, their mode of transmission and pertinent diagnostic procedures.   Table 16-2 lists the drugs commonly used for treatment of parasitic diseases.

16.1:   NEMATODES

1.   ENTEROBIUS VERMICULARIS (PINWORMS):   Pinworms are the most prevalent helminthic infection in this country and are among the top four parasitic diseases in the world (Jansen, 1974).   Children are primarily affected, particularly those who live in crowded quarters, or attend nursery schools.   It is not confined to lower socioeconomic groups or to areas of poor sanitation.   Transmission is hand to mouth, from eggs deposited on toys or other fomites.   Reinfection often occurs in the child who scratches the perianal area where eggs have been laid and then sucks the thumb or places the fingers in the mouth.   However, infection may also be transmitted by the air-borne route when eggs from infected clothing or bedding are inhaled and subsequently swallowed.   For this reason, infections are often difficult to eradicate, unless the initial treatment involves the entire family (particularly children occupying the same bed).   Clothing and linens must be laundered at the same time since eggs may live for a long period and are infective within two hours of being laid.

The female pinworm is larger than the male, being 8-13 mm in length, and is yellowish-white with a sharp point posteriorly.   It can occasionally be identified in the perianal area early in the morning following its nocturnal egg-laying missions.   Pinworms live free within the rectum and colon and can be found in the cecum and appendix.

TABLE 16-1: TRANSMISSION AND DIAGNOSIS OF PARASITIC DISEASES

PARASITE	TRANSMISSION	DIAGNOSIS
E. vermicularis (pinworm)	a) Hand to mouth after scratching perianal area b) Swallow airborne eggs	a) Identify worm during night-time migration b) Collect eggs on cellulose tape first thing in the morning
A. lumbricoides	Swallow eggs in soil contaminated with human feces	Identify worm; stool for ova
Toxocara (Visceral larva migrans)	Swallow eggs in soil contaminated with dog or cat feces	Difficult - identify larvae in biopsy specimens. Presumptive diagnosis by clinical syndrome with eosinophilia, elevated IgE, IgG, isohemagglutinins, serology
N. americanus & A. duodenale (hookworm)	Penetration of skin by larvae in soil contaminated by human feces	Identification of ova in stool
S. stercoralis	a) Penetration of skin by larvae in soil contaminated by human feces b) Hyperinfection as larvae penetrate the colonic mucosa in an immune deficient host	Stool for larvae

TABLE 16-1 (Continued)

PARASITE	TRANSMISSION	DIAGNOSIS
T. trichiura (whipworm)	Swallow eggs in soil contaminated by human feces	Stool for ova
T. spiralis	Ingestion of larvae encysted in poorly cooked pork or bear meat	Skin test, serology, muscle biopsy.
T. solium or saginata (pork and beef tapeworm)	Ingestion of scolex encysted in poorly cooked pork or beef	Stool for ova or proglottids
Diphyllobothrium (fish tapeworm)	Ingestion of scolex in insufficiently cooked fish	Stool for ova or proglottids
Hymenolepsis (dwarf tapeworm)	Swallow eggs in soil contaminated by human feces	Stool for ova or proglottids
Echinococcus granulosus (dog tapeworm)	Ingestion of eggs in soil contaminated by dog feces	Stool test, serology
S. mansoni or japonicum	Penetration of skin or oral mucosa by larvae in fresh water	Concentrated stool or rectal biopsy for ova, determine viability

S. hematobium	Same as above	Concentrated urine for ova; biopsy bladder mucosa or polyp; determine viability
E. histolytica	Ingestion of food or water contaminated with human feces	Identify trophozoites or cysts in warm fresh stool
Naegleria (primary amoebic encephalitis)	Penetration of nasal passages by larvae in infested fresh water	Identify amoeba in nasal secretions or cerebrospinal fluid
G. lamblia	Ingestion of cysts in water contaminated with human feces	Identify trophozoites or cysts in stool, duodenal aspirate or duodenal biopsy
Malaria	Transmission of infected erythrocytes through bite of female anopheles mosquito	Identify parasites in erythrocytes of blood smear

TABLE 16-2: TREATMENT OF PARASITIC DISEASES

PARASITE	DRUG	DOSE	SIDE EFFECTS
E. vermicularis (pinworm)	*Pyrantel pamoate	11 mg/kg p.o. (max. 1 gm) as single dose. Repeat in 2-3 weeks.	Nausea, vomiting, diarrhea
	Pyrvinum pamoate	5 mg/kg p.o. as single dose. Repeat in 2-3 wks.	Stains red. Nausea, vomiting.
	*Mebendazole	100 mg p.o. as single dose over 2 years of age. May repeat in 3 weeks.	Contraindicated in pregnancy
	*Piperazine citrate	50 mg/kg/d p.o. (max. 2.5 gm) for 7 days. Repeat in 3 weeks.	Urticaria, cerebellar ataxia Avoid phenothiazines
A. lumbricoides	*Pyrantel pamoate	11 mg/kg p.o. (max. 1 gm) as single dose	Nausea, vomiting, diarrhea
	*Mebendazole	100 mg p.o. daily for 3 days over 2 yrs of age	Contraindicated in pregnancy
	*Piperazine citrate	50 mg/kg/d p.o. for 7 days	Urticaria, cerebellar ataxia

Toxocara (Visceral larva migrans)	No therapy in mild cases		
	Severe-Thiabendazole	25-50 mg/kg (max. 3 gm) p.o. for 10 days	Dizziness, nausea, vomiting, fatigue, headaches, rash, abdominal cramps
	Plus Prednisone	1-2 mg/kg p.o. daily	
N. Americanus	*Mebendazole	100 mg p.o. b.i.d. for 3 days all ages over 2	Contraindicated in pregnancy
N. Americanus	Tetrachlorethylene	0.12 ml/kg/d (max. 5 ml) in fasting state as single dose	Nausea, headaches, dizziness
	Pyrantel pamoate	11 mg/kg/d p.o. for 3 days (max. 1 gm)	
A. duodenale	*Mebendazole	100 mg p.o. b.i.d. for 3 days over 2 years of age	Contraindicated in pregnancy
	Bephenium	5 gm p.o. single dose over 20 kg. 2.5 gm 20 kg	Give after overnight fast

* Drug of Choice

(Cont'd)

TABLE 16-2 (Continued)

PARASITE	DRUG	DOSE	SIDE EFFECTS
Creeping eruption	Pyrantel pamoate	11 mg/kg p.o. (max 1 gm) as single dose	
	Thiabendazole ointment	Apply locally	
	plus		
	Tablets or suspension	25 mg/kg p.o.b.i.d. for 2 days	see under Toxocara
S. stercoarlis (threadworm)	Thiabendazole	25 mg/kg p.o. b.i.d. for 2 days	see under Toxocara
T. trichiura (whipworm)	Mebendazole	100 mg p.o. b.i.d. for 3 days over 2 years of age	Contraindicated in pregnancy
T. spiralis (trichinosis)	None unless CNS or cardiac symptoms. Then Prednisone.	20-40 mg daily for 2-3 days	
T. saginata	*Niclosamide	Over 40 kg: 2 gms p.o. as single dose	Chew to paste before swallowing

T. saginata	Quinacrine	Under 40 kg: 1 gm p.o. as single dose Over 6 years: 200 mg with fruit juice every 20-30 min. times four. Under 6 years: 100 mg with fruit juice every 5-10 min. times five.	See text also. Contraindicated in emotional instability. May cause vomiting.
	Paromomycin	25 mg/kg/d p.o. for 5-7 days	Nausea, abdominal cramps
T. solium	*Quinacrine Paromomycin	See above See above	See above See above
Hymenolepsis	*Niclosamide	500 mg p.o. under 2 yrs. for 5 days 1 gm ages 2-8 daily for 5 days 2 gms ages 8-adult daily for 5 days	See text under T. saginata
	Paromomycin	See T. saginata	See T. saginata

* Drug of Choice

(Cont'd)

TABLE 16-2 (Continued)

PARASITE	DRUG	DOSE	SIDE EFFECTS
D. latum (fish tapeworm)	Niclosamide	See T. saginata	See T. saginata
E. granulosus (hydatid disease)	Surgical aspiration		See text
S. mansoni	*Stibophen	Adults: Day 1- 1.5 ml IM Day 3- 3.5 ml IM Day 5 and q.o.d. 5 ml IM (total 80 ml)	Abdominal pain, nausea, headache, fatigue, vomiting and joint pain: (reduce dose 1/3)
		Children: Day 1- 0.033 ml/kg IM Day 2- 0.066 ml/kg IM Day 3- 0.1 ml/kg IM and three times a week to a total of 2 ml/kg (max. 100 ml)	Contraindications: renal, cardiac or hepatic disease
	Niridazole	25 mg/kg p.o. daily for 7 days	Headaches, anorexia, abdominal pain

S. haemotobium	*Niridazole Stibophen	See above	See above
S. japonicum	*Antimony K tartrate	Day 1- 8 ml of 0.5% solution IV slowly. Give therapy every other day increasing dose by 4 ml each time until 28 ml. Then give 10 doses of 28 ml (max. 360 ml for adult) Children - reduce dose proportionately.	Cough, nausea, vomiting, hypotension. Contraindicated in heart, renal or hepatic disease
E. histolytica (amebiasis)	Asymptomatic: diodohydroxyquin	30 mg/kg/d p.o. in three doses for 20 days (max. 1.95 g/d)	Dermatitis. May rarely cause optic atrophy with prolonged use.
	Colitis or hepatic abscess: *Metronidazole	40 mg/kg/d in three doses for 5-10 days	Nausea, anorexia, metallic taste. Tumors have been reported in mice.
	Emetine hydrochloride	1 mg/kg/d in two doses deep SC for 4-6 days	Severe cardiac toxicity - arrhythmias, cardiac arrest may occur.

* Drug of Choice

(Cont'd)

TABLE 16-2 (Continued)

PARASITE	DRUG	DOSE	SIDE EFFECTS
Naegleria (primary amoebic encephalitis)	Chloroquine	12 mg/kg/d p.o. in two doses for two days. Then 6 mg/kg/d p.o. in single dose daily for 12 days.	
	Amphotericin B	0.25 mg/kg by slow IV infusion. May increase daily dose as tolerated up to 1 mg/kg/d	Fever, headaches, nausea, vomiting. Has renal toxicity.
Giardia lamblia	Quinacrine	8 mg/kg/d p.o. in 3 doses for 5–7 days (max. 300 mg/d)	Stains skin and sclera yellow. Nausea, vomiting, dermatitis
	Metronidazole	Adults: 250 mg p.o. t.i.d. for X–10 days Children: <2 yrs. – 125 mg p.o. daily for X–10 days 2–4 yrs. – 125 mg p.o. b.i.d. for X–10 days 4–8 yrs. 125 mg p.o. t.i.d. for X–10 days	See amoebiasis above. Side effects less common at lower doses.

Malaria	*Chloroquine	>9–250 mg p.o. b.i.d. for X-10 days. First dose: 10 mg/kg/p.o. (max. 600 mg) Second dose: 5 mg/kg p.o. in 6 hrs. Third dose: 5 mg/kg p.o. 18 hr. after second Fourth dose: 5 mg/kg p.o. 24 hrs. after third	See text also
Malaria	Primaquine	Adults: 15 mg/24 hrs. daily for 2 weeks Children: 0.25 mg/kg/d daily for 2 weeks (max. 15 mg/d)	Begin on 2nd day of chloroquine therapy. Prevents late relapse. Toxicity: Methemoglobinemia, hemolytic anemia, renal dysfunction, Hemolysis in G6PD deficiency
	Amodiaquine	First dose: 5 mg/kg p.o. Second dose: 5 mg/kg p.o. (Max. 600 mg 1st day) Third and fourth dose: 7mg/kg/d daily (max. 400 mg/d)	Doses given in same time sequence as chloroquine

* Drug of Choice

(Cont'd)

TABLE 16-2 (Continued)

PARASITE	DRUG	DOSE	SIDE EFFECTS
	Quinine	Up to 1 year: 100-200 mg p.o. daily 1-3 yr - 200-300 mg daily 4-6 yr - 300-500 mg daily 7-11 yr - 500-1000 mg daily 12-15 yr - 1000-2000 mg daily	Drug of choice for chloro-quine resistance
	Pyrimethamine	0-2 yrs.: 6.25 mg p.o. 2-6 yrs.: 12.5 mg p.o. over 6 yrs.: 25 mg p.o. (all are given as a single dose)	For chloroquine resistant strains. Many strains are also resistant to pyrimethamine

Females migrate down the bowel when gravid, producing 5-15,000 eggs which are deposited on the perianal skin and buttocks. The eggs may cause intense itching. If transmitted to the mouth, swallowed eggs will hatch in the duodenum in two to four weeks to begin the cycle again.

Many adults and children who harbor pinworms may have no symptoms at all. The list of symptoms and behavior changes caused by pinworms is extensive and for the most part undocumented. There is no documentation that pinworms cause enuresis. Pruritus ani is the most frequent finding and scratching may cause severe excoriation and secondary infection. A nonspecific vaginitis may occur if worms migrate there. During nocturnal migration sleep may be disturbed. Pinworms have been found in the appendix, but a causative role in appendicitis has not been substantiated (Most and Shookhoff, 1975). Granulomas of the perineum have also been found, but these are clinically insignificant.

Diagnosis is made by finding the adult female during migration or identifying the eggs collected on a piece of cellophane tape. Usually eggs are not found in the stool. The easiest method of collection is to wrap a piece of cellophane tape around a finger or tongue blade, sticky side out, separate the buttocks and press the tape against the perianal folds first thing in the morning before washing. The tape is then placed sticky side down on a slide and examined microscopically by allowing a drop of toluene to enter the tape. Eggs are flattened on one side and have a thick translucent shell with the coiled larvae inside. Without symptoms, routine screening for eggs by the cellophane tape method should be discouraged. Other laboratory tests are of little value in making the diagnosis. Since there is no tissue migration, there is no peripheral eosinophilia.

Treatment should first involve reassurance of the parent that the finding of pinworms is not a reflection on his or her housekeeping or parenting abilities. There are four effective drugs available for pinworms and three of the drugs use single dose therapy. Pyrvinum pamoate is a cyanine dye which will stain the stool red. It is given in a single dose (see Table 16-2). Nausea and vomiting are frequent side effects. Pyrantel pamoate generally causes nausea less frequently and is nonstaining. It is also given as a single dose. Mebendazole has recently been introduced and is reported to be virtually 100 percent effective in a single dose (Jansen, 1974). It has not been sufficiently studied in persons under two years of age and should not be given to pregnant women, as teratogenesis has been reported in rats (Shirkey, 1975). Piperazine citrate is generally given daily for a week, but good results have recently been reported with two days treatment (Most and Shokoff, 1975). Symptoms of cerebellar ataxia with piperazine, known as "worm wobble," have been reported in England (Most, 1972). It should not be used in patients receiving phenothiazines or in those with seizure disorders.

It is often recommended that all members of a family be treated simultaneously and, although this is probably the most effective method, compliance is often poor. Certainly, all children or adults sharing the same bed or toys, and any symptomatic adults, should be treated.

2. ASCARIS LUMBRICOIDES (ASCARIASIS): Ascariasis is the most common parasitic disease of man with an estimated one billion cases (Jansen, 1974), several million of which occur in the United States. The highest incidence is in the southeastern states where 10-25 percent of all children are infected (Most and Shookhoff, 1975). In areas of poor sanitation, where children can ingest eggs in soil contaminated with human feces, infection may reach nearly 100 percent. Eggs resist drying and cold and will survive for long periods in the soil.

Ascaris is a large creamy-white roundworm. The female ranges from 20 to 35 cm. in length; males are shorter, more slender and have an incurved tail. Females lay several hundred thousand eggs per day, which are passed in the stool. The eggs incubate two to three weeks in the soil before they are infective. When swallowed, they hatch in the duodenum, the larvae penetrate the intestinal wall, enter the portal circulation, cross the liver and are carried to the capillaries of the lungs. Here they rupture into the alveoli, grow and molt over approximately 10 days, migrate up the bronchi and trachea, pass over the epiglottis and are swallowed to reside in the jejunum and ileum where mating and egg-laying take place. The entire cycle takes two to three months.

Clinical symptoms are generally not present unless there are large numbers of worms. In heavy infections, fever, malaise and vague abdominal pain may be present. Occasionally, obstruction of the bile or pancreatic ducts may occur. Moderate eosinophilia generally develops and immunoglobulin E (IgE) may reach high levels. As large numbers of worms rupture into the alveoli, Loeffler's syndrome, a hypersensitivity pneumonitis, may develop (Piggott, et al., 1970). The x-ray shows patchy infiltrates with prominent hilar shadows.

Often, the apparently well patient will present at the doctor's office with a container carrying a worm passed into the stool or vomited. Ova are readily seen in the stools. Barium studies of the small intestine may reveal radiolucent areas outlining the worms, or even outline the worm's own intestinal tract. A moderate eosinophilia and elevated IgE may aid in the diagnosis.

Pyrantel pamoate in a single dose is 90 percent effective (Villarejos, et al., 1971). Mebendazole is also effective but requires three days of therapy (Jansen, 1974). Piperazine citrate requires one week of treatment. Whatever drug is used, stool concentrates should be re-examined in one to two weeks. If eggs are present, the treatment is repeated. The patient may not notice the passage of worms during treatment.

3. TOXOCARA CANIS OR CATI (TOXOCARIASIS, VISCERAL
LARVA MIGRANS): Visceral larva migrans occurs primarily in
children one to four years of age with a 2:1 male predominance. It
is generally a self-limited disease with good prognosis for recovery
in six to 12 months, if further exposure can be prevented (Huntley,
et al., 1965).

The causative agents, Toxocara canis or T. cati, are related to
Ascaris and are the corresponding roundworms of dogs or cats.
Toxacariasis occurs mainly in the U.S. and Europe. Public parks
are a common repository of dog feces, and children playing in the
dirt and then placing fingers in the mouth are readily infected.
Young puppies may be infected at birth, having acquired the larvae
prenatally by virtue of their migration from maternal tissues to the
pup in utero (Woodruff, 1970). Cats do not acquire the infection prenatally. Dogs or cats may also ingest contaminated soil or small
mammals infected with the larvae. Prevention involves periodic
deworming of dogs and cats and keeping children away from areas
heavily contaminated by dog or cat feces.

The mature worm does not develop in man. The eggs are swallowed,
larvae hatch in the intestine, penetrate the bowel wall and travel
through the portal system to the liver, lungs and other tissues. Final tissue location of the larvae depends upon their size and shape
relative to that of the blood vessel. They are generally filtered out
in the liver, lungs, retinal vessels and brain, forming granulomas.
Presenting symptoms are pica in 90 percent; chronic paroxysmal
cough, more severe at night, in 86 percent; and convulsions in 28
percent, with 1/5 of these associated with fever. Signs include
hepatomegaly in 65 percent; rales in 43 percent, malnourishment in
39 percent, and skin lesions in 22 percent. A leukocytosis of
$20,000/mm^3$ occurs in 55 percent of patients, with an eosinophilia
often greater than 50 percent (Huntley, et al., 1965). Bilateral peribronchial infiltrates characterize the hypersensitivity pneumonitis.
Retinal vessel involvement creates an endophthalmitis with occasional loss of vision.

Definitive diagnosis is made by finding larvae or granulomas in tissue biopsy. However, since involvement is patchy, a liver biopsy
may fail to demonstrate the larvae. The combination of fever, pulmonary infiltrates, hepatomegaly and an eosinophilia of greater than
30 percent aid in diagnosis. Immunoglobulin G (IgG) and IgE are
elevated, as are isohemagglutinin titers in over 50 percent. Specific
serologic tests and skin tests are unreliable.

Since the disease is self-limited, in most instances no treatment is
necessary. In severe cases with major pulmonary symptoms or
retinal or CNS involvement, thiabendazole may be of value, although
its effectiveness has not been conclusively documented (Nelson, et
al., 1966). As larvae are destroyed by the thiabendazole, pulmonary

symptoms may increase due to release of antigenic substances.
Corticosteroids should be used in conjunction with the thiabendazole
and then the dosage tapered.

4. ANCYLOSTOMA DUODENALE AND NECATOR AMERICANUS
(HOOKWORM): Ancylostoma duodenale occurs primarily in Europe
and Asia. Necator americanus is the only hookworm found extensively in the United States, although it also occurs in Asia, Africa
and South America. It is thought that N. americanus may have been
brought to this country with the slave trade. In the U.S., 10 to 20
percent of individuals under 25 years of age in the southeastern and
Gulf states are, or have been, infected (Most and Shookhoff, 1975).
Distribution is patchy, varying with sanitation, temperature, humidity and socioeconomic conditions. Human feces containing eggs used
as fertilizer or deposited indiscriminately provides a source of larvae. The larvae can penetrate any exposed area of skin. Although
wearing shoes prevents entry though the soles of the feet, it does not
avoid entry through the hands of children at play (Katz, 1975).

N. americanus is approximately 1 cm in length, with the head sharply
bent forming a definite hook anteriorly. It has a pair of cutting plates
in the buccal cavity. Eggs are passed in the feces onto moist sandy
soil and develop in 24 to 48 hours. The larvae feed on bacteria and
organic material in the soil, molt twice and become infective. These
larvae do not feed and if no host is present they will die in two weeks.
They imbed in the cool, moist soil, extending the anterior hooks into
the air and waving to and fro until a host is contacted. Once in the
host, they migrate into cutaneous venules to be carried to the lungs,
where another molt takes place. They rupture into the alveoli, migrate up the trachea to be swallowed, and reside in the duodenum and
jejunum feeding on villi. As they migrate in the small bowel, they
leave lacerations from which bleeding occurs.

Cutaneous larva migrans is caused mainly by A. braziliense, the
hookworm of dogs and cats. Larvae penetrate deep into the epidermis but do not enter the blood vessels. They migrate for days to
months through tunnels in the skin, causing severe pruritus.

Larval penetration of the skin causes an allergic reaction, with pruritus referred to as "ground itch." Occasionally, Necator may migrate through the skin and cause a transient creeping eruption. Heavy
intestinal infection may cause diarrhea, vague abdominal pain, and
nausea approximately one week before eggs are passed in the feces.
The stool contains many Charcot-Leyden crystals and a moderate
eosinophilia occurs. Bleeding from attachment sites in the intestine
may lead to an iron deficiency anemia if iron replacement is not adequate. Hypoproteinemia occasionally occurs, and generally there
are no pulmonary symptoms.

Diagnosis is made by identifying the ovoid thin-shelled eggs in the feces. The eggs of Necator and Ancylostoma are difficult to distinguish. In this country, it is probably safe to assume most are Necator.

The drug of choice for Necator and Ancylostoma is now mebendazole, which is apparently 100 percent effective for hookworm, as well as for Ascaris and Trichuris, all of which make up the worm "trinity" seen in many parts of the world (Chavarria, et al., 1973). An alternative drug for Necator is tetrachlorethylene in a single dose (Most, 1972). It is taken fasting and no purgative is necessary; however, food should not be taken for two to three hours after the dose. The patient should rest for an hour since tetrachlorethylene, which is an anesthetic, has side effects which include nausea, dizziness, and headache. Pyrantel pamoate may be used for three days with 85 percent cure rate (Botero and Castano, 1973). For Ancylostoma, bephenium hydroxynaphthoate is the alternative drug. It has a wide margin of safety and can be given to infants and pregnant women (Scheibel, 1973). It has a very bitter taste and should be mixed with fruit juice. Pyrantel pamoate may also be used as a single dose.

Creeping eruption can be treated with topically applied thiabendazole ointment, or systemically with oral tablets or suspension. The two percent thiabendazole in 90 percent dimethylsulfoxide suspension cannot be used without an investigator's permit in the U.S., but the topical suspension, which has 1 percent dexamethasone cream added, is available (Scheibel, 1973).

5. STRONGYLOIDES STERCORALIS (THREADWORM): Strongyloidiasis occurs commonly in warm, moist climates, primarily in the Gulf Coast areas of the U.S. Threadworms penetrate the skin in the same manner as hookworm, with larvae being passed in human feces to the warm moist soil. Larvae cannot withstand cold or dry soil.

The threadworm is 2 mm long and lives free in the mucosal epithelium of the duodenum and jejunum. The eggs are laid on the mucosa where they hatch and the larvae are passed in the feces. In the soil, the larvae develop to the infective stage in one to two days. They penetrate the skin of the host, migrate through the lungs, reach the intestine, mature and produce eggs parthenogenetically. Internal autoinfection may occur if the larvae penetrate the intestinal wall and are carried to the lungs. It has been suggested that this autoinfective cycle occurs more frequently in hosts with depressed cellular immunity (Katz, 1975).

A mild local reaction occurs at the site of penetration of the skin. During the intestinal stage in heavy infection diarrhea, abdominal pain and malabsorption may occur. Autoinfection can sometimes occur with invasion at the anus, producing a migrating creeping eruption with linear lesions radiating from the anus (Markell and Voge, 1971). Corticosteroids given for other reasons may cause autoinfection to occur. Light infections are generally asymptomatic.

Diagnosis is made by identifying the larvae in the feces or duodenal aspirate.

Thiabendazole is the drug of choice, effecting a cure in almost 100 percent of cases (Most, 1972; Marsden and Schultz, 1969).

6. TRICHURIS TRICHIURA (WHIPWORM): Trichuriasis is the most common nematode infection in tropical regions of the world. Eight percent of children in these areas are infected, the majority being asymptomatic (Katz, 1975). It affects children primarily over five years of age. Whipworm is not a common parasite in the U.S.

The female whipworm is approximately 5 cm long, has a long thin whiplike anterior and a club-shaped posterior. The anterior end is imbedded in the mucosa of the cecum and appendix, but is also found in the colon and rectum. Females lay several thousand barrel-shaped eggs with mucus polar plugs. The eggs are passed in the feces onto warm, moist shaded soil and require 10 to 14 days to develop into the infective stage. The eggs are swallowed in contaminated soil, hatch in the intestine, develop into mature worms in one to three months, and migrate to the cecum to begin the egg-laying phase.

Individuals infected with Trichuris are often asymptomatic unless a heavy infection is present. It may cause a bloody, mucoid diarrhea with tenesmus, weight loss, abdominal distention and rectal prolapse. Blood loss in the stools is estimated to be only 0.005 ml/worm/day (Layrisse, et al., 1967). Thus, if anemia is present, it isn't caused by the parasite alone. The rectal prolapse is due to edema of the rectum produced by worms imbedded there. A moderate eosinophila may be present in heavy infections.

Diagnosis is made by finding the characteristic egg in the feces. Sigmoidoscopy may reveal worms in the lower colon.

Mebendazole is the treatment of choice (Most and Shookhoff, 1975). Total elimination of the worms is not necessary to relieve symptoms. Enemas with hexylresorcinol were previously recommended but are unnecessary since mebendazole has become available.

7. TRICHINELLA SPIRALIS (TRICHINOSIS): T. spiralis infects any carnivorous or omnivorous animal and is found primarily in rats or pigs in the U.S. It is becoming increasingly uncommon in this country, but still exists where raw or poorly cooked pork is eaten, particularly if uncooked garbage has been fed to the hogs. Bears are also heavily infected. Meat inspection does not necessarily identify infected meat and infection is best prevented by thorough cooking. Freezing at -20ºC. for three days also kills the larvae.

Larvae encysted in the skeletal muscle of poorly cooked meat are ingested. The cysts are digested in the upper small intestine to release the larvae and the worms mature in two days and mate. The
female can produce larvae by the fifth day and continues to do so as
long as it remains in the intestine. The larvae penetrate the lymph
vessels and enter the general circulation, passing through the liver
and lungs. They leave the capillaries in striated muscle primarily
in the diaphragm, penetrating the fibers and producing degeneration
and inflammation. They coil and become surrounded by a sheath derived from muscle fiber. The larvae remain viable for years even
if the capsule calcifies.

In the intestinal phase, a gastroenteritis with nausea, vomiting, abdominal pain, and diarrhea can occur. During migration and muscle
entry, fever, periorbital edema, muscle weakness and pain may occur. Symptoms reach maximum intensity by 12-20 days. Splinter
hemorrhages due to a vasculitis may occur in the subungal regions.
More severe complications include pulmonary edema, focal or diffuse myocarditis, and meningoencephalitis.

The most reliable means of diagnosis is by muscle biopsy after the
larvae become coiled and encapsulated. The tissue should be fresh
and unstained. The Bachman skin test involves intracutaneous administration of 0.1 ml of dried, powered Trichinella larvae (trichi-
nellin). If the infection has been present for two weeks, there should
be a positive reaction indicated by a wheal (5 mm or larger) and
erythema in 15 to 30 minutes (Katz, 1975). The antigen is prepared
by the Center for Disease Control in Atlanta, Georgia. A positive
skin response lasts several years and does not necessarily indicate
an active process. Bentonite flocculation and counter current immunoelectrophoresis (CIE) tests are generally positive by the second
to fourth week and remain so for several years. The CIE test has no
false positives. However, in patients with rheumatoid arthritis, the
bentonite flocculation test may be falsely positive (Katz, 1975).

This disease is better prevented than treated. Thorough cooking of
meat and cooking garbage fed to hogs is essential. Treatment is
symptomatic. Only if there are severe life-threatening symptoms
involving the heart or central nervous system should steroids be used.
Steroids relieve symptoms, but in experimentally induced infections,
increase the number of invading larvae. There is a recent report
that mebendazole both prevents and cures the intestinal as well as the
muscular phases of trichinosis in experimental infections in rats
(Jansen, 1974).

16.2: TAPEWORMS

Tapeworms are more frequent in Asia, South America and Europe
than in the United States. Taenia saginata, the beef tapeworm, is

most common in this country, and the dwarf tapeworm, Hymenolepsis, is prevalent only in the southeastern states. Taenia solium,
the pork tapeworm, is no longer indigenous in the U.S. but is found
in Mexico, and the fish tapeworm, Diphyllobothrium latum, is found
in the northern U.S. Man, as an incidental host, may be infected by
the dog tapeworm, Echinococcus granulosus, which is also found in
the U.S. All tapeworms are hermaphrodites, have a scolex or head
with suckers, a neck or growth region, and a series of proglottids
or segments each containing a full set of male and female genitalia.

1. TAENIA SAGINATA AND TAENIA SOLIUM (Beef and Pork
Tapeworm): Man acquires beef or pork tapeworms by eating poorly
cooked beef or pork with cysticercosis of the muscle. Once ingested, the tapeworm can live for ten years in the intestine if not
treated. Storage of beef at -10° for five days inactivates the larva
as does heating to 56°C.

T. saginata has a length of 15 feet or more with up to 2,000 proglottids, four suckers, and no hooks. T. solium is smaller, only five
to eight feet, with fewer than 1,000 proglottids, four suckers and a
ring of rostellar hooks. Mature proglottids containing eggs break
off and are passed in the human stool as flat white objects which
move actively and change shape due to muscle contractions. These
eggs are ingested by cattle or hogs in which the larvae encyst in
muscle tissue. Man eats inadequately cooked meat and the larvae
are digested out in the stomach and become attached to the mucosa
of the upper small intestine, developing into mature worms in three
months. Cysticercosis may develop in man with T. solium, but not
with T. saginata. This occurs when contaminated food or water,
autoinfection, or retrograde peristalsis deposits larvae in the duodenum where they burrow into the intestinal wall, enter the blood vessels and are carried to all parts of the body. They lodge most frequently in striated muscle and develop into cysticerci or bladder
worms. These larvae are semilucent white, oval bladders filled with
fluid containing the scolex (Markel and Voge, 1971).

Most Taenia infections are asymptomatic, except for the annoying
occurrence of gravid proglottids migrating from the anus down the
leg. Loss of weight due to tapeworms is an old wives' tale. Symptoms of abdominal cramps and false hunger pains have been reported
more frequently in those who know they have the infection than in
those who don't know. Cysticercosis causes symptoms only if localized in a vital area, such as the brain or eye. Calcification of the
cysts in muscle occurs without symptoms.

Diagnosis is made by recovery of the eggs or proglottids in the stool.
The proglottids should be examined in fresh condition and free of
debris, counting the number of lateral arms in the uterus. T. saginata has 15 to 21 arms and T. solium seven to 13.

Niclosamide is generally recommended as the drug of choice but is
available only from the Parasitic Disease Branch of the Center for
Disease Control in Atlanta, Georgia. It is available in 500 mg tablets which must be chewed to a paste before swallowing. Niclosamide is odorless and the tablets are vanilla flavored. Taken in the
fasting state as a single dose, niclosamide is almost 100 percent effective. No purgative is necessary. The stool should be rechecked
in six to 12 weeks and, if proglottids are present, the treatment may
be repeated. An alternative drug is quinacrine. Treatment requires
a liquid diet for 24 hours prior to giving the drug and a saline cathartic the night before. The tablets are given in the fasting state with
30 cc of fruit juice every 20 to 30 minutes until the total dose is
consumed (four divided doses), and then another saline cathartic is
given in one to two hours. Quinacrine should not be used with patients who have psychosis or emotional instability, and it may induce
severe vomiting (Most, 1972). Theoretically, niclosamide could
cause release of eggs and the development of cysticercosis if used
with T. solium, though this has not been reported. Therefore,
niclosamide is available for treatment of T. solium, only if quinacrine has failed to effect a cure. Paromomycin, an antibiotic, has
also been found effective in tapeworm infections (Shirkey, 1975).

2. HYMENOLEPSIS NANA (Dwarf Tapeworm): The dwarf tapeworm
is prevalent in children age four to nine in the southeastern states.
Between 0.2 percent and 3.0 percent of children in certain areas may
be infected (Most and Shookhoff, 1975). Man is the principal host.
Human infection occurs directly by hand to mouth via contaminated
soil, food, or water.

H. nana is one to two cm long with 200 proglottids, four suckers and
rostellar hooks. The gravid proglottids disintegrate as they ripen,
the eggs are released and passed in the feces. Man becomes directly
infected when the eggs are swallowed and hatch in the small intestine. Here they bore into the villi of the mucosa and transform into
larvae. When fully grown, the larvae break into the lumen again,
become attached and mature in a few weeks.

Light infections are usually asymptomatic, but in heavy infections
autoinfection occurs, causing mucosal damage with symptoms of
gastroenteritis and allergy. Diagnosis is made by identifying eggs
in the stool.

Niclosamide repeated daily for five days is effective in clearing both
adults in the lumen and larvae in the villi. It may be repeated in two
weeks.

3. DIPHYLLOBOTHRIUM LATUM (Fish Tapeworm): The fish tape-
worm is prevalent in the lake districts of the northern U.S. and
Canada, as well as in other areas of Europe, South America and the
Middle East. Infection occurs by ingesting insufficiently cooked

fresh-water fish. In the northern U.S., 20 percent of the freshwater fish, particularly pike and pickerel, are infected (Most and Shookhoff, 1975). Man is the principal host, contaminating lakes with feces or raw sewage. Other fish-eating mammals play only minor roles in the spread of the tapeworm. Freezing the fish at -10°C or cooking 15 minutes at 60 to 65°C. inactivates the larvae.

D. latum grows up to 30 feet long with 3,000 to 5,000 proglottids. It has a pair of longitudinal sucking grooves. Eggs are discharged into cold, fresh water where they hatch into ciliated embryos which are consumed by the "water fleas" (cyclops).

Within the cyclops they transform into first stage larvae. The water fleas are eaten by small fish in whom the second stage develops. Finally, larger fish consume the smaller, and the larvae enter the muscle tissue. Man eats the raw fish and the larvae mature in the ileum and jejunum. In six to 12 weeks, eggs are passed in the stool.

The tapeworms may absorb unsaturated fatty acids, particularly if the worms are attached to the duodenal mucosa. Vitamin B_{12} is selectively absorbed by the tapeworm from the host's intestinal tract and a macrocytic anemia may develop. This is most often seen in Finland, where there is also a genetic tendency to pernicious anemia, and rarely occurs in the U.S. Usually, the tapeworm causes no symptoms and it is the passing of a length of the worm which brings the patient to the doctor.

The eggs are present in the stool in large numbers, making diagnosis relatively easy.

Therapy is with Niclosamide in the same dosage as for T. saginata.

4. ECHINOCOCCUS GRANULOSUS (Dog Tapeworm: Hydatid Disease): The dog tapeworm is widely distributed in areas where there are sheep, cattle, or hogs associated with dogs. The most important host is the sheep. Dogs become infected by eating the carcasses of animals who have died from the disease. Man acquires the infection accidentally by ingesting water or food contaminated with dog feces.

The adult worm does not develop in man. The eggs are ingested in contaminated food or water, and are digested in the intestine. The larvae burrow into the mucosa, enter the mesenteric circulation and are carried throughout the body. They are filtered out in liver, lungs, brain, peritoneal cavity and bone, in order of frequency. They form cysts and continue to grow for many years undetected if not in a vital organ. A germinative layer buds into the cyst and scolices develop. Cysts may rupture, releasing toxic fluid, causing anaphylaxis or releasing scolices to imbed elsewhere.

Clinical symptoms, which vary with the location of the cysts, are generally those related to a growing mass. Rupture of the cyst may cause anaphylaxis or an acute abdomen; if in the bile passages, obstructive jaundice may develop. Chemical pneumonitis may develop if rupture occurs in the lungs. Eosinophilia is present if cysts rupture or leak.

Serology is the most reliable method of diagnosis. The Casoni skin test uses an intracutaneous injection of 0.1 ml of antigen from sterile hydatid fluid (Katz, 1975). A positive reaction occurs in 15 minutes. Cross reactions occur in cysticercosis from T. solium. Cysts may calcify and be visible on x-ray or be detected by liver scan or sonography if large.

The only available treatment is surgical aspiration of the cysts. Since showers of scolices may be released, the cyst is carefully aspirated, and formalin is injected to sterilize the germinal layer and the contents. Then, after 15 minutes, it is aspirated again (Markel and Voge, 1971).

:::

16.3: SCHISTOSOMES (BLOOD FLUKES)

Only Schistosoma mansoni is important in the U.S., and infections occur mainly in immigrants from Puerto Rico and the Caribbean. S. haemotobium and S. japonicum are rarely seen. Snails are obligatory vectors, and there are several mammalian reservoir hosts, such as the monkey, which aid spread. Use of human excreta as fertilizer contributes to the prevalence of these infections.

Life cycles of all the blood flukes are similar. S. mansoni inhabit veins which drain the small intestine, and S. haemotobium inhabit those of the urinary bladder. The eggs are deposited in the submucosal vessels and develop into ciliated larvae, gradually moving through the tissues to the mucosal surface and into the lumen. The eggs are deposited in fresh water contaminated with feces or urine, hatch and enter the appropriate snail for two generations of asexual development forming free swimming larvae (cercariae). These penetrate the skin or oral mucosa of man during bathing, washing clothes, or drinking. They are carried via blood and lymph to the right heart and lungs, where they develop further and move to the liver sinusoids, finally reaching maturity. As mature flukes, they migrate against the portal blood flow and move to the vesical or intestinal veins to repeat the cycle.

When the cercariae penetrate the skin, there may be a transient sharp pain. With migration, hypereosinophilia and urticaria may develop. Late afternoon fever and night sweats often occur at the end of the incubation period. Generally, however, there are few symptoms until eggs accumulate in the tissues. The wall of the intestine or bladder becomes inflamed and thickened. Granulomas form and cirrhosis, hepatosplenomegaly, and ascites can develop. In the intestine or bladder, normal passage of stool and urine may be inhibited. As eggs are discharged, diarrhea or hematuria often occurs. A pronounced eosinophilia occurs in the acute stage, followed later by neutropenia with moderate eosinophilia and monocytosis.

Eggs can be identified in the stool or urine if concentrated or multiple specimens are examined, since only a few eggs reach the lumen. Viability of eggs should be determined by examining the activity of the excretory system or allowing eggs to hatch. Treatment should be used only if viable eggs are present.

Niridazole is the treatment of choice for S. haemotobium and perhaps also S. mansoni. It is available through the Parasitic Diseases Service at the Center for Disease Control in Atlanta with proof of viable eggs. Niridazole is contraindicated in the presence of hepatic disease. Adverse effects are headaches, anorexia, and abdominal pain. Spermatogenesis is decreased in 50 percent of those receiving the drug (Scheibel, 1973).

For S. mansoni, and as an alternative for S. haemotobium and S. japonicum, stibophen is given intramuscularly. It has numerous adverse effects. Dosage should be reduced by one-third if vomiting or joint pains occur. When rashes, purpura, or hemolysis occur, the drug should be discontinued. Treatment may be continued, however, when abdominal pain, nausea, headache, or fatigue occur (Shirkey, 1975).

Antimony potassium tartrate (tartar emetic) is the best drug for S. japonicum, which is the most difficult to cure. It is given intravenously every other day in increasing doses, and has cardiac, renal and hepatic toxicity.

16.4: PROTOZOA

1. ENTAMOEBA HISTOLYTICA (Amoebiasis): E. histolytica is found all over the world, but prevalence is directly related to poor sanitary conditions. In the U.S., prevalence varies from one to five percent, occurring most frequently in the south central states (Juniper, 1971). Amoebiasis is more difficult to diagnose in children and, perhaps for this reason, the incidence is reportedly higher in adults. Acute amoebic dysentery does not transmit the disease since the trophozoites which are passed in the stools do not survive outside the body. The cyst is the infective form which is passed in the stools of the chronic carrier. Cysts can be killed by drying, temperatures greater than 55°, and strong disinfectants, but not by ordinary chlorination of water. They can survive for months in water at temperatures greater than 20°C. Cysts are transmitted to man in contaminated water and in food by food handlers, houseflies and cockroaches. Fortunately, only 20 percent of ingested cysts develop into mature protozoa.

Ingested cysts are digested in the stomach and duodenum, liberating
the trophozoites which reach the colon and penetrate the bowel wall
primarily at the cecal and sigmoidorectal levels. Here they live
symbiotically with the anaerobic bacterial flora, which may supply
a factor necessary for virulence. Amoebae often live in the intestinal lumen without invasion or producing symptoms, and subsequently,
under some unidentified stimulus, change to an invasive form (Neal,
1971). Invasive amoebae penetrate into the intestinal capillaries
and may be transported to the liver, resulting in an hepatic abscess,
but these are rare in children.

Eighty-five to 95 percent of those harboring the protozoa are asymptomatic carriers, but these may later develop into frank dysentery
and, therefore, should be treated. Invasive amoebiasis has an insidious onset of cramping abdominal pain and bloody mucoid diarrhea. These symptoms mimic ulcerative colitis and can vary from
mild local irritation to severe involvement of the entire colon. Severe disease may cause loss of weight, low grade fever, anemia,
and leukocytosis. Dehydration or electrolyte imbalance are uncommon unless bacterial dysentery is secondarily present. Amebomas
may be produced by smoldering subclinical infection in the cecum
and can cause symptoms of intestinal obstruction. Hepatic abscesses
cause chills and fever each afternoon to 102°, followed by profuse
night sweats. Leukocytosis and right upper quadrant pain are frequent. However, liver function tests are normal (Markel and Voge,
1971).

Diagnosis is made by identifying cysts or trophozoites in the fresh
stool. Trophozoite motility may be observed if the slide is warmed
slightly. If the stool cannot be examined immediately, it should be
refrigerated. When no convenient lab is available, the stool may be
preserved for transport in both formalin (for cysts) and polyvinyl
alcohol (for trophozoites) (Katz, 1975). Other substances in the stool
may decrease chances of identification. If no amoebae are found, a
non-oily saline cathartic can be used to attempt to get material from
the cecum. Sigmoidoscopy may permit direct aspiration from involved areas of the colon. Swabs should not be used since cotton
strands obscure the organisms. Serologic tests may be helpful but
remain positive for years and often reflect past disease. Hepatic abscesses are identified on technetium scan.

Asymptomatic carriers should be treated with the luminal amebicide,
diiodohydroxyquin, except in highly endemic areas where reinfection
readily occurs. Recently, this drug has been shown to be rarely associated with optic atrophy when high doses have been given for several months. This has not been reported with the doses used for amoebiasis (Katz, 1975). A seven-day course of tetracycline is often given
in conjunction with droxyquin (Most, 1972).

If colitis is present, metronidazole appears to be the best drug (Powell, 1971). It effectively controls the colitis, but does not eradicate

the infection. Supplementation with diiodohydroxyquin may be helpful. Metronidazole is probably the drug of choice for liver abscess.
Anorexia and a metallic taste in the mouth frequently occur with
metronidazole. Recent reports have shown that metronidazole can
induce pulmonary tumors and lymphomas in mice. Another study
reported mutagenic properties of this drug on bacteria (Katz, 1975).

An older drug, emetine hydrochloride, is effective in all forms of
Amebiasis and should probably be used in severe infections. It had
been the drug of choice for hepatic abscess before metronidazole became available. It does have cardiotoxicity, can cause arrhythmias
and even cardiac arrest. These effects can develop up to two weeks
following cessation of therapy. Emetine is given by deep subcutaneous injection and is very painful. Emetine may be supplemented
with chloroquine.

A liver abscess should not be aspirated unless clinically significant
and there is no receding of the mass with drug therapy. This may
be done percutaneously unless the abscess is in the left lobe which
may necessitate open drainage.

2. NAEGLERIA (Primary Amoebic Encephalitis): The first cases of
primary amoebic encephalitis were reported in 1961 but the disease
was present at least as early as 1909 (Carter, 1972). The disease
is caused by the limax amoeba Naebleria. Infection is apparently
acquired by swimming in fresh water. There are also some cases
reported from Australia in persons who swam only in salt water
where the amoebae can't live. Airborne infection seems unlikely as
cysts are not isolated from the nasopharynx. It is possible that septic tanks or waste water may be involved in spread.

The sexes are equally affected and it is primarily a disease of the
young, ages 7 through 20. Incubation period may be three to seven
days.

The free living larvae of the limax amoebae live in fresh water,
moist soil, sewage, or decaying organic matter and feed on fecal
bacteria. They apparently enter man through the nose and cribriform
plate and directly invade the brain causing a purulent meningitis and
an encephalitis. The olfactory mucosa may be ulcerated and inflamed
and often contains amoebae.

Symptoms appear abruptly with the onset of fever, headaches and
occasionally, sore throat and rhinitis. The symptoms are rapidly
progressive over the next three days to vomiting, neck rigidity, disorientation and coma. The majority of cases have died from cerebral
edema and herniation.

The cerebrospinal fluid shows a pleocytosis generally greater than
1,000 cells with 90-100 percent polys, protein is greater than 100

and sugar is normal or slightly decreased (Carter, 1972). However, the bacterial culture is negative and these findings should suggest amoebae may be present. They should be looked for in the cerebrospinal fluid and in nasal secretions.

The only treatment which has been effective is amphotericin B. Two cases have survived with treatment. It is given intravenously and there is no evidence that intrathecal or intraventricular therapy is of any more value than intravenous therapy alone. Other antiprotozoan drugs have no effect.

3. GIARDIA LAMBLIA (Giardiasis): Giardia is an intestinal flagellate of major importance throughout the world. It is a probable cause of many cases of traveler's diarrhea, and is both endemic and epidemic in the United States. The prevalence of Giardia infections in the U.S. is 7.4 percent, and infections occur more commonly in children than adults (Burke, 1975). The mountainous areas of Colorado have a high incidence of giardiasis. The parasite is spread through cysts passed in human feces which contaminate drinking water and possibly also food. The cysts can survive for several months in cold water, but temperatures greater than 50°C. kill the organism. Tap water in endemic areas should be treated with iodine compounds (Wolfe, 1975).

Man ingests the cysts in contaminated water which make their way to the duodenum, are digested and liberate a trophozoite which divides into two organisms. These are pear-shaped with four flagella and two prominent nuclei. On the ventral surface is a large sucking disk by which it attaches to the intestinal mucosa and absorbs food. Few trophozoites are passed in stools and they do not survive outside the host. Cysts are formed as the stool moves through the colon and these are passed in the feces.

Host susceptibility to infection is variable, some remaining asymptomatic and others becoming acutely ill. Ingestion of 100 or more cysts invariably produces infection but often only mild symptoms such as loose stools. It is known that achlorhydria and immunoglobulin deficiencies, particularly decreased IgA and IgM, are associated with symptomatic giardiasis (Burke, 1975).

Most individuals with Giardia are asymptomatic. The clinical spectrum varies from an acute self-limited diarrhea to a chronic intermittent one. The acute episodes are abrupt in onset with a watery, explosive, foul-smelling, mucoid but not bloody, diarrhea. This may be accompanied by epigastric cramps, flatulence and abdominal distention. More frequently, children have a chronic intermittent diarrhea with anorexia, malaise, abdominal cramps and frequently mushy, foul-smelling stools. Occasionally, growth retardation can occur secondary to malabsorption.

Diagnosis is made by finding the cysts or trophozoites in stool, duodenal aspirate or duodenal biopsy. Stool examinations are least reliable because of the intermittent shedding of cysts. Duodenal aspirates are approximately 85 percent reliable and small bowel biopsy 100 percent (Burke, 1975).

There are two effective drugs available. Quinacrine can cause dermatitis, psychotic symptoms, vomiting, and headache, and stains urine, and occasionally skin and sclera, yellow. Metronidazole is used in smaller doses than for amoebiasis but is given over a period of ten days. Side effects are not as frequent. Both drugs are about 80 percent effective following a single course of treatment. Since stool exam may not be indicative of treatment success, subsidence of clinical symptoms is the major criterion used. Relapses are common and the treatment can be repeated.

4. PLASMODIUM (Malaria): Malaria is no longer indigenous to the United States. However, travelers, servicemen, and refugees from Southeast Asia have caused occasional localized outbreaks. Malaria is still a major health problem in warm climates despite extensive efforts to eradicate it.

Four species infect man: P. malariae, P. vivax, and P. ovale all produce milder disease. P. falciparum (malignant tertian malaria) causes severe disease and often death. The life cycles are similar. The parasite is injected into man by the bite of the infected female anopheles mosquito. The pre-erythrocytic development takes place in the hepatic cells and these merozoites then invade red blood cells. Certain of the parasites develop into gametocytes which can infect mosquitoes biting the host.

Infection of erythrocytes leads to destruction of the cell as well as hemolysis of other red cells. The red cells become sticky and adhere to the endothelium of blood vessels causing occlusion and even rupture. Certain hemoglobinopathies may be protective. P. falciparum does not mature in those with sickle cell trait and seems unable to develop high densities of red cell invasion in G6PD deficiency. P. vivax does not mature in thalassemia (Markel and Voge, 1971).

Clinical symptoms generally appear in eight to 15 days after the mosquito bite in the child who has had no previous immunity to malaria. There may be prodromal emotional and behavioral changes such as sleep disturbances, drowsiness, and crying. The hallmark of malaria is fever, which accompanies the erythrocytic phase of the disease. The onset may be gradual or abrupt, with or without prodromal chills, and may reach 104° to 105°. Fever duration varies from 2 to 12 hours. The younger the child the less likely the fever course will be classical. Intermittent fevers every 48 hours are characteristic of P. vivax and every 72 hours in P. malariae infections. The fever of P. falciparum is less characteristic and sometimes continuous. Headaches, generalized myalgia, and abdominal pain often accompany the fever (Vaughn and McKay, 1975).

The spleen becomes large and tender, particularly in P. vivax, and infarction, perisplenitis and even rupture may occur. The liver may be tender and jaundice progressive. Nausea and vomiting may accompany this process, and occasionally severe diarrhea. Convulsions occur occasionally with no focal neurological signs and a normal cerebrospinal fluid.

Generally, P. falciparum has the most severe clinical course. P. vivax generally presents with a milder course of fever every 48 hours, splenic enlargement and some anemia without severe complications. P. malariae has a longer incubation period, up to 30 days or more, has a course similar to P. vivax with fevers every 72 hours, but is more frequently associated with nephrotic syndrome. P. ovale is similar to P. vivax (Gilles, 1966).

Anemia accompanies malaria attacks and is normocytic. The hemoglobin levels may decrease rapidly with hemolysis. Monocytosis is common and leukopenia may occur.

Relapses are uncommon with quartan malaria, due to P. malaria, but do occur with P. falciparum, P. vivax, and P. ovale infections.

Diagnosis depends on identifying the parasite in the peripheral blood. In P. falciparum, the ring form is seen initially, but after ten days crescents (gametocytes) appear in up to 20 percent of erythrocytes. In infections due to the other species of Plasmodia, all forms are present in the erythrocyte but only two percent of red cells are affected (Markel and Voge, 1971).

Management includes treatment of the acute attack, treatment of complications, therapy for late relapses, and destruction of gametocytes. The drug of choice for the acute episode is chloroquine, which can be given orally unless severe vomiting or cerebral malaria occur. If given parenterally, preferably intramuscularly, only 5 mg/kg doses should be used. Response is usually seen in 24 to 36 hours and the patient will become afebrile in 48 hours. Supportive treatment is given for complications: sponging for hyperpyrexia, attention to nutrition since glucose and vitamins are depleted by the parasite, iron therapy, fluids for dehydration and shock, attention to renal function, and treatment of cerebral edema and seizures. Late relapses of P. vivax and P. ovale can be prevented by the addition of primaquine beginning on the second day of chloroquine therapy. Patients should be observed closely for methemoglobinemia, hemolysis (particularly in the presence of G6PD deficiency), neutropenia, and renal dysfunction. Patients should be tested for G6PD deficiency prior to use. Primaquine is not necessary for P. falciparum or P. malariae infections. Destruction of gametocytes occurs following a single dose of primaquine, and asexual precursors are killed by chloroquine. Chloroquine given once a week is used prophylactically to prevent malaria.

Drug resistance to chloroquine is becoming a problem, particularly with strains from Southeast Asia or the West Coast of South America. Patients from these areas with severe infections should probably be treated with an alternative drug regimen. Resistant strains are treated with quinine or a combination of pyrimethamine and a sulfonamide. Unfortunately, many strains are also becoming resistant to pyrimethamine, making quinine the drug of choice for chloroquine-resistant strains.

REFERENCES

Botero, D. and Castano, A.: Comparative study of pyrantel pamoate bephenium hydroxymaphthoate and tetrachlorethylene in the treatment of Necator americanus infections. Am. J. Trop. Med. Hyg. 22:45-52, 1973.

Burke, J.A.: Giardiasis in childhood. Am. J. Dis. Child. 129: 1304-1310, 1975.

Carter, R.F.: Primary amoebic meningo-encephalitis. Roy. Soc. Trop. Med. Hyg. 66 (1):193-208, 1972.

Chavarria, A.P. et al.: Mebendazole: An effective broad spectrum antihelmintic. Am. J. Trop. Med. Hyg. 22:592-595, 1973.

Gilles, H.M.: Malaria in children. Brit. Med. J. 2:1375-1377, 1966.

Huntley, C.C., Costas, M.C., and Lyerly, A.: Visceral larva migrans syndrome. Pediatrics 36 (4) 523-536, 1965.

Jansen, P.A.J.: Recent advances in the treatment of parasitic infections in man. Prog. Drug Res. 18:191-203, 1974.

Juniper, K.: Amebiasis in the United States. Bull. N.Y. Acad. Med. 47:448-459, 1971.

Katz, M.: Parasitic infections. J. Pediatr. 87 (2):165-178, 1975.

Layrisse, M., Aparcedo, L., Martinez-Torres, C., and Roche, M.: Blood loss due to infection with Trichuris trichiura. Am. J. Trop. Med. Hyg. 16:613-619, 1967.

Markell, E.K. and Voge, M.: Medical Parasitology. 3rd Ed. W.B. Saunders Co., Philadelphia, 1971.

Marsden, P.D. and Schultz, M.G.: Intestinal parasites. Gastroenterology 57(6):724-750, 1969.

Most, H. and Shookhoff, H.B.: Helminthic infections. Forum on Infection 2: (1), June 1975.

Most, H.: Treatment of common parasitic infections of man encountered in the United States. NEJM 287 (10:495-498, 698-702, 1972.

Neal, R.A.: Pathogenesis of amebiasis. Bull. N.Y. Acad. Med. 47:469-477, 1971.

Nelson, J.D., McConnel, T.H. and Moore, D.V.: Thiabendazole therapy of visceral larva migrans: A case report. Am. J. Trop. Med. Hyg. 15:930, 1966.

Piggott, J., Hansbarger, E.A., and Heafie, R.C.: Human ascariasis. Am. J. Clin. Path. 53:223-234, 1970.

Powell, S.J.: Therapy of amebiasis. Bull. N.Y. Acad. Med. 47: 469-477, 1971.

Scheibel, L.W.: Chemotherapy of parasitic diseases commonly seen in the United States. J. Flor. Med. Assn. 60 (10):17-24, 1973.

Shirkey, H.C., ed.: Parasitic Diseases. Pediatric Therapy. 5th ed. C.V. Mosby Co., St. Louis, 1975.

Vaughn, V.C. and McKay, R.J., eds.: Parasitic Infections. Nelson Textbook of Pediatrics. 10th Ed. W.B. Saunders Co., Philadelphia, 1975.

Villarejas, V.M. et al.: Experiences with the antihelminthic pyrantel pamoate. Am. J. Trop. Med. Hyg. 20:842-845, 1971.

Wolfe, M.S.: Giardiasis. JAMA 233 (13):1362-1365, 1975.

Woodruff, A.W.: Toxocariasis. Brit. Med. J. 3:663-669, 1970.

CHAPTER 17.   MISCELLANEOUS INFECTIONS

17.1: TUBERCULOSIS

INTRODUCTION: Tuberculosis, once known as "the white plague"
and "the captain of the men of death," has been a leading cause of
death in man for centuries. The disease is caused primarily by
Mycobacterium tuberculosis and M. bovis, and it has served as a
prototype of human infections for epidemiologists, immunologists
and clinicians. Recently, new significance has been attached to
other mycobacteria (atypical mycobacteria) capable of producing
disease indistinguishable from that caused by M. tuberculosis.

The incidence of tuberculosis in the United States has declined stead-
ily, but the disease continues to be a cause of significant morbidity
and mortality. In recent years, approximately 30,000 to 40,000 new
cases and 4,000 deaths have been reported to the Center for Disease
Control. This represents a rate of about 15 new cases and 2 deaths
per 100,000 population per year. Most cases of tuberculosis occur
in adults; less than 10% of cases are seen in the pediatric age group
(Table 17-1).

TABLE 17-1: REPORTED NEW ACTIVE CASES OF TUBERCULOSIS, U.S.A., 1973		
AGE (Years)	CASES PER 100,000 POPULATION	NO. OF CASES (%)
0-4	7.4	1,242 (4)
5-14	2.8	1,081 (4)
15-24	6.4	2,482 (8)
25-44	15.9	8,153 (26)
45-64	25.3	10,916 (35)
65 +	33.4	7,124 (23)
All ages	14.8	30,998 (100)

Modified from MMWR, July 5, 1975, Center for Disease Control,
Atlanta, Georgia.

The incidence of and mortality from tuberculosis are higher in geographic areas where crowding and poor living conditions exist. In
western nations, the pathogenicity of M. tuberculosis has been altered remarkably. The decline in incidence and fatality rates has
been attributed to the improved socioeconomic conditions, case finding and reporting, and chemotherapy.

1. ETIOLOGY AND PATHOGENESIS

<u>1.1: Agent</u>: The mycobacteria are considered transition forms between eubacteria and actinomycetes. They are difficult to stain with usual stains for bacteria (acid-fastness), and some may exhibit branching. The principal pathogenic species include <u>M. tuberculosis</u> (man), <u>M. bovis</u> (cattle and man), <u>M. avium</u> (birds and swine), <u>M. microti</u> (field mouse), unclassified (atypical) mycobacteria, <u>M. leprae</u> (man), <u>M. leprae murium</u> (rat), and <u>M. paratuberculosis</u> (cattle, sheep: Johne's disease).

<u>M. tuberculosis</u> is a strict aerobic, intracellular, and facultative bacterium. It has a thick cell wall containing a high content (20 to 40%) of lipid which facilitates lumping (hydrophobic character) and resistance to acids and many antibiotics. Although <u>M. tuberculosis</u> can survive in a dried state for a prolonged period of time, it is inactivated rapidly by direct sunlight or UV-light.

<u>1.2: Transmission</u>: Tuberculosis is transmitted to susceptible children primarily from infected, untreated adults and adolescents with whom they are in close contact. Dissemination is mainly by means of airborne droplets produced by coughing or sneezing, less frequently by unpasteurized milk, and rarely by direct inoculation of the skin and conjunctiva. In airborne infection, adults and adolescents with large cavitary lesions and chronic coughs are highly contagious. The infectivity is directly proportional to the degree and extent of exposure, as well as to the size of inoculum contained within the droplets. The upper respiratory tract is relatively resistant to airborne infection, but the lower respiratory tract serves as a good portal of entry leading to a primary infection in the lung parenchyma.

Generally, children with pulmonary tuberculosis are not considered contagious because of minimal parenchymal lesions which contain relatively small numbers of bacilli. Furthermore, children usually swallow their secretions, thus preventing airborne dissemination.

Before the institution of strict codes for the pasteurization of milk and milk products, tuberculosis due to <u>M. bovis</u> was common. Although the gastrointestinal tract is the usual portal of entry, the tonsils and adenoids often serve as the primary site of infection.

<u>1.3: Predisposing Factors</u>: Adverse environmental factors (e.g. poor living conditions, poor ventilation, crowding, etc.) increase the susceptibility to infection. Host factors (e.g. age and sex) also affect host suceptibility. Children less than 3 years of age appear to be more susceptible to infection than older children. If untreated, younger children with tuberculosis also have a higher mortality, despite the fact that they respond equally as well to chemotherapy as do older children. Females are more susceptible to infection during the adolescent years prior to the onset of menarche.

The majority of infected individuals are asymptomatic. Factors predisposing to clinical disease include malnutrition, immunosuppressive therapy, diseases affecting the cell-mediated immunity, uncontrolled diabetes and alcoholism.

1.4: Pathogenesis: The respiratory tract is the major portal of entry and the lung is the most common site of infection. The primary focus in adults frequently involves the superior and posterior portions of the lungs, but it may occur anywhere in the lung parenchyma in infants and young children.

Before cell-mediated immunity can effectively contain the infection, the mycobacteria are phagocytized by the alveolar macrophages where they may successfully multiply, and spread into the lung parenchyma creating a nonspecific and nonlocalized inflammatory reaction. Macrophages and lymphocytes infiltrate the area, leading to the formation of microscopic granulomas which consist of an outer zone of epithelioid histiocytes and an inner zone of Langhans' giant cells. Mycobacteria may spill into the lymphatics and channel into the hilar and mediastinal lymph nodes. If excessive numbers of bacilli are not contained in these lymph nodes, some bacilli may reach the venous system via the thoracic duct leading to hematogenous spread. The latter mode of spread may also occur directly from lung parenchymal spilling into the pulmonary venous system. This early lympho-hematogenous dissemination, occurring prior to the appearance of cell-mediated immunity, characteristically occurs in infants and children. At approximately 6 weeks after the onset of infection, the delayed hypersensitivity reaction to tuberculoproteins occurs and the skin test becomes positive.

2. CLINICAL MANIFESTATIONS

The clinical spectrum of tuberculosis ranges from subclinical infection to acute or chronic disease capable of causing death. The majority of infected individuals are asymptomatic; only about 5% of all infected cases develop clinical disease. Of all the clinically recognized tuberculosis in children, over 90% of cases involve intrathoracic (especially pulmonary) sites, and only a small number involve extrathoracic sites. The clinical patterns of intrathoracic or extrathoracic tuberculosis are shown in Table 17-2.

Most patients (except some infants and adolescents) do not develop symptoms immediately after the primary infection; a latency period of varying duration elapses before clinical findings and/or roentgenographic changes are manifest. Tuberculosis may involve any organ or tissue and the clinical patterns are variable, largely depending upon the extent of tissue involvement. In some cases, such as in infants and adolescents, the disease may develop soon after primary infection, occurring as an acute disease. In some adolescent patients, particularly with poorly controlled diabetes, there may be a chronic or adult-type pulmonary tuberculosis with cavitary lesions.

TABLE 17-2: CLINICAL SPECTRUM OF TUBERCULOSIS

A. INTRATHORACIC TUBERCULOSIS:

1. Positive TB skin test only
2. Pulmonary lesions
    2.1. Inactive (calcified or fibrotic)
    2.2. Focal (noncalcified)
    2.3. Extensive infiltration
    2.4. Caseous bronchopneumonia (bronchogenic or hematogenic)
    2.5. Miliary tuberculosis (hematogenic)
3. Lesions of tracheobronchial lymph nodes
    3.1. Inactive (calcified or fibrotic)
    3.2. Hilar lesions
    3.3. Bronchial lesions
        - intraluminal (ulcerative or granulomatous)
        - extraluminal (atelectasis, emphysema, and/or pneumonitis)
4. Combination of pulmonary and tracheobronchial lesions (active or inactive)
5. Pleurisy

B. EXTRATHORACIC TUBERCULOSIS:

1. Cervical lymph nodes and tonsils
2. Middle ear
3. Eye (phlyctenular keratitis, chorioretinitis)
4. Skin
5. Bones and joints
6. Central nervous system (meningitis, tuberculoma)
7. Intra-abdominal (lymphadenopathy, peritonitis, liver, enteritis, fistula ani)
8. Genito-urinary (bladder, kidney, genital organs)
9. Heart (pericarditis)

2.1: Primary Pulmonary Tuberculosis: The incubation period (from infection to development of demonstrable primary lesion with positive skin test) is 2 to 10 weeks. Pulmonary tuberculosis in children is usually asymptomatic; some children may have insidious onset of fever, mild anorexia, or symptoms of upper respiratory infection. The pulmonary lesion is usually confined to a small localized area (2 or 3 cm) and the hilar nodes are often involved. The two lesions (parenchymal and regional lymph node) have been termed as the "primary complex." In the majority of cases, healing occurs with formation of calcified lesions (Ghon complex) within 1 to 2 years. These lesions are considered inactive, but exacerbation may occur. On occasion, the primary lung lesion does not resolve spontaneously, and infection spreads to the surrounding lung tissues resulting in progressive primary tuberculosis. Then the roentgenographic findings resemble bronchopneumonia and lobar pneumonia, but clinically the child may or may not be symptomatic.

In chronic pulmonary tuberculosis with cavitary lesions, particularly in adolescents and adults, patients may have a chronic cough with production of large amounts of purulent sputum. Hemoptysis is associated with bronchial erosions, and pleuritic pain and effusions may occur when the pleura is involved. Chronic expectoration and swallowing of sputum may result in laryngeal involvement, which is manifested by pain and hoarseness.

Tuberculous involvement of tracheobronchial lymph nodes is relatively common. Occasionally, the nodes enlarge and erode or obstruct a bronchus, and the patient will show signs of chronic bronchitis and respiratory distress. The cough may be persistent and may even resemble pertussis. When lymph-hematogenous spread occurs, they may show signs of systemic disease, such as anorexia, weight loss, pallor, and fatigue.

Signs and symptoms due to metastatic spread are referable to the organ system involved. Tuberculous meningitis manifests with fever, signs of meningeal irritation and increased intracranial pressure. Lesions of the bones and joints are highlighted by swelling, limitation of range of motion and pain. The involved peripheral lymph nodes are usually fixed, tender, and may suppurate and cause draining cutaneous tracts. Skin manifestations may include erythema nodosum, varicella-like lesions, chronic ulcers, etc. Tuberculous enteritis may manifest with ulcers, anemia, diarrhea and/or constipation, and involvement of abdominal nodes may result in ascites and peritonitis.

3. DIAGNOSIS

The general approach to diagnosis and management of tuberculosis is outlined in Fig. 17.1.

Tuberculosis should be suspected in patients with history of unexplained fever of extended duration, persistent cough and/or unresolving pneumonia. In such patients, history of contact should be sought. If there is a strong history of intimate contact or exposure, then the presence of infection should be proven. The presence of infection and the activity of the disease can be established by: 1) tuberculin skin test, 2) roentgenographic studies, 3) identification of the tubercle bacilli by smear and culture, and 4) erythrocyte sedimentation rate (a nonspecific test).

3.1: Tuberculin Skin Test: The presence of infection can be established by means of a tuberculin skin test. The most appropriate method of skin testing utilizes the Mantoux test, in which 5 tuberculin units (0.1 ml) of purified protein derivatives (PPD) are inoculated.

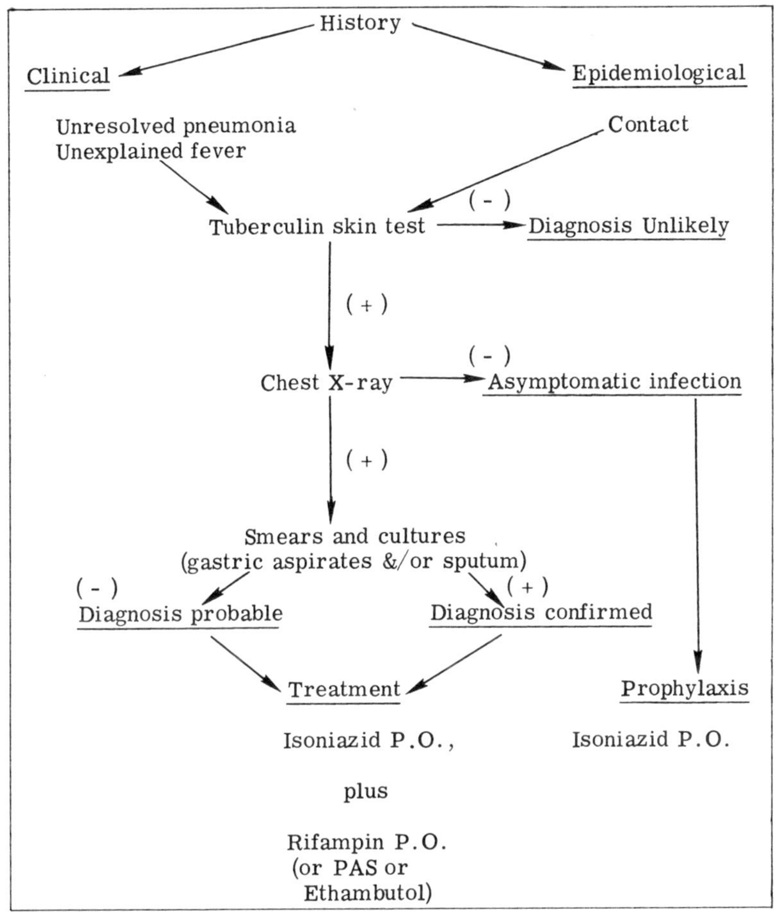

FIG. 17.1: Approach to Pulmonary Tuberculosis in Children

intradermally into the skin of the forearm. The degree of induration
(not erythema) is measured at 48, and again at 72, hours. The interpretation of skin testing results is summarized in Table 17-3.
The skin test, a cell-mediated response or delayed hypersensitivity
reaction, generally becomes positive in 6 weeks (ranges from 2 to
10 weeks) following infection and is positive in 95% of patients infected with M. tuberculosis. False negative reactions can occur in
patients with: 1) malnutrition, 2) overwhelming miliary infection,
3) immunosuppressive therapy, 4) absolute lymphopenia, 5) deficiency
in cell-mediated immunity, 6) concurrent viral infections (such as
measles, mumps, rubella, varicella, or influenza), and 7) recently
received measles vaccine.

TABLE 17-3: INTERPRETATION OF REACTIONS TO SKIN TESTS PERFORMED WITH 5 TEST UNITS OF TUBERCULIN PURIFIED PROTEIN DERIVATIVE GIVEN INTRADERMALLY	
DIAMETER OF REACTION AT 48-72 HR (MM)	INTERPRETATION
0-4	Negative. Patient probably not infected with Mycobacterium tuberculosis.
5-9	Equivocal. Hypersensitivity may be due to Mycobacterium other than M. tuberculosis
≥ 10	Positive. Patient probably infected with M. tuberculosis

3.2: Roentgenographic Studies: Once there is indication of infection (positive skin test), one must look for disease. Tuberculosis, when present, is primarily pulmonic in origin, therefore, a chest roentgenogram is most helpful. In infants, pulmonary infiltrates (a nonspecific consolidation) may be located in any lobe and are usually associated with a hilar lymphadenopathy (Fig. 17.2). In contrast, the infiltrates or cavitary lesions of adolescents and adults are usually located posteriorly in the apices. Calcified encapsulated tubercles may appear, and fluffy infiltrates may also occur in patients with bronchogenic dissemination. Tuberculous meningitis in young infants is often manifested by separation of cranial sutures. In rare cases, radiographic evidence of bone or renal involvement may be present.

3.3: Smear and Cultures: Presumptive diagnosis can be made by microscopic demonstration of acid-fast organisms from discharges of tuberculous lesions such as sputum, gastric washing, spinal fluid, draining sinus, biopsy tissues, pleural or ascitic fluid, urinary sediment, etc. utilizing either the Ziehl-Neelson or Truants or fluorochrome method. Demonstration of organisms by stained smear is usually not successful, and furthermore, specimens may be contaminated with saprophytes or atypical mycobacteria yielding false positive results. Therefore, definitive diagnosis lies in isolation of the organisms by culture. In all cases, multiple specimens should be collected for culture as the number of bacilli excreted may be small. Growth of M. tuberculosis is extremely slow, generally requiring approximately 8 weeks (3 weeks to 3 months) for proper growth and identification.

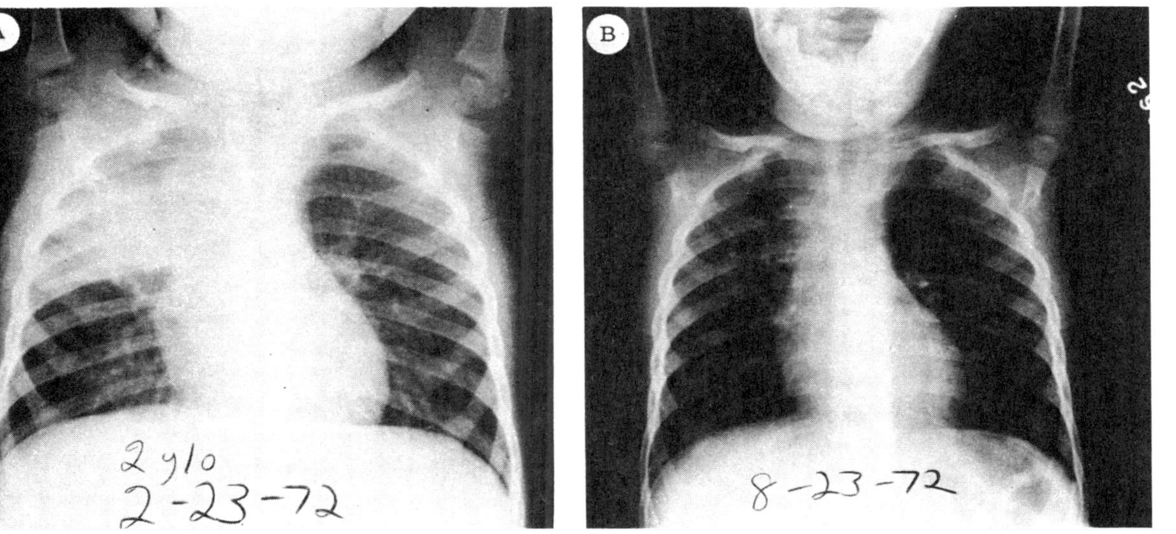

FIG. 17.2 A,B: Pulmonary tuberculosis in a 2-year-old boy.   A) Involvement of the right upper lobe and hilar nodes.   B) Six months after the initiation of chemotherapy, showing significant improvement of infiltrations and adenopathy.

4. MANAGEMENT

<u>4.1: Chemotherapy</u>: Chemotherapy for tuberculosis is very effective and will cure most patients with the disease. The aims of chemotherapy include: 1) preventing the complications that may result from early hematogenous spread, 2) eradicating as many bacilli as possible to lessen the chance of forming dormant foci that serve as sources for late chronic pulmonary tuberculosis, and 3) eliminating infectious human sources of transmission. The approach to chemotherapy varies with the stages of the infection. In general, single drug therapy with isoniazid (INH) is used to treat infection without disease, prevent the development of disease, and prevent a contact from becoming infected.

The kinds of patients who required single drug therapy are listed in the following section entitled "Chemoprophylaxis." Concurrent use of two or three drugs is required for treatment of tuberculous disease, mainly to prevent the development of resistant organisms and to achieve maximum therapeutic effect. A double drug regimen (isoniazid plus another drug) is used for most patients with pulmonary tuberculosis. Triple drug therapy is reserved for the serious forms of disease, such as advanced cavitary pulmonary tuberculosis, disease involving other organs (bone, kidney, etc.), miliary tuberculosis, and tuberculous meningitis.

The types and dosages of antituberculous drugs used in children and their adverse side effects are listed in Table 17-4.

Double drug therapy usually consists of isoniazid plus one other drug (rifampin, ethambutol, or aminosalicylic acid - PAS). Ethambutol is not recommended for use in children under 13 years of age since drug safety has not been established in children. Experience with ethionamide in children is also limited. Pyridoxine 25 to 50 mg. daily may minimize the risk of polyneuritis from isonazid-induced pyridoxine deficiency, particularly in malnourished infants and children.

Triple drug regimen usually consists of isoniazid plus two other drugs (rifampin-streptomycin, rifampin-ethambutol, rifampin-PAS, etc.). When streptomycin is used in initial treatment, it should be discontinued after 8 weeks of therapy in order to avoid the side effects associated with long-term use.

Corticosteroids are added to the therapeutic regimen in patients with severe disease, such as tuberculous meningitis, pericarditis, and peritonitis. In these situations, steroid therapy is usually maintained for the initial 2 to 3 weeks of therapy.

The appropriate duration of chemotherapy for tuberculous disease is not known. The usual duration of therapy is 18 to 24 months and the treatment should be given without interruption. Treatment failure or

TABLE 17-4: ANTITUBERCULOUS DRUGS		
DRUG	DAILY DOSE (mg/kg/24 hrs)	POSSIBLE ADVERSE EFFECTS
Isoniazid (INH)	10-30 (500 mg maximum) in 1 or 2 doses, PO, IM, IV	Peripheral neuropathy, liver damage
Para amino salicylic acid (PAS)	200-300 mg (12 gm maximum) in 2 or 3 doses, PO, IM	Gastric irritation, fever, rash, jaundice
Streptomycin	20-40 (1 gm maximum) single dose initially, then 3 times weekly, IM	Ototoxicity, vestibular damage
Rifampin	15-20 (600 mg maximum) in 1 dose PO	Liver damage
Ethionamide	15-20 in 2-3 doses, PO	Gastric irritation liver damage
Ethambutol	15-20 in 2-3 doses, PO	Optic neuritis

* The higher dose in the range is used in the first few weeks of therapy for severe infection.

relapse is rare in patients receiving uninterrupted treatment with appropriate agents. The usual reasons for failure include: 1) interruption of therapy, and 2) the infecting strain of M. tuberculosis is drug-resistant. Drug resistance may be either primary or develop during therapy. Retreatment always presents a difficult problem, often requiring multiple drug therapy with newer antituberculous agents, as well as data from in vitro drug susceptibility tests of the organisms.

4.2: Chemoprophylaxis: The majority of primary M. tuberculosis infections are asymptomatic. Once infected, but untreated, the risk of developing active tuberculous disease or reactivation continues for many years and may well be lifelong. The effectiveness of isoniazid in preventing complications of primary tuberculosis has been well documented. Curry (1967) reported that the risk for the development of tuberculosis in the untreated, young, tuberculin reactors is 60 times greater than that for the treated group (Table 17-5).

Isoniazid (INH) alone is used for preventive therapy in a dose of 10 mg/kg (maximum 300 mg) once daily for 12 months. Approximately 10 to 20% of adults may develop mild hepatic dysfunction (elevation of transaminase) when taking isoniazid, but such side effects are rare in children.

TABLE 17-5: THE PROTECTIVE VALUE OF ISONIAZID PROPHYLAXIS IN YOUNG TUBERCULIN REACTORS			
Group	No. of Students	No. of Case of Tuberculosis	Risk Ratio
Received prophylaxis	2,910	1	1
No prophylaxis	1,192	25	61
Modified from Curry F.J. (N. Eng. J. Med. 277:562, 1967).			

Preventive therapy is recommended for the following groups as listed in order of priority:

1) Household contacts of infectious cases (household contacts with negative skin test should receive preventive therapy for 3 months and then be skin tested again).

2) Recent converters.

3) Tuberculin reactors, untreated, with abnormal chest x-ray (inactive disease).

4) Tuberculin reactors under age 35 (the risk of tuberculosis is highest in infancy, high again in adolescence and early adulthood).

5) Tuberculin reactors in special clinical situations (patients receiving prolonged therapy with corticosteroids or immunosupressive therapy; patients with certain hematologic and reticuloendothelial diseases, such as leukemia, Hodgkin's disease, diabetes mellitus, silicosis; and after gastrectomy).

6) Tuberculin reactors with measles (or in patients who have recently received live measles vaccine); those undergoing a major surgical procedure (preventive therapy for 8 weeks).

4.3: Active Immunization: Bacillus Calmette-Geurin (BCG) vaccine, derived from a live attenuated strain of M. bovis, confers varying degrees of protection to M. tuberculosis infection. BCG has been used extensively in countries with high prevalence of tuberculosis, but its use in countries with a low incidence of tuberculosis is limited. The use of BCG is discussed in Chapter 25.

ATYPICAL MYCOBACTERIAL INFECTIONS

In contrast to M. tuberculosis, atypical mycobacteria are ubiquitous in nature, commonly found in soil, water, milk and food. They have been isolated all over the world but with greater frequency in subtropical and tropical environments. Several species are saprophytes,

both in man and lower animals. Some of these agents are found to
be pathogenic for man. Subclinical infections are highly prevalent,
as demonstrated by the skin tests. Runyon, in 1959, classified these
agents according to growth rates, pigmentation and colony morphology. The organisms that are pathogenic for man and the diseases
produced by them are summarized in Table 17-6.

TABLE 17-6: ATYPICAL MYCOBACTERIA PATHOGENIC TO MAN		
RUNYON GROUP	**SPECIES**	**DISEASE**
I. Photo- chromogens	M. kansasii	Tuberculosis-like Swimming pool granu- loma and subcutane- ous abscess
II. Scoto- chromogens	M. scrofulaceum	Lymphadenitis
III. Non- chromogens	M. avium M. intracellulare (Battey bacillus)	Tuberculosis (rare) Lymphadenitis, tuberculosis-like
IV. Rapid growers	M. fortuitum	Local abscess, tuberculosis-like
Others	M. ulcerans	Skin ulcers

Atypical mycobacteria, unlike M. tuberculosis or M. bovis, do not
produce disease in guinea pigs and are of low pathogenicity in man.
Human infections are generally acquired by contamination from an
environmental source and are not considered contagious. The portals
of entry are probably oral mucosa, conjunctivae, skin and respiratory tract. The clinical presentation of atypical mycobacteria infections appears to be directly related to the portal of entry.

1. CLINICAL MANIFESTATIONS

Granulomatous cervical adenitis is the most common presentation in
infants and children. Submandibular, submaxillary, and preauricular glands are often involved. The organisms enter these nodes
probably through the oral mucosa and conjunctivae. Unlike M. tuberculosis infections, the anterior cervical chain is rarely involved.
Typically, the disease is characterized by unilateral node enlargement and an acute suppurative process with or without salivary gland
involvement or formation of a nodal-cutaneous fistula. M. scrofulaceum is the most commonly isolated agent. M. kansasii, M. intracellulare, M. fortuitum and other species may also cause the disease.

Swimming pool granuloma, caused by M. marinum, is characterized by benign self-limited ulcerating papules of skin. The lesions appear approximately 3-4 weeks after having suffered an abrasion while swimming in water contaminated with the organism. These lesions heal slowly over months and leave a scar. Chemotherapy is generally not required. M. ulcerans causes rapid, progressive ulcerations confined to the skin, and has a predilection for the distal portion of the extremities. These ulcers heal spontaneously over an 8 to 10 month period. Response to chemotherapy is poor and excision of the ulcer may be recommended.

Pulmonary involvement with atypical mycobacteria, more commonly seen in adults, is uncommon in children. The disease may be identical to the ordinary pulmonary tuberculosis. Causative agents include M. kansasii, M. avium, and M. intracellulare.

Disseminated disease has been reported but is extremely rare and has invariably been fatal. The disease has generally occurred in young children and is overwhelming and rapidly progressive.

2. DIAGNOSIS

Atypical mycobacterial infection is suspected when there is a disease compatible with tuberculosis, but with a negative history of exposure and a small or intermediate reaction to tuberculin skin test. In such a situation, the skin test should be repeated in conjunction with other available atypical mycobacterial antigens.

Definitive diagnosis is made by culturing and identifying the causative agent from a surgical specimen, sputum, gastric washings, or a draining sinus. Multiple specimens should be collected for culture, since the yield of organisms from a single specimen may be very small.

3. THERAPY

Atypical mycobacterial infections are usually resistant to therapy with available antituberculous regimens. M. kansasii is somewhat responsive to multiple drug therapy. Lesions caused by M. scrofulaceum and M. ulcerans are responsive to surgical excision. The cutaneous lesions due to M. marinum usually do not require therapy.

When drug therapy is indicated, it should consist of multiple drugs (such as isoniazid, streptomycin, and para-aminosalicylic acid). Rifampin or cycloserine is often added. Second-line drugs may be necessary if response does not occur or if progression of the disease occurs.

REFERENCES

American Thoracic Society, Committee on Therapy, National Tuberculosis and Respiratory Disease Association, Center for Disease Control: Joint statement on the preventive treatment of tuberculosis. Am. Rev. Respor. Dis. 110:371, 1974.

Black, B.G., Chapman, J.S.: Cervical adenitis in children due to human and unclassified mycobacteria. Pediatr. 33:887, 1964.

Brody, J., Overfield, J., Hammes, L.M.: Depression of the tuberculin reaction by viral vaccines. NEJM 271:1294, 1964.

David, S.D., Comstock, G.W.: Mycobacterial cervical adenitis in children. J. Pediatr. 58:771, 1961.

D'Souza, B.J., Lanksy, L.L., Cho, C.T.: Tuberculous meningitis developing after six months of treatment of pulmonary tuberculosis. A complication of infection with a drug-resistant stain in a two-year-old child. Clin. Pediatr. 14:729, 1975.

Edwards, L.B.: Current status of the tuberculin test. Ann. N.Y. Acad. Sci. 106:32, 1963.

Gunnels, J.J., Bates, J.H., Swindoll, H.: Infectiousness of culture positive tuberculosis patients on chemotherapy. Am. Rev. Respir. Dis. 105:989, 1972.

Kending, E.L., Jr.: Unclassified mycobacteria in children. Am. J. Dis. Child. 101:749, 1961.

Light, I.J., Saidlemon, M., Sutherland, J.M.: Management of newborns after nursery exposure to tuberculosis. Am. Rev. Respir. Dis. 109:415, 1974.

Lincoln, E.M., Sewell, E.M.: Tuberculosis, in Infectious Diseases of Children and Adults. Krugman, S., Ward, R., eds. The C.V. Mosby Co., St. Louis, 1973.

Lincoln, E.M.: Course and prognosis of tuberculosis in children. Am. J. Med. 9:623, 1950.

Morrison, J.B.: Natural history of segmental lesions in primary pulmonary tuberculosis. Arch. Dis. Child. 48:90, 1973.

Steiner, M., Cosio, A.: Primary tuberculosis in children. Incidence of primary drug-resistant disease in 332 children observed between the years 1961 and 1964 at the Kings County Medical Center of Brooklyn. NEJM 274:755, 1966.

Sumaya, C.V., Simek, M., Smith, M.H.D., et al.: Tuberculosis meningitis in children during the isoniazid era. J. Pediatr. 87:43, 1975.

Wolinsky, E.: Nontuberculous mycobacterial infection of man. Med. Clin. N.A. 58:697, 1974.

Zarabi, M., Sane, S., Gerdanig, B.R.: The chest roentgenogram in the early diagnosis of tuberculous meningitis in children. Am. J. Dis. Child. 121:389, 1971.

::

17.2: HEPATITIS

INTRODUCTION: Hepatitis in children and adolescents is generally attributed to two specific, communicable viral syndromes: hepatitis A (or infectious hepatitis) and hepatitis B (or serum hepatitis). The clinical spectrum of both of these entities may include acute and chronic phases, which may be subclinical, clinical, or even fulminant in nature. In general, the clinical spectrum of both entities in children differs from that seen in older adults; therefore, each entity will be discussed separately. The clinical aspects of hepatitis A and B are compared in Table 17-7. Other causes of infectious hepatitis in children are listed in Table 17-8.

1. HEPATITIS A

1.1: EPIDEMIOLOGY: Until recently, all information concerning hepatitis A infection was based on epidemiological data because the virus could not be propagated in in vitro systems and no specific infection-associated antigens had been detected.

The overall incidence of hepatitis A is difficult to compute, as many cases are not reported. However, the annual reported incidence is approximately 40-50 thousand cases per year with 50-80% of cases occurring in children under 15 years. Total annual number of reported deaths in the United States ranges between 600-1000 cases/year (0.3-0.5/100,000 population). Death rates due to hepatitis A in children under 15 years have been estimated to be 0.1/100,000 population of that age group, demonstrating low virulence in that affected population. Epidemics generally occur in children, and are not associated with increased death rates, while the infection is more endemic in adult populations.

Hepatitis A occurs primarily in the 0-14 years age group and may be transmitted by a common source, person to person, or by shellfish ingestion. The fecal-oral route is most common, but infection may rarely occur via parenteral transmission.

TABLE 17-7: COMPARISON OF HEPATITIS A AND B		
	HEPATITIS A	HEPATITIS B
AGENT	probable RNA virus	DNA virus
AGE AND SEX DISTRIBUTION	no sex predilection school age (0-14 yrs.)	slight male sex predilection (5-9 yrs.) (15-30 yrs.)
INCUBATION PERIOD	15-40 days-varies with inoculum	50-180 days-varies with inoculum and route of transmission
TRANSMISSION:		
1) <u>Horizontal</u>:	yes	yes
a) oral-fecal	1°	2°
b) parenteral	2°	1°
2) <u>Vertical</u>:	no	yes
CLINICAL FEATURES:		
1) <u>Pre-icteric</u>:		
a) onset	usually acute	usually insidious
b) fever	common 101°-104°	rare-low grade
c) G.I. symptoms	common	rare
d) rashes	rare	5%
e) serum sickness	rare	10-15%
2) <u>Icteric</u>:		
a) course	rapid	insidious
b) bilirubin levels elevated		
age 6-15	duration 10 days	duration 19 days
age 16-25	duration 17 days	duration 25 days
age 26-40	duration 19 days	duration 32 days
c) SGPT levels elevated		
age 6-15	duration 14 days	duration 27 days
age 16-25	duration 19 days	duration 30 days
age 26-40	duration 24 days	duration 36 days

Table 17-7 (Continued)

	HEPATITIS A	HEPATITIS B
d) infectivity		
stools	8 days after onset jaundice	---
urine	3 days after onset jaundice	---
blood	3 days after onset jaundice	(HBsAg) 50% - 3 weeks 10% - 7 weeks
LAB FEATURES:		
IgM levels (anic-teric/icteric	yes/yes	no/+ or -
Thymol Turbidity	yes/yes	no/+ or -
Antigens	HA-Ag	HBs-Ag HBc-Ag
Immunity	Homologous	??
Active	no vaccine	vaccine experimental
Passive	ISG (immune serum globulin)	a) ISG-small inoc exposure b) hepatitis B im-mune globulin-large inoc exposure

Hepatitis A affects both sexes equally, with the highest incidence of
infections occurring in low socioeconomic populations. Overcrowding and poor sanitation tend to facilitate the spread of common
source and person-to-person infections. In higher socioeconomic
groups, the incidence of childhood infections is lower, which results
in a proportionately higher percentage of susceptible adults.

AGENT: Feinstone (1973), using immune electron microscopy, described a 27 nanometer virus-like particle which proved serologically
to be related to hepatitis A. This particle could be redemonstrated
in the stool specimens of volunteers inoculated with stool filtrates
from known cases of hepatitis A infection. The presence of the
virus-like particles was associated with clinical evidence of infection and the development of specific antibody in convalescent sera.
The antigen (HA-Ag) is detectable in stools five to six days prior to
the onset of liver enzyme elevations, and generally disappears as the

TABLE 17-8: INFECTIOUS CAUSES OF HEPATITIS IN CHILDREN

VIRAL:	Cytomegalovirus Epstein-Barr virus Yellow fever Adenovirus Varicella Rubella Coxsackie viruses Echo viruses
PROTOZOA:	Toxoplasmosis
PARASITES:	Toxocariasis Amoebiasis Schistosomiasis
FUNGI:	Actinomycosis Blastomycosis
OTHERS:	Tuberculosis Brucellosis Syphilis

enzyme levels reach a peak. Provost et al. (1975) have recently described the biochemical and biophysical properties of a human hepatitis virus (CR 326 strain) recovered from clinical cases of human infections and subsequently recovered from marmosets infected with the agent. Physical and chemical characteristics closely relate it to the RNA containing enterovirus group. The host response to infection involves the early development of immune adherence and complement-fixing antibodies, both of which have been demonstrated to persist for up to ten years following infection, and are protective to reinfection with hepatitis A, even if the primary infection was subclinical in nature. Antibody prevalence is almost universal among endemic populations in low socioeconomic settings but approximates less than 50% in middle-class American populations.

1.2: PATHOGENESIS AND PATHOLOGY: The specific mechanisms involved in the production of hepatic damage during the course of hepatitis are not completely defined. However, the pathology is similar for the acute process seen in both hepatitis A and hepatitis B. Trump et al. (1976) have hypothesized that, following an interaction of the virus and the plasma membrane of the hepatocyte, there is an increased permeability to ions at the membrane level. This results in an influx of sodium and water, causing ballooning degeneration the cell with subsequent obstruction of adjacent canaliculi, leading to bile stasis. Ballooning of the endoplasmic reticulum also occurs, and protein synthesis decreases. An exaggerated efflux of potassium may also occur, resulting in cell shrinkage and acidophilic degeneration. Intracellular calcium flux results in alteration of mitochondrial function, while lysosomal alterations and autophagic vacuolation occur in severely altered cells. To a degree, all changes are reversible; however, when they become irreversible, cell death ensues. The extent of quantitative and qualitative cellular involvement determines the pathological staging of the process.

The classic histological picture of acute viral hepatitis is characterized by: 1) a periportal inflammation made up of histiocytes, lymphocytes, plasma cells and occasionally eosinophils, 2) hepato-cellular disarray with varying degrees of cellular necrosis; some cells display ballooning degeneration while others shrink up, forming "Councilman bodies," and 3) hyperplasia and hypertrophy of Kupffer cells and other cells of the reticulo-endothelial system. Grossly, the liver may be bile stained, slightly edematous and mildly enlarged. However, in general, it is normal in size, color and consistency.

In fulminant hepatitis, there is massive cellular necrosis, first involving the centrilobular zones with sparing of the portal structures. Collapse of the reticular framework follows the massive necrosis, and since cellular regeneration is minimal, fibrous tissue replacement of these areas results in a picture of post-necrotic cirrhosis.

1.3: CLINICAL MANIFESTATIONS: The incubation period ranges between 15-40 days (mean 30 days) and is inversely related to the dose of infectious inoculum, but not the mode of infection. Hepatitis A most commonly occurs as a subclinical infection in children, with an anicteric to icteric case ratio of 10:1. In epidemic settings, anicteric cases will generally account for 50-90% of cases, primarily in children. This anicteric population then serves as the mode of maintaining the epidemic, as contact with anicteric cases often goes unnoticed. Anicteric infections are manifested only by anorexia, malaise, nausea, vomiting, headaches, low-grade fevers, abdominal discomfort and occasionally hepatic tenderness. Diagnosis is confirmed only by abnormal liver function tests which are seldom done, unless there is a strong suspicion in an epidemic setting.

The clinical presentation of icteric hepatitis A in adolescents and adults consists of pre-icteric and icteric phases. The pre-icteric phase occurs 3-10 days prior to the onset of jaundice and is manifested by fever (ranging from 100-104°F), vague neuromuscular complaints, and in particular, nausea, vomiting and diarrhea. The liver becomes progressively enlarged and tender, with a rapid rise in SGOT and SGPT which peak prior to the onset of jaundice and remain elevated for about 1-3 weeks. Darkening of the urine due to bilirubin and urobilinogen also occurs during this phase. Mild splenomegaly and lymphadenopathy are occasionally noted.

Jaundice, which marks the onset of the icteric phase, occurs first in the sclerae and then in the skin as bilirubin levels reach 3.5-5.0 mg%.

The bilirubin rises to peak levels within 4-5 days, during which time stools become lighter in color. Elevated levels generally persist for not more than 12-14 days. Paradoxically, as the bilirubin reaches peak levels, the patient begins to feel better; despite the worsening of the jaundice, complaints of anorexia, vomiting, and malaise decrease. In the small percentage of cases that develop fulminating hepatitis, patients experience a progressive worsening of their initial symptoms, jaundice deepens, the liver reduces in size without clinical improvement, and ascites may occur. When hepatic coma occurs, deterioration in mental status may progress from disorientation to lethargy, stupor and finally coma.

In greater than 95% of childhood cases, complete recovery without sequelae occurs within 6 weeks. Relapse occurs in about 2% of all childhood cases. This may simply be associated with a subclinical recurrence of liver function abnormalities, or may also be associated with a recurrence of clinical symptoms. In general, these relapses resolve without sequelae. There is no real evidence to date to suggest that there is an increased incidence of chronic disease associated with hepatitis A infections. In less than .01% of all cases of acute viral hepatitis, fulminating hepatitis may be a consequence. Survival rates in these particular cases range from 20-40%, depending upon the patient's age, level of coma and the extent of hepatic necrosis. Mortality appears to be higher in children than in adults. Post-necrotic cirrhosis may complicate the few cases that do survive the insult of hepatic failure.

1.4: DIAGNOSIS: Diagnosis is primarily based on epidemiologic criteria, i.e.: 1) complaints of anorexia, malaise, nausea and vomiting with or without jaundice, associated with 2) a history of either contact with infected persons, ingestion of potentially contaminated material or inoculation with blood products, in the presence of 3) elevated levels of SGOT and SGPT. Krugman and Giles (1972) feel that there is always an elevation of IgM in hepatitis A and usually an abnormal thymol turbidity. Antibody detection by immune adherence and complement fixation techniques are not available in most laboratories but are promising.

In case of fulminating hepatitis, the SGOT and SGPT levels may reach values of greater than 3000 I.U. very rapidly, but may fall precipitously as the liver rapidly shrinks. These patients may also have a prolongation of the prothrombin time that does not correct with vitamin K supplementation, which further suggests severe hepatic damage. Patients in hepatic coma may also have elevated arterial ammonia levels and abnormalities on an electroencephalogram.

In general, a liver biopsy will give a definitive diagnosis in cases where a specific diagnosis cannot be made on the basis of epidemiological, clinical and simple laboratory findings. Biopsy will also distinguish hepatitis from Reye's syndrome, and serve to define the extent of hepatic necrosis in cases of fulminating hepatitis. In many cases, this may determine the extent to which therapeutic modalities are used in case management.

1.5: MANAGEMENT AND PREVENTION: In the majority of cases, therapy is limited to bed rest, restriction of strenuous activity while symptomatic, and maintenance of adequate caloric intake. High protein intake is recommended except in fulminant cases.

In fulminating cases, medical therapy includes careful monitoring of fluids, electrolytes, and acid-base balance. Maintenance of an alkalotic state appears to improve cerebral blood flow and enhance cerebral oxygenation. Maintenance of adequate caloric intake is important, with emphasis on vitamin supplementation and the limitation of protein intake. Bowel sterilization with neomycin and transfusion of fresh whole blood and fresh frozen plasma to correct coagulation abnormalities is commonly necessary. Systemic antibiotics are used in cases of superinfection, which is common, and adequate coverage usually entails the use of a penicillin and an aminoglycoside. The biologic support methods that are used vary according to regional facilities and experience. They range from single or multiple two volume exchange transfusions, to dialysis and even cross-circulation with human volunteers.

Prevention is directed at identifying and controlling the source of an epidemic. Where person-person spread is suspected, anicteric cases must be identified as potential sources of spread. In common source epidemics, where water, refuse and sewage are sources of infection, sanitation and hygiene must be enforced. In hospitals and institutions, disposal of contaminated materials must be enforced as blood, urine and stools remain infectious for variable periods.

Adult patients are usually not isolated within a hospital setting, as hygiene and contaminant disposal can be enforced. Children, however, need to be isolated, as strict enforcement of hand washing is impossible, as is the guarantee that fecal-oral contamination will not occur among ward mates if isolation is not practiced.

Prevention in the form of passive immunization with immune serum globulin will modify disease or result in an inapparent infection. When administered in appropriate doses (Table 17-9) at least 6 days prior to the onset of symptoms, protection will result in 80-90% of cases for up to 6 months. Krugman (1976) determined that preparations of commercial immune serum globulin had an anti-HA titer of 1:3200 as determined by immune adherence hemagglutination. None of 8 susceptible patients who received an MS-1 (hepatitis A) serum-immune serum globulin mixture developed biochemical evidence of hepatic dysfunction, while only two showed immunologic evidence of an inapparent infection. Meanwhile, 8 of 14 (57%) controls who received only the inoculation of MS-1 serum developed hepatitis, as

<table>
<tr><td colspan="2" align="center">TABLE 17-9: IMMUNE SERUM GLOBULIN PROPHYLAXIS
FOR HEPATITIS A</td></tr>
</table>

1. CONDITION OF EXPOSURE (0.02 ml/pound intramuscularly):

   a) Exposure to common sources of infection such as contaminated food or water.

   b) Exposure via inoculation with contaminated needles or blood itself.

   c) Exposure to household members with hepatitis.

2. TRAVEL TO ENDEMIC AREAS:

   a) Length of stay less than 3 months:

less than 50 pounds	0.5 ml
50-100 pounds	1.0 ml
greater than 100 pounds	2.0 ml

   b) Length of stay greater than 3 months:

less than 50 pounds	1.0 ml
50-100 pounds	2.5 ml
greater than 100 pounds	5.0 ml

   c) People residing in developing countries or endemic tropical countries. (Doses in section 2.b should be repeated every 4-6 months).

Adapted from: 1) PHS Advisory Committee on Immunization practices. Ann. Int. Med. 77:427, 1972. 2) Center for Disease Control. Health information for international travel 1975. Morbidity and Mortality Weekly Rep. 24 (suppl):55, 1975.

evidenced by abnormal elevations of liver enzymes after an incubation of 29-42 days and an eight-fold rise in the convalescence antibody titer. Although active immunization is not possible at present, the isolation of the hepatitis A antigen should lead to the development of vaccines in the future.

2. HEPATITIS B

2.1: EPIDEMIOLOGY: There has been a marked increase in the annual occurrence of cases of hepatitis B. In 1966 there were 1,497 reported cases, while in 1976 there were 14,850 reported cases. Where hepatitis B accounted for 4% of all specified reported hepatitis cases in 1966, it accounted for 31% of all specified reported cases in 1976. The incidence rate of hepatitis B in 1966 was 1.79 per 100,000 population, and in 1976 it was 6.92 per 100,000 population. The highest case concentration occurs in the 15-29 year age group with a slight male predominance. A smaller concentration occurs between the ages of 5-9 years (Fig. 17.3).

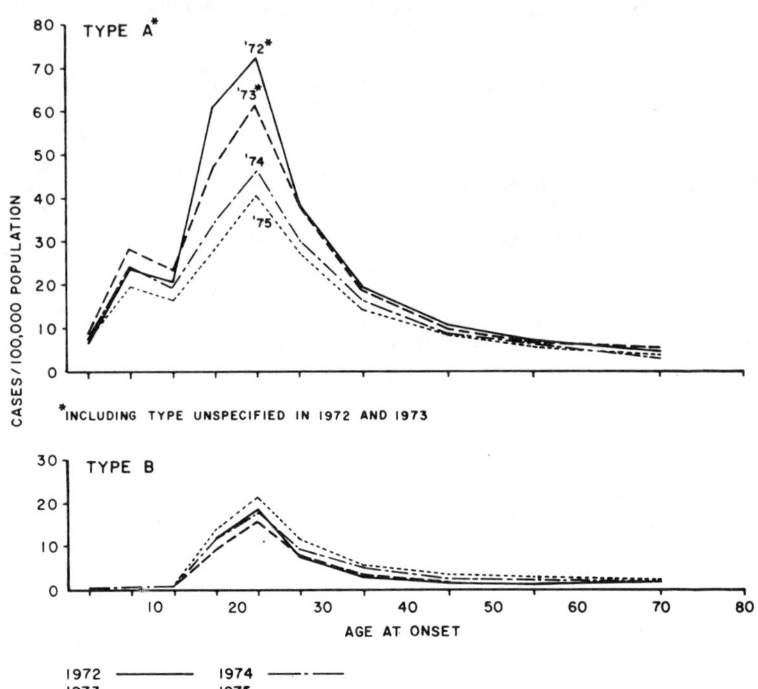

FIG. 17.3: Age specific rates for hepatitis in the U.S. 1972-75. Adapted from: Center for Disease Control. Hepatitis Surveilance. Report No. 40, March 1977.

Certain aspects in the natural history of the disease tend to account for this increase and explain transmission trends. These are: 1) a high rate of subclinical infections (50-90%), 2) a relatively longer period of infectivity than is seen in hepatitis A, and 3) a tendency toward chronicity and carrier states which varies from 0.1% in the U.S. to as high as 10% in tropical areas. Hepatitis B may be transmitted both parenterally and non-parenterally. The primary modes of parenteral transmission are: blood and blood products, hemodialysis units, and contaminated needles among drug abusers. Percutaneous contamination via the communal use of razors, toothbrushes and scrub brushes has been reported. Non-parenteral transmission may be oral, via saliva and/or nasopharyngeal secretions, or sexual, as both semen and menstrual blood have been shown to contain HBsAg. In addition, vertical transmission has been reported. Transplacental transmission varies from 0-40% in cases of asymptomatic female carriers and in cases of maternal hepatitis early in pregnancy. Transmission as high as 70-100% has been reported in cases where maternal infection occurred late in gestation.

AGENT: Viral hepatitis B is synonymous with serum hepatitis. It is caused by the hepatitis B virus which to date has not been grown in in vitro systems. Blumberg et al. were the first to demonstrate the association of the Australia antigen or hepatitis B antigen (HB-Ag) with hepatitis B infection. Since then, the hepatitis B antigen has been found to consist of two components which possess antigenically distinct characteristics that are genetically determined by the genome of the hepatitis B virus. The first of these is the hepatitis B surface antigen (HBsAg), which has been found on various particulate forms in the sera of antigen carriers. These particles are felt to be the products of infection and include: 1) filamentous structures of variable length which are 22 nanometers in diameter, 2) spherical particles which are 22 nanometers in diameter, and 3) the surface coating of the Dane particle. These surface antigens have been demonstrated to be structurally composed of polypeptides which possess group (a) and sub-type (dw/yw) (dr/yr) antigenic specificities. These characteristics are virus specific and have been useful in epidemiological studies, as the various subtypes have varying population frequencies and geographic distributions.

The second distinct component of the HB-Ag is the core antigen (HBcAg), which is a 28 nanometer particle found in the nuclei of hepatocytes in hepatitis B infected patients. The core antigen is not found circulating freely in the sera, but may be chemically dislodged from freely circulating Dane particles. This core contains a small, circular double-strand of DNA with a closely attached molecule of DNA polymerase. By its DNA character and morphology, this virus falls into a previously unclassified group of viruses.

The Dane particle, first described in 1970, is a 42 nanometer particle found in relatively small amounts in the sera of hepatitis B.

It is felt by some to represent the hepatitis B virus itself, but the infectious nature of pure samples remains to be proven. The HBcAg is present on the core of the Dane particle and the HBsAg is present on the envelope of the Dane particle.

2.2: HOST RESPONSE: The host response to hepatitis B infection involves both cellular and humoral components. The humoral response involves anti-HBsAg antibodies which appear prior to hepatocellular damage, just as the HBsAg begins to disappear. These antibodies usually persist for long periods of time, except in chronic carriers. Later in convalescence, anti-HBcAg antibodies appear. These antibodies decrease in titer as infection resolves but almost universally persist in chronic carriers. The cellular response is less well defined. However, during infection, a T-cell lymphopenia exists and parallels the appearance of null cells, which are usually detectable during periods of enzyme elevations and in the case of chronic hepatitis. Whether this determines the eventual outcome of infection, i.e. resolution versus chronicity, remains to be seen.

2.3: CLINICAL MANIFESTATIONS: Hepatitis B, like hepatitis A, generally causes a benign infection in childhood, with a high proportion of anicteric cases. The onset is generally insidious except in rare cases of acute fulminating hepatitis, where mental confusion and combativeness rapidly progress to a comatose state in the face of acute hepatic failure. The incubation period may span 40-180 days (average 70 days) and is probably inversely related to the dose of inoculum. In general, parenteral transmission is associated with a shorter incubation than is non-parenteral transmission.

Clinically, anicteric cases are indistinguishable from anicteric cases of hepatitis A. In icteric cases, there is a 5-8 day pre-icteric period not characterized by gastrointestinal symptoms, and fevers are low grade in nature. Rashes occur in 5% of cases, and urticaria in 3%. Gianotti has described a papular erythematous rash with follicular hyperplasia which involves the face, limbs and buttocks in selective cases of hepatitis B. A systemic serum sickness syndrome of approximately 7 days duration occurs in 10-12% of cases. It is characterized clinically by arthritis, arthralgias, urticaria and angioedema, and biochemically by decreased serum levels of complement components. Hepatomegaly and hepatic tenderness occur in 70-90% of cases, and splenomegaly in 25-30%.

Jaundice marks the onset of the icteric phase and is usually preceded by bilirubinuria. The bilirubin rises comparatively slower than in hepatitis A, reaching a maximum in 10-30 days (average 14), and lasts an average of 25 days in patients 16-25 years of age. Stools now become acholic. As the bilirubin slowly rises, the patient may experience an initial period of well-being. However, he may re-experience symptoms of fatigue and malaise as bilirubin levels finally peak. Serum SGOT and SGPT begin to rise in the pre-icteric period, slowly

peak and remain elevated for a relatively longer period than in
hepatitis A. The duration of bilirubin and liver enzyme elevation
appears to increase with age. In children, however, complete recovery within 4-6 weeks occurs in 90-95% of cases.

Between 5-10% of all cases of hepatitis develop some form of chronic
process. This generally takes one of two forms: chronic persistent
hepatitis or chronic active hepatitis. Chronic persistent hepatitis
primarily affects adolescent males who are chronic HBsAg carriers.
The disease process is usually benign and self-limiting in nature.
Symptomatology may or may not exist, and usually consists only of
mild fatigue, hepatic tenderness and intermittent mild icterus.
Characterized clinically by persistent serum transaminase elevations that may last up to several years, pathological data reveal
only minimal necrosis, a mild manonuclear infiltrate and ballooning
of hepatocytes, set against a normal hepatic architecture.

Chronic active hepatitis, however, is of a much more severe nature
and is associated with the presence of HBsAg in less than 25% of
cases. Severe hepatic disease following acute hepatitis may be totally asymptomatic in some cases, but in others may be associated
with hepato-splenomegaly, jaundice, ascites, arthritis, rashes and
nephritis. On biopsy, hepatic histology shows piecemeal necrosis
and portal inflammation, primarily mononuclear in nature. Laboratory abnormalities include markedly elevated serum transaminases,
elevated bilirubins, hypergammaglobulinemia and depletion of liver
dependent coagulation factors.

2.4: DIAGNOSIS: Diagnosis is based primarily on epidemiologic
parameters, i.e. natural history and laboratory findings. The hepatitis B surface antigen (HBsAg) may be detectable as early as 30
days after exposure and peaks in prevalence as symptoms occur.
Persistence is variable, occurring in 50% of cases at 3 weeks, 10%
at 7 weeks and indefinitely in 0.1% of cases in the U.S. Antibody to
the core antigen appears in convalescence, disappears with clinical
recovery and/or persists in chronic carriers.

2.5: MANAGEMENT AND PREVENTION: Hepatitis B is generally
a benign disease in pediatric populations and therapy is usually limited to bed rest and adequate caloric intake during the acute stage.
Steroids are not indicated in uncomplicated cases of acute hepatitis
or in chronic persistent hepatitis, and may even perpetuate the process by causing a relapse. However, in the face of clinical deterioration with markedly abnormal serum transaminase levels, steroids
are indicated when dealing with chronic active hepatitis. Prednisone (2 mg/kg/day) is recommended for approximately one month,
then the patient is placed on a maintenance regimen of 10 mg/qd,
once a clinical remission is achieved. This maintenance regimen is
then continued for at least six more months of therapy. As relapses
may occur, any individual patient may require reinduction of therapy

with high dose prednisone; at times, the addition of azothioprine is
necessary. Silverberg (1977) estimates five-year survival rates
at 50-80%.

Preventive measures include: 1) cooperation with the Public Health
Service in reporting all detected cases, and 2) proper follow-up of
clinical cases and known carriers. Prevention of equipment contamination must be practiced in barber shops, beauty salons, and
even tattoo parlors where percutaneous transmission may occur.
In hospitals, physician and dental offices, and extended care facilities or institutions, scrupulous hygiene must be practiced. Disposal of needles and syringes is mandatory and precaution should be
exercised when drawing bloods. Blood banks have become much
more efficient in screening donors and blood donations. The new
radioimmunoassay technique has shown that contamination may be
reduced by 90%. At the same time, periodic screening of household
contacts, especially spouses, and high risk hospital personnel should
be practiced.

Passive immunization for hepatitis B, using either conventional immune serum globulin or high titer hepatitis B immune globulin, has
proven to be safe, as there is no increased rate of HBsAg carrier
states or evidence of infectivity. With regard to efficacy, conventional gamma globulin appears effective where exposure is non-
parenteral and the inoculum is small. Hepatitis B immune globulin
appears more efficacious where parenteral exposure occurs or the
inoculum is large. However, use of hepatitis B immune globulin
may, in some cases, prolong the incubation period of hepatitis B; at
the same time, it may affect the development of passive-active immunity in some recipients.

Active immunity following hepatitis B infection is generally homolo-
gous; however, this is not universal and may possibly be explained
on the basis of several existing subtypes. There is no heterologous
immunity between hepatitis A and hepatitis B infections.

REFERENCES

Barker, L.F., Peterson, M.R., Shulman, N.R., et al.: Antibody
responses in viral hepatitis type B. JAMA 223:1005-1008, 1973.

Blumberg, B.S.: Polymorphisms of the serum proteins and the development of iso-precipitins in transfused patients. Bull. N.Y.
Acad. Med. 40:377-386, 1964.

Blumberg, B.S., Gerstley, B.J., Hungerford, D.A.: A serum antigen in Down's syndrome, leukemia and hepatitis. Ann. Intern.
Med. 924-931, 1967.

Center for Disease Control: Hepatitis Surveillance. Report No. 39:
Feb. 1977.

Center for Disease Control: Hepatitis Surveillance. Report No. 40: 24-26, 1977.

Courouce-Panty, A.M., Delons, S., Soulier, J.P.: Attempts to prevent hepatitis B by using specific anti-HBs immunization. Am. J. Med. Sci. 270:375-383, 1975.

Dane, D.S., Cameron, C.H., Briggs, M.: Virus-like particles in serum of patients with Australia-antigen associated hepatitis. Lancet 1:695-698, 1970.

Deinhardt, F.: Recent hepatitis type A virus (HAV) candidates, in Hepatitis and Blood Transfusion. Vyas, G.N., Perkins, H.A., Schmid, R., eds. Grune and Stratton, New York, 1972, pp. 383-385.

Edgington, T.S., Chisari, F.V.: Immunological aspects of hepatitis B virus infection. Am. J. Med. Sci. 270:213, 1975.

Feinstone, S.M., Kepikian, A.Z., Purcell, R.H.: Hepatitis A detection by immune electron microscopy of a virus-like antigen associated with acute illness. Science 182:1026-1028, 1973.

Gerin, J.L., Shih, J.W.K., Kaplan, P.M.: Biophysical and biochemical characterizations of hepatitis B antigen. Am. J. Med. Sci. 270:115-121, 1975.

Gianotti, F.: The Australian Antigen in infantile papular acrodermatitis. Proceedings of the 6th meeting of the European Association of the Liver. London, No. 16.

Giles, J.P., Krugman, S.: Viral hepatitis. Differential diagnostic features between infections with type A and B viruses. Am. J. Dis. Child. 123:281, 1972.

Hilleman, M.R., Provost, P.J., Miller, W.J.: Development and utilization of complement-fixation and immune adherence tests for human hepatitis A virus and antibody. Am. J. Med. Sci. 270:93-98, 1975.

Hoofnagle, J.H., Gerety, R.J., Barker, L.F.: Antibody to hepatitis B virus core in man. Lancet 2:869-873, 1973.

Kaplan, P.M., Gerin, J.L., Alter, J.H.: Hepatic B specific DNA polymerase activity during post-transfusion hepatitis. Nature (Lond) 249:762-764, 1973.

Kaplan, P.M., Greenman, R.L., Gerin, J.L., et al.: DNA polymerase associated with human hepatitis B antigen. J. Virol. 12:995-1005, 1973.

Kaprikiam, A.Z., Wyatt, R G., Dolin, R., et al.: Visualization by immunoelectron microscopy of a 27-nm. particle associated with acute infectious nonbacterial gastroenteritis. Virology 10: 1075-1081, 1972.

Krugman, S., Ward, R., Giles, J.P.: The natural history of infectious hepatitis. Am. J. Med. 32:717-718, 1962.

Krugman, S., Giles, J.P., Hammond, J.: Infectious hepatitis: Evidence for two distinctive clinical, epidemiological, and immunological types of infection. JAMA 200:365-373, 1967.

Krugman, S., Giles, J.P.: Viral hepatitis. JAMA 212:1019-1029, 1970.

Krugman, S., Giles, J.P.: Viral hepatitis: New light on an old disease. JAMA 212:1019-1029, 1970.

Krugman, S., Friedman, H., Lattimer, C.: Viral hepatitis, type A. Identification by specific complement-fixation and immune adherence tests. NEJM 292:1141, 1975.

Krugman, S : Effect of human immune serum globulin on infectivity of hepatitis A virus. J. Inf. Dis. 134:70, 1976.

LeBouvier, G.L.: The heterogenicity of Australian antigen. J. Infect. Dis. 123:671-675, 1971.

Marston, H.Q.: Inaugural remarks, in Hepatitis and Blood Transfusion. Vyas, G.N., Perkins, H.A., Schmid, R., eds. Grune and Stratton, New York, 1972, pp. 3-7.

Provost, P.J., Wolanski, B.S., Miller, W.J., et al.: Biophysical and biochemical properties of CR326 human hepatitis A virus. Proceedings of a Symposium on Viral Hepatitis. Natl. Acad. Sci. USA, Washington, D.C., March 17-19, 1975. Am. J. Med. Sci. 270:87-92, 1975.

Provost, P.J., Ittensohn, O.L., Villarejos, V.M., et al.: Etiologic relationship of marmoset-propagated CR326 hepatitis A virus to hepatitis in man. Proc. Soc. Exp. Biol. Med. 142:1257-1267, 1973.

Provost, P.J., Ittensohn, O.L., Villarejos, V.M., et al.: Biologic relationship of marmoset-propagated CR326 hepatitis A virus to hepatitis in man. Proc. Soc. Exp. Biol. Med. 142:1257-1267, 1973.

Purcell, R.H., Holland, P.V., Walsh, J.H., et al.: A complement-fixation test for measuring Australia antigen and antibody. J. Infect. Dis. 120:383-386, 1969.

Purcell, R.H.: Current understanding of hepatitis B virus infection
and its implications for immunoprophylaxis, The Gustave Stern
Symposium. Antiviral Mechanisms. Perspectives in Virology IX.
Pollard, M., ed., Academic Press, New York, 1975, pp. 49-76.

Reid, D.: Prevention of hepatitis with immunoglobulin. Postgrad.
Med. J. 47:488-489, 1971.

Silverberg, M.: Chronic hepatitis in childhood. Pediatr. Ann. 6:
311, 1977.

Stevens, C.E., Beasley, R.P., Tsui, J., et al.: Vertical transmission of hepatitis B antigen in Taiwan. NEJM 292:771-774, 1975.

Trump, B.F., Kim, M.D., Iseri, O.A.: Cellular pathophysiology
of hepatitis. Am. J. Clin. Path. 65:828, 1976.

Vyas, G.N., Shulman, N.R.: Hemagglutination assay for antigen
and antibody associated with viral hepatitis. Science 170:332-330,
1970.

Wewalka, F.G.: Protracted and recurrent forms of viral hepatitis.
Am. J. Dis. Child. 123:283-286, 1972.

::

17.3: INFECTIOUS MONONUCLEOSIS

INTRODUCTION: Infectious mononucleosis is an acute infectious disease most likely caused by Epstein-Barr virus (EBV). The disease
is characterized by: 1) clinical features of fever, exudative or membranous pharyngitis, generalized lymphadenopathy and splenomegaly,
2) absolute atypical lymphocytosis, 3) development of heterophile
antibody, and 4) development of antibodies to EBV.

The syndrome of infectious mononucleosis was first described as
"glandular fever" by Pfeiffer (1889) in Germany. Sprunt and Evans
(1920) introduced the term "infectious mononucleosis," distinguishing it from leukemia. In 1932, Paul and Bunnell detected heterophile
antibody response associated with mononucleosis. A few years later,
Davidsohn provided differential absorption to make the serology more
specific (the Paul-Bunnell-Davidsohn test). In 1952, Bender and
Hoagland independently suggested that a valid diagnosis of infectious
mononucleosis must fulfill three criteria: clinical, hematologic and
serologic. Henle et al. (1968) first described the association of infectious mononucleosis and EBV infection, and this finding was subsequently supported by others. At the present time, it is generally
believed that infectious mononucleosis is either caused by EBV or by
a closely related agent.

EPIDEMIOLOGY: EBV infections, which are most commonly asymptomatic, are widely distributed throughout the world. Like other herpesviruses (such as cytomegalovirus and herpes simplex), EBV infections are acquired earlier in life among members of lower socioeconomic groups than those of higher socioeconomic groups. In developing countries, approximately 95% of children are seropositive before reaching school age. However, in the United States, 50 to 60% of students entering college have been infected, and during the college years an additional 10% become infected each year.

Contrary to the epidemiology of EBV infection in general populations, as mentioned above, the clinical syndrome of infectious mononucleosis occurs most commonly in well-developed countries and is not well recognized in developing countries. This finding is probably related to the high rate of subclinical infection and acquisition of immunity occurring early in life in developing countries. In the United States, the incidence of clinical infectious mononucleosis is approximately 25 to 50 cases per 100,000 population and the majority (80%) occurs in older children and young adults (15 to 25 years). The disease is less often seen in individuals under 5 or over 35 years of age.

Transmission of the disease is probably by close personal contact (such as kissing) via oropharyngeal secretions and, in rare cases, by blood transfusion. The agent is probably not very contagious because secondary attack rates on hospital wards and in college dormitorites are very low.

1. ETIOLOGY AND PATHOLOGY

1.1: Agent: EBV, a herpesvirus, was originally detected by electron microscopy in cell cultures derived from Burkitt lymphoma. The causal relationship between EBV and infectious mononucleosis was first recognized by Henle et al. (1968). Now there is sufficient evidence to suggest that EBV is the etiologic agent of infectious mononucleosis (Evans, 1971). For example, antibodies to EBV: 1) are absent before illness, 2) appear during illness, 3) persist for years after illness, 4) show no such relation to any other disease, 5) when present indicate immunity to the disease, and 6) when absent indicate susceptibility to the disease. Furthermore, EBV: 1) is regularly present in cultured lymphocytes from patients with infectious mononucleosis, 2) persists in lymphocytes for years after the illness, 3) may be necessary for lymphocyte proliferation in vitro, 4) produces,the disease in susceptible recipients via blood transfusion, and 5) has produced mononucleosis in one transmission experiment.

Several investigators have isolated leukocyte-transforming agents from the oropharyngeal secretions of patients with infectious mononucleosis and these agents may persist for months after the acute illness. The agents appear to be lymphotropic for B lymphocytes and have been cultivated primarily in human lymphocytes. It is believed that these agents are either identical to or closely related to EBV. In addition, there is some epidemiologic evidence to suggest the possible relation between EBV and Burkitt lymphoma, nasopharyngeal cancer, Hodgkin's disease, Boeck's sarcoid and systemic lupus erythematosus (Evans, 1971).

1.2: Pathology: Infectious mononucleosis involves primarily the lymphoid tissues and peripheral blood. There is a generalized enlargement of lymph nodes, tonsils, spleen and liver accompanied by many atypical lymphocytes in peripheral blood. Other organs may also be involved, but with a lesser frequency and severity. These include lungs, heart, kidneys, adrenals, central nervous system and skin. Histologically, there is nonspecific lymphoid hyperplasia with varying degrees of focal infiltration with atypical mononuclear cells.

2. CLINICAL MANIFESTATIONS

The clinical features of infectious mononucleosis vary from mild to severe. The age of the infected individual appears to affect the host responses (Table 17-10). Older children and young adults tend to have a more severe and characteristic disease, whereas young children often have an asymptomatic or mild infection with pharyngitis as the only manifestation.

The incubation period for infectious mononucleosis varies from 2 to 8 weeks (about 30-50 days in young adults). The typical case in the young adult usually presents with 2 to 5 days of nonspecific generalized symptoms such as headache, malaise, chills, sweats, anorexia, nausea and vomiting. This is followed by the more characteristic symptoms such as fever, sore throat, lymphadenopathy and splenomegaly.

Fever is a constant finding. There is a daily temperature elevation up to 38.5°C (or higher) lasting for 1 to 3 weeks. Sore throat is also a prominent symptom and begins within a few days after the onset of the illness. There is a rapid increase in intensity of the sore throat which lasts for about one week. On examination one finds hyperplasia of the pharyngeal lymphoid tissues and not infrequently, exudative tonsillitis or pharyngitis. Ulceration with formation of pseudomembranes may be seen in the tonsillar tissues in some cases. A petechial enanthem on the soft palate is often seen.

Lymphadenopathy, particularly the anterior and posterior cervical nodes, are present in most patients. The nodes are moderately enlarged, discrete, tender and symmetrical. Generalized lymphadenopathy may also develop.

Splenomegaly of mild to moderate degrees is present in 50-75% of cases. Rupture of the spleen, a fatal complication of infectious mononucleosis, is rare.

TABLE 17-10: THE SPECTRUM OF PRIMARY EPSTEIN-BARR VIRUS (EBV) INFECTION

INFECTION	ANTIBODY TO EBV		HETEROPHILE ANTIBODY	LYMPHO-CYTOSIS	AGE* (Years)	COMMENT
	BEFORE INFECTION	AFTER INFECTION				
Asymptomatic infection	-	+	0	0	1-5	...
Mild pharyngitis and tonsillitis	-	+	0	+/-	5-15	...
Infectious mononucleosis	-	+	60%	+	15-25	Other HA [†] negative cases due to CMV
Transfusion mononucleosis	-	+	Some cases	+	Any	Most cases due to CMV

* Age of highest frequency. The older the age on primary infection, the more severe and characteristic the illness. Heterophile negative infectious mononucleosis is most common in childhood.

[†] HA = heterophile antibody.

(Evans, A.S., J. Infect. Dis. 124:330, 1971)

Hepatomegaly is relatively uncommon, occurring in approximately 10% of cases, and half of these patients may develop jaundice. However, elevation of serum transaminase can be detected in almost all patients with "classical" infectious mononucleosis.

Skin rashes of various types have been seen in about 5% of patients. Usually the rash is a faint, erythematous or maculopapular eruption appearing on the trunk and proximal extremities (Fig. 17.4), but it may be urticarial, scarlatiniform or hemorrhagic. Ampicillin administration in patients with sore throat due to infectious mononucleosis increases the incidence of the rash and intensifies the cutaneous manifestations.

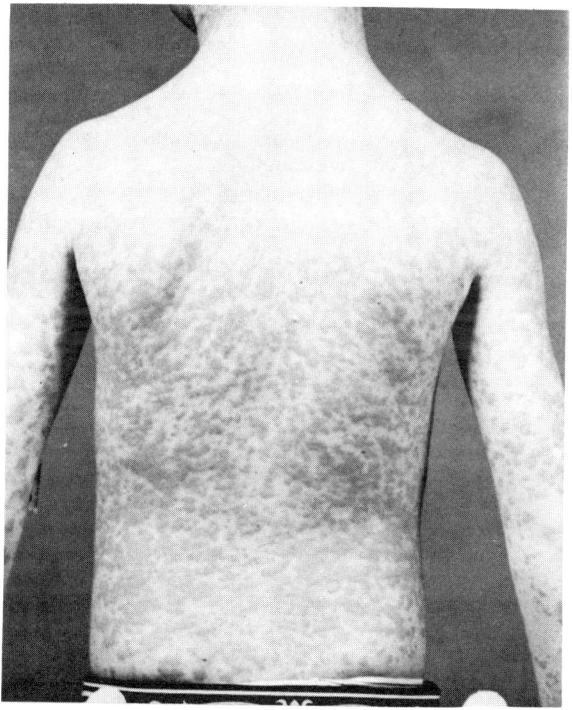

FIG. 17.4: Generalized maculo-papular rash in
a boy with infectious mononucleosis.

Bilateral periorbital edema is seen in about one-third of the patients. Other features which occur less frequently include myalgia, arthralgia, chest pain, ocular pain, photophobia, conjunctivitis, gingivitis, abdominal pain, diarrhea, cough, pneumonitis, rhinitis, epistaxis, bradycardia, etc. Complications of infectious mononucleosis may develop in rare cases, and involve any organ. A list of the complications is shown in Table 17-11.

TABLE 17-11: INFECTIOUS MONONUCLEOSIS: REPORTED COMPLICATIONS	
TYPE OF COMPLICATION	**DIAGNOSIS OR DESCRIPTION OF ABNORMALITY**
NEUROLOGICAL	Bell's palsy, cerebellar syndrome, encephalitis, encephalomyelitis, encephalomyelopathy, Guillain-Barre syndrome, meningitis, meningoencephalitis, myelitis, optic neuritis, peripheral neuritis, psychosis, radiculoneuritis. Ataxia, positive Babinski sign, coma, convulsions, diplopia, extraocular palsy, facial diplegia, hemiplegia, hyperaesthesia, meningismus, mental confusion, nystagmus, papilloedema, psychotic reaction, ptosis, respiratory paralysis, positive Romberg sign, seizures, status epilepticus, scotomata
CARDIAC	ECG changes, myocarditis, pericarditis
OCULAR	Conjunctivitis, diplopia, eyelid oedema, hemianopsia, lacrimal pericyclitis, nystagmus, optic neuritis, ptosis, retinal oedema, retinal haemorrhage, retro-orbital pain, scotomata, uveitis
RESPIRATORY	Laryngeal obstruction, peritonsillar abscess, pharyngeal oedema, pleural effusion, pleuritis, pneumonitis
HAEMATOLOGICAL	Acquired haemolytic anaemia, agranulocytosis, eosinophilia, fibrinolysis, pancytopenia, splenic rupture, thrombocytopenia
DIGESTIVE	Oesophageal varices, gingivitis, hepatic dysfunction, hepatic necrosis, jaundice, melaena
RENAL	Haematuria, haemoglobinuria, nephritis, nephrotic syndrome, porphyrinuria, proteinuria
OTHER	Bullous myringitis, endocervicitis, orchitis, otitis media, pancreatitis, parotitis, porphyria, skin rashes
From "Infectious Mononucleosis," Carter RL, Penman HG (eds), Blackwell Scientific Pub., 1969.	

3. DIAGNOSIS

The diagnosis of infectious mononucleosis is based on: 1) clinical
features, 2) hematologic changes, 3) heterophile antibodies, and
4) antibody responses to EBV. As indicated earlier, the clinical
presentation, hematologic changes and heterophile responses vary
with the age of the patient. The typical features of infectious mononucleosis discussed here may not be present in young children; in
such cases antibody responses to EBV may be the only indication of
EBV infection.

3.1: <u>Hematologic Finding</u>: The characteristic changes in peripheral
blood occur after the first week of the illness and persist for 2-3
weeks or longer. These changes include: 1) absolute lymphocytosis
(greater than 4,500 per cu. mm.), 2) relative lymphocytosis (more
than 50% of leukocytes are lymphocyte), and 3) presence of atypical
lymphocytes or Downey cells (usually more than 20%).

Other less frequent hematologic changes or complications in mononucleosis include hemolytic anemia associated with positive Coomb's
test and elevated anti-i cold agglutinins, aplastic anemia, thrombocytopenia, and disseminated intravascular coagulation.

The presence of atypical lymphocytes is not a specific finding of infectious mononucleosis. This type of cell may also be seen in patients with viral hepatitis, rubella, rubeola, cytomegalovirus
infection and many other infections, as well as in certain lympho-
proliferative disorders.

3.2: <u>Heterophile Antibodies</u>: The heterophile agglutination test
(Paul-Bunnell) is the most commonly used laboratory tool in the diagnosis of infectious mononucleosis. Patients with infectious mononucleosis usually develop heterophile antibodies during the first or
second weeks of the illness. Heterophile antibodies may persist for
varying periods of time (2 to 10 weeks or longer); generally the
higher the titer the longer the persistence. These antibodies are
present in the majority (90%) of adolescent and adult patients and are
often negative in young children.

Heterophile antibodies are nonspecific agglutinins for sheep red blood
cells and are predominantly of the IgM class. These antibodies may
occur in patients with infectious mononucleosis, serum sickness,
hepatitis, rubella, leukemia, and Hodgkin's disease, as well as normal persons (Forssman antibodies). Differential absorption test
(Paul-Bunnell-Davidsohn) has been used to differentiate various
types of agglutinins (Table 17-12). Agglutinins associated with infectious mononucleosis are completely absorbed by beef red cells
and are not affected by guinea pig kidney cells; agglutinins of serum
sickness are absorbed by both antigens; agglutinins of normal serum
are absorbed by guinea pig kidney but not by beef red cells. Variations between laboratories exist as to their interpretation of the

<table>
<tr><td colspan="3" align="center">TABLE 17-12: DIFFERENTIAL ABSORPTION OF
HETEROPHILE ANTIBODIES IN HUMAN SERUM</td></tr>
<tr><td><u>SERUM</u></td><td><u>Guinea Pig Kidney</u></td><td><u>Beef Red Cells</u></td></tr>
<tr><td>Infectious mononucleosis</td><td>-</td><td>+</td></tr>
<tr><td>Serum sickness</td><td>+</td><td>+</td></tr>
<tr><td>Normal (Forssman)</td><td>+</td><td>-</td></tr>
<tr><td colspan="3">+ = absorption, - = no absorption</td></tr>
</table>

antibody titer. Most laboratories consider a heterophile titer of 1:40 or greater (Paul-Bunnell-Davidsohn) to be positive for infectious mononucleosis. In the standard Paul-Bunnell test (without guinea pig kidney absorption), a titer of 1:40 or less is considered negative, 1:80 to 1:160 as presumptive and 1:320 or greater as positive.

There are several rapid slide tests ("spot test," "mono test") that have become available in recent years. The differential absorption with guinea pig kidney and beef red cells is included in some of these tests. The serum is first mixed with guinea pig kidney, and the mixture is then added to the formalinized horse red cells. If mononucleosis is present, agglutination of the horse red cells occurs within a few minutes. The test is generally accurate, rapid and inexpensive, but false positive tests have been reported.

The Ox-cell hemolysin test has also been introduced recently. This test does not require guinea pig kidney absorption. A hemolysin titer of 1:240 or greater is considered positive for infectious mononucleosis.

Other nonspecific reactions have also been demonstrated in the patients with infectious mononucleosis, including elevation of total serum IgM, cold agglutinins, rheumatoid factors, serologic response for syphilis and agglutinins for other red cells antigens.

3.3: Specific Antibodies Against EBV: Antibodies to EBV antigens (such as viral capsid antigens, viral nuclear antigens, complement-fixing antigens, etc.) develop during the course of the disease and persist for varying periods. Antibodies to viral capsid antigens, as tested by immunofluorescent staining of EB-3 or HRIK cells which contain EBV antigens, usually reach peak levels (1:40 to 1:320) by the time infectious mononucleosis is suspected; therefore, rise in antibody titer is usually not encountered. Such antibodies tend to persist for years, making measurement of these antibodies more useful in epidemiologic studies and less practical in routine clinical diagnosis.

Other antibodies, such as those directed against EBV nuclear antigens and complement-fixing antigens, appear later, and an antibody
rise may be demonstrated between acute and convalescent sera.
Specific EBV IgM antibodies directed against viral capsid antigens
have been shown to correlate well with the presence of heterophile
antibodies. At the present time, measurement of various EBV antibodies has not been adopted for routine use in most clinical laboratories simply because of technical difficulty.

The patient with a typical clinical presentation, hematologic picture
and serologic response seldom presents a problem in diagnosis.
Other diseases most often considered in the differential diagnosis
include streptococcal tonsillitis or pharyngitis, diphtheria, blood
dyscrasias, rubella, rubeola, hepatitis, aseptic meningitis and
toxoplasmosis.

4. MANAGEMENT

The treatment of uncomplicated cases of infectious mononucleosis
includes supportive care, symptomatic relief and bed rest during the
acute phase of the disease. Recovery is generally complete within
3 to 4 weeks and the outcome is usually good. In some icteric cases,
malaise may persist and convalescence may take an additional 6 to 8
weeks. Patients can usually determine their activity by their own
feeling of well being.

Corticosteroids are reserved for treatment of some of the complications of infectious mononucleosis, such as severe pharyngeal edema
with airway obstruction, hemolytic anemia, thrombocytopenia, central nervous system involvement and toxemia. Corticosteroids are
not recommended for symptomatic relief of the common signs and
symptoms of fever and adenopathy.

REFERENCES

Chang, R.S., Golden, H.D.: Transformation of human leukocytes
by throat washing from infectious mononucleosis patients. Nature
234:359, 1971.

Evans, A.S., Niederman, J.C., McCollum, R.W.: Seroepidemio-
logic studies of infectious mononucleosis with EB virus. NEJM 279:
1121-1127, 1968.

Evans, A.S.: The spectrum of infections with Epstein-Barr virus:
A hypothesis. J. Infect. Dis. 124:330, 1971.

Finch, S.C.: Clinical symptoms and signs of infectious mononucleosis, in Infectious Mononucleosis. Carter, R.L., Penman, H.G.,
eds. Blackwell Scientific Publications, Oxford and Edinburgh, 1969,
pp. 19-46.

Gerber, P., Walsh, J.H., Rosenblum, E.N., et al.: Association of EB-virus infection with the post-perfusion syndrome. Lancet 1: 593, 1969.

Gerber, P., Nonoyama, M., Lucas, S., et al.: Oral excretion of Epstein-Barr virus by healthy subjects and patients with infectious mononucleosis. Lancet 2:988, 1972.

Henle, G., Henle, W., Diehl, V.: Relation of Burkitt's tumor-associated herpes-type virus to infectious mononucleosis. Proc. Nat. Acad. Sci. USA 59:94, 1968.

Heath, C.W., Jr., Brodsky, A.L., Potolsky, A.I.: Infectious mononucleosis in a general population. Am. J. Epidem. 95:38, 1972.

Hoagland, R.J.: Infectious Mononucleosis. Grune and Stratton, Inc., New York, 1967.

Jordan, M.C., Rousseau, W.E., Stewart, J.A., et al.: Spontaneous cytomegalovirus mononucleosis. Clinical and laboratory observations in nine cases. Ann. Int. Med. 79:153, 1973.

Klemola, E., von Essen, R., Henle, G., et al.: Infectious mono-nucleosis-like disease with negative heterophile agglutination test. Clinical features in relation to Epstein-Barr virus and cytomegalo-virus antibodies. J. Infect. Dis. 121:608, 1970.

Miller, G., Niederman, J.C., Andrews, L.L.: Prolonged orophar-yngeal excretion of Epstein-Barr virus after infectious mononucleosis. NEJM 288:229, 1973.

Niederman, J.C., McCollum, R.W., Henle, G., et al.: Infectious mononucleosis. Clinical manifestations in relation to EB virus an-tibodies. JAMA 203:205, 1968.

/ SECTION II. DIAGNOSTIC AND MANAGEMENT PROBLEMS

CHAPTER 18. LABORATORY APPROACHES

INTRODUCTION: For diagnosis of pediatric infectious diseases, the
physician must know what constitutes an adequate specimen for microbiological studies and should provide an adequate specimen. Information concerning the source of specimen, brief history, and
suspected infection are helpful to the microbiologist in selecting appropriate tests. The physician should also know what microbial
agents any specific laboratory regards as routine and which tests
require a special request.

Pitfalls are numerous in clinical reliance upon laboratory services.
Probably the most dangerous would be excessive dependence. The
success probability of most detection, culture and identification systems may be as high as 95%; some are known to be lower, but none
are 100%. Another danger is that the microbiologist may not be able
to detect an unsatisfactory specimen because it is not visibly different from a satisfactory one. Further, a microbiologist who fails to
report explicitly that a culture result, particularly if negative, was
derived from a known unsatisfactory specimen, is derelict; yet such
dereliction occurs, especially in large and busy laboratories. The
final most prominent hazard is the telephoned preliminary report,
which is often uncomfortably and dangerously confused at some point
between the microbiologist and the physician, even when they are
speaking to each other. Precision of speech by each person cannot
be overemphasized.

1. BACTERIOLOGY

1.1: Nose and Throat Cultures: Nose specimens from children are
useful only if a localized infection exists. Staphylococcus aureus is
a transient normal in at least 25% of healthy children and adults and
its isolation, except in localized infection or in carrier searches, is
not helpful. If pertussis is suspected, the best specimen is a nasopharyngeal swab, though a careful oropharyngeal swab may be used
for infants too small for a safe nasopharyngeal swab. Because Bordetella pertussis is extremely fastidious and is so rare as not to be
generally regarded as routine, advance notice to the laboratory is
very helpful.

The dry cotton or rayon swab should be used for all throat specimens
except when Neisseria gonorrhoeae is suspected, in which case a
swab in transport medium designed specifically for the gonococcus
(commercially available) must be used. Each laboratory will have a

policy regarding throat cultures, which is probably one of the following three: 1) it may identify and report all growth without comment, 2) it may report a "normal microbial population" or a similar phrase, or 3) it may report only the presence or absence of beta-hemolytic streptococci, Group A or non-Group A. Gram stain is inappropriate, since pathogenic bacteria are morphologically indistinguishable from the normal flora. Isolation medium will consist of a good blood agar base with 5-6% defibrinated sheep blood. Whether a second plate, enriched chocolate agar, or horse or rabbit blood agar is added depends upon whether the laboratory identifies all growth or only screens for beta-hemolytic streptococci.

The clinician should understand the reliability of identification of the hemolytic streptococci: bacitracin susceptibility discs are not suitable. Limit of accuracy of the bacitracin test is about 85-90%, but error is conservative in that the test is more likely to identify a nonmember of Group A as Group A than it is to fail to identify a member of Group A. The fluorescent antibody (FA) test is technically demanding but agrees with the precipitin test about 99% of the time if done correctly. Groups B and D can presumptively be identified by rather simple biochemical tests, and specific identification of groups C, F and G, occasional agents of pharyngitis, is not routinely necessary.

<u>Corynebacterium diphtheriae</u> and <u>Neisseria meningitidis</u> always require specific requests. Each will grow on most media but neither is readily distinguished from normal populations of coryneforms and Neisseria species. The only suitable confirmation of a diphtheria diagnosis is demonstration of toxin production by Corynebacterium diphtheriae, for which the in vitro precipitin test is very reliable. Throat cultures for <u>N. meningitidis</u> are generally not helpful except in carrier and contact studies but, if isolated, must be serogrouped if the result is to be useful.

<u>1.2: Lower Respiratory Secretions</u>: The standard specimen for aerobic and facultative bacteria is expectorated sputum, which is not easy to obtain in young children or infants. Specimens from hospitalized children can be collected by tracheal or bronchial aspiration and, in some cases, by lung aspiration. An aspirated specimen must be clearly so marked. All lower respiratory secretions should be studied by Gram stain for bacterial distribution, polymorphonuclear neutrophils, and squamous epithelial cells. Expectorated sputum having more than 10-20 squamous epithelial cells and fewer than 20-30 PMN's per high dry microscopic field is probably saliva.

<u>1.3: Ear and Eye Cultures</u>: Any ear drainage or purulent conjunctivitis should be sampled by the cotton or rayon swab, except that if neonatal ophthalmic gonorrhea is being considered the transport system for the gonococcus should be used. This specimen will probably not be adequate for a Gram stain unless two swabs are used. Because of the high association of <u>Haemophilus influenzae</u> with childhood

otitis, the primary isolation media used will amost certainly include
an agar capable of supporting Haemophilus species, such as enriched chocolate, rabbit, or horse blood agar, and may include EMB
or MacConkey's agar to permit more rapid identification of other
Gram negative bacilli.

1.4: Skin Lesions and Wounds: Culture from any abscess, draining
sinus, purulent exudate, or wound which looks infected may be of
value. The sterile swab is convenient and suitable for the specimen,
though an aspirate is more convenient for the laboratory. The swab
should be applied at or near the advancing margin of the infection and
a generous amount of material collected. If volume permits, a direct Gram stain should be done. The laboratory will make no as-
sumptions about etiology but will inoculate several agars and broths
calculated to recover the most probable bacteria except anaerobes.
If the clinician suspects a specific bacterium and does not know with
certainty that it is among those likely to be recovered by the routine procedure, he or she should cite the agent by name on the request. Cultures for anaerobic bacteria, mycobacteria, and fungi can
be done only if they are specifically requested.

1.5: Urine Cultures: Clean voided midstream collection of urine
into a sterile vessel is desirable if the child is old enough to cooperate. Suprapubic bladder aspiration is suitable for infants and young
children. A sterile plastic bag may be affixed to the infant or very
young child. Catheterization for the sole purpose of specimen collection is discouraged unless no other recourse is available. Urine
from an open catheter will yield urethral and environmental bacteria
in mixed culture, possibly in large enough numbers to confuse interpretation of the report. Urine from a closed drainage system is
quite satisfactory if collected from the line anterior to the collection
bag and without urinary tract irrigation solutions. Culture of catheter tips has been shown to reflect only the microbial population of the
urethra and is not generally done.

Prompt delivery of the urine specimen is mandatory as most laboratories reject as unsuitable specimens showing no collection time
(note that this refers to exit from the patient, not to time retrieved
from a bedside table) or specimens more than 1 or 2 hours old. It
is safe, however, to refrigerate specimens up to 8-10 hours (a specimen marked "refrigerated" which does not feel cold should be
rejected).

Valuable preliminary information may be gained from Gram stain
examination of well-mixed, not centrifuged, urine. Finding of more
than 1 bacterium per oil immersion field (average of 50 fields), with
or without leukocytes, corresponds well with counts of more than
10^5 bacteria/ml of urine.

Specimens are inoculated to a good non-selective medium. All clean-
voided or catheter specimens must have colony counts derived from

serial dilution (actually little used), wire loops calibrated to deliver 0.01 or 0.001 ml, or equivalent systems. All bacteria present at more than 10^5/ml must be identified, counts between 10^4 and 10^5 should be so reported, and counts less than 10^3/ml are rarely other than contaminants and need not be identified routinely. On the other hand, all growth from bladder and renal aspirates, ostensibly sterile sources, must be identified and reported. Interpretation of reports must give heavy consideration to the handling history of the specimens, and in pediatrics a strict interpretation according to colony count may not always be possible, inasmuch as many specimens are collected at random times rather than after overnight concentration and incubation in the bladder.

Several satisfactory commercial systems for detection of urinary tract infection are available. They must be interpreted strictly according to the manufacturers' schemes. Most of these are miniature culture systems in plastic cups or wells, slides or paddles coated with agar, or roll tubes, and permit both enumeration and conventional identification. Certain others depend upon direct detection of chemical reactions, in reagent-impregnated papers, of the bacteria most expected in urinary tract infection. It should be noted that occasional infections may be caused by bacteria lacking the pathways for these reactions.

1.6: <u>Cerebrospinal Fluids</u>: Direct examination of CSF is mandatory. If multiple tubes are collected, the tubes with the least visible blood should be centrifuged and the sediment examined by Gram stain. Presence of numerous leukocytes justifies a lengthy search for bacteria; excessive protein debris may make detection of small numbers of gram-negative rods difficult for an inexperienced microscopist. The Gram stain can be expected to be positive for about half of the cases with positive cultures. If small, pleomorphic gram-negative rods, suggesting <u>H. influenzae</u>, are seen. A direct Neufeld (capsular swelling) test against specific high titered antiserum, most frequently group B, may enable a direct presumptive diagnosis. Interpretation of this test requires substantial experience. If the Gram stain is positive, one should proceed directly to the culture. If negative, direct counterimmunoelectrophoresis (CIE) of the fluid may detect 20 to 30% more infections than the Gram stain alone. CIE is not yet routine in many hospital laboratories. CIE detects the circulating antigens, not antibodies, of a limited number of bacteria and requires meticulous evaluation of commercial antisera, many of which are of too low titer to be useful. Antisera can be found for all groups of <u>H. influenzae</u> and <u>Neisseria meningitidis</u> and most groups of <u>Streptococcus pneumoniae</u>, but not for <u>Escherichia coli</u>. Antigen concentrations of Group B streptococci make the test unsatisfactory for these bacteria at this time.

Cultures must be done whether direct examinations are positive or negative. The primary inoculation battery will include 2 or 3 agar media and 1 or more broths selected around the growth requirements

of the most likely bacteria. Anaerobes need not be considered unless specific evidence incriminates them. If Leptospira are being
considered in diagnosis, special mention must be made as they do
not grow in routine bacteriological media. Spinal fluid sediments
should be inoculated and, if sediment is sparse, a portion of super-
natant should be inoculated to broth or incubated. Isolates from
spinal fluid are tested for antimicrobial sensitivity by the usual
methods and criteria except that H. influenzae must be tested for
beta-lactamase (penicillinase) production and ampicillin susceptibility by one of several methods specific for this organism.

1.7: Blood Cultures: It appears that 3 blood specimens in one day,
randomly spaced or adjusted to temperature fluctuations, will permit recovery of the agent of 90% of bacteremias and septicemias.
More than three per day should not be needed except in the face of
negative cultures with good clinical suspicion of bacteremia. The
need for simultaneous submission of two specimens from separate
puncture sites, as a control of contamination by skin bacteria, is
eliminated by scrupulous attention to cleaning and disinfection of the
puncture site. The recommended method is essentially as thorough
as a surgical scrub and consists of soap and water or alcohol scrubbing, application of an iodophor for at least 1 minute, and then removal of the iodophor with 70% alcohol in a gauze or pledget.

Blood cultures after an agent has been isolated can be used for evaluation of therapy efficacy but probably are not routinely necessary.

For an older child, 10 ml of blood is desirable, but specimens as
small as 3 ml are productive. The success rate with 1 or 2 ml specimens may not be as low as formerly believed.

The blood specimen may be inoculated directly to sealed bottles of
blood culture broth by means of a sterile collecting set or syringe,
or may be collected into a tube containing anticoagulants not toxic
for bacteria (only sodium polyanethol sulfonate "SPS" and sodium
anethol sulfonate "SAS" are suitable). Even in specimens inoculated
directly from vein to bottle, SPS is frequently included in the culture
broth for inactivation of the antibacterial capacity of blood or of
amino-glycoside, tetracycline or polymixin antibiotics. Several
studies show increased bacterial isolations when 0.025-0.03% SPS
is included in the blood culture medium; a few studies show no such
increase. Maximum recovery is achieved when each blood specimen
is inoculated to two bottles, one incubated anaerobically (sealed,
oxygen-free CO_2 in the head space), the other containing a sterile
airway to permit aerobic growth. Some laboratories may use a
single bottle system, in which case the selection of medium must
specifically exclude broths designed primarily for anaerobes, e.g.
thioglycollate.

Blood cultures must be examined daily for visible evidence of growth,
beginning the first day after inoculation. The examination must include

subculture or Gram stain and subculture after 24, 48, or 72 hours,
incubation must be continued for 7 to 14 days, and terminal examination of visibly negative cultures should include subculture to an
aerobic and an anaerobic agar plate. A few strains of Brucella
species may require 3 to 4 weeks incubation. The use of rapid detection instruments does not cancel the need for terminal subculture
of blood cultures.

1.8: Stool Cultures: Feces or rectal swab is generally adequate for
isolation of Salmonella, Shigella, and E. coli. A generous amount
of fecal material should be visible on the swab, which should reach
the laboratory while still moist. Transport kits containing bacterial
preservative are available from laboratories which regularly receive specimens by mail. Multiple (2 to 4) specimens are desirable,
even though acute diarrhea specimens may yield Shigella or enteropathogenic E. coli from the first culture.

The Gram stain is of no value relative to the usual gastroenteritis
or diarrhea, since pathogens are indistinguishable from normal bacteria. Very rarely an exception might be justified.

The policies of most laboratories will fall in one of two categories.
Most public health laboratories will evaluate only the presence or
absence of Salmonella sp. and Shigella sp. and, only for children
less than $1\frac{1}{2}$ to 2 years old, of enteropathogenic serotypes of E. coli.
Most hospital laboratories will include the foregoing plus inoculation
of a nonselective medium for evaluation of the total nonanaerobic
flora. In the latter laboratories, a collection of growth including,
except in neonates, E. coli, Klebsiella and Enterobacter species,
Streptococcus species, and a few Micrococcus and Staphylococcus
species may be reported as "normal population." A pronounced
shift in distribution will be reported specifically by most laboratories.

Fecal specimens are inoculated to one or more selective and differential agars, such as Hektoen, SS, MacConkey's, XLD, and to a
selective broth, such as selenite. A blood agar plate is added if
total population is to be evaluated. All colonies resembling Salmonella or Shigella will be identified. Enteropathogenic E. coli need
not be sought in children older than 2 years, and typing of E. coli
as to toxigenic type is not generally available at this time.

Direct detection of enteropathogenic E. coli by direct immunofluorescent (FA) examination of slides made from rectal swabs is possible, but the number of bacteria required for detection is sufficiently
large that culture is simpler and equally reliable; thus, FA is not
widely used except when speed of detection is critical.

1.9: Anaerobic Bacteriology: Data citing anaerobes as the agents of
about 8% of infections at deep body sites do not distinguish effectively
between adults and children. It might be presumed that aspiration
pneumonia caused by anaerobic bacteria would be less likely in

infants prior to tooth eruption than in older children and adults, because of the association between dentition and oral anaerobic bacteria. In other cases, the following partial list might be applied:

Likely sites for anaerobic infections: any deep body abscess (thoracic, intracranial, intraabdominal); aspiration pneumonia; surface wounds sustained in a soil or sewage-rich environment, inadequately cleaned and sustaining interrupted blood flow; septicemia in connection with proved anaerobic cause of any of the preceding; sinus tract infections.

Unlikely sites for anaerobic infection: any surface wound adequately cleaned and debrided; urinary tract in absence of abscess; cerebrospinal fluid.

Botulism and tetanus: Refrigerated, not frozen, sera should be sent by the swiftest means to a reference laboratory for toxins demonstration. In infant botulism feces also should be tested for toxin. Cultures are of no use in classical botulism but wound cultures are needed in wound botulism and fecal cultures are needed in infant botulism.

Anaerobic culture of feces is not indicated, as anaerobic bacteria comprise about 80% to 90% of the bacterial population. Anaerobic culture from fresh wounds sustained in a soil or sewage rich environment will yield the anaerobes of the environment and has no value in predicting subsequent infection.

Opinions differ as to the degree of care needed in protection of specimens for anaerobic culture. Many of the proven anaerobic pathogens can be isolated in only moderately protected systems, but many of these bacteria are not very exacting in their sensitivity to oxygen and an oxidized environment. Laboratories employing the most sophisticated anaerobic culture practices isolate numerous anaerobic bacteria not previously detected, but many of these may be nonpathogenic. Agreement does exist, however, that some degree of special attention is required and that most anaerobic bacteriology should be done in laboratories having some special equipment.

The ideal anaerobic specimen is an aspirate, collected by surface puncture or surgical procedure, from a confined abscess. Air should be expelled from the syringe, covering the needle with an alcohol-soaked pledget, and the needle should be sealed by plunging the tip into any available rubber stopper. This specimen will retain the original population of bacteria for 2 to 4 hours if kept at room temperature, and is equally suitable for aerobic culture. If an aspirate is impossible, a swab sterilized in a tube of oxygen-free CO_2 may be used and delivered in a second tube of oxygen-free CO_2. This specimen will retain the original population and distribution well, though it may be inadequate for a good Gram stain. Biopsy and surgical tissues and bone marrow aspirates can be delivered in the wide-mouth oxygen-free tube prepared for the swab. Lower respiratory secretions should be aspirated by some means which prevents introduction of anaerobic mouth flora to the specimen.

Two transport systems for anaerobics have been recently marketed and may be found satisfactory; other systems will probably follow. Should these be used, the transport system must be selected specially for anaerobes; the transport vials and tubes used for gonococci and general bacteriology are unsuitable.

Gram stains are done on all specimens for anaerobic culture, because they may permit tentative clinical interpretation and because the bacteria isolated from culture ought to reflect the morphological types seen in the Gram stain.

Specimens should be inoculated to enriched media, solid and liquid, of low oxidation-reduction potential (Eh). The system of medium preparation, inoculation technique, and incubation will vary with the resources of the laboratory but will probably consist of one of three. Simplest is conventional streaking of plates and their incubation in sealed jars, in which air is replaced by evacuation and filling with inert gas and carbon dioxide, or by addition of reagents and catalysts which generate inert gas and water from the air (e.g., Gas Pak, trademark of Bioquest). Another system involves inoculation of agar tubes by use of a mechanism which maintains an oxygen-free environment in the tubes during inoculation and incubation (developed at Virginia Polytechnic Institute). The final likely system employs conventional streaking techniques done within a large sealed chamber containing an oxygen-free atmosphere, by means of glove portholes. In all these cases, broths inoculated will be of low Eh. Clinical value compared to cost is debated for all these systems but, in general, the speed of isolation and number of genera recovered per specimen are directly proportional to the degree to which the system protects the specimen and culture from oxidation and oxygen. Isolates obtained by any system are identified by colony morphology, Gram stain, biochemical reactions (carbohydrate fermentation, enzyme patterns, etc.) and gas-liquid chromatographic identification of metabolic end products. Time required for final identification varies both with technical adequacy and bacterial identity, and may be as little as 48 hours under the best possible conditions or as much as 7 or 8 days if difficulties are encountered, with the usual being 4 to 5 days.

2. BACTERIOLOGY IN THE OFFICE

A limited number of procedures can be done in the office to good advantage. Direct Gram stains are quite popular and very useful if the clinician is careful to use good reagents, observe staining times carefully, limit specimen selection, and practice extensively. Commercial Gram stain reagents are available and recommended and will

give good results if the recommended procedure and expiration dates
are rigidly honored. Several gram-positive bacteria, including
Streptococcus, Clostridium, and Bacillus species, are unpredictable in Gram stains directly from the specimen. Reliability of the
Gram reaction can be judged by the appearance of mammalian cells,
which ought to be pink, and by including a stain of a known Staphylococcus epidermidis culture, which ought to be blue to purple. The
Gram stain is probably very useful for urines and in simple uncomplicated infected wounds and abscesses; additional material for culture should be collected simultaneously.

Throat cultures for isolation and presumptive identification of Group
A streptococci may be practical. Fresh sheep blood agar plates
are available commercially and are reliable so long as they are
fresh and not outdated. A cut deep into the agar with the bacteriologically charged inoculating loop should be made on each plate to
ensure detection of the 0.5-1.0% of Group A streptococci, which are
beta-hemolytic only in reduced oxygen.

Urine cultures using the commercial culture sets already described
may be practical. Negative results usually require no further work,
while positive cultures can be sent to a bacteriology laboratory if
firm identification and antibiotic susceptibility tests are necessary.

Time and expense required to maintain proficiency and to test media
and reagents for adequacy of quality imply that most other bacteriological work should be sent to a competent laboratory.

Private physicians should be alert to the microbiological services
available to them at modest or no charge from local and state public health laboratories. These services are frequently, but not always, limited to the diseases of public health significance for that
locality.

3. ANTIMICROBIAL SUSCEPTIBILITY TESTS

**3.1: Rapidly Growing, Non-fastidious, Aerobic and Facultative
Bacteria:** The most widely used tests for susceptibility to antimicrobial agents are the disc diffusion tests of Bauer, Kirby, Sherris,
and Turk (Bauer-Kirby) and of Barry. Both are interpreted tests
rather than quantitative reports, interpretation depending upon di-
ameters of bacterial growth inhibition. Useful working definitions
of the interpretive criteria might be these: Sensitive - 95% or more
of isolates of this bacterium will respond to the usual doses of this
antibiotic; Intermediate - most isolates of this bacterium will not
respond to the usual doses of this antibiotic but might respond if
higher than usual body concentrations can be attained; Resistant -
95% or more of isolates of this bacterium will not respond to the
serum and tissue concentrations normally attainable with this
antibiotic.

In practice, specific limitations should be applied to routine antibiotic susceptibility testing. Bacteria which cannot grow at the
standardized Bauer-Kirby conditions cannot be tested by this method.
Bacteria whose antibiotic susceptibility pattern is known not to vary
as, for example, Group A beta-hemolytic streptococci, need not be
tested. Antibiotics are selected for testing as families of antibiotics, which are alike with respect to mode of antibacterial action,
even if different pharmacologically. The current recommended
practices are that only one penicillinase-sensitive and one penicillinase resistant penicillin be tested, except for the special cases of
ampicillin and carbenicillin for specific gram-negative rods, and
that only one cephalosporin, one tetracycline, one polymixin, one
sulfa, each aminoglycoside, each macrolide (erythromycin and tro-
leandomycin), lincomycin, and clindamycin be tested.

Susceptibility testing directly from a specimen is not done. The effects of probable mixed bacterial populations, lack of control of
inoculum density, and effect of residual tissue material on bacterial
growth or antibiotic diffusion are not predictable. Probably the
clinical efficacy of relying upon published probabilities or frequencies of susceptibility of the suspected infecting bacterium is superior
to direct testing. However, in the extraordinary case, direct testing might be tolerated if a direct Gram stain or specimen source
permits strong inference that only one species is present. Results
are then interpreted conservatively, and the test is repeated as soon
as the agent is isolated.

Standardization of the Bauer-Kirby test implies that results from
different laboratories should be interchangeable; this is usually, but
not always true. The specifics of the method require that an inoculum of a pure culture of logarithmic phase bacteria be adjusted to a
specific turbidity and swabbed in a particular way onto a plate of
Mueller-Hinton agar of prescribed composition, pH, depth, and ma-
trix character. Antibiotic discs standardized at a high content, ostensibly exceeding the amount which will diffuse through the agar
during 16-20 hours of incubation, are placed on the surface. Plates
are incubated at 36C in air and the zones of inhibition are measured
and interpreted.

Use of control organisms is obligatory. The strains currently in
use are S. aureus American Type Culture Collection (ATCC) 25923,
E. coli ATCC 25922, and P. aeruginosa 27853.

The Barry agar-overlay test employs essentially the same zone diameter interpretive criteria as the Bauer-Kirby method. It differs
from the Bauer-Kirby principally in that bacteria are applied to the
agar plate surface as a lawn of bacteria, of prescribed density, in
melted and cooled agar.

Recent appearance of ampicillin resistant strains of Haemophilus
influenzae type B dictates testing at least of isolates from blood and

spinal fluid. The Bauer-Kirby test cannot be used. Presumptive susceptibility can be judged quickly by a simple test for beta-lactamase (penicillinase) production but this result, whether positive or negative, must be confirmed by either a disc diffusion test or a dilution test. Each method has been modified specifically for this organism, and zone diameter interpretations which apply to no other bacteria have been developed for the disc method.

Instrument dependent (or automated) systems have recently come into use as alternatives to the standard disc tests. They are quite expensive, but in some settings the expense can be justified by the fact that interpreted sensitivity results for rapidly growing aerobic and facultative bacteria can be available within a few hours after bacterial isolation, rather than on the day following. Extended evaluation shows that they are reliable when operated within their recognized limitations.

Dilution susceptibility tests are used instead of disc diffusion tests as routine in a few laboratories and are available as special tests in most larger laboratories. Opinions differ as to their value as a routine test, but they are doubtless useful in complicated therapy decisions. End points of these tests are the familiar Minimum Inhibitory Concentration (MIC) and Minimum Bactericidal Concentration (MBC). The procedure involves inoculation of bacteria isolated from an infection to graded concentration of an antibiotic in a broth or agar quantitation of the inoculum, incubation, examination for inhibition of visible growth, subculture from tubes showing no growth, counting of colonies in sub-culture and calculation of the MBC at some arbitrary level (proportion of the inoculum killed by the antibiotic, e.g. 95%, 99%, etc.). Enumeration of inoculum is important and, for most bacteria, 10^4-10^6 bacteria/ml is recommended. Microdilution systems are available to decrease technical complexity of the test.

Therapeutic preparations of antibiotics from pharmacy generally should not be used either for dilution susceptibility tests or as standards in antibiotic assays of serum. Some antibiotics for human administration bear molecular substitutents which must be removed metabolically before they are microbiologically active; some preparations contain minuscule amounts of preservative which are harmless to the person but are, or might be, inhibitory to bacteria; and the drug weights in pharmacy preparations are not accurate enough to permit dilution to the microgram levels needed for in vitro tests.

Assays of antibiotics in body fluids: The simplest test is an estimate of antibiotics in body fluids, known as the serum antibacterial, serum bactericidal, or serum inhibition test, in which sera from a person receiving antibiotics are tested against the infecting bacterium isolated from that person. Technically it is exactly like the dilution susceptibility test. End points are the Maximum Inhibitory Dilution

and the Maximum Bactericidal Dilution. Maximum active dilutions
of sera collected at the time of expected maximum and minimum
serum antibiotic concentration may provide adequate information for
clinical decisions. If antibiotic concentration must be estimated,
and only one antibiotic is being given, M.I.C. of the organism mul-
tiplied by maximum inhibitory dilution of the serum approximates
antibiotic concentration.

For very toxic antibiotics, or in a limited number of other cases,
specific assay of antibiotic concentration is possible for any single
antibiotic case. The most straightforward assays are done by agar
diffusion and can be done for any single antibiotic, employing the
test serum and standard antibiotic concentrations in agar defined
for that antibiotic, and standard bacterial strains. This technique
cannot accommodate multiple antibiotics except in a few situations.
Enzymatic or immunologic assays by radiometric detection are available for some of the aminoglycoside antibiotics and chloramphenicol,
while chemical methods are generally used for assay of sulfas and
sometimes of chloramphenicol.

3.2: Anaerobic Bacteria: Susceptibility testing of anaerobic bacteria enjoys no standard method, hence interlaboratory agreement
cannot be expected. Generally, adequate guidance can be had by
careful attention to published frequencies of effectiveness from institutions testing by dilution technique, the method of choice. Two
test methods of promise are available in some laboratories. The
Sutter-Finegold disc diffusion test, specifically for anaerobes, is
conceptually analogous to the Bauer-Kirby method, but special anaerobic media, incubation, and different interpretations of zone di-
ameters are used. Wilkins' method employs antibiotics eluted from
discs into anaerobically prepared broths inoculated with bacteria.
It should be noted that these two methods may disagree.

3.3: Mycobacteria: Technical complexity limits susceptibility testing of mycobacteria to reference laboratories and larger institutions.
Many physicians treat tuberculosis successfully with a limited number of antituberculous drugs, but the existence of drug resistant mycobacteria justifies susceptibility testing. The direct and indirect
tests differ only in that the direct is done with specimen material before mycobacterial isolation and the indirect with isolated pure cultures. In each, a measured inoculum is placed on a set of mycobacterial media containing drugs at specific concentrations and on a
drug-free medium. After 2 to 4 weeks, incubation growth in the
presence of drug is evaluated relative to growth on the drug-free control. Criteria for judging whether or not an isolate is resistant to a
drug are not standardized at this time. Clearly, equivalent growth
with and without drug implies resistance, complete suppression of
growth implies susceptibility, and it is generally agreed that resistance exists if growth in the presence of drug is more than 50% of
those without drug. Whether clinical resistance is implied by 1%, 5%,
10% or some other fraction of in vitro resitance by an isolate is not
yet clear.

3.4: Fungi: Testing of antifungal agents is likely to vary greatly
between laboratories. Broth dilution testing of yeasts and yeast-like
fungi seems simple, but important variables as to choice of broth,
incubation temperature, inoculum size and atmosphere of incubation
greatly influence test results. Increasing numbers of laboratories
are attempting testing of 5-fluorocytosine simply because it is less
predictable in use than other antifungal drugs, but it is still by no
means a universal test. A semisolid agar method has been suggested
for filamentous fungi. Two vital precautions regarding this last
must be mentioned. Multiple inhibitory end points are common for
a single isolate tested simultaneously in multiple tubes, and it is
obligatory that this procedure be done only in a biological safety
cabinet.

4. MYCOLOGY

4.1: Dermatomycoses: Some of the dermatomycoses may be examined by Wood's lamp (2200-3700 nm) in a darkened room. Tinea
versicolor due to Pityrosporum furfur shows red to orange fluorescence. Yellow-green fluorescence suggests ringworm as being
caused by Microsporum audouinii, M. canis, M. distortum, M. fer-
rugineum or rarely, Trichophyton schoenleinii. Absence of such
fluorescence means either that the disease is not ringworm or, more
likely, that the agent is a non-fluorescent dermatophyte, in which
case hairs or skin scrapings may be collected for microscopic examination and culture. Customarily, skin scrapings and broken, dull
hairs are treated with potassium hydroxide to remove keratin, and
are examined microscopically for hyphae, spores, and spore arrange-
ment. Definitive identification, if needed, is attained by cultivation
on mycological media, but one should keep in mind that dermatophytes
are unpredictable in vitro and a negative culture is possible even from
a specimen which is positive microscopically. There are no demonstrable circulating antibodies produced in dermatomycosis.

4.2: Yeasts and Yeastlike Fungi: Candida species will usually be
detected and reported in specimens submitted for routine bacterial
culture, but is usually identified only as C. albicans or not C. albicans. Though this level of identification is adequate in most cases
of uncomplicated infections, definitive identification can be secured
by submission of specimens specifically for culture on fungal media.
This latter course may be recommended from sites other than mouth,
rectum, and external genitourinary systems. C. albicans can be recovered and identified in as little as 3 to 4 days, but 2 to 4 weeks
should be allowed for identification of other yeasts, and it should be
noted that recovery of Cryptococcus neoformans from spinal fluid
may be especially troublesome and may require several cultures.

Yeasts and their pseudohyphae can be detected by direct examination
of specimens by Gram stain, periodic acid Schiff stain, or wet mount
(least effective). Inclusion of a contrast wet-mount-nigrosin or India

ink in examination of spinal fluid sediments permits presumptive identification of C. neoformans only if an encapsulated strain is present.

Serologic tests are not available for Candida, Trichosporon or Geotrichum but are available for C. neoformans, which are generally available only in larger or reference laboratories.

4.3: Systemic Mycoses: Systemic mycoses in the United States are usually thought of as disease due to Histoplasma capsulatum, Coccidioides immitis, and Blastomyces dermatitidis, but Paracoccidioides brasiliensis and Sporothrix schenckii are occasionally recovered. Fortunately the same systems of specimen selection, cultivation, and incubation are adequate for all.

Most frequently, sputum is the specimen needed but aspirated respiratory secretions are good substitutes. If tissue is to be submitted, part of the tissue should go to the histology laboratory and part to the microbiology laboratory for culture. Direct examination of respiratory secretions by wet mount, with or without lactophenol cotton blue due, is fairly productive in active pulmonary disease but should not be expected as part of the routine examination of every sputum specimen. Microscopic identification of the spherules of C. immitis or of the tuberculate spores of H. capsulatum is diagnostically reliable, but the frequency of their occurrence in atypical form is high. Other genera are not distinctive in appearance. Cytochemical stains, such as periodic acid Schiff or methenamine silver, may be very helpful. All specimens, positive or negative by direct examination, must be inoculated to mycological media. Absolute identification requires that dimorphism be shown (yeast-like at 36-37°C, filamentous at 20-25°C), but occasional strains cannot be made to convert.

A word of caution: No petri dish or tube containing filamentous growth may ever be opened in a laboratory or office, only in a biological hood.

In addition to skin tests for systemic fungi serologic tests may be very useful. Methods are available for invasive Aspergillus, C. inimitis, B. dermatitidis, P. brasiliensis, H. capsulatum, and the yeast C. neoformans. Test systems include immunodiffusion, precipitin, complement fixation, and passive hemagglutination. Because of shared antigens and similarity of primary disease, batteries of tests, rather than tests for individual fungi, are usual. If properly interpreted, most of these have good diagnostic value and a few have prognostic utility. The tests are most often reserved for large laboratories and reference institutions.

5. THE MYCOBACTERIA

Species other than Mycobacterium tuberculosis known to be either
opportunistically or intrinsically pathogenic include at least M. bovis,
M. africanum (not native to the U.S.), Group I members M. kansasii
and M. marinum, Group II members M. serofulaceum and M. szul-
gai, Group III members M. xenopi, M. avium, and M. intracellulare, and Group IV members M. fortuitum and M. chelonei. Whether
an isolate of any of these is indeed a pathogen in a particular patient
should be evaluated with especial care. The list of species consti-
tuting normal microbial population of the human body or of the environment is long.

If mycobacterial skin disease, including "swimming pool granuloma,"
is suspected, skin scrapings should be submitted for culture, but not
direct examination. For systemic disease the following scheme of
specimen selection is generally adequate. All specimens are collected in sterile vessels. Throat swabs, rectal swabs, or feces are
unacceptable. In pulmonary disease, sputum (not saliva) is preferred, two or more early morning specimens on separate days;
these specimens will tolerate delay up to 48 hours. Alternatives of
sputum include both bronchial aspirates and gastric washings. The
gastric washings must be aseptically neutralized to pH 7 if transpor-
tation delay of more than one hour is expected. Urine specimens
must not be pooled; the first morning specimen is submitted on two
or more separate days, neutralized to pH 7 if delay is expected. Disseminated mycobacterial disease is studied from specimens of whatever tissues are involved-blood, urine or cerebrospinal fluid. Mycobacteria may survive in these specimens but the imperatives of
diagnosis suggest that they be delivered promptly.

Specimens from sources normally sterile are inoculated without treatment, except for grinding of solid tissues, to multiple tubes or plates
of mycobacterium media, and slides are made from all but blood.
Respiratory secretions, gastric washings, and urines are treated by
one of several methods designed to kill bacteria but not mycobacteria, to solubilize mucus and protein, and to collect the mycobacteria
in a centrifuged sediment. The sediment is inoculated to multiple
tubes or plates of mycobacteriological media and slides are made
from all but gastric washings, and in some laboratories, urines.
Slides are stained either by a fluorochrome technique or by the acid-
fast stain. Slides from blood are not done because the number of organisms expected is below the limit of microscopic detection, and
are not made from gastric washings or urines because of the probability that acid fast bacilli seen represent normal body or environmental mycobacteria, indistinguishable from pathogens.

All cultures are incubated at 35-37°C (adding 25-30°C for skin specimens) in CO_2 until growth is detected, or for 6 to 8 weeks. M. tuberculosis is generally detected after 2 to 4 weeks, occasionally

later, and most members of Group IV are detected in 1 or 2 weeks.
Growth may be identified by the laboratory or may be sent to a reference laboratory. Presumptive identification of M. tuberculosis
solely by niacin production (98% of strains are positive) is the minimum acceptable level of identification. Whether other isolates are
identified merely as "other than M. tuberculosis" to Runyon group,
or to species, will governed by a particular laboratory's capabilities.

6. PARASITOLOGY

The intestinal parasite most frequently encountered is the pinworm,
Enterobius vermicularis. The best specimen is collected in the
early morning before the child defecates or bathes. Although commercial collection kits are available, a tongue depressor blade with
cellophane tape attached to the end so that the sticky side is out is
entirely suitable. The anal folds are spread, the sticky tape touched
firmly to several areas of skin, then the tape is removed from the
blade and fastened firmly and flatly to a clean microscope slide. If
opaque, so-called "transparent" tape is used, a small drop of xylene
is required under the tape. The slide is examined for the characteristic ovum, frequently containing a gently motile larva in fresh specimens, occasionally seeing free larvae as well. The principal precaution is that inexperienced microscopists seem to mistake other
fecal particles for ova more often than to overlook ova. A slide prepared as described is stable for weeks.

Other intestinal parasites are usually sought from fecal specimens,
with occasional need to examine duodenal aspirates for Giardia
lamblia and rarely, biopsy. Careful, explicit instructions about
collection of feces should be given parents and guardians, primarily
because feces mixed with urine, water, or soil are not suitable for
examination.

Because excretion of parasites may be irregular, therefore, multiple specimens (3 to 4) should be submitted unless the first specimen is positive. Ideally, one specimen a day on successive days is
examined. Generally, one expects a predominance of amoebic trophozoites (which rapidly degenerate) in watery and loose feces and
a predominance of amoebic cysts in formed feces. A specimen delivered to the laboratory more than one hour after excretion cannot
be examined for trophozoites but is satisfactory for cysts and ova.
The following specimens are unreliable: (1) the first evacuation after an enema, (2) specimens collected less than 7 to 10 days after
either barium or bismuth is given, (3) specimens collected while
anti-diarrhea drugs are being given, and (4) specimens collected
less than 10 to 14 days after antibiotic therapy.

Specimens from hospitalized children may or may not be mixed with
preservative immediately after excretion and before delivery to the
laboratory, depending upon local preference, but specimens from

outpatient children should be preserved if at all possible. Some laboratories provide collection kits, each kit containing a vial of buffered formalin, a vial of Schaudinn's fixative in polyvinyl alcohol, and an empty vial. This assortment permits examination of direct and concentrated preparations from the formalin-preserved specimen for cysts and ova, examination of the PVA-preserved specimen for trophozoites and cysts, and if needed, examination of the unpreserved specimen for ova and adult worms. It should be noted that the low incidence of parasitic diseases in the United States provokes many laboratories to adopt a less extensive protocol.

Specialized references and consultation should be sought for the examination of blood and hematopoietic parasites, toxoplasmosis, Pneumocystis and the pathogenic soil amoebae (Hartmanella, Acanthamoeba and Naegleria). Serologic tests for every parasitic disease, using one or more methods, have been described but not all have been reliable even in the hands of experts. The three tests in widest use in this country are those for amoebiasis, toxoplasmosis, and trichinosis. The potential for a positive immunofluorescence or indirect hemagglutination test for amoebiasis is high in extraintestinal amoebic disease, moderate in acute diarrheal disease, and negligible in the asymptomatic carrier stage. Demonstration of an elevated titer for toxoplasmosis by methylene blue dye or indirect immunofluorescent test may not reflect active disease unless the elevation is very great. Bentonite or cholesterol-lecithin tests or latex agglutination methods may become reactive early in trichinosis and revert to nonreactivity a few years later.

REFERENCES

Attebery, H.R., Sutter, V.L., and Finegold, S.M.: Normal human intestinal flora. In, Anaerobic Bacteria: Role in Disease. Balows, A., Dehaan, R.M., Dowell, V.R., and Guze, L.B., eds. Charles C Thomas, Springfield, 1974, p. 81.

Bailey, W.R. and Scott, E.G.: Diagnostic Microbiology. 4th ed. C.V. Mosby, St. Louis, 1975.

Barry, A.L., Smith, P.B., and Turck, M.: Laboratory diagnosis of urinary tract infections. Cumitech 2. American Society for Microbiology, Washington, D.C., 1975.

Committee. Performance standards for antimicrobial disc susceptibility tests. Approved Standard ASM-2. National Committee for Clinical Laboratory Standards, Villanova, 1975.

Lennette, E.H., Spaulding, E.H., and Truant, J.P.: Manual of Clinical Microbiology. 2nd ed. American Society for Microbiology, Washington, D.C., 1974.

Moore, W.E C., Cato, E.P., and Holdeman, L.V.: Review: Anaerobic bacteria of the gastrointestinal flora and their occurrence in clinical infections. J. Infect. Dis. 119:641, 1969.

Murray, P.R. and Washington, J.A. II.: Microscopic and bacteriologic analysis of expectorated sputum. Mayo Clin. Proc. 50: 339, 1975.

Smith, D.T.: Microbiologic ecology and flora of the normal human body. In, Zinsser's Microbiology. 15th ed. Joklik, W.K and Smith, D.T., eds. Appleton-Century-Crofts, New York, 1972, p. 355.

Sutter, V.L., and Finegold, S.M.: Antibiotic susceptibility testing of anaerobes. In, Current Techniques for Antibiotic Susceptibility Testing. Balows, A., ed. Charles C Thomas, Springfield, 1974, p. 109.

Thornsberry, C. and Kirven, L.A.: Ampicillin resistance in Haemophilus influenzae as determined by a rapid test for beta-lactamase production. Antimicrobe. Ag. Chemother. 6:653, 1974.

INTRODUCTION: Children with unusually frequent or severe infections should be evaluated for alterations in host defense (also see
Chapter 20). The alterations may involve: (1) <u>primary defect</u> of
specific immune function (e.g. antibody production, cellular immunity, phagocytosis-complement, and combined abnormalities),
or (2) <u>secondary defect</u> resulting from an underlying disease, immunosuppressive therapy or a combination of both.

A list of specific defects (Table 19-1) which result in altered host
defense is provided in this chapter. A more comprehensive discussion on this subject can be found elsewhere (Stiehm and Fulginiti,
1973; Bellanti, 1973). The rapidly changing approaches to prevention and management of infection in children with altered host defense
are briefly discussed here.

TABLE 19-1: TYPES OF ALTERED HOST DEFENSES
1. Alterations of protective barrier
2. Phagocytic defects
3. Immune deficiency disorders
4. Secondary alterations of host defenses

1. INFECTIONS ASSOCIATED WITH PRIMARY ALTERATIONS OF HOST DEFENSE

<u>1.1: Alteration of Protective Barriers</u>: Patients with alteration of
protective barriers, either mechanical or anatomic-physiologic, are
more susceptible to infections. These infections are usually caused
by normal skin flora (S. epidermidis and S. aureus) and by other
low virulence agents such as diphtheroids, serratia, mimae,
pseudomonas and candida. The types of defects in barriers and the
mechanisms involved in enhanced susceptibility are listed in Table
19-2.

<u>1.2: Defects in Phagocytes and Complement</u>: Deficiency in number
and function of wandering phagocytes is often associated with a local
pyogenic infection, whereas deficiency in fixed phagocytes (i.e.
splenectomy) may result in systemic infections as manifested by
septicemia, meningitis, pneumonia and osteomyelitis. High mortality is associated with pneumococcal sepsis in post-splenectomy
patients (Balfanz, 1976). The specific defects involved in various

TABLE 19-2: ALTERATIONS OF PROTECTIVE BARRIER	
DEFECTS	POSSIBLE MECHANISMS

1. MECHANICAL:
a. Surgery:
    General
    Cardiac
	
	Bypass skin barrier
	Foreign body as a nidus of infection

b. Skin: Burn	 Altered flora and physiochemical properties of skin Neutrophil dysfunction Abnormal responses to antigenic stimulation Impairment of delayed hypersensitivity Altered homograft rejection

Disease
    pemphigus,
    ulcers, eczema
	
	Bypass skin barrier

c. Others:
    Ventricular shunts
    Catheters
      Intravenous
      Urinary
    Inhalation
	
	Nidus for infection
	
	Nidus for infection
	New portal of entry
	New portal of entry, contaminated equipment

2. ANATOMIC-PHYSIOLOGIC: Dermal tracts	 Skin bypasses as a barrier to infection
Congenital heart disease	Damaged tissue as a nidus of infection
Congenital genito-urinary abnormalities	New portal of entry
Cystic fibrosis	Presence of ciliary dyskinesia factor Impaired phagocytosis of pseudomonas

types of phagocytic dysfunction are shown in Table 19-3. The common infecting agents seen in patients with defects in wandering phagocytes are staphylococci, anaerobic bacteria, E. coli, pseudomonas, serratia, H. influenzae, nocardia, candida, and aspergillus. Deficiency of fixed phagocytes is often associated with pneumococcal infection; however, salmonella and H. influenzae may also be involved.

Complement deficiency can result in pyogenic infections with pneumococci, streptococci, meningococci, klebsiella and H. influenzae. The mechanisms of increased susceptibility to these infections in patients with deficiency of complement are shown in Table 19-3.

1.3: Defects in Cellular Immunity: Patients with cellular immunodeficiency often have local, as well as systemic infections caused by viral, fungal or mycobacterial agents. Mucocutaneous tissues, respiratory tract and gastrointestinal tract are most often affected. Common agents include candida, herpes simplex virus, cytomegalovirus, varicella zoster virus, pneumocystis, listeria, nocardia, mycobacteria and cryptococcus. Bacterial agents (such as pseudomonas) may also cause severe infection in these patients The reasons for increased susceptibility in these patients are listed in Table 19-3.

1.4: Defects in Humoral Immunity: Immune deficiency states associated with humoral immunodeficiency syndromes (Table 19-4) often lead to pyogenic bacterial respiratory infection, as well as septicemia and meningitis. Bronchiectasis may develop as a complication of recurrent or severe pneumonia. Pseudomonas, staphylococci, pneumococci, meningococci, H. influenzae are the common organisms affecting this group of patients.

1.5: Combined Immunodeficiency: Patients with combined immunodeficiency syndromes are susceptible to bacterial infections with both gram positive and gram negative agents, as well as viral and fungal agents as discussed in the previous sections.

2. INFECTIONS ASSOCIATED WITH SECONDARY ALTERATIONS OF HOST DEFENSE

Patients with various forms of secondary alterations of host defense and their reasons for enhanced susceptibility to infection are listed in Table 19-5.

2.1: Cancer: Cancer patients are prone to develop septicemia, pneumonia and gastrointestinal infections. In general, bacterial and fungal infections are found in patients in relapse. Viral infections and unusual organisms such as pneumocystis and toxoplasma usually occur during remission. Leukemic patients have many more infections than those patients with solid tumors (Bodey, 1974).

TABLE 19-3: PHAGOCYTIC DEFECTS

DEFECTS	POSSIBLE MECHANISMS
1. WANDERING PHAGOCYTE: 　a. Neutropenia: 　　<u>Primary</u>[1] 　　Secondary[2]	Insufficient number of neutrophils
b. <u>Defective function:</u> 　　Chronic granulomatous disease	Impaired H_2O_2 production with defective bactericidal function Myeloperoxidase deficiency with failure to kill (candida)
Chediak-Higashi syndrome	Defective bactericidal activity Impaired chemotaxis Neutropenia Intact lysosomal inclusions
Job syndrome	Unknown
Glucose-6-phosphate dehydrogenase 　　　deficiency	Deficiency cellular NADH and NADPH Deficient HMPS activity Decreased H_2O_2 production Defect in bacterial killing
Lazy leukocyte syndrome	Defective neutrophil mobility, random and directed
Intrinsic chemotaxis defects	Intrinsic cellular defects in chemotaxis and migration; may be associated with failure of response to MIF,

	decreased delayed cutaneous response or defective response to candida antigen
2. FIXED PHAGOCYTE:	
a. <u>Splenic deficiency</u>:	Defective opsonization Defective clearing of organisms

Congenital absence
    Familial hypoplasia
    Post-splenectomy syndrome[3]	

b. <u>Functional Asplenia</u>:
    <u>Sickle cell disease</u>
    Other hemoglobinopathies, Thalassemia
      major
	Reticuloendothelial blockade

[1]Congenital (reticular dysgenesis), familial, cyclic; associated with pancreatic insufficiency, aplastic anemia, and any agammaglobulinemia or immune deficiency disease.

[2]Immune, associated with maternal-child incompatibility, drugs, infection, collagen disease; myelophthisic, associated with tumor, irradiation, chemotherapy; hypersplenism.

[3]Trauma, portal vein thrombosis, congenital hemolytic anemia, ITP, Wiskott-Aldrich, Thalassemia major, portal vein hypertension.

TABLE 19-4: IMMUNE DEFICIENCY DISORDERS

DEFECTS	POSSIBLE MECHANISMS
1. Cellular immunodeficiency syndromes:	Impaired delayed hypersensitivity response
a. Predominantly T cell defects	Absence of T cell cooperation for B cell synthesis of antibodies to T cell specific antigens Lymphopenia
b. Thymic hypoplasia (DiGeorge)	Defective T cell function Decreased skin reactivity Decreased T lymphocytes
2. Complement deficiency states:	Defective chemotaxis Impaired opsonization, failure to promote phagocytosis Absence of total hemolytic complement Absence of C_3
b. C_3 hypercatabolism	Absence of C_3 inactivator Defective chemotaxis Decreased bactericidal activity Decreased hemolytic activity
3. Humoral immunodeficiency syndrome:	Defective phagocytosis
a. Predominantly B cell defects	Failure of lysis and agglutination of bacteria Inadequate neutralization of bacterial toxins Decreased antibody response to antigens or infection

b. Transient hypogammaglobulinemia of infancy	Delayed synthesis of immunoglobulin with infection or antigen
c. X-linked agammaglobulinemia, Bruton's	Decrease in plasma cells Decrease in lymphocytes Absence of B cells Decreased immunoglobulins Decreased naturally occurring antibodies Decreased antibody production Late loss of lymphocyte number and function
d. Others X-linked with increased IgM Selective immunoglobulin deficiency, (IgM and IgA, IgG light chain, Igm) Selective deficiencies of IgG subclasses Selective IgA deficiency	Partial immunoglobulin deficiency
4. <u>Combined immunodeficiency syndromes:</u>	Absence of T and B cell responses
a. Severe combined immune deficiency* (SCID), Swiss type agammaglobulinemia	Delayed hypersensitivity Decreased lymphocyte response to phytohemagglutinin Decreased skin graft rejection Neutropenia (±) Immunoglobulins (±)

* Also associated with dysostosis (short limb dwarfism), Adenosine deaminase deficiency, and congenital neutropenia (reticular dysgenesis).

TABLE 19-4 (Continued)

DEFECTS	POSSIBLE MECHANISMS
b. Ataxia-Telangiectasia	Decreased T cells number and function Late loss of lymphocyte number and function IgA ($\pm$)
c. Wiskott-Aldrich syndrome	Lymphopenia Decreased cellular immunity Low IgM Lack of "natural" antibodies Failure to respond to polysaccharide antigens
d. Thymoma	
e. Mucocutaneous candidiasis	Lack of response to candida antigens
5. Variable unclassified immunodeficiency: (acquired hypogammaglobulinemia)	

TABLE 19-5: SECONDARY ALTERATIONS OF HOST DEFENSES

CONDITIONS	POSSIBLE MECHANISMS
1. CANCER:	Granulocytopenia Decreased neutrophil chemotaxis Decreased neutrophil bactericidal activity Decreased digestive capacity of neutrophils Lymphopenia Decreased cellular immunity Impaired specific antigenic response Deficient immunoglobulin synthesis Decreased RE phagocytosis Decreased macrophage function
2. IMMUNOSUPPRESSION, CHEMOTHERAPY:	Decreased local inflammatory response Decreased lymphocyte function Decreased T cells Decreased cellular immunity Neutropenia Decreased size of thymus and nodes Lymphopenia Deficient monocyte release and adherence Decreased chemotaxis Decreased release of kinins Neutropenia Decreased T and B cell function Decreased specific immune response, primary and secondary

TABLE 19-5 (Continued)

CONDITIONS	POSSIBLE MECHANISMS
	Decreased cell replication Decreased delayed hypersensitivity Decreased skin graft rejection
3. RADIATION:	Neutropenia Decreased T and B cell function Decrease in specific immune response Neutrophil function
4. TRANSPLANTATION:	Decreased specific immune response
5. MALNUTRITION:	Impaired T cell function Decreased protein synthesis and reduced complement activity Impaired migration of phagocytes Reduced bactericidal activity of neutrophils Reduced specific antibody response
6. GASTROINTESTINAL DISEASE:	
a. Protein losing enteropathy	Low levels of IgG
b. Lymphangiectasia of the bowel	Decreased T cell function Lymphopenia, loss of lymphocytes Loss of immunoglobulin

7. INFECTION:	
a. Leprosy	Anergy, decreased skin reactivity
b. Measles	Depressed T cell functions
c. Congenital rubella	As above
d. Congenital cytomegalovirus infection	As above
8. ENDOCRINE:	
a. Diabetes mellitus	Impaired phagocytosis Decreased serum opsonizing capacity Decreased chemotaxis of neutrophils Decreased fibroblast proliferation
b. Other Endocrinopathies	
Hypothyroidism	Unknown
Adrenal insufficiency	Unknown
Hypoparathyroidism	Absence of candidacidal factor (?)
Multiple endocrine gland abnormalities	Absence of candidacidal factor (?)

TABLE 19-5 (Continued)

CONDITIONS	POSSIBLE MECHANISMS
9. OTHER:	
a. Immunologic amnesia	Delayed hypersensitivity not retained No accelerated rejection of allografts Primary antibody response instead of secondary antibody response Loss of circulating lymphocytes
b. Sarcoidosis	Anergy
c. Nephrotic syndrome	Loss of immunoglobulins
d. Uremia	Defects in early phases of inflammatory response Lymphopenia Impaired T cell function

The single most important finding associated with an infection in a cancer patient is granulocytopenia. The presence of granulocytopenia markedly increases the likelihood of a gram-negative infection. Greater than 60% of the infections in such patients are secondary to bacterial sepsis which carries a 60% mortality. Fever in a granulocytopenic patient with cancer is an important sign of infection. Appropriate cultures and early antibiotic therapy are essential.

The most common bacteria causing such infections are staphylococci, E. coli, klebsiella, pseudomonas. Herpes simplex virus, varicella zoster virus, cytomegalovirus, pneumocystis candida and aspergillus are also common.

Hodgkin's Disease patients seem to have a somewhat different pattern of infection (Sim, 1975). These patients have a high incidence of cryptococcal infection as well as mycobacterial and brucella infections. They also have an increased incidence of varicella zoster and Pneumocystis carinii infections.

2.2: Immunosuppressive Therapy: Patients experiencing various forms of immunosuppression (steroids, chemotherapeutic agents, radiation and transplantation) are susceptible to a wide variety of infections. The most common bacterial organisms are staphylococci, E. coli, klebsiella, pseudomonas, serratia and enterobacter species. Pneumocystis carinii infections are common. The most common cause of viral infection by far is CMV. Herpes simplex and varicella zoster viruses are common viral pathogens. Other organisms causing infection include candida, aspergillus, mucor and cryptococcus. The location of the infection and the organism causing the infection depend somewhat on the underlying disease for which immunosuppression is being used. Patients with cardiac problems may experience pneumonia, whereas those patients with liver disease experience primarily septicemia. Patients with acute leukemia and lymphoma also experience septicemia. There is a notably decreased incidence of infections due to enteroviruses or respiratory viruses.

Transplantation patients undergoing immunosuppressive chemotherapy experience both pneumonia and septicemia. CMV is a common viral infection. It is important to note that patients undergoing transplant have an altered defense mechanism, even in the absence of immunosuppressive chemotherapy, and are susceptible to such organisms as CMV, nocardia, staphylococcus and streptococcus.

2.3: Infection and Malnutrition: Transient immunosuppression may occur in systemic viral infections (e.g. measles, congenital rubella and congenital cytomegalovirus infections) and perhaps also in severe bacterial infections.

Malnutrition may result in alteration of host defenses (see Chapter 21). Gastrointestinal disease may also alter the host defense and patients are more susceptible to pneumococci, enteric bacteria and giardia lamblia.

2.4: Endocrinopathy: Endocrine abnormalities may result in altered host defense leading to infection. Patients with diabetes mellitus are subject to bacterial and fungal infections. Septicemia, pyelonephritis and perinephric abscesses may occur. Common organisms include S. aureus, E. coli, proteus, clostridia, actinomyces, candida, mucor and torulopsis. Other endocrine abnormalities have been associated with increased incidence of infection, especially Candida albicans (Richman et al., 1975).

2.5: Others: Secondary alterations in host defense may occur with certain other disease entities. Nephrotic syndrome patients have been observed to be at high risk for peritonitis, especially with pneumococci, and for infections secondary to group A streptococci. Infections secondary to staphylococci, H. influenzae and enteric bacteria also occur. Patients with uremia have been reported to be subject to bacterial fungal and viral infections. Common organisms include bacteroides, serratia, enterobacter, staphylococcus, candida and mucor. Patients with sarcoidosis have been reported to have an increased incidence of tuberculosis and fungal infections.

3. PREVENTION AND TREATMENT

Management of patients with altered host defense involves: (1) modification of the host's defect, and (2) control of infection. Modulation of the defect in host response is necessary since without such a treatment measure, failure is increased in any given infection. Control of infection in patients with altered host defense includes preventive measures (e.g. active immunization, isolation, prophylactic antibiotics, etc.) and appropriate antimicrobial therapy. Modification of the host's defect consists of correction of the defect in the protective barrier, replacement therapy (e.g. immunoglobulin replacement, plasma infusion, granulocyte transfusion, etc.) and reconstitution therapy (e.g. transplantation of bone marrow, thymus and liver, thymosin, transfer factor, etc.).

3.1: Immunization: Children receiving long-term immunosuppressive therapy or with cellular immunodeficiency should avoid BCG or live virus vaccine because of the aberrant responses and the risk of overwhelming infection. These children may be protected by inactivated vaccines (e.g. DPT). Active immunization for children under short-term immunosuppressive therapy should be deferred until treatment has been discontinued. Although attenuated live virus vaccines (e.g. polio, vaccinia) are generally not contagious, they may produce disease in an abnormal host who has been exposed to the vaccine recipient (e.g. vaccinia in a child with skin disorders; polio in an infant

with severe cellular immunodeficiency). Thus, special precautions
should be taken in administering live virus vaccines to infants and
children with immune deficiency diseases and to their siblings (see
Chapter 25).

Active immunization against pseudomonas in patients with severe
burns has reduced deaths from pseudomonas sepsis (Alexander et
al., 1974). The use of such vaccinations in patients such as cancer patients who are at risk for pseudomonas infection has not been
definitely effective (Haghbin, 1973).

3.2: Isolation: The general approach to the control of infection and
isolation measures in the hospital is discussed in Chapter 24.

Efforts to prevent infection in patients with severe immunodeficiency
or immunosuppression have included the use of antibiotics to reduce
the bacterial flora and the use of isolation units in a hospital setting.
Both of these techniques tend to decrease the bacterial burden. Combined use of laminar air flow units and antibiotic sterilization has
reduced infectious death in cancer patients at high risk for infection
(Levine et al., 1974). There is also some evidence that either the
use of flora alteration or laminar air flow units alone would decrease
infectious complications. Techniques other than these extensive and
expensive methods have not proven effective. Attempts should be
made to minimize the chance of exposure to certain contagious diseases (e.g. chicken pox) in patients with cellular immunity defects.

3.3: Antimicrobial Therapy: Prophylactic use of penicillin or rapid
antibiotic therapy is recommended in splenic deficient (splenectomy)
patients because of the risk of overwhelming pneumococcal sepsis.
The value of prophylactic antibiotics in children with chronic granulomatous disease is less well defined. In many situations, the use of
prophylactic antibiotics will merely add to the difficulty in choosing
appropriate therapy when severe infection is present.

Determination of the causative agent, by extensive culturing, and its
antibiotic sensitivities are of great importance in the treatment of
infection in a compromised host. Infections in these patients often
present with a paucity of clinical findings in the presence of early
dissemination. Therefore, therapy must be instituted as early as
possible, even before culture results and sensitivity results are
available. Early use of antibiotics will reduce the mortality associated with septicemia in neutropenic cancer patients (Schimpff et al.,
1971). The choice of antibiotics may be based on the typical organisms that usually infect patients with specific immune deficiencies.
However, it must be noted that there is a constantly changing picture
of organisms which are responsible for infection. In addition, these
patients are at risk for having infections with greater than one organism. The organisms causing infection may exist in the patient's

own flora, having been acquired during the disease, and in many
cases the organisms may be resistant to usual or previously used
antibiotics. Therefore, the choice of antibiotics must be governed
by these findings. Correction of the specific alteration of host defense must always be considered in treating an infection with
antibiotics.

3.4: Granulocyte Transfusion: The transfusion of granulocytes has
been suggested as a form of therapy for patients with deficiency in
granulocyte number or granulocyte function. This type of therapy
has been best studied in patients with acute leukemia and neutropenia.
Daily transfusion of these patients with granulocytes has resulted in
a decreased mortality from infection (Higby et al., 1975). This type
of therapy is reserved for patients who are neutropenic with documented infection resistant to conventional treatment.

Blood transfusions should be avoided in patients with immunodeficiency
because of the risk of a graft versus host reaction from heterologous
lymphocytes.

3.5: Immunoglobulin: Immunoglobulin therapy has been used to correct deficient humoral immunity in patients with B cell dysfunction
or combined B and T cell dysfunction. It also has been effective in
patients with deficiencies of specific antibody production. Conventional immunoglobulin therapy has been somewhat restricted by the
inability to use preparations intravenously because of the induction of
shock secondary to the anti-complement effect of aggregated IgG.
The use of irradiated plasma from a related donor avoids the anaphy-
lactoid phenomena associated with intravenous immunoglobulin use;
however, it carries with it the risk of hepatitis. Both immunoglobulin
and plasma therapy have been used successfully in patients with agammaglobulinemia, Wiskott-Aldrich syndrome, Ataxia-Telangiectasia,
and certain conditions with opsonin deficiencies. More recently, investigation regarding the intravenous use of altered gamma globulin
preparations has resulted in the successful use of plasmin-treated
gamma globulin without evidence of the anti-complement effect
(Barandun et al., 1975).

3.6: Bone Marrow Transplantation: Bone marrow transplantation
has been used to reconstitute host defenses compromised by decrease
in circulating phagocytes and combined immunodeficiencies. This
type of therapy has a high degree of complications such as graft rejection, graft vs. host disease caused by the donor T cells and severe, often fatal, infection. Neutropenia secondary to aplastic anemia can be corrected in approximately 40% of cases; however,
one-half of the patients undergo severe graft vs. host reactions and
one-half of those die (van Bekkum, 1974). Bone marrow transplant
has also been used in patients with acute leukemia who are resistant
to other forms of therapy; the procedure allows the restoration of

normal marrow following attempts at complete eradication of the affected marrow. This therapy has a high degree of morbidity and mortality and recurrence of the leukemia. Bone marrow transplantation is more effective in patients with severe combined immune deficiency; these patients are better candidates since the immune response involved in graft rejection is defective. Accurate histo-compatibility typing is the most important correlate with successful bone marrow transplantation. The need for histo-compatibility usually limits the patient to sibling donors. Very few histo-incompatible transplants have been effective. Investigation is under way to make use of histo-incompatible marrow in transplantation by using stem cell suspensions, plasma blocking antibodies, clonal destruction following transplantation, pre-treatment with iso-antibodies or anti-lymphocyte globulin incubations, and techniques of gradual transplantation. In addition to histo-compatibility, suppression and aggressive treatment of infection seems to be critically important to a successful transplantation. Investigation is also under way in the use of other tissue for transplantation, such as fetal liver, that has not undergone differentiation of the T lymphocytes.

3.7: Thymus Transplantation: Transplantation of fetal thymus has been used to reconstitute cellular immunity. Successful reconstitution of cellular immunity by thymus transplantation was first accomplished in patients with the typical DiGeorge Syndrome. This syndrome is highly variable; however, those patients with purely defects in T cell function or cellular immunity have undergone successful correction of the immune defect following thymus transplantation (Rachelefsky et al., 1975). This therapy has been limited by difficulties with histocompatibility and subsequent graft vs. host reactions. Attempts have been made to reconstitute cellular immunity in patients with severe combined immune deficiency and mucocutaneous candidadiasis. Transplantation has been of little success in these patients. The major restriction has been graft vs. host reaction secondary to HLA and MLC histoincompatibility. Adjuncts to transplantation being investigated include transplantation within milliporefilters, the use of transfer factor or thymosin in conjunction with transplantation, and the use of other tissue for transplantation, such as liver and spleen.

3.8: Thymosin: Thymosin has been used to reconstitute cellular immunity in patients with defective T cell function. Successful restoration of cellular immunity by thymus transplants in milliporefilters indicated the presence of a thymus hormone. Thymosin from calf thymus has been used in vitro to induce T cell function. In addition, calf thymus has been used in vivo to reconstitute T cell function and cellular immunity in a patient. This hormone may induce maturation of T cell function and is presently being investigated (Wara et al., 1975).

3.9: Transfer Factor: Cell-free dialyzable transfer factor has been used to reconstitute cellular immunity in patients. Being cell-free, transfer factor has the advantage of not being involved in graft vs. host disease. Transfer factor has been used in patients with T cell dysfunction most often associated with some form of combined immunodeficiency (Ammann et al., 1976). It has been most effective in patients with mucocutaneous candidiasis, especially the granulomatous variety, and patients with Wiskott-Aldrich syndrome who have IgG monocyte receptors. It has had variable effectiveness in other immune deficiency states, such as severe combined immune deficiency, ataxia telangiectasia and variable immune deficiency. It also has been effective in altering the decreased delayed hypersensitivity seen as either primary or secondary phenomena with certain infections such as lepromatous leprosy, tuberculosis and coccidioidomycosis, and in patients with malignancy. Transfer factor may be synergistic with thymus tissue and has been used in conjunction with thymic transplantation. Its effect may be associated with induced maturation of lymphocyte function (Rachelefsky et al., 1975).

3.10: C_3b Inactivator: A clinical immune deficiency state may exist with C-3 deficiency. This deficiency may be the result of hypercatabolism of C-3 because of absence of C3b inactivator in some cases. Plasma infusion may partially or completely correct the abnormalities of complement-mediated function in patients with C_3b inactivator deficiency. C_3b inactivator has been purified and infused with resultant correction of complement-mediated function abnormalities in a patient (Ziegler et al., 1975).

REFERENCES

Alexander, J.M. and Fischer, M.W.: Immunization against pseudomonas in infections after thermal injury. J. Infect. Dis. 130:152 (Suppl.), 1974.

Ammann, A.J., Wara, D. and Salmon, S.: Transfer factor-therapy in patients with deficient cell-mediated immunity and deficient antibody-mediated immunity. Cell. Immuno. 12:94, 1974.

Balfanz, J.R., Nesbit, M.E., Jarvis, C., and Krivit, W.: Overwhelming sepsis following splenectomy for trauma. J. Pediat. 88: 458, 1976.

Barandun, S., Castel, V., Makula, M F., Morell, A., Plan, R. and Skvaril, F.: Clinical tolerance and catabolism of plasmin-treated Y-globulin for intravenous application. Vox. Sang. 28:157, 1975.

Bellanti, J.A.: Immunology. W.B. Saunders Co., Philadelphia, 1973.

Bergsma, D., Good, R.A., Finstad, J., and Paul, N.W.: Birth Defects XI. Sinauer Associates Inc., Sunderland, 1975.

Bodey, G.P.: Antibiotic therapy of infections in patients undergoing cancer chemotherapy, in Antibiotics and Chemotherapy. S. Karger, New York, 1974.

Boggs, D R.: Transfusion of neutrophils as prevention or treatment of infection in patients with neutropenia. NEJM 209:1055, 1974.

Feigin, R.D., Shearer, W T.: Opportunistic infection in children - in the compromised host I. J. Pediat. 87:507, 1975.

Feigin, R.D., Shearer, W.T.: Opportunistic infection in children - in the compromised host II. J. Pediat. 87:677, 1975.

Haghbin, M., Armstrong, D. and Murphy, M.L.: Controlled prospective trial of pseudomonas aeruginosa vaccine in children with acute leukemia. Cancer 32:761, 1973.

Higby, D.J., Yates, J.W., Henderson, E.S. and Holland, J.F.: Filtration leukapheresis for granulocyte transfusion therapy. NEJM 292:761, 1975.

Janeway, C.A.: Immunity and Allergy, in Textbook of Pediatrics, Vaughan and McKay, eds., W.B. Saunders Co., Philadelphia, 1975.

Levine, A.S., Schimpff, S.C., Graw, R.G. and Young, R.C.: Hematologic malignancies and other marrow failure states: Progress in the management of complicating infections. Sem. Hem. 11:141, 1974.

Park, B.H., Biggar, W.D. and Good, R.A.: Transplantation of Incompatible Bone Marrow in Infants with Severe Combined Immunodeficiency Disease. Birth Defects: Orig. Art. Series XI, Sinauer Associates, Inc., Sunderland, 1975.

Rachelefsky, G.S., Stiehm, E.R., Ammann, A.J., Cederbaum, S.D., Opelz, G., and Terasaki, P.I.: T-cell reconstitution by thymus transplantation and transfer factor in severe combined immunodeficiency. Pediatrics 55:1, 1975.

Richman, R.A., Rosenthal, I.M., Solomon, L.M. and Karachorlu, K.V.: Candidiasis and multiple endocrinopathy. Arch. Dermatol. 111:625, 1975.

Rodriguez, V., Burgess, J., and Bodey, G.P.: Management of fever of unknown origin in patients with neoplasms and neutropenia. Cancer 32:4, 1973.

Schimpff, S., Satterlee, W., Young, V.M., and Serpick, A.: Empiric therapy with carbenicillin and gentamicin for febrile patients with cancer and granulocytopenia. NEJM 284:3, 1971.

Sim, S.: Chemotherapy of infections in cancer patients: A review. Am. J. Hosp. Pharm. 32:35, 1975.

Smith, C.H.: Blood Diseases of Infancy and Childhood. C.V. Mosby Company, St. Louis, 1972.

Stiehm, E.R. and Fulginiti, V.A.: Immunologic Disorders in Infants and Children. W.B. Saunders Company, Philadelphia, 1973.

Van Bekkum, D.W.: Strategy of clinical bone marrow transplantations with emphasis on treatment of combined immune deficiency. Trans. Pro. 6:373, 1974.

Wara, D.W., Goldstein, A.L., Doyle, N.E. and Ammann, A.J.: Thymosin activity in patients with cellular immunodeficiency. NEJM 292:70, 1975.

Ziegler, J.B., Alper, C.A., Rosen, F.S., Lachmann, P.J. and Sherington, L.: Restoration by purified C_3b inactivator of complement-mediated function in vivo in a patient with C_3b inactivator deficiency. J. Clin. Invest. 55:668, 1975.

CHAPTER 20. THE CHILD WITH FREQUENT INFECTIONS

INTRODUCTION: The problem of a child with frequent or recurrent
infections is commonly encountered in pediatrics. Since Bruton
first described a case of agammaglobulinemia in 1952, many forms
of immune deficiency diseases and their minor variants have been
recognized. Recent advances in immunology have provided new
techniques enabling the clinician to evaluate patients with recurrent
infections and enlarging the scope of immunological disorders. The
general diagnostic plans and approaches to evaluate the child with
frequent infections are discussed in this chapter.

Normal infants and children are often afflicted with minor respiratory infections. Therefore, it is important to determine whether
the patient is having more frequent infections than normal children.
The average child has approximately 6 to 8 respiratory infections
per year the first several years of life. This incidence is greatly
influenced by: (1) the activity and mobility of the child, (2) the presence of other siblings in the family, and (3) the age as related to
school attendance. These infections are usually mild, lasting for
a few days to a week, and are resolved spontaneously without complications. The majority of these respiratory infections are caused by
viruses and are self-limited. These children are growing and developing normally and have periods of well-being between these infections. If the child in question fits this description, then it is unlikely that the child has an underlying immune defect. A problem of
greater concern requiring careful evaluation is the child who appears
chronically ill, who is not growing, and who has recurrent infections
of unusual severity with unusual microorganisms in a restricted location. Specifically, the following groups of children should receive
a thorough evaluation: (1) infants under 3 months of age with repeated respiratory infections, (2) infants under 9 months of age with
no exposure to other sources of infection who have repeated infections, (3) children at any age with repeated infections and resulting
in complications (e.g. chronic draining ears, chronic diarrhea, and
candidiasis unresponsive to therapy), and (4) children with two or
more episodes of severe pyogenic infections (e.g. sepsis, meningitis,
abscess, osteomyelitis, pneumonia with empyema).

1. HISTORY

The importance of the history in evaluating a child with frequent infection cannot be overemphasized. The specific data needed for evaluation are listed in Table 20-1. From the clinical history one may
place the child's defect in one of the four major categories (Table
20-2), namely: (1) physio-anatomy, (2) phagocytosis-complement,
(3) humoral immunity, and (4) cellular immunity.

<table>
<tr><td colspan="1" align="center">TABLE 20-1: HISTORICAL FEATURES IN
RECURRENT INFECTIONS</td></tr>
<tr><td>

1. Prenatal history: maternal illness, gestation period
2. Neonatal history: birth weight and length, illness, hypocalcemia, tetany
3. Past medical history: immunization history and any adverse reactions, illnesses, medications, allergies, surgery performed (splenectomy, T & A)
4. Family history: consanguinity, early infant deaths, increased susceptibility to infection, collagen, or autoimmune diseases, malignancy, endocrine diseases, heart disease
5. Age at onset of infection
6. Location and type of infection
7. Interval between infections

</td></tr>
</table>

<table>
<tr><td align="center">TABLE 20-2: DEFECTS IN IMMUNE DEFENSES</td></tr>
<tr><td>

1. Physio-anatomic
2. Phagocytosis - Complement system defects
3. Immunodeficiency disorders:
    a. Humoral immunity defects
    b. Cell-mediated immunity defects
    c. Combined immunodefects

</td></tr>
</table>

The immunizations previously received provide the basis for selecting appropriate studies concerning function of humoral immunity and for selecting the proper antigens to test delayed hypersensitivity. A normal response to smallpox vaccination generally indicates intact cellular immunity. The presence of neonatal hypocalcemia or tetany may suggest the presence of DiGeorge syndrome (thymic hypoplasia with absent parathyroid glands).

Family history is of key importance, as many of the immunodeficiency diseases are genetically determined. The pattern of illness in affected relatives may be a clue to the specific disorder in the patient. Disorders that are X-linked, such as Bruton's agammaglobulinemia, thymic dysplasia, and certain types of chronic granulomatous disease, are suggested by evidence of involvement of maternal uncles or cousins. Autosomal recessive disorders occur in siblings of both sexes. In many instances, however, no identifiable family pattern of inheritance is found. This is probably related to lack of complete information on highly mobile families or to new mutational events.

The age of onset is directly related to the severity of the immune deficiency. Infants with congenital hypogammaglobulinemia usually remain asymptomatic until the passively transferred maternal IgG is no longer present by the age of 5-6 months. On the other hand, disorders such as DiGeorge syndrome and severe combined immuno-deficiency (Swiss-type) usually do not have adequate protection from maternal antibody alone, and these infants become severely ill from bacterial and viral infections in the first three months of life. Infections secondary to physio-anatomic defects may occur at any age. These defects include burns, malnutrition, cystic fibrosis, foreign body, skull fracture with silent CSF leak, midline sinus tracts, diabetes, nephrosis, obstructive uropathy, and splenectomy. These disorders can usually be excluded by careful history and physical examination, and appropriate laboratory evaluation (Table 20-3).

The site and type of infection are important. An infection recurring at one site with the same organism is often associated with a physio-anatomic problem such as cystic fibrosis, sickle cell disease, or foreign body. A child who has suffered significant head trauma may develop recurrent pneumococcal meningitis, as a result of cerebro-spinal fluid leakage from the fractured cribriform plate. By contrast, systemic immunodeficiency, either from humoral or cellular defects or both, is characterized by multiple sites of infection with different organisms. A child with chronic candida infections of the nails or mouth, liver abscess, or osteomyelitis without an antecedent cause may have a defect in host defensive mechanisms.

The type of organisms causing infection also provides some clues to the defect. Commonly, recurrent infections may be caused by: (1) bacteria of high virulence (e.g. Staphylococcus aureus, and Hemophilus influenzae, or (2) microorganisms of low virulence. An important clue to immunodeficiency is the presence of unusual or opportunistic organisms. The presence of Pneumocystis carinii, aspergillus or serratia should suggest a thorough immunologic evaluation. For example, a recurrent infection resistant to appropriate antimicrobial therapy may signal the presence of a cellular defect in immunity. Infection with organisms of usual low pathogenicity, such as Staphylococcus albus or Serratia marcescens, suggests the presence of a possible phagocyte defect. In general, those children with hypogammaglobulinemia or defects in phagocytosis do not generally have problems with viral illnesses or immunizations with a live virus vaccine, but instead may develop devastating bacterial infections such as pneumococcal or H. influenzae meningitis or sepsis. On the other hand, a child with defective cellular immunity may have chronic candidiasis and when given a live virus vaccine (i.e. polio or vaccinia) may have a fatal consequence. Chronic pyogenic abscesses may signal phagocytic defect or complement defects.

The state of well-being between infections is also an important factor to consider in the history. Most normal infants and children, in spite of repeated respiratory infections, have periods of well-being between these episodes. In contrast, the immunodeficient child appears to be chronically ill, exhibits failure to thrive and growth retardation. The importance of growth as an indicator of well-being or illness cannot be overlooked. Children who fail to thrive may present

TABLE 20-3: PHYSIO-ANATOMIC DEFECTS WITH INCREASED SUSCEPTIBILITY TO INFECTION	
TYPE OF DEFECT	DISORDER
Integument defect	Trauma, burns, skull fractures, mid-line sinus tract to CNS, eczema, Needles, catheters, shunts, prosthesis, inhalation therapy equipment
Systemic defect	Sickle cell disease Diabetes, splenectomy Nephrosis
Obstructive defect	Ureteral or urethral stenosis, bronchial asthma, cystic fibrosis Foreign bodies
Miscellaneous defects	Malnutrition, uremia, prematurity, malignancy, protein losing entero-pathies, immunosuppressive therapy

with associated gastrointestinal symptoms, such as malabsorption and chronic diarrhea; in such patients, the diagnosis of cystic fibrosis should always be considered. Delayed developmental milestones can also be a manifestation of immune deficiency.

2. PHYSICAL EXAMINATION

Physical examination provides important clues to the diagnosis of a child with frequent infections. Certain physical findings may be associated with specific immunodeficiency disorders (Table 20-4), and these may help to give the clinician direction in further testing. In

TABLE 20-4: CLINICAL FEATURES IN RECURRENT INFECTIONS SUGGESTIVE OF IMMUNE DEFICIENCY
1. Chronic infection, recurrent or resistant to therapy 2. Unusual organisms 3. Skin rash (eczema, monilia, other fungi) 4. Growth failure 5. Chronic diarrhea 6. Hepatosplenomegaly 7. Recurrent severe infection (meningitis, osteomyelitis, septicemia)

essence, the physical examination should be directed toward answering four major questions: (1) is there evidence of failure to thrive? (2) are there other signs of chronic infection? (3) what is the status of the visible or palpable lymphoid tissues? and (4) are the associated physical signs suggesting a specific disorder? The presence of poor growth, failure to thrive, and development delay may also suggest an immune defect. Patients with immunodeficiency generally appear chronically ill with pallor, irritability and poor subcutaneous fat. Chronic mucocutaneous candidiasis, chronically draining ears, or the presence of multiple abscesses usually indicates some defect in host defensive mechanisms. It is not uncommon to find hepatomegaly or splenomegaly in altered immune hosts. Severe hepatosplenomegaly is found in patients with Chediak-Higashi syndrome, graft-versus-host reaction, and chronic granulomatous disease. The absence of palpable lymph nodes in the cervical, inguinal or submandibular areas in a chronically ill-looking child should lead the clinician to suspect an immune deficiency state. Tonsillar or other lymphoid tissues are absent in patients with congenital sex-linked hypogammaglobulinemia and severe combined immunodeficiency disease (Swiss-type).

The cutaneous signs of immune deficiency are useful and can provide the clinician important clues (Table 20-5). Petechiae, chronic eczema and thrombocytopenia in a male infant suggest the diagnosis of Wiskott-Aldrich syndrome. Neurologic signs such as ataxia in a patient with repeated sino-pulmonary infections and telangiectasis alert the clinician to the diagnosis of ataxia telangiectasia. Hypocalcemia, tetany, cardiac anomalies and hypoplastic mandible may be seen in the DiGeorge syndrome. An autoimmune phenomenon associated with idiopathic hypoparathyroidism, Addison's disease, or pernicious anemia may precede other manifestations of chronic muco-cutaneous candidiasis. The association of partial albinism with Chediak-Higashi syndrome and short-limbed dwarfism with both antibody and cellular immunodeficiency can lead the clinician to the correct diagnosis.

With the information obtained from the history and physical examination, the clinician is able to categorize the patient into the four major areas mentioned earlier, namely: physio-anatomic defects, defects in phagocytosis or complement system, defects in humoral immunity, or defects in cellular immunity. Defects in physio-anatomic barriers have been mentioned previously and in general are nonimmunologic. These anatomically confined disorders, such as cystic fibrosis, urethral stenosis, foreign bodies, skull fractures, and sickle cell disease, are well recognized and will not be considered further. Their importance is derived from the fact that they can be easily overlooked while the clinician is trying to define more complex and unusual disorders.

TABLE 20-5: CUTANEOUS SIGNS OF IMMUNE DEFICIENCY	
FEATURES	**DISORDERS**
Petechiae	Wiskott-Aldrich syndrome
Chronic eczema	Wiskott-Aldrich syndrome; Job's syndrome
Telangiectasia (conjunctiva, ears)	Ataxia-telangiectasia
Total alopecia	Severe combined immunodeficiency (Swiss-type)
Onychomycosis	Chronic mucocutaneous candidiasis
Monilia (recurrent or re-sistant to therapy)	Chronic mucocutaneous candidiasis; severe combined immunodefi-ciency; DiGeorge syndrome
Maculopapular rash with erythema, ulcer forma-tion, desquamation	Graft-versus-host reaction; Di-George syndrome
Recurrent abscesses (pyogenic)	Chronic granulomatous disease; Job's syndrome, humoral immunity disorders (Bruton's)
Partial albinism	Chediak-Higashi syndrome
Cartilage-hair hypoplasia	Cellular immunodeficiency

3. LABORATORY EVALUATION

3.1: INITIAL EVALUATION:

Regardless of which diagnostic category the patient is placed in following the history and physical examination, the initial laboratory
investigation is of great importance and it can usually be carried out
without special facilities. A complete blood count (hemoglobin, hematocrit, total white blood cell with differential, and platelet count)
can provide information on the quantitative adequacy of the lymphocytes and neutrophils. An absolute neutrophil count of less than
$1200/mm^3$ may indicate a less than adequate number of phagocytes.
The absolute number of lymphocytes should also be greater than
$1200/mm^3$. A low platelet count suggests the diagnosis of Wiskott-
Aldrich syndrome. Anemia in the presence of repeated infections is
suggestive of an immune defect, but may also be compatible with
other chronic illnesses. A peripheral blood smear under a Wright
stain may show the characteristic giant cytoplasmic granules in the

neutrophils as seen in Chediak-Higashi syndrome. Howell-Jolly bodies and bizarre fragmented red blood cells may be seen in patients with functional or congenital absence of the spleen. Eosinophilia or monocytosis may be seen in congenital hypogammaglobulinemia. Estimation of serum proteins (albumin and globulin) and erythrocyte sedimentation rate (ESR) and c-reactive protein (CRP) are helpful as screening procedures. The documentation of chronic infection by appropriate cultures and radiographic means is necessary. A radiographic examination of lateral neck and chest is helpful to document the presence or absence of lymphoid tissue, but absence does not preclude its adequate functional status. The presence of a right-sided aortic arch or cardiomegaly and absent thymic shadow on chest x-ray suggests DiGeorge syndrome. Monilial esophagitis demonstrated by a barium swallow study points toward thymic dysplasia or a combined immune defect. Abnormalities of any of these screening tests should lead the clinician to evaluate more specifically the areas of immune dysfunction.

3.2: SPECIFIC EVALUATION:

<u>Phagocytosis - Complement System</u>: The types of defects in phagocytosis-complement system are summarized in Table 20-6. The presence of neutropenia (less than $1200/\text{mm}^3$ neutrophils) may

TABLE 20-6: DEFECTS OF PHAGOCYTOSIS - COMPLEMENT SYSTEM	
QUANTITATIVE	Cyclic neutropenia, leukopenia, hyposplenism (congenital or acquired)
QUALITATIVE	Chronic granulomatous disease Chediak-Higashi syndrome Job's syndrome Lazy leukocyte syndrome Glucose-6 phosphate dehydrogenase deficiency Myeloperoxidase deficiency Defective leukocyte chemotaxis
COMPLEMENT	C1Q, C1R, C1S deficiency C3 C5

indicate a specific quantitative defect in phagocytes. Because of
inadequate numbers of phagocytes, bacteria introduced beneath the
skin are not cleared, thus preparing the way for development of
furunculosis, cellulitis, and abscess formation. Frequently, neutropenia may be caused by severe septicemia or viremia, or it may
be produced by drug reactions or use of immunosuppressive agents.
Cyclic neutropenia should be ruled out by obtaining serial counts
over a four- to six-week period, as the typical interval between
episodes is usually about 3 weeks. Any black child who has a history of frequent pneumonia and is noted to have Howell-Jolly bodies
on a peripheral smear should have sickle cell preparation done.
Chediak-Higashi syndrome can be detected by examining a peripheral
blood smear for large inclusions in white blood cells. If there is any
question about the presence of a spleen, a radioactive spleen scan
can be done.

To detect a qualitative defect in phagocytosis, such as chronic granulomatous disease (CGD), in which phagocytic cells ingest bacteria
but fail to kill them, the nitroblue tetrazolium test (NBT) is useful.
The NBT test is based on the ability of normal metabolically active
neutrophils to reduce the colorless NBT dye to a blue-colored compound when ingested. Normally greater than 10% of the neutrophils
become NBT positive after ingestion of the dye. In patients with
CGD, there are very few NBT positive cells. Even after stimulation of these leukocytes with endotoxin, most of the CGD leukocytes
remain NBT negative. Other more specific tests may be done in
specialized laboratories to determine enzyme activities as well as
the ability for phagocytic killing, chemotaxis, and migration.

Several defects in phagocytosis are associated with complement deficiencies. The measurement of total complement and the C_3 component is a good screening test for these rare disorders. Quantitative or qualitative defects of complement components require further
studies in specialized laboratories.

<u>Humoral Immunity</u>: Disorders of humoral antibody system represent
by far the most common cause of immune defects in children and infants (Table 20-7). These disorders usually present with severe
pyogenic infections late in the first year of life. The best initial
test is an immunoglobulin assay (IgG, IgA, IgM) by radial diffusion.
The test is much more specific and sensitive than the protein electrophoresis. The immunoglobulin values, which vary with age,
must be at least two standard deviations from the mean before they
can be considered abnormal. Most laboratories accept a lower limit
for IgG of 250 mg/dl and for IgM and IgA of less than 10 mg/dl. Diffuse elevation of immunoglobulins may be seen in chronic infections
or chronic disease states such as cystic fibrosis, chronic osteomyelitis, lupus, and other auto-immune disorders. Depressed levels
are seen in the congenital hypogammaglobulinemias, which may be
generalized or selective (e.g. IgA deficiency). Secretory IgA is the
major immunoglobulin in secretions, and is absent in most of those

TABLE 20-7: IMMUNODEFICIENCY DISORDERS
HUMORAL IMMUNITY DEFECTS: 1. Transient hypogammaglobulinemia of infancy 2. Congenital sex-linked hypogammaglobulinemia (Bruton's) 3. Acquired variable-onset hypogammaglobulinemia 4. Selective IgA deficiency 5. Selective IgM deficiency **CELL-MEDIATED IMMUNITY DEFECTS:** 1. Thymic hypoplasia (DiGeorge syndrome) 2. Chronic mucocutaneous candidiasis **COMBINED IMMUNODEFECTS:** 1. Severe combined immunodeficiency (Swiss-type) 2. Nezelof's syndrome autosomal recessive, normal immunoglobulins, deficient cell immunity 3. Ataxia-telangiectasia 4. Wiskott-Aldrich syndrome 5. Immunodeficiency with short-limbed dwarfism 6. Combined immunodeficiency with adenosine deaminase deficiency

patients with selective IgA deficiency. The findings of a normal IgA
by immunoglobulin assay excludes the presence of isolated secretory
IgA deficiency. Clinical use of IgD and IgE have not presently been
as helpful as other immunoglobulins in the diagnosis of immune
disorders.

In addition to the quantitative determination of immunoglobulins, the
child's ability to produce specific and effective antibody response to
an antigenic stimulation must be assessed. Since antibody to diphtheria toxin is in the IgG class, those infants who have been immunized
with diphtheria should have sufficient antibody to neutralize the Schick
test antigen. Thus, a positive Schick test in a fully immunized child
is evidence for functional defect in humoral immunity. The Schick
test is subject to error if DPT immunizations are not complete, if
the child is under 6 months of age, or in those who have received
gamma globulin within 30 days. The presence of isohemagglutinin
may be used to indicate IgM antibody formation. A child aged one
year or older should have a titer of $>1{:}4$ of anti-A and/or anti-B substances. Specific antibody titers to tetanus, diphtheria, mumps,
polio, and typhoid may be measured if immunization or clinical disease has occurred. Another test of humoral function includes the
quantitation of B lymphocytes which can be identified either by immunofluorescence using anti-immunoglobulins or by their formation
of rosettes with mouse erythrocytes. Normal values are approximately

5-20%. A lymph node biopsy can be performed after antigen stimulation, in order to determine the presence of new germinal follicles
and plasma cells. If there is an immunoglobulin loss through gastrointestinal tract, kidney, or other secretions, immunoglobulin
levels and their half-life can be determined.

<u>Cell-Mediated Immunity</u>: The final component of the immune sys-
tem to be evaluated is cell-mediated immunity, which is directly
dependent upon the small lymphocyte (see Table 20-7). The small
lymphocyte is important in recognizing the foreign antigen, remem-
bering whether there has been previous contact and then initiating
the events to limit the invasiveness of the antigen. As previously
mentioned, a good initial screening test is the absolute number of
lymphocytes, which should be greater than $1200/mm^3$. However,
it is important to note that the lymphocyte count may on occasion be
normal, or even elevated in the presence of severe immunodeficiency. In order to measure the function of the small lymphocytes,
skin tests for delayed hypersensitivity are most useful. The intradermal injection of an antigen to which the patient has been previously exposed produces an area of induration and erythema at the
site of skin testing within 48 to 72 hours. The usual battery of skin
tests used in the pediatric population consists of Candida (Dermato-
phyton O), streptokinase-streptodornase (SKSD), and purified-protein
derivative (PPD). In addition, other skin test antigens such as tetanus,
mumps, trichophyton, histoplasmin and coccidioidomycin may be used,
depending on the child's previous exposure. Since most of these antigens are ubiquitous in the environment, one or more of these tests
should be positive in the immunocompetent individual older than one
year of age. The most consistently positive antigen is Candida. In
the child less than one year of age it is possible to be skin test negative to all of these antigens because exposure has not yet taken place.
However, in an infant with history of thrush, the Candida skin test is
usually positive. Another method of testing delayed hypersensitivity
is sensitization with dinitrochlorbenzene (DNCB). At this time, use
of DNCB is not recommended as an initial test because of the probable sensitization of infants and children who prove to have normal
intact immunity. Also, it is frequently difficult to standardize the
test dose concentration because of the instability of this compound in
acetone solution. However, if all previous skin tests have been negative after second strength testing, sensitization with DNCB may be
attempted. Skin grafting is not recommended because of the possibility of sensitizing the patient to foreign histocompatibility antigens
which may make future transplantation impossible.

More specific tests for determining lymphocyte function are now
available in specialized laboratories. The lymphocyte stimulation
with phytohemagglutinin (PHA) evaluates the ability of thymus derived
lymphocytes to proliferate and undergo blast transformation after being stimulated by this mitogen. Lymphocytes from normal persons
will show 90-98% conversion to blast forms while cells from patients

with cell-mediated immune deficiency demonstrate little or no transformation. Chronic or debilitating disease may result in depressed lymphocyte transformation, but absent transformation is seen only in congenital cellular immunodeficiency (DiGeorge syndrome). Congenital viral infections (e.g. rubella) also exhibit severe depression of lymphocyte transformation. Lymphocytes can also be stimulated by specific antigens such as PPD and Candida. Lymphocyte stimulation tests are useful in patients who are thought to have intact cellular immunity response to a specific antigen, but who demonstrate a negative delayed hypersensitivity response. If the patient's lymphocytes are incubated with the antigen and transformation occurs, this illustrates a specific defect in recognition of the antigen, as might be found in chronic mucocutaneous candidiasis. Foreign cells from mixed lymphocytes cultures can also be used to stimulate lymphocytes and study their ability to recognize foreign cells.

The measurement of thymic-derived lymphocytes (T cells) is possible because of their peculiar property of permitting the binding of sheep red blood cells to their surface membranes, forming what is termed T cell rosettes. Normally, 60-70% of the peripheral blood mononuclear cells undergo this reaction. Severely depressed numbers of T cells (less than 20%) are seen in most cellular immunodeficiency disorders, but have also been observed in acute and chronic viral infection, malignancy, and during immunosuppressive therapy.

Another specialized test that may be performed is the measurement of lymphokines such as migration inhibitory factor (MIF) produced by T cell lymphocytes following exposure to specific antigen or mitogen. This lymphokine prevents migration of macrophages from an area surrounding the lymphocytes in the presence of antigen. Production of MIF is felt to correlate well with delayed hypersensitivity and the presence of intact cell-mediated immunity.

4. SUMMARY

Infants and children with frequent infections requiring special attention are easily identified by history and physical examination. The defect in host defense, if present, can be evaluated according to the following systems: physioanatomic, phagocytosis-complement, humoral immunity and cellular immunity. The majority of patients with frequent infections do not have an identifiable cause, even with the extensive evaluation. However, every effort should be made to diagnose the child who has an underlying defect which may be amenable to therapy. Infections associated with primary and secondary alterations of host defense and their therapy are discussed in Chapter 19.

REFERENCES

Alper, C.A., Abramson, N., Johnston, R.B., Jr., Jandl, J.H. and Rosen, F.S.: Increased susceptibility to infection associated with abnormalities of complement mediated functions and of the third component of complement (C3). NEJM 282:349, 1970.

Ammann, A.J. and Hong, R.: Selective IgA deficiency: Presentation of 30 cases and a review of the literature. Medicine 50:223, 1971.

Ammann, A.J. and Wara, D.W.: Evaluation of Infants and Children With Recurrent Infection. Current Problems in Pediatrics. Yearbook Med. Publishers, Chicago, 1975.

Bellanti, J.A. and Schlegal, R.J.: The diagnosis of immune deficiency diseases. Pediatr. Clin. N.A. 18:49, 1971.

Bergsma, D., ed.: Immunodeficiency in man and animals. Birth Defects, Original Article Series. Vol. 11, No. 1. The National Foundation, 1975.

Buckley, R.H , Dees, S.C., and O'Fallon, W.M.: Serum immunoglobulins. II. Levels in children subject to recurrent infection. Pediatrics 42:50, 1968.

David, J.R.: Lymphocyte mediators and cellular hypersensitivity. NEJM 288:143, 1973.

Edelson, P.J.: Diagnosis of immunologic deficiency in childhood. Calif. Med. 116:19, 1972.

Fudenberg, H., Good, R.A., Goodman, H.C., Hitzig, W., Kunkel, H.G., Roitt, I.M., Rosen, F.S., Rowe, D.S., Seligmann, M., and Soothill, J.R.: Primary immunodeficiencies. Reports of a World Health Organization committee. Pediatrics 47:927-946, 1971.

Geha, R.F., Schneeberger, E., Merler, E., and Rosen, F.S.: Heterogeneity of "acquired" or common variable agammaglobulinemia. NEJM 291:1-6, 1974.

Hill, H.R., Ochs, H.D., Quie, P.G., Clark, R.A., Pabst, H.F., Klebanoff, S.J , and Wedgwood, R.J.: Defect in neutrophil granulocyte chemotaxis in Job's syndrome or recurrent "cold" staphylococcal abscesses. Lancet 2:617-623, 1974.

Johnston, R.B., Jr. and Baehner, R.L.: Chronic granulomatous disease: Correlation between pathogenesis and clinical findings. Pediatrics 48:730-739, 1971.

Johnston, R.B., Jr. and Janeway, C.A.: The child with frequent infections: diagnostic considerations. Pediatrics 43:596-600, 1969.

Miller, M.E.: Enhanced susceptibility to infection. Med. Clin. N.A. 54:713-722, 1970.

Norman, M.E. and South, M.A.: Evaluation of children for immunologic deficiency disease. Clin. Pediatr. 13:644, 1974.

Quie, P.G.: Infections due to neutrophil malfunction. Medicine 52:411, 1973.

Robbins, J.B., Eitzman, D.V., and Ellis, E.F.: Immunochemical evidence for the development of an "acquired" hypogammaglobulinemic state. NEJM 274:607, 1966.

Schlegel, R.J.: Chronic granulomatous disease, 1974. JAMA 231:615, 1975.

Schur, P.H., Borel, H., Gelfand, E.W., Alper, C.A., and Rosen, R.S.: Selective gamma-G globulin deficiencies in patients with recurrent pyogenic infections. NEJM 283:631, 1970.

Seeger, R.C. and Stiehm, E.R.: T and B lymphocyte populations. Pediatrics 55:157, 1975.

Stiehm, E.R. and Fulginiti, V.A., eds.: Immunologic Disorders in Infants and Children. W.B. Saunders Co., Philadelphia, 1973.

Stossel, T.P.: Phagocytosis. NEJM 290:717, 774, 833, 1974.

Tomasi, T.B., Jr.: Secretory immunoglobulins. NEJM 287:500, 1972.

Waldman, R.H. and Ganguly, R.: Immunity to infections on secretory surfaces. J. Infect. Dis. 130:419, 1974.

Winkelstein, J.A.: Opsonins: Their function, identity, and clinical significance. J. Pediatr. 82:747, 1973.

INTRODUCTION: "A full stomach is like Heaven, everything else
is luxury." This Chinese proverb supports the fact that throughout
a large part of the world malnutrition and infection are the two most
important factors determining the health of infants and children.

Nutritional factors play a significant role in resistance to infection.
Epidemics of contagious diseases occurred repeatedly after war and
famine in human history. It is believed that the well-nourished host
is more resistant to infection than the malnourished, and the clinical course and severity of infection are more severe in an under-
nourished host. Although data from controlled experiments in humans are not available, epidemiological studies and animal experiments provide evidence that depletion of protein, vitamins, iron,
or other nutritive elements is often associated with increased vul-
nerability to infections.

Infections in infants and children often lead to malnutrition. Many
infections, either symptomatic or asymptomatic, are capable of inducing negative nitrogen balance, anorexia, and dietary restriction.
The synergy of malnutrition and infection contribute to subsequent
impaired learning in older children and to excess mortality in infants
and young children. The possibility of synergy is always present
whenever malnutrition and infection coexist. Thus, treatment of infectious disease in infants and children with nutritional deficiency
should always consider the potential interaction of the two processes.

The growing interest in nutrition and infection is underpinned by the
realization that primary health problems of the foreseeable future
for a majority of the world population will relate directly to the
quantity and quality of the food supply. Public health policy as well
as medical practice will be profoundly affected. It must be remem-
bered that while it is most convenient to discuss "the infectious agent"
in relation to a specific clinical complex, what is actually occurring
is a multi-causal chain of events which are rooted in both sociocultural and biomedical spheres (Kass, 1971). In order to adequately
describe, prevent, and treat disease, all links in the chain must be
considered. The interactions of nutritional disorders with infectious
disease, the understanding of which is at this time merely beginning,
will certainly prove basic to any effort to improve the health of the
world's children.

1. INTERACTION OF NUTRITION AND INFECTION

The low prevalence of both malnutrition and infectious disease in the
industrialized world does not often provide an opportunity to observe

their interaction. However, in developing countries and in poverty regions of the industrialized world, clinicians are impressed by the frequent association of the two conditions.

Studies isolating deficiencies of one nutrient and one infectious agent are limited to laboratory animals except under unusual circumstances. Thus, most of the knowledge about the interactions of nutrition and infection has developed from epidemiologic studies of children with protein-calorie malnutrition.

Animal experiments have demonstrated that the interaction of malnutrition and infection may be synergistic or antagonistic; in other words, the resulting morbidity and mortality are greater (synergism) or less (antagonism) than the sum of disease from malnutrition and infection acting separately. The usual effect of the interaction of malnutrition and infection is that of synergism. Clinically, antagonism between malnutrition and infection is of only theoretical importance, because when the host suffers from a nutrient deficiency severe enough to suppress the growth of a microbial agent, the deficiency itself will result in interference with host defense to such an extent that the expected antagonism will not be seen (Scrimshaw, et al., 1968).

A disorder known as weaning diarrhea demonstrates how the interaction of infection with malnutrition occurring at the time of weaning results in synergism. Recurrent bouts of infectious diarrhea in these infants will precipitate acute episodes of protein-calorie malnutrition, which in turn can cause malabsorption and further malnourishment. If this cycle is uninterrupted, death or severe growth retardation is the outcome. As reported by Scrimshaw and colleagues (1968), death from diarrheal diseases among the preschool age group in a Guatemalan population was 500 times that of a corresponding age group in the U.S.A. Alteration of intestinal flora may be responsible for the high incidence of diarrheal diseases in malnourished children. Mata and colleagues (1971) studied the indigenous flora of healthy children and those suffering from protein-calorie malnutrition in the same ecosystem. They found no difference in total bacterial counts from stomach, jejunal or ileal aspirates or fecal specimens, but the children suffering from protein-calorie malnutrition had less variety in their flora and more colonization with Proteus, Pseudomonas and other gram-negative bacilli.

Two basic types of protein-calorie malnutrition are seen: (1) Kwashiorkor is a severe protein deficiency with or without caloric depletion in which high carbohydrate foods (such as gruels deficient in protein, essential fatty acids and other nutrients) are consumed nearly exclusively, resulting in growth failure. Clinically, kwashiorkor is characterized by pitting edema, hyperpigmented, hyperkeratotic skin lesions (especially of the lower extremities and trunk), anorexia, diarrhea and vomiting, and a unique demeanor of apathy, indifference and lethargy when undisturbed, changing to irritability when stimulated. (2) <u>Marasmus</u> is a disorder in which a deficiency of all essential nutrients produce caloric depletion and growth failure accompanied by generalized wasting of fat and muscle, loss of skin turgor, abdominal distension, alert behavior and good appetite.

2. EFFECTS OF NUTRITIONAL STATUS ON SUSCEPTIBILITY TO INFECTION

It is generally believed that malnutrition increases the host's susceptibility to infectious diseases. Varying degrees of nutritional deficiency are frequently seen in infants and children with chronic diseases, and in hospitalized children who have debilitating diseases with prolonged inadequate nutrition (e.g. patients requiring extended intensive care, disease of the central nervous system, postoperative states, gastrointestinal disease, etc.). Nutritional deficiency may adversely affect host defense mechanisms. Deficiency of some proteins, amino acids, and vitamins are known to alter the host functions (Table 21-1).

TABLE 21-1: HOST DEFENSE FACTORS AFFECTED BY VARIOUS NUTRITIONAL DEFICIENCIES

HOST FACTORS	NUTRITIONAL DEFICIENCIES
1. Suppression of antibody formation	Protein, vitamins A and C, riboflavin, thiamine, pantothenic acid, biotin, niacin, tryptophan, pyroxidine
2. Depression of phagocytic activity	Kwashiorkor, vitamins A and C, riboflavin, thiamine, folic acid
3. Loss of tissue integrity*	Vitamins A and C, niacin and protein
4. Impaired formation of collagen**	Protein, methionine, vitamin C
5. Alteration of intestinal flora	Protein, calories

* Reduced mucus secretions, increased mucosa permeability, epithelial metaplasia, edema.

**Necessary for localizing infections.

Recently, various immunologic functions have been studied in children with protein-calorie malnutrition. Studies on the mechanisms of enhanced susceptibility to infection in protein-calorie malnutrition show that these patients demonstrate defects in host resistance factors, including cell-mediated immunity, phagocytic functions and perhaps humoral immunity.

2.1: Cell-Mediated Immunity (T-Cell Function): Malnourished children, including newborn infants, are prone to certain infections that are seen in a variety of conditions, such as some reticuloses, Hodgkin's disease, burn patients, and patients receiving immunosuppressive therapy. Malnourished children are more susceptible to gram-negative septicemia, disseminated herpesvirus infection, and have a tendency to develop gangrene rather than suppuration. Responses to skin tests are diminished (Edelman et al., 1973). Negative tuberculin skin tests are seen in face of active pulmonary and joint tuberculosis (Harland et al., 1965; Geefhuysen et al., 1971; and Chandra, 1972). Children with protein-calorie malnutrition are found to have depletion of T cells in the thymo-lymphatic tissues and depressed T cell function by in vitro studies (Smythe et al., 1971).

2.2: Phagocytosis: Phagocytosis is the process whereby the invading organisms are ingested and killed by the host's leukocytes. The four steps involved are chemotaxis, opsonization, ingestion and killing. Chemotaxis and opsonization are enhanced by the factors present in the complement cascade. Serum levels of complement and its components are markedly reduced in individuals with protein-calorie malnutrition, and these levels return toward normal with adequate dietary therapy (Chandra, 1975a, Sirishana et al., 1973). Ingestion and killing of bacteria are energy-dependent processes (i.e., engulfment of bacteria requires the glycolytic energy and destruction of bacteria needs the oxidative metabolic energy). Malnourished patients have derangement of these energy processes, which improve following dietary therapy (Selvaraj et al., 1972; Arbeter et al., 1971).

2.3: Humoral Immunity: The role of immunoglobulin in resistance to infection in the malnourished is less clear. Serum immunoglobulin levels in malnourished children are variable. Some studies showed nearly adult levels of IgG and IgM by the first year of life. Others have reported nearly absent levels in their malnourished populations. Secretory IgA is shown to be reduced in malnourished children (Chandra, 1975b).

2.4: Iron-Deficiency Anemia and Infection: Iron-deficiency anemia, a common nutritional problem among infants and children, is thought to predispose to an increased incidence of infectious diseases (Mackay, 1928; Andelman et al., 1966). The frequency of respiratory infections and gastroenteritis is said to be reduced through improving the nutritional status by feeding a formula containing iron. The possible relationship between a severe vital infection and malnutrition associated with iron-deficiency among socially less privileged populations has also been suggested (Lang et al., 1969). Contrary to the above suggestions, other studies have failed to identify a relationship between iron-deficiency anemia and the risk of infection (Burman, 1972; Masawe et al., 1974). The varying severity of anemia and the presence or absence of concomitant deficiency of other nutrients may be responsible for the variable clinical observations.

Assessments of host defense mechanisms in children with iron-deficiency anemia have also yielded contradictory results. Some investigators have found that iron-deficiency anemia is associated with reduction of bactericidal capacity of leukocytes and a diminished lymphocyte responsiveness, but others have failed to find such a relationship. The controversy over the clinical and laboratory aspects of iron-deficiency and infection has been reviewed recently (Lukens, 1975; Buckley, 1975).

Weinberg suggested (1974) that iron-deficiency exerts a beneficial effect in defense against bacterial infection. There are in vitro and animal data that demonstrate impaired growth of bacterial pathogens in iron-deficient environments and sequestering of serum iron in infected animals.

Thus, available data suggest there are both synergistic (depressed host defense) as well as antagonistic (impaired microbial growth) effects of iron-deficiency on infectious disease. Further study may provide answers as to which effect is most important in a given clinical situation.

3. EFFECTS OF INFECTION ON NUTRITIONAL STATUS

The effects of nutritional status on susceptibility to infections are mediated primarily through biochemical and physiologic processes discussed in the previous section. In contrast, the effects of infections on the host's nutritional status are mediated through anatomic, physiologic, and sociocultural processes.

Anatomic processes involving the effects of infection on nutrition include diarrhea, tissue inflammation and necrosis, increased mucus secretion, fatty changes in the liver, as well as skin and hair changes. Many of these changes lead to malabsorption and maldigestion.

The physiological processes mediating the effects of infections on nutrition are: (1) hypermetabolism (fever, leukocytosis, increased secretion, adrenal corticosteroids, alteration of nitrogen, folate, iron, etc.), and (2) decreased intake secondary to anorexia.

The sociocultural dimension of the effects of nutrition on infection are food habits and folk-medical beliefs and practices. ("He that eats till he is sick must fast till he is well" - English proverb.) The catabolic effects of infectious diseases may be intensified by dietary practices that restrict intake of nutrients or fluids during illness.

Other processes that are essentially developmental can be of significance. The effects of infection on nutrition are more profound for mother and fetus or infant than at later stages in their lives (Mata et al., 1972; Lee and Dubos, 1968).

In considering specific nutrients, protein and nitrogen have been the earliest and most extensively studied. Increase in nitrogen excretion in the urine in patients with typhoid fever was described over a century ago and even with chloramphenicol treatment, this is still a major feature of the disease (Woodward and Smadel, 1964). Many clinical and epidemiological studies emphasize the role of infection in precipitating kwashiorkor in children with chronic, subclinical malnutrition. Nitrogen loss is related to two factors: (1) decreased absorption in the gut, probably secondary to decreased transit time or local mucosal alterations, and (2) altered catabolism resulting in markedly increased urinary excretion. The latter effect is more pronounced in well-nourished subjects, while those malnourished with a reduced nitrogen reserve show less excretion. Dietary increase in nitrogen intake will overcome the effects of decreased absorption (Scrimshaw et al., 1968). Specific microbial agents known to affect the nitrogen metabolism in humans and in animals adversely are shown in Table 21-2. In addition to the effect on nitrogen metabolism, infection may induce deficiency of various nutrients (Table 21-3).

4. TOTAL PARENTERAL NUTRITION AND SEPSIS

The provision of amino acids, lipids, vitamins, minerals and glucose in the form of hyperosmolar solutions by venous infusion to debilitated and post-surgical infants and children has become a widely accepted form of therapy. Total parenteral nutrition (TPN) allows many patients to grow and develop despite major conditions previously associated with inanition and death. Accompanying the therapeutic benefits of this procedure are the complications of sepsis, venous thrombosis, and the increased risk of metabolic derangements. The incidence of septicemia complicating TPN has varied from 6 to 27 percent (Goldman and Maki, 1973). Candida septicemia is most often encountered in sepsis associated with in-dwelling catheters. Other agents involved are _Staphylococcus aureus_, _Staphylococcus epidermidis_ and gram-negative bacilli.

		DATA FROM	
MICROORGANISM	AGENT	HUMANS	ANIMALS
Bacteria	Mycobacterium tuberculosis	+	+
	Salmonella species	+	+
	Pasturella tularensis	+	+
	Staphylococcus	+	
	Bacillus abortus		+
Viruses	Venezuelan encephalomyelitis		+
	Newcastle disease		+
	Poliovirus	+	
	Chicken pox	+	
	Measles	+	
	Rubella	+	
	Influenza	+	
	Yellow fever and smallpox	+	
Rickettsiae	Rocky mountain spotted fever	+	
	Q-fever	+	
Protozoa	Plasmodium berghei		+
	P. gallinaceum		+
	P. vivax	+	
	Giardia lamblia	+	
	Trypanosoma species		+

TABLE 21-2: SPECIFIC INFECTIONS WHICH ADVERSELY AFFECT THE NITROGEN METABOLISM IN HUMANS AND ANIMALS

Data from Scrimshaw et al. 1968.

There are several reasons for the increased incidence of sepsis in patients receiving TPN:

1. Use of broad spectrum antibiotics that alter the patient's flora prior to or during TPN and thus predispose patients to sepsis by fungi.

2. Contamination of the catheter at the time of placement, secondary to breaks in sterile technique.

3. Radiation, corticosteroid therapy and immunosuppressants.

TABLE 21-3: SPECIFIC NUTRIENTS ADVERSELY AFFECTED BY INFECTIONS			
	IN SPECIFIED STUDY		
NUTRIENTS	CLINICAL*	FIELD**	ANIMAL
Vitamin A	+	+	+
Thiamine	+	+	+
Other B complex vitamins		+	+
Vitamin C	+	+	+
Vitamin D	+		
Vitamin K			+
Glucose	+		+

*Clinical study here means retrospective or prospective study carried out with small group of designated patients.

**Field study here means study designed with epidemiologic methods in large population usually sampling techniques.

Data from Schrimshaw et al. 1968, Cook et al. 1974, Rayfield et al. 1973, and Yueng et al. 1973.

4. Bacterial and fungal contamination of TPN solutions.

5. Immune deficiency secondary to the malnourished state which makes a patient a candidate for TPN.

Because of the high risk of sepsis in TPN, several principles should be followed in its use (Goldman and Malki, 1973; Ryan et al., 1974):

1. TPN should be initiated only after careful weighing of potential benefits versus potential risk by a physician knowledgeable in its techniques and complications.

2. A team of physicians, nurses and pharmacists with particular interest and expertise should be responsible for overseeing TPN therapy.

3. A detailed protocol for preparation, administration and maintenance of TPN solutions and catheters, emphasizing adequate infection control measures, should be instituted.

4. The TPN catheter should be placed in the standard fashion (Dudrick, 1968; Ryan et al., 1974).

5. Frequent inspection of insertion site with sterile technique should be instituted. Any signs of local inflammation, thrombosis or leakage should result in immediate withdrawal.

6. Infections via TPN catheters should be considered in the differential diagnosis of unexplained fever. If no other source of infection is found, the catheter should be removed. Once removed it should not be replaced for 24 hours, but the patient should be maintained on peripheral glucose and electrolyte solution.

7. The catheter should not be used for withdrawal of blood samples, administration of medication, monitoring of central venous pressures or anything else but TPN.

5. THE NEONATE

The neonate differs from the adult as well as from the child in that it is in a transitional state between complete maternal dependence and complete independence. The neonate's defense mechanisms, responses to infection, and nutritional needs are sufficiently different that a separate brief consideration is warranted (also see Chapter 8).

The manner whereby the factors of maternal infection and maternal malnutrition effect the nutritional status and susceptibility to infection of the fetus and neonate is not completely understood (Beisel, 1975). It is clear that maternal infection by various agents (e.g. rubella, cytomegalovirus, toxoplasma, herpes simplex, syphilis) may result in fetal and neonatal malnutrition and growth retardation. It is also known that neonatal infection may induce a compromised nutritional status through malabsorption, maldigestion, or inability to feed. Neonatal malnutrition is frequently seen in infants under prolonged intensive care for debilitating conditions and in congenital or acquired neonatal infections. Studies on the host defensive factors in these malnourished neonates have shown some defects involving the functions of T cells, B cells, and phagocytes (Chandra, 1975c). What part of these findings is due to infection (pre- or postnatal), malnutrition, or a synergy of the two conditions is unknown. There is little doubt that neonatal malnutrition may result in decreased immunocompetence and hence susceptibility to infection.

REFERENCES

Andelman, M.B. and Sered, B.E.: Utilization of dietary iron by term infants. Am. J. Dis. Child. 111:45, 1966.

Arbeter, A., Echevarri, L., Franco, D., Munson, D., Velex, H., and Vitalet, J.: Nutrition and infection. Fred. Proc. 30:1421, 1971.

Awdeh, S.L., et al.: A survey of nutritional immunological interactions. Bull. WHO 46:537, 1972.

Beisel, W.R.: Synergistic effects of maternal malnutrition and infection on the neonate. Am. J. Dis. Child. 129:571, 1975.

Buckley, R.H.: Iron deficiency anemia: Its relationship to infection susceptibility and host defense. J. Pediatr. 86:993, 1975.

Burman, D.: Hemoglobin levels in normal infants aged 3 to 4 months and the effect of iron. Arch. Dis. Child. 47:261, 1972.

Chandra, R.K.: Immunocompetence in undernutrition. J. Pediatr. 81:1194, 1972.

Chandra, R.K.: Serum complement and immunocongluttinin malnutrition. Arch. Dis. Child. 50:225, 1975 (a).

Chandra, R.K.: Reduced secretory antibody response to live attenuated measles and poliovirus vaccines in malnourished children. Brit. Med. J. 2:583, 1975 (b).

Chandra, R.K.: Fetal malnutrition and postnatal immunocompetence. Am. J. Dis. Child. 129:450, 1975 (c).

Cook, G.C., Morgan, V.O. and Hoffman, A.V.: Impairment of folate absorption by systemic bacterial infections. Lancet 2:1416, 1974.

Edelman, R., Suskind, R., Olsen, R.E. and Sirishana, S.: Mechanisms of defective delayed cutaneous hypersensitivity in children with PCM. Lancet 1:506, 1973.

Geefhuysen, J., Rosen, E.U., Katz, J., Ipp, T., and Metz, J.: Impaired cellular immunity in kwashiorkor with improvement after therapy. Brit. Med. J. 4:527, 1971.

Goldman, D.A. and Maki, D.G.: Infection control in total parenteral nutrition. JAMA 223:1360, 1973.

Gordon, J.E. and Scrimshaw, N.S.: Infectious disease in the malnourished. Med. Clin. N.A. 54:1495, 1970.

Harland, P.S.: Tuberculin reactions in malnourished children. Lancet 2:719, 1965.

Kass, E.H.: Infectious disease and social change. J. Inf. Dis. 123:110, 1971.

Lang, W.R., Howden, C.W., Laws, J., and Burton, J.F.: Bronchopneumonia with serious sequelae in children with evidence of adenovirus type 21 infection. Brit. Med. J. 1:73, 1969.

Lee, C. and Dubos, R.: Lasting biologic effects of early environmental influences. J. Exp. Med. 128:753, 1968.

Lukens, J.N.: Iron deficiency and infection. Am. J. Dis. Child. 129:160, 1975.

Mackay, H.M.M.: Anaemia in infancy: Its prevalence and prevention. Arch. Dis. Child. 3:117, 1928.

Masawe, A.E.J., Miundi, J.M. and Swai, G.B.R.: Infections in iron deficiency and other types of anemia in the tropics. Lancet 2: 314, 1974.

Mata, L.J. and Urrutia, J.J.: Intestinal colonization of children in a rural area of low socioeconomic level. Ann. N.Y. Acad. Sci. 176:93, 1971.

Mata, L.J., Urrutia, J.J., Albertoz, C., Pellecer, D., and Arellano, E.: Influence of recurrent infection on nutrition and growth of children in Guatemala. Am. J. Clin. Nutr. 25:1267, 1972.

Rayfield, E.J., Curnow, R.T., George, D.T., and Biesel, W.R.: Impaired carbohydrate metabolism during a mild viral illness. NEJM 289:618, 1973.

Ryan, J.A. et al.: Catheter complications in total parenteral nutrition. NEJM 290:757, 1974.

Scrimshaw, N.S., Taylor, C.E. and Gordon, J.E.: Interactions of nutrition and infection. WHO, Geneva, 1968.

Selvaraj, R.J. and Bhat, K.S.: Metabolic and bacteriocidal activities of leukocytes in PCM. Am. J. Clin. Nutr. 25:166, 1972.

Sirishana, S., Suskind, R., Edelman, R., Charuptana, C., and Olsen, R.E.: Complement and C3 proactivator levels in children with PCM and the effect of dietary treatment. Lancet 1:1016, 1973.

Smythe, P.M., Schonland, M., Breteton-Stiles, G.G., Coovadia, H.M., Grace, H.J., Loening, W.E.K., Mafoyane, A., Parent, M.A., and Vos, G.H.: Thymolymphatic deficiency and depression of cell-mediated immunity in PCM. Lancet 2:939, 1971.

Weinberg, E.D.: Iron and susceptibility to infectious disease. Science 184:952, 1974.

Woodward, T.E., and Smadel, J.E.: Management of typhoid fever and its complications. Ann. Int. Med. 60:144, 1964.

Yeung, C.Y , Lee, V.M.Y. and Yeung, C.M.: Glucose disappearance rate in neonatal infection. J. Pediatr. 82:486, 1973.

Walker, W.A.: Host defense mechanisms in the gastrointestinal tract. Pediatrics 57:901, 1976.

CHAPTER 22. SEPSIS AND SEPTIC SHOCK

INTRODUCTION: Sepsis (septicemia) represents a systemic disease associated with the presence and persistence of microorganisms or their toxins in the blood. Clinically, septicemia differs
from bacteremia in that the latter implies only the presence of bacteria in the bloodstream, either transient or persistent, without an
associated systemic illness. Septic shock is a clinical feature of
overwhelming infection and is manifested by shock, hemorrhagic
diathesis, and often death. The majority of patients with sepsis or
septic shock have bacterial infections. Other infecting agents such
as viruses, fungi, and rickettsiae may also produce septic manifestations indistinguishable from those caused by bacteria, but they
play a less important role. The chapter deals primarily with bacterial sepsis and septic shock.

In hospitalized patients, the incidence of gram-negative septicemia
has increased over the past 20 years. This is in large part due to
improved survival among patients with chronic diseases associated
with unusual susceptibility to severe infection. Recent surveys indicate that approximately 1% of hospital patients have gram-negative
bacteremia and a significant number of these patients have clinical
sepsis. Fatality rates from septicemia are 30 to 50% (higher for
septic shock) in most series. Early recognition of sepsis and septic
shock, appropriate monitoring of vital functions, and prompt specific and supportive therapy are essential in preventing the fatal outcome. Thus, sepsis and septic shock constitute an important problem in infectious diseases. Although sepsis and septic shock in the
neonate are considered briefly in this chapter, neonatal sepsis is
dealt with more extensively in the chapter entitled "Neonatal
Infections."

1. ETIOLOGY AND PATHOGENESIS

1.1: Etiology: The bacteria involved in sepsis and septic shock vary
with the age of the patient and the presence or absence of underlying
disease (Table 22-1). In newborn infants, E. coli, group B streptococci are the most common agents causing bacterial sepsis. Other
bacteria encountered include klebsiella-aerobacter, enterococci,
pseudomonas, proteus, salmonella, listeria, serratia, pneumococci,
and meningococci. Almost any organism can cause sepsis during
the newborn period. Beyond the neonatal age, the agents involved in
sepsis in children differ, depending upon the status of the child's
host defense mechanisms. In previously well infants and children,
pneumococci, meningococci, group A streptococci, staphylococci,
and Hemophilus influenzae are the most frequent causes of septicemia. E. coli, klebsiella-aerobacter, proteus, pseudomonas,

TABLE 22-1: BACTERIAL AGENTS ASSOCIATED WITH SEPSIS		
	AGENT	
GROUP	**COMMON**	**LESS COMMON**
Newborn	E. coli, group B strep-tococci, staphylococci	Klebsiella, entero-cocci, pseudomonas, proteus, salmonella, listeria, serattia, pneumococci, meningococci
No underlying disease (be-yond newborn age)	Pneumococci, H. in-fluenzae, meningococci, group A streptococci, staphylococci	E. coli, Klebsiella, proteus, pseudomo-nas, salmonella, bacteroides
With under-lying disease:	Staphylococci, E. coli, Klebsiella, Pseudomonas	

salmonella, and bacteroides occur less frequently. However, children with altered host defense mechanisms often encounter septicemia due to staphylococci, E. coli, klebsiella-aerobacter, pseudomonas, and other bacteria with low virulence.

1.2: Pathogenesis: Bacteremia or septicemia represents failure of
the host's defense mechanisms to restrict invading microorganisms
to a local site. Transient bacteremia may be induced by: 1) mechanical manipulation, 2) urologic instrumentation, and 3) manipulation of such foci as infected tonsils, furuncles and carbuncles. On
the other hand, septicemia is often associated with severe localized
infections such as pneumonia, septic arthritis, osteomyelitis, and
meningitis.

Studies on the mechanism of removal of bacteria from the circulating
blood in animals and humans indicate that lymph nodes, liver, spleen,
bone marrow, lung and skeletal muscles may effectively remove the
microorganisms. In extravascular infections, bacteria enter into the
lymphatics and are filtered through the local lymph nodes, which remove 99% of streptococci, with the remaining 1% escaping into the
circulating blood as detected by blood cultures (Drinker, 1934).

In intravascular infections (e.g. septic thrombophlebitis, endocarditis), bacteria enter into the blood stream from the vegetations at a
rather constant rate, and a large number (up to 95%) of bacteria are
removed in the liver during a single circuit of blood (Beeson, 1945).
Thus, varying organs and tissues have a high degree of filtering ef-
ficiency. Factors determining the development of sepsis or septic
shock, though not well defined, include nutritional status of the child,

general immunologic competency, local susceptibility, number as well as virulence of the infecting agent, and presence or absence of immunity to the infecting organism.

2. CLINICAL MANIFESTATIONS

2.1: Sepsis: The severity and clinical features of sepsis vary considerably. If infective foci are present, the clinical presentations are generally those manifestations associated with the primary infection, e.g. meningitis, pneumonia, empyema, gastroenteritis, endocarditis, or pyelonephritis. Newborn infants and patients with chronic debilitating disease such as leukemia and aplastic anemia, often reveal an overwhelming "septic" condition without having a recognizable localized focus of infection.

The clinical manifestations of sepsis do not differ significantly with the etiologic agent. However, some clinical features of sepsis are helpful in distinguishing certain bacterial pathogens (Table 22-2). Sepsis due to Pseudomonas aeruginosa is often associated with ecthyma gangrenosum which is characterized by tender, indurated or ulcerative lesions with necrotic dark centers, or by vesicular lesions filled with cloudy fluid and with an erythematous margin.

2.2: Septic Shock: Septic shock is manifested by an initial vasoconstriction followed by (or alternating with) vasodilatation, venous pooling of blood and peripheral vascular collapse. Early, the extremities may be well perfused and warm, the pulse full, and the blood pressure normal. Later, the classic signs of shock appear, consisting of decreased alertness and responsiveness, pallor, clamminess, sweating, cyanosis, tachypnea, rapid and weak pulse, hypotension, and diminished urinary output. In neonates and very young infants, additional indicators are diminished muscle tone, weak cry, poor suck, anorexia, and minimal deviation of the vital signs from the baseline values. In older children, septic shock should always be suspected when a febrile patient has chills associated with hypotension.

3. DIAGNOSIS AND MONITORING OF VITAL FUNCTIONS

3.1: Laboratory Diagnosis: Blood cultures are the single most important test in establishing the diagnosis. Urine, stool, and other exudates should be submitted for bacterial cultures. Cerebral spinal fluid examination and cultures are often necessary, particularly if the child shows signs of CNS involvement. Roentgenographic examination is needed if the primary infection involves the lungs, intraabdominal structures or bones and joints. Other tests are often useful, and these include serum bilirubin, complete blood count including platelets, urinalysis, blood sugar, blood urea nitrogen and creatinine, serum electrolytes and coagulation studies, including fibrinogen. Appropriate Limulus test for detection of endotoxin in blood has been found useful by some investigators.

ORGANISM	CLUES
TABLE 22-2: CLINICAL CLUES TO THE BACTERIOLOGIC DIAGNOSIS IN SEPTICEMIA AND SEPTIC SHOCK BEYOND THE NEWBORN PERIOD	
1. Staphylococcus aureus	Skin lesions (boils or carbuncles), infected wounds; erythematous rash; recent cardiac operations
2. Streptococcus group A or Staphylococcus aureus	Extensive skin lesion (burn, epidermolysis, exudative erythema multiforme)
3. Streptococcus pneumoniae	Presence of lobar pneumonia; splenectomy, sickle cell, nephritic syndrome, liver cirrhosis
4. Neisseria meningitidis	Multiple petechial skin lesions,* meningitis, shock
5. Hemophilus influenzae	Meningitis, cellulitis, arthritis, epiglottitis
6. Pseudomonas aeruginosa	Severe burns; hematologic disorders, altered immunity as a result of the primary disease or therapy. Ecthyma gangrenosa
7. E. coli, Klebsiella, Enterobacter	Altered immunity, urinary tract infection
8. Bacteroides	Intra-abdominal infection, foul pus, recent abdominal surgery

* Also seen in pseudomonas, pneumococci, hemophilus, streptococci, staphylococci, rickettsiae, viruses.

<u>3.2: Monitoring of Vital Functions</u>: Continuous monitoring of vital functions is essential in following the clinical course and in providing appropriate therapy.

a) <u>Arterial Blood Gas</u>: Blood gas monitoring is essential for provision of respiratory support, oxygen administration, assessment of acid base balance and its correction. Cannulation of the peripheral arteries (umbilical, femoral, brachial) may be necessary. Open-end catheters should be used and flushed continuously with heparinized solution to prevent clotting.

b) <u>Respiratory and Heart Rates</u>: Increasing respiratory rates, grunting respirations and large alveolar-arterial oxygen tension gradients indicate the onset of shock lung, a most serious complication of shock. Tachycardia (200 beats per minute) is a normal response of the cardiovascular system to catecholamine stimulation in an attempt to maintain adequate cardiac output (cardiac output = heart rate X stroke volume). Bradycardia indicates marked anoxia and carries a very poor prognosis.

c) <u>Inspired Oxygen Concentration</u>: The inspired oxygen concentration should be continuously monitored and adjusted to maintain an arterial PaO_2 of 70-80 mmHg (TORR). In the presence of a large right-to-left intrapulmonary shunt (shock lung), this level may not be reached even though the inspired oxygen concentration is 100%. The toxic effects of oxygen on the lungs are minimized if the ambient oxygen concentration is kept below 60%. Recently, the application of continuous positive airway pressure (CPAP) or positive end-expiratory pressure (PEEP) have been used to obviate the need for high oxygen concentration.

d) <u>Urinary Output and Osmolarity</u>: This is the best parameter of adequate renal perfusion. The patient should be promptly catheterized to determine minute-by-minute urine volume. In small infants, a #5 plastic feeding tube should be employed rather than a Foley balloon catheter.

e) <u>Central Venous Pressure (CVP)</u>: Measurement of CVP allows an assessment of functional intravascular volume and the ability of the heart to handle the load. Directional changes are more important than absolute values. Thus, a falling CVP indicates the need for rapid volume replacement whereas a rising CVP in face of inadequate peripheral perfusion suggests the need for inotropic support and/or the use of drugs which improve vascular compliance. In recent years, the Swan-Ganz flow directed catheter has been used to measure pulmonary arterial and wedge pressures. As pulmonary wedge pressure closely reflects left atrial pressure, this measurement allows administration of large volumes of fluids in hypovolemic states more safely. Although pulmonary wedge pressure is superior to CVP in the presence of decreased left ventricular performance (cardiogenic shock), in septic shock the CVP has been found to be a reliable index of left ventricular filling pressure.

f) <u>Blood Pressure</u>: The blood pressure is a function of both cardiac output and peripheral resistance. Thus, it can be maintained in the normal range by intense vasoconstriction in the presence of low cardiac output. One should not rely heavily on this parameter in assessing trends in shock, as it indicates neither blood flow nor its distribution to vital organs. The arterial blood pressure should be measured by direct arterial cannulation as centrally as possible (descending aorta in newborns), since there is an amplification of systolic pressures from the central aorta to the peripheral arteries. Auscultatory methods are particularly unreliable in shock because the intense peripheral vasoconstriction reduces the threshold of the Korotoff sounds, and because of the difficulty in selecting the appropriate sized cuffs, especially in small infants.

g) <u>Body Temperature</u>: Both core and skin temperature should be monitored to prevent heat loss which increases oxygen consumption and further increases oxygen demand. The skin temperature also suggests clinical trends - a rewarming skin during volume replacement indicates that the microcirculation is recovering.

h) <u>Blood Chemistry</u>: Sodium, potassium, chloride, carbon dioxide content, pH, calcium, BUN, lactate, creatinine, serum osmolarity and glucose should be followed at close intervals. Hypoglycemia should be corrected by rapid infusion of 50% glucose.

i) <u>Blood Cell Indices</u>: Hemoglobin, hematocrit and white cell count and differential should be monitored as indices of volume changes and of infections. Early detection of disseminated intravascular coagulation is accomplished by determination of the platelet count, fibrinogen level, presence of fibrin split products, prothrombin time and partial thromboplastin time.

4. MANAGEMENT

<u>4.1: Antibiotic Therapy</u>: Appropriate antibiotic therapy should be instituted upon the suspicion of sepsis and administered generously by the intravenous route. Selection of antibiotics prior to culture reports is based on the possible source of primary infection and clinical clues listed in Table 22-2. Broad spectrum coverage with antibiotics is generally necessary. A combination of one of the penicillins (penicillin G, ampicillin, nafcillin or related drug) and an aminoglycoside (kanamycin or gentamicin) is widely used (dosage and schedule see page 571). Chloramphenicol plus penicillin (or ampicillin) is commonly given to patients with meningitis or brain abscess. A penicillinase-resistant penicillin such as nafcillin is administered if <u>S. aureus</u> is suspected. Gentamicin and/or carbenicillin are given if the clinical condition suggests a pseudomonas infection.

<u>4.2: Respiratory Support</u>: Apnea often complicates severe infections of the newborn and young infant. Shock lung is a life-threatening complication of all forms of shock. Oxygen administration, continuous positive airway pressure breathing and mechanical ventilation represent very important aspects of the therapy in septic shock. Oxygen should be administered with appropriate humidification, and monitoring of arterial oxygen tension is essential. Changes in the physical properties of pulmonary capillary membranes in shock lung allow edema formation to occur at normal capillary hydrostatic pressures. It is vital, therefore, that noncolloid solutions be given carefully. Diuretic and steroid therapy may be necessary as adjuncts to respiratory support if pulmonary edema complicates septic shock.

<u>4.3: Circulatory Support</u>: This includes volume expansion and
treatment of microcirculatory failure by steroids and vasoactive
substances. Volume expansion is of primary importance in the
early phase of shock even if clinical evidence of external fluid loss
is lacking. Unless the CVP exceeds 10 cm of water, 10-20 cc/kg
body weight of crystalloid solution (5% dextrose and 1/2 normal saline) should be infused over a 10-minute period. Often this volume
suffices to **restore adequate tissue perfusion**. The CVP serves as a
useful guide for further fluid administration (blood, plasma, plas-
manate). The aim of the therapy is to restore vital organ perfusion.
Pharmacological doses of hydrocortisone have been shown to enhance
survival in several forms of shock (including endotoxic) in animals
and humans, although data on controlled clinical studies are lacking.
Steroids are generally given as soon as a diagnosis of septic shock is
made and before irreversible changes have occurred. The recommended dose is 35-50 mg/kg body weight of hydrocortisone for four
doses, if necessary (Hodes, 1969). Vasoconstrictive drugs are usually contraindicated in shock because of the generalized marked peripheral vasoconstriction. Vasodilator drugs remain in the experimental stage and no experience is available in children with septic
shock. Isoproterenol, a beta-receptor stimulating drug, has been
widely used in adults. Its mechanism of action of combined vaso-
dilatory effect on the peripheral arteries and of positive inotropic
effect has prompted its use in shock. In children, isoproterenol is
of relatively limited value because of the marked tachycardia which
is present in shock. More recently, dopamine has been successfully
employed in the treatment of cardiogenic and septic shock in adults
(Winslow, et al., 1973). Dopamine has a unique property of increasing renal perfusion in addition to increasing cardiac contractility, and
cardiac output. Dopamine should not be used until adequate trial of
volume expansion has been tried. The dose of dopamine varies from
1 μg/kg/min to as high as 15 μg/kg/min (Goldberg, 1974).

<u>4.4: Correction of Metabolic Acidosis</u>: Endotoxic shock in infants,
particularly when associated with severe diarrhea, is complicated by
severe metabolic acidemia. Sodium bicarbonate infusion should be
carried out promptly and pH monitored frequently. The dose of bicarbonate is calculated on the basis of the estimated base deficit.
The extracellular fluid space in infants is estimated at 20% of the body
weight.

<u>4.5: Anticoagulant Therapy with Heparin</u>: Septic shock in infants is
often associated with disseminated intravascular coagulation (DIC).
When either clinical or laboratory evidence of DIC is obtained, heparin may be given. The recommended dose is 1 mg/kg body weight
every 4 hours. The whole blood clotting time should be kept at $2\frac{1}{2}$
times normal or around 30 minutes. Heparin treatment should be
continued until coagulation values have returned to normal or until
the patient has recovered from the infection which has caused the
shock (Hodes, 1969)

4.6: Therapy Directed to Improve Oxygen Release: In endotoxic shock, there is a shift of the oxygen dissociation curve to the left with increased affinity of the hemoglobin for oxygen and further compromising oxygen delivery to the tissues. This is particularly true in infants with large concentrations of fetal hemoglobin. To improve oxygen release in the young infant during endotoxic shock, exchange transfusion with freshly heparinized adult blood has been proposed and has been used in the treatment of septicemia (Prod' hom, et al., 1974). This form of therapy, however, deserves further evaluation.

REFERENCES

Ayres, S.M., Giannelli, S., and Mueller, H.S.: Shock, In Care of the Critically Ill. Appleton-Century-Crofts, New York, Div. of Prentice-Hall, Inc., 1974, pp. 258-301.

Balagtas, R.C., Bell, C.E., Edwards, L.D. and Levin, S.: Risk of local and systemic infections associated with umbilical vein catheterization: A prospective study in 86 newborn patients. Pediatrics 48:359, 1971.

Barnes, J.M. and Trueta, J : Absorption of bacteria, toxins and snake venoms from the tissues: Importance of the lymphatic circulation. Lancet 1:623, 1941.

Berry, L.J. and Smythe, D.S.: Effects of bacterial endotoxin on metabolism. J. Exp. Med. VII-120:721, 1964.

Berry, L.J., Smythe, D.S. and Young, L.G.: Effects of bacterial endotoxin on metabolism. J. Exp. Med. I-110:389, 1959.

Burke, J.P., Klein, J.O., Gezon, H.M. and Finland, M.: Pneumococcal bacteremia. Am. J. Dis. Child. 121:353, 1971.

Cobe, W.: Transient bacteremia. J. Oral Surg. 7:609, 1954.

Cohn, J.N., Tristani, F.E., and Khatri, I.M.: Studies in clinical shock and hypotension: relationship between left and right ventricular function. J. Clin. Invest. 48:2008, 1969.

Collins, R.N., Braun, P.A., Zinner, S.H. and Kass, E.H.: Risk of local and systemic infection with polyethylene intravenous catheters. NEJM 279:340, 1968.

Corrigan, J.J.: Thrombocytopenia and sepsis. J. Pediatr. 85:219-221, 1974.

Curti, J.T.: Antibiotics and gram-negative bacteremia. JAMA 231:1361, 1975.

Drinker, C.K., Field, M.E. and Ward, H.K.: The filtering capacity of lymph nodes. J. Exp. Med. 59:393, 1934.

Findland, M.: Treatment of pneumonia and other serious infections. NEJM 263:207, 1960.

Freid, M.A. and Vosti, K.L.: The importance of underlying disease in patients with gram-negative bacteremia. Arch. Intern. Med. 121:418, 1968.

Goldberg, L.I.: Dopamine: clinical uses of an endogenous catecholamine. NEJM 291:707, 1974.

Hardaway, R.M.: Overwhelming bacterial infections in childhood. Report of the 55th Ross Conference on Pediatric Research, Ross Laboratories, Columbus, Ohio, 1966.

Harris, J.A. and Cobbs, C.G.: Persistent gram-negative bacteremia. Am. J. Surg. 125:705, 1973.

Heldrich, F.J. Jr.: Diplococcus pneumoniae bacteremia. Am. J. Dis. Child 119:12, 1970.

Hinshaw, L.B., Peyton, M.D., Archer, L.T., et al.: Prevention of death in endotoxic shock by glucose administration. Surg. Gynec. Obstet. 139:851-859, 1974.

Hodes, H.L., Care of the critically ill child: endotoxin shock (diagnosis and treatment). Pediatrics 44:248-260, 1969.

Johnson, D.G.: Shock and its management in pediatrics. Hosp. Med. 11:22-41, August, 1975.

Johnson, R.B., Jr. and Sell, S.H.: Septicemia in infants and children. Pediatrics 34:473, 1969.

Kamada, R.O. and Smith, J.R.: The phenomenon of respiratory failure in shock: the genesis of shock lung. Am. Heart J. 83:1-4, 1972.

Kun, E. and Abood, L.G.: Mechanisms of inhibition of glycogen synthesis by endotoxins of salmonella aertrycke and type I meningococcus. Proc. Soc. Exp. Biol. Med. 71:362, 1949.

Levin, J., Poore, T.E., Young, N.S., et al.: Gram-negative sepsis: detection of endotoxemia with the limulus test. Ann. Int. Med. 76:1, 1972.

Martin, C.M., Cuomo, A.J., Geraghty, M.J., Zager, J.R., and Mandes, T.C.: Gram-negative rod bacteremia. J. Infect. Dis. 119: 506, 1969.

McCabe, W.R.: Gram-negative bacteremia. Arch. Int. Med. 19: 135, 1974.

McGowan, J.E., Jr., Bratton, L., Klein, J.O., and Finland, M.: Bacteremia in febrile children seen in a "walk-in" pediatric clinic. NEJM 288:1310, 1973.

McGowan, J.R., Jr., Klein, J.O., Bratton, L., Barnes, M.W., and Finland, M.: Meningitis and bacteremia due to Haemophilus influenzae: occurrence and mortality at Boston City Hospital. J. Infect. Dis. 130:119, 1974.

Motsay, G.J , Alho, A., Dietzman, R., et al.: Forelimb, small intestine, and pulmonary vascular beds in canine endotoxin shock, in Steroids and Shock, Glenn, T.M., Ph.D., ed. University Park Press, Baltimore, 1974, pp. 151-163.

Myerowitz, R.L., Medeiros, A.A., and O'Brien, T.F.: Recent experience with bacillemia due to gram-negative organisms. J. Infect. Dis. 124:239, 1971.

Myers, M.G., Wright, P.F., Smith, A.L., and Smith, D.H.: Complications of occult pneumococcal bacteremia in children. J. Pediatr. 84:656, 1974.

Nies, A.S., Forsyth, R.P., Williams, H.E., et al.: Contribution of kinines to endotoxic shock in unanesthetized Rhesus monkey. Circ. Res. 22:155, 1968.

Nolan, C.M. and Beaty, H.N.: Staphylococcus aureus bacteremia - current clinical pattern. Am. J. Med. 60:495, 1976.

Prod'hom, L.S., Choffat, J.M., Frenck, N., et al.: Care of the seriously ill neonate with hyaline membrane disease and with sepsis (sclerema neonatorum). Pediatrics, Vol. 53, #2:170-181, 1974.

Skilman, J.J.: Treatment of acute respiratory distress syndrome: role of albumin and diuretics (shock in low and high flow states). Excerpta Medica, 1972, p. 196.

Smits, H. and Freedman, L.R.: Prolonged venous catheterization as a cause of sepsis. NEJM 276:1229, 1967.

Stiehm, E.R. and Damroch, D.S.: Factors in prognosis of meningococcal infections: review of 63 cases with emphasis on recognition and management of severely ill patients. J. Pediatr. 68:457, 1966.

Watkins, F.M., Rabelo, A., Plzak, L.F. and Sheldon, G.F.: The left-shifted oxyhemoglobin curve in sepsis: a preventable defect. Ann. Surg., August, 1974, pp. 213-220.

Weil, M.H. and Shubin, H.: Monitoring and measurements during shock, in Treatment of Shock: Principles and Practice, Schumer, W., M.D. and Nyhus, L.M., M.D., eds. Lea & Febiger, Philadelphia, 1974, pp. 3-22.

Winslow, E.J., Loeb, H.S., Rahintoola, S.H., et al.: Hemodynamic studies and results of therapy in 50 patients with bacteremic shock. Am. J. Med. 54:421, 1973.

Schumer, W.: Steroids in the treatment of clinical septic shock. Ann. Surg. 184:333, 1976.

CHAPTER 23. ANAEROBIC INFECTIONS

GENERAL CONSIDERATIONS: Anaerobic bacteria were first described by Louis Pasteur, and the fetid odor of purulent exudates
was attributed to anaerobes prior to 1900. Anaerobic production of
the fecal odor was demonstrated in the 1930's by showing that growth
of E. coli in pleural fluid does not smell fetid, while anaerobic organisms grown under identical conditions do. Despite a recent growing awareness of anaerobic pathogens causing adult infections, only
recently have a few reports considered the special problems of anaerobes in neonates and children. This chapter deals with anaerobic infections in general and special attention is given to pediatric
problems.

Anaerobes are difficult to isolate from clinical specimens because
exposure to oxygen is lethal to some bacteria. Extremely oxygen-
sensitive organisms are seldom isolated from clinical specimens,
even with the most sophisticated methods presently available. Less
oxygen sensitive anaerobes may survive in the presence of oxygen
and even proliferate, provided the Eh (oxidation-reduction potential)
of the environment is lowered. Eh reduction is found in body folds,
crevices (e.g. gingival crevices), and orifices where aerobic organisms proliferate. Normal body tissues have an Eh of +0.126 to
0.246, but in circumstances allowing reduction from -0.100 to
-0.250 anaerobic bacteria will multiply. Reduction of Eh may be
created by aerobic bacterial growth or by processes which interrupt capillary blood flow (e.g. surgical procedures, trauma, severe
atherosclerosis, etc.). Tetanus spores do not form in vivo unless
there is reduction of the Eh to less than +0.01 volts. Germination of
tetanus spores can be induced by the presence of sterile earth,
$CaCl_2$, or interruption of capillary blood flow (Fildes, 1929).

The mechanisms of oxygen toxicity to anaerobes has not been fully
defined. It is postulated to be related to oxygen binding to chemical
components in growth media, or lack of production of superoxide
dismutase by strict anaerobes.

Anaerobic organisms outnumber aerobes on most body surfaces, as
shown in Table 23-1. Hence, any infectious process adjacent to
body surfaces is likely to have pathogens which include anaerobes.

1. SPECIMEN COLLECTION

Principles of bacterial isolation in suspected anaerobic infections are
as follows: 1) Collect the specimen by a technique which will minimize or avoid oxygen exposure. This can be readily accomplished
by using a needle and syringe for aspiration of purulent material.

TABLE 23-1: ANAEROBIC AND AEROBIC ORGANISMS
ISOLATED FROM BODY SURFACES AND FLUIDS

SPECIMEN	NO. ANAEROBES	NO. AEROBES
Nasal washings	10^{2-5}	10^{1-4}
Saliva	10^{8-9}	10^{7-8}
Tooth surfaces	10^6	10^6
Gingival scrapings	10^7	10^7
Skin	10^3	10^2
Colon	10^{10-11}	10^{7-8}
Vagina	10^3	10^2

Any air present should be excluded. When this is not possible, a
swab moistened with saline which contains no benzyl alcohol or other
bacteriostatic substance can be used to collect infected material. If
pre-reduced swabs and oxygen depleted (gassed out) tubes containing
a gas other than air are available, these should be used for collection and transport. In each clinical situation, caution should be exercised to avoid contamination by contiguous normal flora. (2) Transport and process rapidly. (3) Allow anaerobic incubation at 37C for
at least 48 hours. Exposure to atmospheric oxygen prior to 48 hours
has been shown to reduce the number of anerobic pathogens isolated.
After colonial growth is obtained, most organisms are more resistant
to brief oxygen exposure so that subculturing can be performed more
leisurely.

2. CLINICAL MICROBIOLOGY

Bacteriologic findings which implicate anaerobes in infectious problems are listed in Table 23-2. Clinically important anaerobes are
shown in Table 23-3.

Peptostreptococcus and Peptococcus are found in the normal flora of
the mouth, upper respiratory tract, feces, vagina, and skin. They
may be primary pathogens in endocarditis, brain abscess, puerperal
sepsis, traumatic wounds, and postoperative necrotizing fasciitis.

Cl. perfringens, Cl. tetani, and Cl. septicum are soil inhabitants,
and are occasionally found in man. Several types of each species
may produce similar patterns of disease.

The Actinomyces inhabit the mouth and throat. Sulfur granules are
filamentous masses recovered from purulent exudates. Actinomyces
israelii and Arachnia proprionica may cause identical syndromes.

TABLE 23-2: BACTERIOLOGIC FINDINGS IMPLICATING ANAEROBES

1. Negative cultures with organisms on gram stain

2. Gram stain morphology of certain organisms

3. Failure of organisms to grow aerobically

4. Growth only in depths (anaerobic zone) of fluid media

5. Characteristic colonies on agar

6. Fluorescence (red) of B. melaninogenicus under ultraviolet light

TABLE 23-3: CLINICALLY IMPORTANT ANAEROBIC GENERA

GRAM-POSITIVE	cocci	Peptostreptococcus Peptococcus
	bacilli	Clostridium* Actinomyces Arachnia Propionibacterium
GRAM-NEGATIVE	cocci	Veillonella
	bacilli	Bacteroides Fusobacterium

* Spore formers

The anaerobic gram-negative cocci are of three genera: Veillonella, Acidaminococcus, and Megasphera. Although they too are inhabitants of the normal gastrointestinal tract, they seldom are incriminated in producing disease.

Bacteroides and Fusobacterium are the most important genera of gram-negative rods. Bacteroides fragilis, ss. fragilis, one of 5 subspecies of B. fragilis, is the anaerobe most frequently isolated from clinical specimens. B. fragilis, ss. vulgatus, is the organism isolated from stools in highest number. In fact, this anaerobe alone comprises 16% of the dry weight of feces. All Bacteroides species together constitute 20% of the usual fecal weight, and fecal anaerobes outnumber aerobes by a factor of nearly 10^3, as shown in Table 23-1. Typical Gram stain appearance of B. fragilis is described as bipolar staining or "safety pin"-like.

Species of Fusobacterium most often isolated from infected specimens are F. nucleatum (fusiforme), F. necrophorium (formerly Sphaerophorus necrophorus), and F. mortiferium. F. nucleatum is the predominant fusobacterium from clinical specimens involving mouth, lung, pleural cavity, and brain.

Laboratory identification of anaerobes, as with aerobes, makes use of: (1) gram stain, (2) colony morphology on growth media, and (3) biochemical reactions. Extensive descriptions of reactions are available (Holdeman et al., 1972).

3. CLINICAL SYNDROMES

Clinical findings that suggest a particular infection caused by anaerobic pathogens are listed in Table 23-4 and are for the most part, self-explanatory.

TABLE 23-4: CLINICAL FINDINGS IMPLICATING ANAEROBIC ORGANISMS IN INFECTIONS
1. Foul-smelling discharge
2. Black discoloration of hemorrhagic exudate (B. melaninogenicus)
3. "Sulfur granules" in tissues (actinomycosis)
4. Infection site adjacent to areas with normal anaerobic flora (near mucosal surfaces)
5. Necrotic tissue or gas in tissue
6. A clinically apparent infection with negative cultures
7. Infection occurring after abdominal trauma or surgery
8. Bacteremia with jaundice (B. fragilis)
9. Infection following aminoglycoside use
10. Human or animal bites

Bacteroides species, Clostridium species and anaerobic cocci comprise approximately 80% of significant anaerobic isolates from infants and children (Dunkle et al., 1976). Peritonitis, septicemia, abscesses, and wounds are the most common clinical problems from which these pathogens are recovered (Table 23-5).

3.1: ABDOMINAL INFECTIONS: The clinical setting for anaerobic intraabdominal infections includes appendicitis, inflammatory bowel disease, trauma, and post-gastrointestinal surgery. Purulent material can collect in any site intraperitoneally, retroperitoneally, or within the viscera. Children treated for both aerobes and anaerobes have a high overall cure rate, although a few cases are described in which a satisfactory outcome is seen with treatment of aerobes alone (Dunkle et al., 1976). Studies of infection in animal models indicate that therapy should be directed towards both aerobes and anaerobes (Weinstein et al., 1975).

3.2: BACTEREMIA: Anaerobic bacteremia has been shown to be less common in children than adults, accounting for one in 1700 pediatric admission compared to one in 300 medical-surgical admissions

TABLE 23-5: ANAEROBES ASSOCIATED WITH CLINICALLY SIGNIFICANT INFECTIONS OF CHILDREN*

INFECTION	MAJOR ORGANISMS
Peritonitis	B. fragilis and spp., Clostridium, Peptococcus, Fusobacterium
Septicemia	Clostridium, Fusobacterium, B. fragilis, Propionibacterium
Abscesses	Bacteroides, Clostridium, Peptostreptococcus, Peptococcus
Wounds	B. fragilis, Clostridium
Cellulitis	Bacteroides, Fusobacterium, Peptococcus, Peptostreptococcus

* From Dunkle et al., 1976.

and one in 50 gynecologic admissions (Gorbach et al., 1974). Anaerobic organisms have been recovered from one in 133 (0.75%) pediatric blood cultures (Dunkle et al., 1976). In contrast, aerobes were recovered from 9% of all blood cultures. Both anaerobic and aerobic isolated from blood cultures were twice as common in the newborn as in children over 1 month of age (Dunkle et al., 1976).

Neonatal bacteremia has occurred in 1.8 newborns per 1,000 live births (Chow et al., 1974). Pathogens may be recovered from peripheral or cord blood. Multiple organisms are isolated from one-third of neonates. The clinical settings which are apt to be associated with anaerobic infections are identical to those associated with other neonatal sepsis: prolonged rupture of membranes, maternal amnionitis, foul-smelling amniotic fluid, prematurity, and respiratory distress. One series has shown a favorable prognosis with only one death in 23 cases, despite the fact that 9 neonates received no antimicrobial therapy and 5 received antibiotics not usually effective against the pathogen recovered from the blood (Chow et al., 1974). A more recent study showed a mortality rate of 37.5% in neonates with clinically significant bacteremia, which suggests that many of the isolates of the previous study reflected transient bacteremias and not septicemia (Dunkle et al., 1976).

Propionibacterium acnes is a frequent blood isolate but is rarely a pathogen. P. acnes is a common skin inhabitant. It has comprised over one-fifth of all anaerobes recovered from all sites and 66% (27 of 41) of all blood isolates (Dunkle et al., 1976). However, it rarely can be incriminated as a pathogen, and only 3 of 27 blood isolates of P. acnes were believed to be of clinical significance. These were associated with the following infections: (1) an abscess in proximity to an infected ventriculoperitoneal shunt, (2) necrotizing enterocolitis, and (3) chronic otitis media following myringotomy.

Although mortality rates for anaerobic bacteremia range between 25 and 35 percent in adults, no deaths were found in 53 maternal bacteroides bacteremias (Pearson et al., 1967). In contrast, septic abortion and fetal or neonatal death were common in this population. In fact, only one twin survived out of 55 fetuses. Other studies of anaerobic bacteremia in children have shown mortality rates of 4% and 37.5% (Chow et al., 1974, and Dunkle et al., 1976).

Anaerobic endocarditis is uncommon, accounting for less than 4% in one series of 1500 cases of endocarditis. Anaerobic cocci accounted for most of these. Reports of other organisms producing endocarditis include Propionibacterium, Bacteroides, and Fusobacterium. Again, most of these patients had gastrointestinal disease as a predisposing cause of bacteremia.

3.3: ORAL INFECTIONS: Fluctuant oral or dental abscesses are usually mixed infections that include a number of species. Most commonly isolated are anaerobic cocci (Peptococcus and Peptostreptococcus) followed by Fusobacterium nucleatum, Bacteroides oralis, B. melaninogenicus, Actinomyces, and Veillonella.

Dental caries occur as a result of solubilization of tooth mineral by acid solutions, especially that produced by bacterial proliferation. Genetic and developmental factors control the dimensions of pits and fissures in teeth. The size of these determine the microbial load retained by them. Streptococcus mutans is one of the most important pathogens that produces caries, and S. mutans requires sucrose to adhere to solid tooth surfaces. Sucrose is present in dental placque, and probably provides the mechanism for adherence by bacteria and subsequent enamel erosion.

Actinomyces viscosus, which is dependent on starch instead of sucrose, is an important cause of root decay. Lactobacillus species have long been associated with dental caries, but a cause and effect relationship has not been determined.

3.4: SINUSITIS: Chronic inflammation of the paranasal sinuses has been shown to be caused by anaerobes alone in 31% of cases, and aerobes associated with anaerobes in an additional 20% (Frederick et al., 1974). The most commonly recovered anaerobes were anaerobic streptococci, corynebacteria (gram-positive rods, not further identified), Bacteroides species, and Veillonella. Staphylococcus aureus, Streptococcus viridans, and Hemophilus influenzae were anaerobes most often isolated. Fully one-fourth of sinus exudates have no culture growth which raises the suspicion of anaerobes, and one-half of these did have organisms apparent on Gram stain.

3.5: VINCENT'S ANGINA: A common anaerobic infection of former days was exudative tonsillitis associated with submandibular cellulitis. This was caused by Fusobacterium necrophorium, but is seldom seen now.

3.6: PLEUROPULMONARY INFECTIONS: Four clinical syndromes are commonly associated with anaerobic involvement of the lungs and pleura: (1) aspiration pneumonia, (2) lung abscess, (3) necrotizing pneumonia, and (4) empyema (Table 23-6).

TABLE 23-6: ANAEROBIC PLEUROPULMONARY INFECTIONS			
TYPE OF INFECTION	ANAEROBES ONLY (%)	ANAEROBES + AEROBES (%)	AEROBES ONLY (%)
Aspiration Pneumonia (70 Cases)	46	41	12
Lung Abscess (26 Cases)	62	31	8
Necrotizing Pneumonia (18 Cases)	66	28	6
Empyema (35 Cases)	37	34	29
From Bartlett and Finegold, Am. Rev. Resp. Dis. 110:56, 1974.			

Frequent conditions which predispose to these infections are periodontitis, altered consciousness, esophageal or swallowing mechanism alterations. Either the right or left lower basilar lobar segments are likely to be involved in pneumonia or abscess, as would be suspected since aspiration is the most frequently incriminated mechanism for production of anaerobic pleuropulmonary infections.

Again, multiple pathogens are the rule, with Fusobacterium nucleatum, Bacteroides melaninogenicus, Peptococcus, Peptostreptococcus, and microaerophilic streptococci being recovered in each type of pleuropulmonary infection. Concomitant aerobes were less often recovered than aerobes: Staphylococcus aureus, Streptococcus pneumoniae, Streptococcus faecalis, and E. coli. In empyema, Haemophilus influenzae is also isolated occasionally.

Clinical suspicion of underlying anaerobic involvement consists of: (1) a history of aspiration, (2) a putrid discharge or sputum, (3) a clinical course that is longer than 7 days prior to presentation, or (4) if tissue necrosis is apparent.

Therapy with penicillin has made a dramatic change in the prognosis of these patients. Nearly all the organisms are sensitive to penicillin,

except for B. fragilis which amounts to less than 10% of these infections. Most investigators feel that parenteral penicillin continues
to be the drug of choice, in combination with the use of aminoglycoside for aerobic gram-negative rods. In lung abscess after the patient becomes afebrile and improves clinically, oral penicillin should
be continued for 6 to 12 weeks or longer until the chest x-ray is clear
or shows a small stable residual lesion. Unless prolonged antimicrobial therapy is administered, relapse may occur.

Drainage is the most important therapeutic maneuver of empyema.
This may be attempted with needle aspiration, but purulent fluid
may be loculated and surgical drainage is frequently required.

3.7: SKIN INFECTION (ACNE): Propionibacterium acnes is the
commonest member of the anaerobic flora of normal skin. It is the
predominant anaerobe in the anterior nares. Some studies implicate
P. acnes in the pathogenesis of acne vulgaris. However, since
P. acnes is sensitive to penicillin, and therapy with penicillin does
not result in improvement of the acne, another mechanism may
therefore be involved.

3.8: SOFT TISSUE INFECTIONS: The indigenous microflora from
intestine, vagina, skin or mouth are responsible for the majority of
mixed aerobic-anaerobic infections involving the soft tissues. Distinctive clinical syndromes have been described.

Progressive bacterial synergistic gangrene is often termed Meleney's
gangrene. Two organisms, microaerophilic streptococci and Staphylococcus aureus, act synergistically to produce gangrene, particularly after laparotomy for intraabdominal infections, especially when
through-and-through stay sutures are used. The gangrene has a
central ulcer and the surrounding area has a purplish hue with an
erythematous margin. The gangrene is quite painful and progresses
centrifugally. There may be little systemic toxicity.

Synergistic necrotizing cellulitis is differentiated from Meleney's
synergistic gangrene in having a rapidly progressive course, usually
occurring in the lower extremities of diabetics, associated with a
thin blood discharge initially, later becoming purulent, extremely
tender wounds, and fever. Most frequently isolated are aerobic
gram-negative rods, Peptostreptococci, and bacteroides species.
The mortality rate is high.

Nonclostridial crepitant cellulitis is associated with abundant gas
formation and little systemic toxicity. It is differentiated from clostridial myonecrosis by gradual onset, less severe pain, and lack of
muscle involvement.

Clostridial myonecrosis (gas gangrene) is an acute illness with sudden onset, extreme toxicity, severe pain, a thin brownish exudate

with a sweet odor and no polymorphonuclear leukocytes. The muscle appears dead or cooked, and even apparently healthy muscle may already be invaded. Death occurs frequently. Therapy must involve radical resection, penicillin, and some authorities recommend hyperbaric oxygen.

Meleney's chronic burrowing ulcer is a deep indolent subcutaneous infection associated with microaerophilic streptococci alone. These may erode the skin to produce secondary ulcers but are slowly progressive over many months.

Necrotizing fasciitis is a life-threatening dissection through deep fascial planes by Peptostreptococci, group A streptococci, or S. aureus. It may follow trauma or surgery, and is associated with undermining of tissue, crepitant cellulitis, cutaneous gangrene, or skin vesicles. Toxicity is severe and mortality is 30%.

Streptococcal myositis is produced by anaerobic streptococci and S. aureus, group A streptococci, etc. The onset is gradual, slight toxicity, increasing pain, a thin discharge, and edematous followed by hemorrhagic muscle. This discharge contains polymorphonuclear cells and gram-positive cocci in chains.

Treatment of syndromes other than the clostridial infections usually need not be so radical. Wide excision, antimicrobials, and supportive measures are appropriate. Prophylactic antitoxin and antimicrobials at the time of injury may not prevent gas gangrene. Clostridia can frequently be recovered from open wounds associated with trauma and usually represent contamination. However, cellulitis has been reported to occur in about 15% of such injuries. Devitalized tissue must therefore be excised in an effort to prevent growth of these organisms with production of clinical disease.

3.9: ACTINOMYCOSIS: Actinomycosis may present as one of three major clinical forms: cervicofacial, pulmonary, and abdominal. The cervicofacial form frequently presents as an abscess following tooth extraction. The mandible may become involved near the angle of the jaw, and the maxillary sinus is also vulnerable. The initial lesion is an extremely hard, indurated area over the site of infection. The area becomes irregularly swollen, and abscesses rupture or become fluctuant and are drained. Sinus tracts can develop from the deeper structures and drain a serosanguinous or purulent fluid which may contain sulfur granules, the tangled forms of Actinomyces israelii, or Arachnia propionica. Multiple other organisms as anaerobic cocci and Bacteroides species may be present.

Pulmonary actinomycosis usually takes the form of necrotizing pneumonia or lung abscesses. Pleural effusions are uncommon but do occur in association. The abdominal actinomycosis usually follows appendicitis, or bowel perforation. Sinus tracts may form.

These organisms are not recovered on occasion due to confusion regarding their status as anaerobes and not fungi (see Chapter 15). Therapy is with penicillins, but may need to be continued for 8 to 12 weeks or longer to insure eradication.

3.10: BOTULISM: Clostridium botulinum produces a toxin that blocks transmission at skeletal neuromuscular junctions. Seven serotypes of Cl. botulinum are known, but only A, B, and E result in human disease (Table 23-7). Clinical symptomatology is caused

TABLE 23-7: EXOTOXINS OF CL. BOTULINUM AND DISEASE EPIDEMIOLOGY			
Type	Species Having Disease	Food Associated With Toxin	Area of Predominant Occurrence
A	Man	Home Canned	Western USA
B	Man	Home Canned	Eastern USA & Europe
E	Man	Fish	Alaska, Great Lakes, Canada, Japan, Scandanavia

by ingestion of preformed toxin. These toxins may be inactivated by heating to 60°C for 30 minutes or boiling for 10 minutes. In contrast to type A or B, type E Cl. botulinum has minimal proteolytic activity, therefore foods do not taste spoiled after contamination by this organism. In addition, the clinical syndrome of type E may mimic acute gastrointestinal disease with intestinal obstruction. Neurologic signs may occur later. Recently, infant botulism has been described (Midura et al., 1976). Type A and type B organisms have been found in feces. It was suspected that toxin was formed in the gastrointestinal tract and then absorbed. A similar phenomenon has been described in older persons in whom Cl. botulinum, growing in wounds, elaborated toxin and resulted in clinical disease. Botulism is further discussed in Chapter 9.

3.11: TETANUS: Clostridium tetani is ubiquitous and is part of the intestinal flora of man and animals. Clinical tetanus develops following contamination of wounds, even of small size. Tetanus is also seen in drug addicts using dirty needles or injecting through contaminated skin surfaces. Neonatal tetanus is now unusual in the United States, but is common in many developing countries. Neonatal tetanus results from contamination of the umbilical cord with tetanus spores. (See Chapter 6 for additional discussion.)

4. ANTIMICROBIAL THERAPY

4.1: ANTIMICROBIAL AGENTS: Penicillin G is considered the drug of choice for all anaerobes except B. fragilis. A few other organisms require high levels of penicillin for inhibition. Ampicillin and cephaloridine are comparable to penicillin G in activity. The semi-synthetic penicillins remain less active. Due to the high serum levels that can be achieved with carbenicillin and cefazolin, these agents may be of value on occasion.

Chloramphenicol is the most active antimicrobial against all types of anaerobes, and very few strains are resistant. It is clinically effective against infection in all sites of the body, including the central nervous system. Available evidence suggests that chloramphenicol should be used intravenously as the irreversible bone marrow toxicity appears less frequently associated with this route. Dose-related bone marrow toxicity is a common feature and can be monitored with frequent blood studies.

In situations in which a bactericidal antibiotic is needed, penicillins or cephalosporins should be chosen, except for infections with B. fagilis. Clindamycin is effective against some B. fragilis strains. Metronidazole (Flagyl) has been shown to have good killing activity in vitro, but it has not been used extensively in clinical infections. Other factors to be considered in antimicrobial choice are drug allergy, drug penetration, toxicity, renal and hepatic function of the patient.

4.2: RESISTANT ANAEROBES: B. fragilis is the most commonly encountered resistant anaerobe. It is relatively resistant to penicillin, cephalosporins, and totally resistant to aminoglycosides. Chloramphenicol and clindamycin are uniformly effective. Tetracycline was once effective, but at present only about 35% of strains remain sensitive. Mixed pleuropulmonary infections involving B. fragilis (15-20%) are still effectively treated with penicillin G. Cl. ramosum, a less frequent isolate, is relatively penicillin resistant; only 15% of these organisms are resistant to penicillin and clindamycin, but sensitive to chloramphenicol.

REFERENCES

Balows, A., DeHann, R.M., Dowell, V.R., Guze, L.G., eds.: Anaerobic Bacteria. Charles C Thomas, Springfield, 1974.

Bartlett, J.G., Finegold, S.M.: Anaerobic infections of the lung and pleural space. Am. Rev. Resp. Dis. 110:56-77, 1974.

Chow, A.W., Leake, R.D., Yamauchi, T., Anthony, B.F., and Guze, L.B.: Significance of anaerobes in neonatal bacteremia: analysis of 23 cases and review of the literature. Pediatrics 54: 736-745, 1974.

Dunkle, L.M., Brotherton, T.J., Feigin, R.D.: Anaerobic infections in children: a prospective study. Pediatrics 57:311-320, 1976.

Dysart, N.K., Griswold, W.R., Schanberger, J.E., Goscienski, P.J., and Chow, A.W.: Meningitis due to Bacteroides fragilis in a newborn infant. J. Pediatr. 89:509, 1975.

Gorbach, S.L., Bartlett, J.G.: Anaerobic infections. NEJM 290: 1177-1184, 1237-1245, 1289-1294, 1974.

Fildes, P.: Tetanus IX. The Oxidation-reduction potential of the subcutaneous tissue fluid on the guinea-pig; its effect on infection. Brit. J. Exp. Path. 10:197-204, 1929.

Finegold, S.M.: Antimicrobial therapy of anaerobic infections. Postgrad. Med. 58:72-78, 1975.

Frederick, J., Braude, A.I.: Anaerobic infection of the paranasal sinuses. NEJM 290:135-137, 1974.

Harrod, J.R., Stevens, D.A.: Anaerobic infections in the newborn infant. J. Pediatr. 85:399-402, 1974.

Holdeman, L.V. and Moore, W.E.C., eds.: Anaerobe Laboratory Manual, V.P.I. Anaerobe Laboratory, Virginia Polytechnic Institute and State University, Blacksburg, 1972.

Midura, T.F., Arnon, S.S.: Infant botulism. Lancet 2:934-935, 1976.

Pearson, H.E., Anderson, G.V.: Perinatal deaths associated with bacteroides infections. Obstet. Gyn. 30:486-492, 1967.

Weinstein, W.M., Onderdonk, A.B., Bartlett, J.G., Louie, T.J., and Gorbach, S.L.: Antimicrobial therapy of experimental intra-abdominal sepsis. J. Infect. Dis. 132:282-286, 1975.

CHAPTER 24. HOSPITAL-ACQUIRED INFECTIONS AND
INFECTION CONTROL

INTRODUCTION: Hospital-acquired or nosocomial infections are
important clinical and epidemiologic problems in most hospitals and
represent potential health hazards to both patients and hospital personnel. They are major causes of morbidity and mortality among
hospitalized patients and contribute directly to the high costs of
medical care. It has been estimated that each year 30 million persons are admitted to acute-care hospitals in the United States. Based
on an average of 5% of patients acquiring infections during hospitalization, approximately 1.5 million patients are thought to develop nosocomial infections each year. It has been estimated that the duration
of hospitalization of each patient with a nosocomial infection is prolonged an average of 7 days. If one assumed a hospitalization cost
of $150 per day, then each hospital-acquired infection would cost
about $1,000. Based on these estimates, infections acquired in hos-
pitals cost Americans approximately 1.5 billion dollars per year
(Schaffner, 1976).

DEFINITION: An infection may be present on admission, appearing
during hospitalization, or appearing after the patient has been discharged from the hospital. A hospital-acquired (nosocomial) infection is one that occurs during hospitalization. It is neither present
nor known to be incubating at the time of admission, unless related
to a previous hospitalization. Thus, a patient who is in the incubation
period of an infection at the time of admission and subsequently develops a clinically active infection does not have a nosocomial infection, unless the infection was acquired during a prior hospitalization.
An infection acquired during hospitalization but is not clinically evident until the patient is discharged from the hospital is also considered a hospital-acquired infection. When the incubation period is
unknown, an infection is regarded hospital-acquired if it develops at
any time after admission. An infection present on admission may be
classified as hospital-acquired only if it is known to have been acquired during a prior hospitalization. However, it is frequently difficult to identify those infections present on admission but in reality
are acquired from a previous hospitalization. Those infections which
are obviously acquired outside the hospital are termed community-
acquired. The term hospital-associated infection is used to encompass those infections acquired in the hospital as well as those present
on admission (Brachmann, 1963).

INCIDENCE AND PREVALENCE: The frequency of hospital-acquired
infections has been reported to vary from 3.5 to 15.5 percent of hospital population. These variations in frequency are dependent to a
large extent on the ways the data are collected. In some studies, the

frequencies are expressed as prevalence rates, in which the data
are obtained by determining the number of patients with nosocomial
infections existing in the hospital at a particular point in time. In
other reports, the data are expressed as incidence rates which represent the number of nosocomial infections occurring among patients
admitted to a hospital during a given period of time. The prevalence
rate of nosocomial infections is generally higher than the incidence
rate.

A review of selected reports published in the literature indicates
that approximately 5 percent of all patients admitted to hospitals
developed an infection during the course of their hospitalization,
with the incidence rates varying from 3.5 to 6.5 percent (Table
24-1). In several prevalent surveys, the proportions of patients
found to have nosocomial infections range from 4.7 to 15.5 percent.
Prevalence surveys conducted on three different occasions at the
Boston City Hospital revealed 12.0 to 15.5 percent of hospitalized
patients having nosocomial infections (Kislak et al., 1964; Barrett
et al., 1967; Adler et al., 1971).

The incidence of infection has been shown to vary according to type
of hospital. In a survey of 68 hospitals participating in the 1970
National Nosocomial Infections Study conducted by the Center for
Disease Control (CDC), the average rate of infections occurring in
all types of hospitals was 5 percent (Bennett et al., 1971). Community hospitals have the lowest rate of infection. Of the 40 community hospitals included in the study, the rate was 2.3 percent,
compared with 4.9 percent for university hospitals and 11.4 percent
for chronic disease hospitals. Community hospitals with less than
300 beds generally have lower incidence of infection than those with
more than 300 beds.

The frequency of nosocomial infection also varies with the type of
hospital service. In the CDC National Nosocomial Infections Study
for the period of January 1970 to December 1973, the incidence of
infection was highest in the surgical services, with the rate of 4.7
per 100 discharges (Stamm et al., 1976). The lowest rates were
seen in pediatrics (1.2%) and nursery (0.9%). In the 1970 Boston
City Hospital survey, the prevalence of infection in the surgical services was twice as high as that in the medical services. The incidence of nosocomial infections for a nine-month period in 1976 by
hospital service at the University of Kansas is summarized in
Table 24-2.

SITES OF INFECTIONS: The various clinical manifestations of nosocomial infections are generally classified according to sites of infection. Most of the infections involve the genitourinary tract, respiratory tract and surgical wounds (Table 24-3). According to the
National Nosocomial Infections Study of CDC, about 80% of all infections acquired in different types of hospitals affect these three sites
(Stamm et al., 1976). Urinary tract infections are most common,

TABLE 24-1: INCIDENCE AND PREVALENCE OF HOSPITAL-ACQUIRED INFECTIONS IN SELECTED HOSPITALS 1959-1976		
SOURCE	INCIDENCE %	PREVALENCE %
Hospital for Sick Children, Toronto, Canada, 1959 (Roy et al. 1962)	6.5	
Boston City Hospital, 1964 (Kislak et al. 1964)		13.5
Boston City Hospital, 1967 (Barrett et al. 1967)		15.5
University of Kentucky, 1965 (Adler et al. 1971)	6.1	
Johns Hopkins Hospital, 1965-1967 (Thoburn et al. 1968)	4.0	4.7
Six U.S. Community Hospitals, 1965-1966 (Eickhoff et al. 1969)	3.5	
Eight U.S. Community Hospitals, 1969-1970 (Scheckler et al. 1971)		5.5
68 U.S. Hospitals, 1970 (Bennett et al. 1971)	5.0	
Brooke Army Medical Center, 1973 (Moore 1974)	5.0	
University of Virginia (Wenzel et al. 1976)	6.0	
University of Kansas, 1976	3.8	

TABLE 24-2: INCIDENCE OF HOSPITAL-ACQUIRED INFECTIONS
BY HOSPITAL SERVICE
UNIVERSITY OF KANSAS MEDICAL CENTER
APRIL - DECEMBER 1976

Hospital Service	Number of Discharges	Number of Infections	Rate per 100 Discharges
Surgery	5,461	312*	5.7
Medicine	3,972	131	3.3
Gynecology	1,308	33	2.5
Obstetrics	1,753	27	1.5
Pediatrics	1,126	17	1.5
Nursery	993	28**	2.8

* Includes Burn Center

** Includes Intensive Care Unit, 0.8% excluding ICU

TABLE 24-3: FREQUENCY OF HOSPITAL-ACQUIRED
INFECTIONS BY SITE OF INFECTION
UNIVERSITY OF KANSAS MEDICAL CENTER
APRIL - DECEMBER 1976

Site of Infection	Number of Infections	Percent of Total	Rate per 1000 Discharges (N=14.613)
Genitourinary tract	258	47.1	18
Surgical wound	77	14.1	5
Respiratory tract	68	12.4	5
Blood	52	9.5	4
Skin and Subcutaneous tissues	50	9.1	3
Gynecological system	16	2.9	1
Gastrointestinal tract	11	2.0	1
Others	16	2.9	1
TOTAL	548	100.0	38

accounting for about 40% of nosocomial infections (Thoburn et al., 1968; Stamm et al., 1976). In most acute-care hospitals, surgical wound infections rank second in frequency, followed by respiratory tract infections. Bacteremia generally occurs in less than 10% of infections; this infection, however, is frequently associated with high fatality (DuPont, 1969). Other infections such as endocarditis, meningitis, osteomyelitis, or intra-abdominal abscess may occur but are relatively uncommon. Gastrointestinal infections due to organisms such as Salmonella, Shigella and enteropathogenic Escherichia coli may be introduced into nurseries and cause extensive epidemics.

FACTORS INFLUENCING INFECTIONS: Many factors can influence the development of hospital infections. Although interrelated and frequently overlapping with each other, the various factors may be grouped under three major categories: microbial agent, host susceptibility, and environment.

Microbial Agents: Infection may be caused by exposure to any potentially pathogenic agent. The most common types of microorganisms involved in hospital infections are bacteria, viruses and fungi. During the 1950's and early 1960's, Staphylococcus aureus was the predominant organism causing hospital infections. However, during the late 1960's, the incidence of staphylococcal infection began to decrease and enteric gram-negative bacilli emerged as the major cause of nosocomial infections. In 1964, for example, Staphylococcus aureus caused about one-third of all infections acquired at the Boston City Hospital, while in 1967 the frequency of infections caused by this organism had decreased to 10 percent. In contrast, between 1964 and 1970, the frequency of infection caused by the gram-negative organisms at this hospital had increased from 22.7 to 37.8 percent (Finland, 1973). Today, gram-negative aerobic bacilli constitute 60-65 percent of all isolates from patients with nosocomial infections (Table 24-4). This change in microbial ecology has been attributed at least in part to the extensive use of penicillinase-resistant penicillins.

The most common gram-negative bacteria isolated from nosocomial infections are Escherichia coli, Pseudomonas aeruginosa, members of the Klebsiella-Enterobacter group, and Proteus species. Many gram-negative bacteria normally considered either nonpathogenic or lowly pathogenic for humans have been found to cause hospital-acquired infections. Serratia marcescens, a gram-negative coccobacterium previously regarded strictly as a non-pathogen, is now isolated with increasing frequency from patients with respiratory and urinary tract infections (Sanders et al., 1970; Maki et al., 1973). Flavobacterium, a gram-negative, yellow pigment-producing organism, has been associated with outbreaks of meningitis and septicemia in newborn infants (Cabrera et al., 1961; Stamm et al., 1975). Achromobacter, a non-pigment producing gram-negative bacterium which

TABLE 24-4: DISTRIBUTION OF MICROORGANISMS ISOLATED FROM PATIENTS WITH HOSPITAL-ACQUIRED INFECTIONS, UNIVERSITY OF KANSAS MEDICAL (KUMC) CENTER AND NATIONAL NOSOCOMIAL INFECTIONS STUDY (CDC)

ORGANISMS	KUMC (%)	BOSTON CITY HOSPITAL (%)	CDC (%)
Staphylococcus (Coag +)	10.0	14.3	9.6
Staphylococcus (Coag -)			3.6
Enterococcus	6.1	7.5	7.7
Streptococcus (Group A)	0.8	0.7	2.2
E. coli	16.7	10.9	20.9
Klebsiella- Enterobacter	13.2	23.1	13.2
Proteus	8.9	11.6	9.6
Pseudomonas	20.5	15.0	8.9
Serratia	1.4	3.4	1.1
Others	22.4	13.5	23.2
TOTAL	100.0	100.0	100.0

can readily grow in distilled water, has also been associated with septicemia in newborn infants (Foley et al., 1961). Infections due to other bacteria such as Listeria monocytogenes, Mima polymorpha, and Vibrio fetus are being recognized with increasing frequency. Viruses such as cytomegalovirus and hepatitis B, fungi such as Candida albicans, Aspergillus species and Nocardia asteroides, and protozoa such as Pneumocystis carinii and Toxoplasma gondii are becoming more important as causes of nosocomial and opportunistic infections (Riley, 1969; Frenkel, 1974).

Host Susceptibility: Host resistance is generally considered a more important determinant of nosocomial infection than the type of organism producing infection. Among the significant factors which influence host resistance are age, immunologic status, type of underlying disease, and effects of diagnostic and therapeutic procedures.

Although hospital-acquired infections are frequently associated with infancy and old age, age itself may not be as important a predisposing factor to infection as the associated conditions prevalent in certain age groups. For example, meningitis caused by gram-negative bacilli is a common complication in infants with meningomyelocele, and urinary tract infection is frequently observed in children with congenital abnormality of the urinary tract. It is well known that premature infants are more susceptible to serious infections than full-term infants. Patients with underlying diseases such as cystic fibrosis, leukemia, lymphoma, agranulocytosis, and dysglobulinemia are more prone to develop nosocomial infections than patients without such conditions.

Many diagnostic procedures such as cardiac catheterization, bone marrow aspirations and cystoscopy tend to increase the risk of infection. The risk of infection is also enhanced by the use of therapeutic procedures such as tracheostomy, endotracheal intubation, use of antibiotics, ionizing radiation, blood transfusions, steroids, cytotoxic agents and immunosuppressive drugs.

Environment: Infections occurring in the hospital environment may arise either exogenously or endogenously. Exogenous infections refer to those infections in which the sources are infected persons or inanimate objects in the hospital environment. Exogenous sources may be patients, visitors or employees and include persons who have active disease, are in the incubation period of an infection or are asymptomatic carriers of an infection. Of the various inanimate sources associated with hospital-acquired infections, indwelling urinary catheters, intravascular devices, inhalation therapy equipment, and contaminated solutions are among the most commonly encountered. Endogenous infections, on the other hand, are derived from the patient's own indigenous microflora which, under normal circumstances, do not cause disease. However, when the patient's host resistance is depressed as a result of certain diagnostic or therapeutic procedures, infection may ensue.

Patients are frequently colonized by pathogenic microorganisms after they are admitted to the hospital. Johanson et al. (1972) showed that respiratory tract colonization occurred in 45% of patients admitted to a medical intensive care unit, with 22% colonized on the first day of admission. Of 26 patients who developed nosocomial infection, 85% were shown to have been colonized with gram-negative bacilli. Twenty-three percent of 95 patients who were colonized with gram-negative bacilli developed respiratory infections, while only 3.3% of 118 noncolonized patients developed infection.

The role of intestinal colonization as a reservoir of nosocomial Klebsiella infection was reported by Selden et al. (1971). Rectal swab culture studies revealed that 25% of 138 patients on the acute-care wards were intestinal carriers of multidrug-resistant Klebsiella. Among 31 patients who became intestinal carriers of Klebsiella during hospitalization, 45% developed nosocomial infection caused by the same serotype. In contrast, only 10% of 101 patients who did not become intestinal carriers developed infection caused by the same serotype. The data indicate that antibiotic therapy was a predisposing factor to intestinal colonization with Klebsiella and had exerted a selective pressure in favor of developing multidrug-resistant Klebsiella.

Studies have shown that microorganisms isolated from hospital personnel or within the hospital are more resistant to antibiotics than those isolated from outside the hospital. Multiple-resistant organisms have been found to be more common in hospital-acquired infections than in community-acquired infections. Lorian et al. (1972) reported that 70% of the strains resistant to 7 drugs were isolated from patients with hospital-acquired infections, compared with 30% from those with community-acquired infections.

Environmental factors such as overcrowding, poor ventilation, contaminated air, poor housekeeping, and inadequate handwashing facilities can influence the spread of microorganisms in the hospital environment.

MECHANISMS OF TRANSMISSION: Infections occurring in the hospital may be spread by the following routes: contact, airborne, common vehicle and vectorborne.

<u>Contact Spread</u>: Spread from person to person is the most common mechanism of transmission. Infections may be spread by direct contact, indirect contact or droplets. Direct contact transmission refers to spread from one person to another directly without an intermediary object. Direct contact by hands has been demonstrated the most important means of spreading infections from one patient to another. Hands of physicians, nurses, and other attendants have been found to be the principal method of transmission of <u>Staphylococcus aureus</u> in newborn nurseries and of <u>Pseudomonas aeruginosa</u> in burn units. Indirect contact involves spread of infection to a susceptible person by coming in contact with contaminated articles such as towels, surgical instruments, catheters, dressings and clothing (fomites). Spread from person to person may also take place by coming in contact with droplets of secretions produced by sneezing, coughing or talking. Transmission by droplets is considered a contact infection rather than an airborne infection because of the close association between the source and the susceptible host, since droplets usually do not travel more than about three feet from the source. Influenza, parainfluenza, measles and streptococcal pharyngitis are examples of infections spread by droplets. Mufson et al. (1973) reported the spread of parainfluenza-3 infection among hospitalized children over a 15-month period. About one-fifth of the 197 contacts of the infected index cases developed evidence of nosocomial infection with parainfluenza-3 virus. An infection may be spread to a susceptible host by more than one way. For example, during endotracheal incubation, pathogens may be transmitted to a patient by the attendant's hands or from a contaminated instrument.

<u>Airborne</u>: Airborne infection occurs when a susceptible person inhales droplet nuclei or suspended dust particles which contain an infectious agent. Droplet nuclei are small residues produced by evaporation of droplets and remain suspended in air for long periods of

time. Tuberculosis and chickenpox are examples of infections transmitted by airborne droplet nuclei. Ehrenkranz et al. (1972) reported an outbreak of tuberculosis in a general hospital in which the source was traced to a 65-year old man initially diagnosed as having acute pulmonary edema. Tuberculous infection was detected in 25 employees, 2 of whom developed active pulmonary tuberculosis. Epidemiologic studies indicated that Mycobacterium tuberculosis spread by the airborne route was the cause of the epidemic.

Common Vehicle: Infection by common vehicle refers to transmission by some contaminated source such as food, water, drugs, blood or blood products. The recent nationwide epidemic of septicemia resulting from infusion of contaminated intravenous products is an example of transmission by this route. A total of 378 patients in 25 U.S. hospitals developed septicemia as a result of receiving intravenous infusion fluid contaminated with either Enterobacter cloacae or Enterobacter agglomerans (Maki et al., 1976). Extensive common source outbreaks of salmonellosis affecting multiple hospitals may occasionally occur. Sanders et al. (1963) investigated an outbreak of Salmonella derby infection involving 53 hospitals in 13 states. The source of infection was raw or undercooked eggs. The primary infections resulted in extensive secondary person-to-person spread which became a major problem in several hospitals.

Vectorborne: Transmission of infections by arthropod vectors, such as mosquitoes, may occur but is of little importance in hospitals of this country.

1. INFECTION CONTROL

The first step in the control of hospital infection is to establish an effective surveillance system. The principal objective of having such a system is to obtain data on infections which normally occur in the hospital. Such data are essential for providing a baseline so that infection control personnel can determine when special investigations are needed, where these investigations are to be conducted, and for providing information to make recommendations and establish policy for prevention and control of nosocomial infections.

Beginning July 1, 1971, the Joint Commission on Accreditation of Hospitals requires each hospital to have an infection control committee for assuming the responsibility of developing an effective infection control program. The elements of the program should include: (1) surveillance of nosocomial infections, (2) isolation policies and procedures, (3) surveillance, prevention and control procedures relating to the inanimate hospital environment, (4) in-service training and education, (5) provision for microbiology laboratory support, (6) an employee health program, and (7) monitoring of antibiotic utilization.

An infection control committee should consist of representatives from the clinical services, administration, and central services. Generally, members should include representatives from internal medicine, pediatrics, obstetrics, surgery, nursing, clinical microbiology and hospital administration. In addition, regular or ad hoc members may also be designated from dietetics, housekeeping, pharmacy, medical records, employee health service, and house staff. The committee should be chaired by an effective leader who has the respect and confidence of the hospital staff. In larger hospitals, the chairman is usually the hospital epidemiologist or a physician who has had special training in infectious diseases. In smaller hospitals, the chairmanship is usually assumed by the hospital pathologist, bacteriologist or a physician who has special interest in infectious diseases. The committee should meet regularly and on special occasions as indicated.

The key to a successful surveillance program is the infection control nurse. Surveillance activities of the infection control nurse vary somewhat, depending on the size and type of hospital and the characteristics of the surveillance program. In general, she should be a registered nurse who has had clinical experience in a hospital and possesses a reasonable knowledge of epidemiology and infectious disease. In hospitals with more than 400 beds, a full-time infection control nurse is usually required. However, in hospitals of lesser size, the position is usually part-time, based on a ratio of 10 hours per 100 beds (Garner et al., 1971).

The infection control nurse is responsible for developing a surveillance program to detect nosocomial infections on a systematic basis. Various methods have been used for the detection of these infections. The most common methods used include:

1. Daily review of microbiology laboratory reports to note positive cultures, and review charts to determine the clinical significance of such cultures.
2. Regular, preferably daily, ward rounds to review patients on isolation, patients with fever and those receiving antibiotics or special treatments.
3. Reports of infections by charge nurse or physicians.
4. Review of infection logs kept on nursing units.
5. Review of nursing care plan (Kardex).
6. Postdischarge follow-up survey by mail or telephone.
7. Review of autopsy reports to detect undiagnosed infections.
8. Prevalence surveys conducted at regular intervals to validate surveillance data.

In addition to case-finding, the infection control nurse is responsible for tabulating and analyzing nosocomial infection data and for preparing a monthly report to be reviewed by the infection control committee. She is also responsible for advising hospital personnel about

the hospital's policy on isolation and disposition of patients admitted
with infection. Together with the hospital epidemiologist, she is
responsible for initiating epidemiologic investigations of outbreaks
or situations in which the level of infections appear to be above
normal.

It is of utmost importance that the data collected by the infection
control nurse be tabulated on a current basis so that the information generated can be periodically examined by and discussed with
the hospital epidemiologist or the chairman of the infection control
committee. The monthly surveillance report should be analyzed and
tabulated according to type of infection, type of service, and type of
microorganisms isolated. The incidence of infection is usually expressed as number of hospital-acquired infections per 100 patient
admissions or discharges. The monthly surveillance report, together with information on antibiotic sensitivity patterns, antibiotic
utilization, environmental microbiology, and other pertinent data
should be distributed to the hospital staff.

2. ISOLATION TECHNIQUES AND PROCEDURES

Preventing the spread of microorganisms among patients, hospital
employees and visitors should be based on sound epidemiologic principles. Since agent and host factors are frequently difficult to control, prevention should be directed toward interrupting the chain of
transmission. Among the various preventive measures, isolation is
one of the best means available. The aim is to create a barrier between the patient and his environment. In general, isolation procedures may be grouped into the following categories:

1) Strict isolation
2) Respiratory isolation
3) Enteric precautions
4) Wound and skin precautions
5) Protective isolation

Strict Isolation: This type of isolation is required to prevent the
transmission of highly communicable diseases that are transmitted
by both the contact and airborne routes. A single room is indicated;
gowns, masks and gloves must be worn by all persons entering the
patient's room. The diseases requiring strict isolation are:

1) Anthrax, inhalation
2) Burn wound, extensive, infected with:
   a) Staphylococcus aureus, or
   b) Group A streptococcus
3) Congenital rubella syndrome
4) Diphtheria
5) Disseminated neonatal Herpesvirus hominis (herpes simplex)
6) Plague, pulmonic

7) Pneumonia, infected with:
   a) Staphylococcus aureus, or
   b) Group A streptococcus
8) Rabies
9) Skin infection, extensive, with:
   a) Staphylococcus aureus, or
   b) Group A streptococcus
10) Smallpox
11) Vaccinia
   a) Generalized and progressive
   b) Eczema vaccinatum
12) Varicella and disseminated herpes zoster

Respiratory Isolation: The aim is to prevent transmission of micro-organisms spread by the respiratory route. This type of isolation generally requires a single room and wearing of a mask. The diseases requiring respiratory isolation are:

1) Measles (rubeola)
2) Meningitis, meningococcal
3) Meningococcemia
4) Mumps
5) Pertussis (whooping cough)
6) Rubella (German measles), except congenital rubella syndrome
7) Tuberculosis, pulmonary - sputum positive or suspect

Enteric Precautions: Transmission of infection in this category depends on ingestion of pathogens transmitted through direct or indirect contact with infected feces of patients or heavily contaminated articles. Viral hepatitis, cholera, typhoid fever, staphylococcal enterocolitis, and gastroenteritis caused by Salmonella, Shigella, enteropathogenic Escherichia coli and Yersinia enterocolitica are some of the infections requiring enteric precautions. Strict handwashing is necessary, as well as wearing of gowns and gloves. Single rooms are required for children with infections in this category.

Wound and Skin Precautions: Precautions required to control cross-infection in this category include adequate handwashing before and after patient contact and proper use of gowns and gloves when indicated. Gloves are used for change of wound dressing, or if the attendant must come in contact with skin or wound lesions that are heavily contaminated. Wearing of a mask is not necessary except for changing dressings. The following diseases require these types of precautions:

1) Burns with excessive purulent drainage, except those with:
   a) Staphylococcus aureus, or
   b) Group A streptococcus
2) Gas gangrene
3) Herpes zoster

4) Melioidosis
5) Plague, bubonic
6) Skin infection, extensive, that cannot be covered by a dressing, except those infected with:
   a) Staphylococcus aureus, or
   b) Group A streptococcus
7) Wound infection with excessive purulent drainage that cannot be covered by a dressing

Protective Isolation: Patients with certain diseases such as leukemia, lymphoma and agranulocytosis, and those who are receiving immunosuppressive therapy are significantly more susceptible to infections than patients without such diseases or conditions. The aim is to prevent patients from coming in contact with potentially pathogenic microorganisms introduced exogenously. This type of isolation has only limited usefulness since patients requiring protective isolation are frequently infected by their own indigenous microflora. In patients with extensive noninfected burns or dermatitis, gowns, masks, and gloves are worn for the protection of the attendant as well as the patient.

Handwashing: Of the various techniques used for preventing spread of infection from one patient to another, handwashing is the single most important. It should be a routine practice of all personnel to wash their hands before and after contact with each patient. There is no uniform policy regarding the use of antiseptic agent in connection with handwashing. Some believe antiseptic agents should be used for all personnel handwashing, while others believe plain soap or other detergents should be used for routine handwashing, and antiseptic agents should be reserved for special purposes. A recent survey of 82 hospitals by the CDC revealed 83% requiring handwashing with an iodophor or some other antiseptic and 47% requiring handwashing with only plain soap between routine patient contact (Steere et al., 1975).

It is probably desirable to use an antiseptic agent in handwashing when heavy contamination is present. However, antiseptic agents may cause excessive drying of skin if used frequently and may cause dermatitis or other undesirable effects. Handwashing with soap containing hexachlorophene is effective in reducing Staphylococcus aureus on the hands, but it may also increase the risk of hand colonization with gram-negative bacilli (Bruun et al., 1973). In view of some of the undesirable properties associated with the use of antiseptics, it has been suggested that its use should be limited to handwashing before surgery and other high risk invasive procedures, and in the care of newborn infants, but soap and water should be used for routine handwashing.

Single Room: Private rooms are indicated for isolation of patients with disease which are highly contagious and airborne. Each room should contain handwashing, bathing and toilet facilities.

Gowns: Individual gown is necessary when pathogenic organisms
from the patient can be transmitted to the attendant's clothing by
direct contact. Gowning is advisable when holding infants in diapers.
However, it is not required for examining an infant in an incubator.
Sterile gowns are recommended for use in caring for patients in protective isolation. They should also be worn for changing dressings
and for caring for patients with extensive burns or extensive wound
infections. Clean, freshly laundered or disposable gowns may be
used for all other purposes.

Masks: A mask is worn to protect the wearer against acquiring an
infection spread by droplets or aerosols. They should cover the nose
and mouth. Masks should be worn only once. They must not be lowered around the neck and then reused. When the mask becomes wet,
it is inefficient and should be discarded in a suitable container before
the user leaves the contaminated area. Filter masks are more effective than paper or standard cotton gauze masks. Masking of hospital
personnel does not seem to affect the colonization of Staphylococcus
aureus among infants in newborn nurseries (Forfar et al., 1958).

Gloves: Gloves are used for the protection of both the attendant and
the patient. They must be worn by all persons having direct contact
with patients requiring strict isolation or with articles contaminated
with pathogenic microorganisms. When contaminated dressings are
changed, two sets of gloves must be used, one set for removing
soiled dressing and the other set for applying new dressings. Hands
should be washed between glove changes.

The attending physician is responsible for placing his or her patient
on isolation. However, a policy should be established to allow a
charge nurse to have a patient placed on isolation for up to 48 hours
if a physician is not available to make a determination. In such an
event, the charge nurse should notify her action to both the attending
physician and the infection control officer as soon as possible. A
card system specifying isolation procedures for various communicable
diseases has been developed by the Center for Disease Control, Public Health Service. By using this card system, exact isolation procedures for a specific infection can be determined directly by reading
the information on the card. After the type of isolation has been determined, the appropriate card should be displayed conspicuously on
the door, foot of the bed, or other area in the immediate vicinity of
the isolated patient (Isolation Techniques for Use in Hospitals, Second Edition, 1975; Infection Control in the Hospital, Third Edition,
1974).

3. INFECTIONS IN NEWBORN NURSERIES

Because of their increased susceptibility to infections, newborn infants present a special challenge to infection control. In the 1950's
and early 1960's, staphylococci replaced streptococci as the chief

cause of infection in newborn nurseries. During that period, Staphylococcus aureus was responsible for serious epidemics throughout
the world. Since that time, however, the prevalence of staphylococcal disease had declined, followed by the emergence of a wide
variety of gram-negative bacterial infections.

Staphylococcal Infections: Newborn infants rapidly become colonized
on their body surfaces by the staphyloccus strain prevalent in the
nursery. By the fifth day, 40 to 90 percent of infants will be colonized with Staphylococcus aureus (Shinefield et al., 1965). Usually,
the umbilical stump becomes colonized first, then the nares, perineum, buttocks and other areas of the skin.

Although a high proportion of infants are colonized by coagulase-
positive staphylococci, only few develop infection with significant
clinical manifestations. The most common clinical manifestations
of staphylococcal infection during the neonatal period are conjunctivitis, skin rashes and paronychiae (Riley, 1969). These lesions
are generally benign and thus are frequently overlooked. The more
serious manifestations are pyoderma, which may progress to extensive cellulitis or occasionally abscess formation, pneumonia and
septicemia, resulting in high fatality. Other manifestations include
meningitis, osteomyelitis, arthritis and intra-abdominal abscess.
Staphylococci acquired in the nursery often do not produce clinical
disease in infants until after they are discharged from the nursery.
Therefore, when an outbreak is suspected, it is essential to have
home follow-up. Follow-up telephone surveys of physicians and
mothers have been found to be a valuable epidemiologic tool for assessing staphylococcal infections acquired in nurseries (Murray et
al., 1958).

Spread of infections by hands of hospital personnel is the primary
mode of transmission within nurseries. Studies of Lipsitz et al.
(1962) have indicated that 92% of newborn infants acquired staphylococci when they were attended by personnel with unwashed hands,
compared with a 53% acquisition rate when the attendants washed
their hands. These studies also indicated that airborne transmission
could occur, but to a much lesser extent than transmission by direct
person-to-person contact.

When an epidemic of staphylococcal disease occurs in a nursery, the
causative organism is usually an epidemic strain. In the past, most
of the nursery outbreaks have been caused by phage type 80/81. The
prevalent strain is usually introduced into the nursery by a nursery
worker who has an overt staphylococcal infection or who is a dis-
seminating carrier. Once the staphylococcus is introduced, transmission is often maintained by infant-to-infant spread.

Although the factors which influence development of disease following colonization are still not fully understood, infants who are heavily colonized and who are colonized during the first few days after birth are more likely to develop staphylococcal disease (Fekety, 1964). Also, colonized male infants appear to be more prone to develop disease than female infants. Therefore, to reduce the risk of epidemic disease, it appears reasonable to reduce the colonization rate in hospital nurseries. Since colonization of newborns is attributable largely to transmission by direct contact, handwashing before and after handling each infant is considered the most effective means of reducing prevalence of colonization.

Bathing of newborn infants with 3% hexachlorophene has been found effective in reducing staphylococcus colonization and thus reducing the risk of infection. However, recent studies of monkeys bathed daily in 3% hexachlorophene for 90 days revealed evidence of neurotoxicity (Lockhart, 1972). Brain lesions similar to those seen in monkeys were found in infants bathed in hexachlorophene (Powell et al., 1973; Shuman et al., 1974). On the basis of these observations, daily bathing of newborn infants with 3% hexachlorophene is no longer recommended as a routine practice.

Shortly after the recommendation to ban the use of hexachlorophene, a number of outbreaks of staphylococcal disease had appeared in nurseries in which hexachlorophene bathing had been discontinued (Kaslow et al., 1973). Because of this, some have suggested single bathing of full-term infants with 3% hexachlorophene for the control of staphylococcal infections in nurseries (Kwong et al., 1973). Since neurotoxicity was observed primarily in very low birth weight infants who had received multiple bathings, it is possible that the concentration of hexachlorophene absorbed by a single bathing would not be sufficient to cause adverse neurotoxic effects. Also, it has been reported by the Australia Drug Evaluation Committee that continued use of hexachlorophene on a limited scale has revealed no evidence of brain disease (Plueckhahn, 1973).

Gram-Negative Rod Infections: Since the 1960's, the use of semi-synthetic penicillinase-resistant penicillins has suppressed hospital epidemics due to Staphylococcus aureus, and enteric gram-negative bacilli have emerged as the predominant cause of hospital-acquired infections. The common use of hexachlorophene for bathing of newborn infants is also thought to have an influential effect on the change of microbial ecology in nurseries. As in other areas of the hospital, many of the gram-negative organisms encountered in nurseries are normally considered not highly pathogenic. Among the variety of gram-negative organisms identified are Klebsiella pneumoniae, Pseudomonas aeruginosa, Escherichia coli, Proteus species, Enterobacter, Salmonella species, Shigella species, Hafnia, Achromobacter, Flavobacterium and Serratia.

Certain organisms such as Salmonella may be transmitted from the mother or from a common source such as contaminated food. However, the sources of most gram-negative rod infections are contaminated equipment, such as humidifying equipment, resuscitators, faucet aerators or other pieces of equipment used in the nursery. Outbreaks caused by these organisms are often serious and highly fatal, particularly in premature infants.

The epidemiology of gram-negative rod infections is different from that of staphylococcus infection. While control of staphylococcus infection depends primarily on adherence to handwashing and other proper nursing techniques, control of gram-negative bacillary infections rests primarily on rigorous sterilization of humidifying apparatus and other equipment used in the nursery.

Viral Infections: Various viruses, including influenza virus, parainfluenza viruses, respiratory syncytial virus, coxsackie viruses and echoviruses have been reported to cause infection in nurseries (Artenstein et al., 1962; Hall et al., 1975). Although infections caused by these agents are usually mild, severe outbreaks with fulminating illnesses have been reported, particularly among premature infants. Infections caused by respiratory viruses, such as influenza virus and respiratory syncytial virus, are difficult to control. However, segregation of clinically infected infants from non-infected infants may be of value. Since coxsackie viruses and echoviruses are transmitted principally by personal contact, handwashing should be effective in limiting the spread of these infections.

4. INHALATION THERAPY-ASSOCIATED INFECTIONS

Widespread use of inhalation therapy equipment in recent years has been considered a major cause of hospital-acquired respiratory infections, particularly necrotizing gram-negative pneumonia. Epidemics have been attributed to contaminated nebulizers, anesthesia machines, resuscitation equipment, and contaminated medications, solutions and other materials used in connection with inhalation therapy (Mertz et al., 1967; Pierce et al., 1970; Sanford et al., 1971).

Inhalation therapy equipment is used to deliver gas mixtures, with or without medications, to the patient's respiratory system. Two methods of delivery are generally used: nebulization and humidification. In nebulization, both water droplets and vapor are produced by a jet of air or gas using the Venturi principle, or by dropping water on a spinning disc or vibrating reed. In humidification, on the other hand, water vapor is created by passing air or gas through water without generating water droplets. Inhalation therapy utilizing nebulizers is more likely to cause infection than therapy utilizing humidifiers. If water in the nebulizer reservoir is contaminated with bacteria, particulate water, together with the bacteria will be delivered

into the effluent stream of gas. When humidifiers are used, it is
likely only water vapor is generated in the bacteria-free gas phase.
Although infections associated with the use of fine-particle humidifiers has been reported (Grieble et al., 1970), ventilators and humidifiers used in connection with inhalation therapy generally provide only minimal risk for transmitting bacteria into the patient's
inspired gas. Small-volume nebulizers used to deliver medications
also seldom present a hazard unless the liquid medication in the reservoir is contaminated. Large-volume nebulizers, on the other hand,
have been found to be a major source of infection. Contamination
of the nebulizers, however, can be readily controlled by appropriate
decontamination procedures. A standardized procedure of decontamination with 0.25 percent acetic acid has been reported by Sanford (1974). Once a day, while the equipment is still in use, the
contents from the reservoir nebulizer jar should be emptied and
rinsed with water, followed by aerosolizing the machine with 0.25
acetic acid. Using this procedure for systematic decontamination
of inhalation therapy equipment, it was possible to reduce the frequency of necrotizing pneumonia mortality from 7.9 percent to 1.8
percent.

5. CATHETER-ASSOCIATED INFECTIONS

Bladder catheterization is a major predisposing factor associated
with urinary tract infection and gram-negative septicemia. It has
been estimated that 10-15% of patients admitted to general hospitals
will have indwelling catheters placed in the bladder sometime during
their hospitalization (Kunin et al., 1966; Garibaldi et al., 1974;
Stamm 1975). The risk of developing urinary tract infection associated with urinary catheters depends on the method and duration of
catheterization. Bacteriuria has been observed in 1-5% of patients
after a single short-term catheterization. A much higher incidence
of infection occurs when indwelling catheters are used. Kass (1956)
has shown that 90% of patients developed bacteriuria within 48 hours
if indwelling catheters were attached to open drainage; bacteriuria
was observed in 95% of patients if the catheter was left in place for
four days. The risk of acquiring bacteriuria with respect to duration
of catheterization is relatively constant, with an increase of 5-10%
for each day of catheterization.

Studies have indicated that undoubtedly indwelling catheters with open
drainage are the most common cause of urinary tract infection;
therefore, a closed system of drainage should always be used. When
such a system is used, the incidence of urinary tract infection can
be reduced to possibly 15-25% if the duration of catheterization does
not exceed two weeks (Stamm, 1975). Kunin and McCormack (1966)
demonstrated that routine use of closed drainage could maintain sterile urine in 50% of males and females for 13.5 and 11.0 days
respectively.

Acquisition of bacteriuria in patients with indwelling catheters can
be reduced by continuous bladder irrigation using a triple-lumen
catheter with either an acetic acid or neomycin-polymyxin solution.
The incidence of infection after ten days of catheterization was reduced to 20% when acetic acid or nitrofurazone was used as bladder
rinse, and to 6% when neomycin-polymyxin solution was used for
irrigation (Andriole, 1975).

To reduce the incidence of hospital-acquired urinary tract infection
to a minimum, indwelling urinary catheters should be used only
when absolutely necessary and catheters should be inserted only by
adequately trained personnel using aseptic techniques. When an indwelling urinary catheter is required, a sterile closed drainage system should always be used. Antibacterial cleansing of the meatal-
catheter junction followed by application of an antimicrobial ointment
may further reduce the incidence of urinary tract infection.

6. INFECTIONS ASSOCIATED WITH INTRAVENOUS THERAPY

Intravenous infusion therapy has become an integral part of modern
hospital practice. It has been estimated that at least 8 million hospitalized patients receive intravenous fluid each year (Maki et al.,
1973). Associated with this usage are the common occurrences of
thrombophlebitis and septicemia. Contaminated intravenous fluids
and indwelling plastic catheters are frequent sources of these infections. It has been reported that one-third to one-fourth of all catheters left in place for 48 hours or more are associated with symptomatic clinical phlebitis. When intravenous plastic catheters are left
in for longer than 48 hours, the incidence of septicemia has generally
ranged between 2 and 5 percent and in some instances the rates may
be as high as 8 percent. The most common microorganisms isolated
from patients with sepsis caused by plastic intravenous catheters are
Staphylococcus epidermidis, Staphylococcus aureus, Klebsiella-
Enterobacter, Enterococcus, Pseudomonas and Proteus. Septicemia
associated with agents such as Mimeae, Herellea, Serratia marcescens, and Candida and other fungi have also been reported (Maki et
al., 1973). Candida and other fungi are most frequently isolated
from patients who develop septicemia in association with total parenteral nutrition therapy (Curry et al., 1971). Recently, nation-wide
epidemics of septicemia caused by contaminated intravenous products
have also been reported. Members of the Klebsiellae are the most
common organisms associated with these outbreaks.

To reduce the incidence of infection associated with intravenous
therapy, stainless steel needles should be used in preference to polyethylene catheters (Goldman et al., 1973). Hands should be thoroughly washed and aseptic techniques should be used for venipuncture. Venipuncture sites should be prepared with an effective
antiseptic such as tincture of iodine, an iodophor solution, or 70%

alcohol. After insertion, the cannula should be securely anchored
and an antimicrobial ointment should be applied to the cannula site.
The date and time of intravenous insertion should be recorded. Each
day the intravenous site should be inspected, and if there is no evidence of infection, an antimicrobial ointment should be reapplied
and the dressing should then be changed. Cannula should be changed
every 24 to 72 hours whenever possible. If evidence of infection
occurs, the cannula should be inserted at a different site. In view
of the fact that antibiotic ointments may selectively encourage growth
of resistant bacteria and Candida, it may be preferable to use antiseptic agents such as iodophor ointment.

7. VIRAL HEPATITIS, TYPE B

Hepatitis B has been recognized as one of the major causes of viral
infections among patients and employees in hospitals. Within the
last decade, there has been a 9-fold increase in the number of cases
of type B hepatitis reported in the United States. In 1975, the number of viral hepatitis cases reported as type B was 13,121. This number represents probably less than 50% of the cases which actually occurred. Hepatitis B virus is most commonly transmitted by blood
transfusion. It has been found that approximately 0.1% of the general population in the United States possess hepatitis B virus in their
blood, as reflected by the presence of HBsAg (Hepatitis B surface
antigen). Hepatitis B virus infection may also be transmitted by inadvertent percutaneous inoculation with contaminated needles or other
instruments, or by accidental splattering of HBsAg-positive blood or
other material onto the skin or mucus membranes. Since hepatitis
B infections could be transmitted experimentally by ingestion of material containing hepatitis B virus (Krugman et al., 1967), it is con-
ceivable that infection could also be acquired by accidental ingestion
of HBsAg-positive blood. The possibility of airborne transmission
of hepatitis B virus has been reported (Almeida et al., 1971), but
transmission by such method is probably unusual and occurs only
under special circumstances.

The incidence of nosocomial hepatitis B virus infection has been found
to be more common in hemodialysis units, hematology-oncology units,
renal transplantation units and clinical pathology laboratories. Therefore, special considerations should be given for the prevention of
nosocomial hepatitis B in such areas (Snydman et al., 1975).

Hemodialysis units are frequent reservoirs of hepatitis B virus and
extensive outbreaks have been reported among personnel working in
such units. William et al. (1974) reported an outbreak of hepatitis
B occurring among personnel at a university hospital. Between
January 1968 and August 1972, 79 cases of type B viral hepatitis
were identified. Thirty-four cases were among staff working on the
renal ward and hemodialysis unit, and 34 among personnel working

in the clinical laboratories. The occurrence of cases among personnel correlated temporally with the prevalence of HBsAg-positive patients undergoing hemodialysis in the hospital. A survey by the CDC in 1970 indicated that 80% of the dialysis units had hepatitis B infection occurring either in patients or staff (Garibaldi et al., 1973). Although the majority of the infected patients were asymptomatic, 75% of them were antigenemic for more than 3 months. In an outbreak of hepatitis B virus infection occurring in an oncology unit (Wands et al., 1974), 29 (32%) of 91 personnel working in the unit developed infection, 9 of whom had clinical hepatitis.

Control of hepatitis B rests on a continuous program of surveillance, education on the basic epidemiologic knowledge of viral hepatitis among staff and appropriate sterilization and disinfection of equipment and material used in high risk areas of the hospital. Overcrowded working conditions should be eliminated. Blood or other potentially contaminated materials spilled in the environment should be immediately cleaned and disinfected with a chemical such as sodium hypochlorite solution. Since the dose of hepatitis B virus required for infection is extremely small, special caution should be taken to cover minor cuts and abrasions on fingers and hands to reduce the risk of contact with infectious material. Gowns and gloves should be worn when working in contaminated areas.

Since the risk of infection is particularly high in hemodialysis and hematology-oncology units, special procedures should be established for detection and prevention of infection to both patients and employees in these areas. All patients scheduled for treatment and persons considered for employment in such units should be screened for HBsAg and anti-HBs before they are admitted to the unit. Patients who are HBsAg carriers should be handled with extreme caution and should be isolated in a separate unit for HBsAg-positive patients. It is preferable that employees who are positive for either antigen or antibody be assigned to care for patients who are HBsAg-positive.

All patients receiving treatments in high risk areas should be tested for hepatitis B antigen once a month. All employees possessing HBsAg should also be tested every month over a period of 6 months to determine whether they are persistent hepatitis B antigen carriers. If antigenemia persists for 6 months or longer, liver function and other studies should be performed to ascertain whether they have chronic active hepatitis. Routine screening of hospital employees is not recommended at present because the role played by employees with antigenemia in dissemination of hepatitis B virus has not yet been delineated. Studies have indicated that transmission of hepatitis B infection from employees to patients can occur; however, available data suggest that such risks are relatively small.

REFERENCES

Adler, J.L., Burke, J.P. and Finland, M.: Infection and antibiotic usage at Boston City Hospital, January 1970. Arch. Intern. Med. 127:460, 1971.

Almeida, J.D., Chrisholm, G.D., Kulatilake, A.E., et al.: Possible airborne spread of serum hepatitis virus within a hemodialysis unit. Lancet 2:849, 1971.

Andriole, T.V.: Hospital-acquired urinary infections and the indwelling catheter. Urol. Clin. N.A. 2:451, 1975.

Artenstein, M.S. and Weinstein, L.: Hospital-acquired enterovirus infections. NEJM 267:1005, 1962.

Barrett, F.F., Casey, J.I. and Finland, M.: Infections and antibiotic use among patients at Boston City Hospital, February, 1967. NEJM 278:5, 1968.

Bassett, D.C.J., Thompson, S.A.S., and Page, B.: Neonatal infections with pseudomonas aeruginosa associated with contaminated resuscitation equipment. Lancet 1:781, 1965.

Bennett, J.V., Scheckler, W.E., Maki, D.G., et al.: Current national patterns. United States. In, Proceedings of the International Conference on Nosocomial Infections. Am. Hosp. Assoc., Chicago, p. 42, 1971.

Brachman, P.S.: Nosocomial respiratory infections. Prev. Med. 3:500, 1974.

Cabrera, H.A. and Davis, G.H.: Epidemic meningitis of the newborn caused by flavobacteria. I. Epidemiology and bacteriology. Am. J. Dis. Child. 101:289, 1961.

Curry, C.R. and Quie, P.G.: Fungal septicemia in patients receiving parenteral hyperalimentation. NEJM 285:1221, 1971.

DuPont, H.L. and Spink, W.W.: Infections due to gram-negative organisms: an analysis of 860 patients with bacteremia at the University of Minnesota Medical Center, 1958-1966. Medicine 48:307, 1969.

Ehrenkranz, J.J. and Kicklighter, J.L.: Tuberculosis outbreak in a general hospital: evidence for airborne spread of infection. Ann. Intern. Med. 77:377, 1971.

Eickoff, T.C., Brachman, P.S., Bennett, J.V., et al.: Surveillance of nosocomial infections in community hospitals. J. Infect. Dis. 120:305, 1969.

Eickoff, T.C.: New antibacterial treatment of nosocomial infections. Bull. N.Y. Acad. Med. 51:1056, 1975.

Feingold, D.S.: Hospital-acquired infections. NEJM 283:1384, 1970.

Fekety, F.R.: The epidemiology and prevention of staphylococcal infection. Medicine 43:593, 1964.

Finland, M.: Excursions into epidemiology: selected studies during the past four decades at Boston City Hospital. J. Infect. Dis. 128: 76, 1973.

Foley, J.F., Gravelle, C.R., Englehard, W.E., et al.: Achromobacter septicemia - fatalities in prematures. I. Clinical and epidemiological study. Am. J. Dis. Child. 101:279, 1961.

Forfar, J.O. and MacCabe, A.F.: Masking and gowning in nurseries for the newborn infant. Effect on staphylococcal carriage and infection. Br. Med. J. 1:76, 1958.

Frenkel, J.K.: Toxoplasmosis and pneumocystosis: clinical and laboratory aspects in immunocompetent and compromised hosts. In, Opportunistic Pathogens, Prier, J.E. and Friedman, H., eds., University Park Press, Baltimore, p. 203, 1974.

Garibaldi, R.A., Forrest, J.N., Bryan, J.A., et al.: Hemodialysis - Associated hepatitis. J. Am. Med. Assoc. 225:384, 1973.

Garibdlai, R.A., Burke, J.P., Dickman, M.L., et al.: Factors predisposing to bacteriuria during indwelling urethral catheterization. NEJM 291:215, 1974.

Garner, J.S., Bennett, J.V., Scheckler, W.E., et al.: Surveillance of nosocomial infections. In, Proceedings of the International Conference on Nosocomial Infections. Am. Hosp. Assoc., Chicago, p. 277, 1971.

Gocke, D.J.: A prospective study of posttransfusion hepatitis. The role of Australian antigen. J. Am. Med. Assoc. 219:1165, 1972.

Goldmann, D.A., Maki, D.G., Rhame, F.S. et al.: Guidelines for infection control in intravenous therapy. Ann. Int. Med. 79:848, 1973.

Graybill, J.R., Marshall, L.W., Charache, R., et al.: Nosocomial pneumonia, a continuing major problem. Am. Rev. Resp. Dis. 108: 1130, 1973.

Grieble, H.G., Colton, F.R., Bird, T.J., et al.: Fine-particle
humidifiers. Source of pseudomonas aeruginosa infections in a re-
spiratory-disease unit. NEJM 282:531, 1970.

Hall, C.B. and Douglas, R.G.: Nosocomial influenza infection as
a cause of intercurrent fevers in infants. Pediatrics 55:673, 1975.

Hall, C.B., Douglas, R.G., Geiman, J.M., et al.: Nosocomial
respiratory syncytial virus infections. NEJM 293:1343, 1975.

Infection Control in the Hospital. Third Ed., Amer. Hosp. Assoc.,
Chicago, 1974.

Isolation Techniques for Use in Hospitals. Second Ed. Center for
Disease Control, Atlanta, 1975.

Johanson, W.G., Jr., Pierce, A.K., Sanford, J.P., et al.: Nosocomial respiratory infections with gram-negative bacilli. Ann. Int.
Med. 77:701, 1972.

Joint Commission on Accreditation of Hospitals, American Hospital
Association: Accreditation Manual for Hospitals. Am. Med. Assoc.,
Chicago, 1976.

Kaslow, R.A., Dixon, R.E., Martin, S.M. et al.: Staphylococcal
diseases related to hospital nursery bathing practices - a nationwide
epidemiologic investigation. Pediatrics 51:418, 1973.

Kass, E.H.: Asymptomatic infections of the urinary tract. Trans.
Assoc. Am. Physicians 69:56, 1956.

Kislak, J.W., Eickhoff, T.C., and Finland, M.: Hospital-acquired
infections and antibiotic usage in the Boston City Hospital - January,
1964. NEJM 271:834, 1964.

Krugman, S., Giles, J.P., and Hammond, J.: Infectious hepatitis.
Evidence for two distinct clinical, epidemiological and immunological types of infection. J. Am. Med. Assoc. 200:369, 1967.

Kunin, C.M. and McCormack, R.C.: Prevention of catheter-induced
urinary tract infections by sterile closed drainage. NEJM 274:1155,
1966.

Kwong, M.S., Loew, A.D., Anthony, B.F., et al.: The effect of
hexachlorophene on staphylococcal colonization rates in the newborn
infant: a controlled study using a single-bath method. J. Pediatr.
82:982, 1973.

Lockhart, J.D.: How toxic is hexachlorophene? Pediatrics 50:229,
1972.

Maki, D.G., Goldmann, D.A., and Rhame, F.S.: Infection control in intravenous therapy. Ann. Int. Med. 79:867, 1973.

Maki, D.G., Hennekens, C.H., Bennett, J.V., et al.: Nosocomial urinary tract infection with serratia marcescens: an epidemiologic study. J. Infect. Dis. 128:579, 1973.

Maki, D.G., Rhame, F.S., Mackel, D.C., et al.: Nationwide epidemic of septicemia caused by contaminated intravenous products. I. Epidemiologic and clinical features. Am. J. Med. 60:471, 1976.

McNamara, M.J., Hill, M.C., Balows, A., et al.: A study of the bacteriologic patterns of hospital infections. Ann. Intern. Med. 66: 480, 1967.

Mertz, J.J., Scharer, L., and McClements, J.H.: A hospital outbreak of Klebsiella pneumonia from inhalation therapy and contaminated aerosol solutions. Am. Rev. Resp. Dis. 95:454, 1967.

Moffet, H.L.: Pediatric Infectious Diseases. J.B. Lippincott Co., Philadelphia, p. 390, 1975.

Moore, W.L., Jr.: Nosocomial infections: an overview. Am. J. Hosp. Pharm. 31:832-838, 1974.

Morse, L.J., Williams, H.L., Grenn, F.P., Jr., et al.: Septicemia due to Klebsiella pneumoniae originating from a hand-cream dispenser. NEJM 277:472, 1967.

Mufson, M.A., Mocega, H.E., and Crause, H.E.: Acquisition of para-influenza-3 virus infections by hospitalized children: I. Frequencies, rates, and temporal data. J. Infect. Dis. 128:141, 1973.

Murray, W.A., McDaniel, G.E., and Reed, M.: Evaluation of the phone survey in an outbreak of staphylococcal infections in a hospital nursery for the newborn. Am. J. Pub. Health 48:310, 1958.

Pattison, C.P., Boyer, K., Maynard, J.E., et al.: Epidemic hepatitis in a clinical laboratory. J. Am. Med. Assoc. 230:854, 1974.

Pierce, A.K., Sanford, J.P., Thomas, G.D., et al.: Long-term evaluation of decontamination of inhalation-therapy equipment and the occurrence of necrotizing pneumonia. NEJM 282:528, 1970.

Plueckhahn, V.S.: Hexachlorophene and the control of staphylococcal sepsis in a maternity unit in Geelong, Australia. Pediatrics 51: 368, 1973.

Powell, H., Swarner, O., Gluck, L., et al.: Hexachlorophene myelinopathy in premature infants. J. Pediat. 82:976, 1973.

Riley, H.D., Jr.: Hospital-associated infections. Pediat. Clin. N.A. 16:701, 1969.

Rogers, L.A. and Osterhout, S.: Pneumonia following tracheostomy. Am. Surg. 36:39, 1970.

Roy, T.E., McDonald, S., Patrick, M.L., et al.: A survey of hospital infection in a pediatric hospital. Canada Med. Assoc. J. 87:531, 592, 656, 1962.

Sanders, E., Sweeney, F.J., Jr., Friedman, E.A., et al.: An outbreak of hospital-associated infections due to salmonella derby. J. Am. Med. Assoc. 186:984, 1963.

Sanders, C.V., Jr., Luby, J.P., Johanson, W.G., et al.: Serratia Marcescens infections from inhalation therapy medications: Nosocomial outbreak. Ann. Intern. Med. 73:15, 1970.

Sanford, J.P. and Pierce, A.K.: Current infection problems - respiratory. In, Proceedings of the International Conference on Nosocomial Infections, Am. Hosp. Assoc., Chicago, p. 77, 1971.

Sanford, J.P.: Infection control in critical care units. Crit. Care Med. 2:211, 1974.

Schaffner, W.: The ongoing problems of hospital infections. Adv. Int. Med. 21:175, 1976.

Scheckler, W.E., Garner, J.S., Kaiser, A.B., et al.: Prevalence of infections and antibiotic usage in eight community hospitals. In, Proceedings of the International Conference on Nosocomial Infections. Am. Hosp. Assoc., Chicago, p. 299, 1971.

Shuman, R.M., Leech, R.W., and Alvord, E.C., Jr.: Neurotoxicity of hexachlorophene in the human. I. A clinicopathologic study of 248 children. Pediatrics 54:689, 1974.

Selden, R., Lee, S., Wang, W.L.L., et al.: Nosocomial Klebsiella infections: intestinal colonization as a reservoir. Ann. Intern. Med. 74:657, 1971.

Sever, J.L.: Possible role of humidifying equipment in spread of infections from newborn nursery. Pediatrics 24:50, 1959.

Shinefield, H.R. and Ribble, J.C.: Current aspects of infections and diseases related to staphylococcus aureus. Ann. Rev. Med. 16: 263, 1965.

Snydman, D.R., Bryan, J.A., and Dixon, R.E.: Prevention of nosocomial viral hepatitis, type B (hepatitis B). Ann. Intern. Med. 83:838, 1975.

Stamm, W.E.: Guidelines for prevention of catheter-associated urinary tract infections. Ann. Intern. Med. 82:386, 1975.

Stamm, W.E. and Bennett, J.V.: Nosocomial infections. In, Communicable and Infectious Diseases. Top, F.H., Sr., and Wehrle, P.F., eds. C.V. Mosby Co., 1976.

Stamm, W.E., Colella, J.J., Anderson, R.L., et al.: Indwelling arterial catheters as a source of nosocomial bacteremia. An outbreak caused by flavobacterium species. NEJM 292:1099, 1975.

Steere, A.C. and Mallison, G.F.: Handwashing practices for the prevention of nosocomial infections. Ann. Intern. Med. 83:683, 1975.

Thoburn, R., Fekety, F.R., Jr., and Cluff, L.E.: Infections acquired by hospitalized patients. Arch. Intern. Med. 121:1, 1968.

Turck, M., Goffe, B. and Petersdorf, R.G.: The urethral catheter and urinary tract infection. J. Urol. 88:834, 1962.

Wands, J.R., Walker, J.A., Davis, T.T., et al.: Hepatitis B in an oncology unit. NEJM 291:1371, 1974.

Wenzel, R.P., Osterman, C.A. and Hunting, K.J.: Hospital-acquired infections. II. Infection rates by site, service and common procedures in a university hospital. Am. J. Epid. 104:645, 1976.

Wenzel, R.P., Osterman, C.A., Hunting, K.J., et al.: Hospital-acquired infections. I. Surveillance in a university hospital. Am. J. Epid. 103:251, 1976.

Williams, S.V., Huff, J.C., Feinglass, E.J., et al.: Epidemic viral hepatitis type B in hospital personnel. Am. J. Med. 57:904, 1974.

CHAPTER 25. ACTIVE IMMUNIZATION FOR INFECTIOUS DISEASES

INTRODUCTION: Routine immunization during infancy against diphtheria, tetanus and pertussis has been common practice in the United States for the past 30 years. Yet in 1975 there were 307 cases of diphtheria, 102 cases of tetanus, and over 1,738 cases of pertussis reported in this country. Following the introduction of inactivated polio virus vaccine (IPV) in 1955 and the live oral polio virus vaccine (OPV) in 1962, the number of cases of paralytic poliomyelitis declined from 18,000 cases in 1954 to 8 cases in 1975. Similarly, but less spectacularly, widespread use of measles (rubeola) vaccines since 1963 has resulted in a 90% reduction in the incidence of measles but there were still 24,000 cases reported in 1975. Thus, despite the availability and use of safe and effective vaccines, we have yet to eradicate any of the infections for which immunization has been routine, although control of these infections has certainly been and/or is being achieved because of available vaccines and immunization programs.

There is some concern that the success achieved to date may be in jeopardy if the results of recent immunization surveys conducted in preschool age children are indicative of current levels of immunization in this country. Very simply, these surveys have shown that many children are not being adequately immunized, if at all. Furthermore, the numbers of adequately immunized children seem to be gradually declining in the populations surveyed. For example, in 1964, 87.6% of children between the ages of 1 and 4 years had received at least 3 doses of either inactivated or oral polio vaccine, whereas in 1970 the percentage had declined to 65.9%.

In poverty areas within large central cities, the percentage of adequately immunized preschoolers is especially low, one survey having shown that fewer than half the children of age 1 to 4 years had received measles vaccine and only slightly over half had received 3 doses each of polio vaccine and DTP. A more recent immunization survey incorporated children from three central city census tracts and one suburban census tract in a large metropolitan area. Again, those children in the inner city were more likely to have low levels of antibody to diphtheria, tetanus, measles, or rubella than their suburban counterparts, although the differences were not great. Of considerable concern were the findings which indicated that in the total study population, 63% of children were susceptible to rubella, 33% had inadequate titers of measles antibody and 57% had serum antibody levels of less than 1:10 to one or more types of poliovirus. Clearly, the availability per se of safe and effective vaccines, which are frequently provided free of cost, will not assure high levels of protection in our preschool populations. Lest we become complacent, increased efforts must be undertaken to assure that all preschool children are immunized, using every available means.

The recommendations made in this chapter concerning both routine and special immunizations, follow in general the recommendations of the Committee on Infectious Diseases of the American Academy of Pediatrics (1974) and the Advisory Committee on Immunization Practice of the Public Health Service (1972). Up-to-date recommendations about immunizations may be obtained from Morbidity and Mortality Weekly Reports, a free publication that can be obtained from the Center for Disease Control, Atlanta, Georgia 30333.

1. ROUTINE IMMUNIZATIONS

It is common practice for children in the United States to be routinely immunized against diphtheria, tetanus, pertussis, poliomyelitis, measles (rubeola), rubella, and mumps. In years past it was also routine to vaccinate against smallpox, but this practice has been discontinued. Smallpox vaccine will be considered under "special" immunizations. The recommended schedule for routine immunizations of normal infants and children is shown in Table 25-1. Before considering each of the vaccines in more detail, some general comments about routine immunization practices may be helpful.

First, the schedule for routine immunizations should be compatible with other schedules for routine health care of infants and children, thus avoiding special trips to the office or clinic for immunizations. There is considerable latitude with respect to timing of immunizations in the recommended schedule as shown in Table 25-1. For example, although the interval between primary DPT and TOPV immunizations should be at least six weeks to assure optimal antibody responses to polioviruses, it may be considerably longer than eight weeks without jeopardizing vaccine efficacy, provided the series is ultimately completed.

Second, the physician administering vaccines should keep detailed records of the vaccines used in his office, including information as to the manufacturer, lot number, volume administered, site of injection, and all reported reactions. Likewise both the physician and parents should keep separate records of the immunizations given to each child.

Third, there are relatively few contraindications to routine immunizations and they may be listed as follows: (1) An acute febrile illness is reason to defer immunization at least until the infection has been controlled; however, minor infections such as colds are not contraindications to routine immunizations. (2) Specific general contraindications to administration of all live virus vaccines (e.g. OPV, Measles, Rubella and Mumps) include a) pregnancy; b) diseases

TABLE 25-1: RECOMMENDED SCHEDULE FOR ACTIVE IMMUNIZATION OF NORMAL INFANTS AND CHILDREN*

2 mo.	DTP[1]	TOPV[2]
4 mo.	DTP	TOPV
6 mo.	DTP	TOPV
15 mo.	Measles[3]	Tuberculin Test[4]
	Rubella[3]	Mumps[3]
$1\frac{1}{2}$ yr.	DTP	TOPV
4-6 yr.	DTP	TOPV
14-16 yr.	Td[5]	and thereafter every 10 yrs.

1. DTP - diphtheria and tetanus toxoids combined with pertussis vaccine.
2. TOPV - trivalent oral poliovirus vaccine. This recommendation is suitable for breast-fed as well as bottle-fed infants.
3. May be given at 15 months as measles-rubella or measles-mumps-rubella combined vaccines.
4. Frequency of repeated tuberculin tests depends on risk of exposure of the child and on the prevalence of tuberculosis in the population group. The initial test should be at the time of, or preceding, the measles immunization.
5. Td - combined tetanus and diphtheria toxoids (adult type) for those more than 6 years of age in contrast to diphtheria and tetanus (DT) which contains a larger amount of diphtheria and antigen.

* Modified from Report of the Commission on Infectious Diseases, Seventeenth Edition, 1974, American Academy of Pediatrics.

associated with impaired host response, such as immunodeficiency diseases, leukemia, lymphoma and other generalized malignancies, and in patients receiving immunosuppressive therapy; c) recent administration of blood or blood products, especially immune serum globulin; and d) hypersensitivity to the animals from which the tissue culture cells are derived for use in vaccine production or to other components of the vaccine.

Fourth, neurological disorders in infants and children do not constitute a valid contraindication to routine immunizations. Children with brain damage or seizure disorders do not have a higher incidence of serious reactions from routine immunizations than do normal children.

Finally, if the immunization schedule is interrupted, regardless of the length of time elapsed, it is not necessary to begin the primary series of immunizations all over again. If the child has not been immunized in infancy, or if the parent is uncertain about the child's immunizations, and/or if no records are available, then the recommended schedule shown in Table 25-2 may be followed.

1.1: DIPHTHERIA AND TETANUS TOXOIDS AND PERTUSSIS VACCINE (DTP):

Preparation: Diphtheria and tetanus toxoids are prepared by formaldehyde treatment of the respective toxins. Pertussis vaccine is a killed suspension of bacteria or a bacterial fraction. Three preparations of these products are currently available: (1) diphtheria and tetanus toxoids and pertussis vaccine (DTP); (2) tetanus and diphtheria toxoids (Td); and (3) tetanus toxoid (T). Td is the preparation recommended for children over 6 years of age and adults; it contains about 15% of the diphtheria toxoid found in the vaccine used in infants, hence, the small "d". Care should be taken to examine the package insert when using any of these preparations, primarily to ensure that the adsorbed form of the vaccine is the one being used. The toxoids (diphtheria and tetanus) are available in both fluid and adsorbed forms. Studies have clearly indicated that the aluminum phosphate adsorbed toxoid is the preparation of choice for both primary and booster immunizations.

Administration: In infancy, the mid-lateral thigh is the preferred site of injection for DTP, and it should be given deep into the muscle mass. In older patients, the deltoid muscle is an acceptable site, as is the upper outer quadrant of the buttock, provided the sciatic nerve is carefully avoided.

There are no specific contraindications other than those previously listed. Although the occurrence of a severe, febrile reaction to DTP is cause for caution in administering subsequent infections, if a febrile reaction does occur, a useful approach is to give fractional doses of DTP and extend the primary immunization schedule by one or two doses.

Complications and Management: The incidence of major reactions to DTP is very low, whereas the number of minor reactions and complications such as a painful, swollen injection site or transient temperature elevation are fairly common. It is a standard practice in our clinic to inform the mother of the possibility of a febrile reaction following the initial and subsequent DTP injections and to instruct her in the use of appropriate antipyretics, such as acetaminophen.

Of the three components of the DTP vaccine, pertussis is the immunogen most likely to produce dramatic complications. Convulsions and encephalopathy have occurred following pertussis vaccine, and this is

TABLE 25-2: PRIMARY IMMUNIZATION FOR CHILDREN NOT IMMUNIZED IN INFANCY*	
1 THROUGH 5 YEARS OF AGE	
First visit	DTP, TOPV, Tuberculin Test
1 mo. later	Measles[1], Rubella[1], Mumps
2 mo later	DTP, TOPV
4 mo later	DTP, TOPV
6 to 12 mo later or preschool	DTP, TOPV
Age 14-16 yr	Td, continue every 10 yr
6 YEARS OF AGE AND OVER	
First visit	Td, TOPV, Tuberculin Test
1 mo later	Measles, Rubella, Mumps
2 mo later	Td, TOPV
6 to 12 mo later	Td, TOPV
Age 14-16 yr	Td, continue every 10 yr

[1] To be given at 15 months of age or later.

* Modified from Report of the Commission on Infectious Diseases, Seventeenth Edition, 1974, American Academy of Pediatrics.

a clear indication to discontinue the use of DTP and to substitute DT and to substitute DT adsorbed for subsequent immunizations. Two other complications are reported less frequently. One is shock, which occurs within 6 hours of the immunization and is described by the mother as "the baby turned white as a sheet," or became ashen. Although the duration of shock symptoms varies from a few minutes to several hours, no fatalities have been reported. The second infrequent complication is "persistent screaming," manifested by a high-pitched scream that may continue for several hours following immunization. This has occurred in the same child when given another dose of the vaccine; like shock, it is an indication for discontinuing the use of DTP and substituting DT for subsequent immunizations.

1.2: POLIO VACCINE:

<u>Preparation</u>: Although inactivated polio vaccines were widely used throughout the United States for a number of years, they have gradually been replaced by oral polio vaccines. Live oral polio vaccines offer several advantages over the inactivated polio vaccine in that fewer booster doses are required for maintenance of adequate immunity. It is thought that one booster dose of trivalent OPV at 18 months and another at 4 or 5 years is sufficient to confer lifetime immunity. On the other hand, the use of inactivated vaccine requires periodic boosters every two to three years. Currently, the live oral polio vaccine most commonly used is a trivalent vaccine (TOPV), containing all three types of attenuated polio viruses. This vaccine has been shown to be efficient and convenient, offering some theoretical advantage over the monovalent vaccines which were used initially. In 1972, oral polio vaccine produced in WI-38 strains of human diploid cells was licensed in the United States. This mode of production will eventually replace the production of oral polio vaccine in primary Rhesus monkey kidney cell cultures and is considered to be its equivalent in safety and effectiveness.

<u>Administration</u>: Trivalent oral polio vaccine (TOPV) is given orally at two months of age, usually at the same time of the first DTP injection. The timing of subsequent doses is shown on the schedules in Tables 25-1 and 25-2. At present, the only indication for use of the inactivated polio vaccine arises when there is a need to immunize infants with immune deficiency diseases and for their siblings. The only contraindications for administration of oral polio vaccines are those mentioned that are applicable to all live virus vaccines. The current trivalent oral polio vaccine is suitable for both bottle and breast fed infants, although for the latter the vaccine should be given midway between feedings, because breast milk does contain polio virus neutralizing antibodies and may interfere with vaccine efficacy.

<u>Complications and Management</u>: The only serious complication of trivalent oral polio vaccine has been the rare occurrence of paralysis in vaccine recipients or in their close contacts within two months of administration. During the eight-year period between 1963 and 1970, 9 cases of "vaccine-associated paralysis" in recipients and 21 cases in contacts of recipients were reported. The evidence that the attenuated viruses used in the vaccine actually caused paralytic disease in the normal infant or child is somewhat tenuous, although this complication has occurred in children with immunodeficiency diseases. However, the complication is most common in individuals immunized after 30 years of age, or in contacts of vaccine recipients over 30 years of age.

1.3: MEASLES VACCINE:

<u>Preparation</u>: Measles vaccines currently available in the United States are attenuated virus vaccines prepared in the cultures of chick embryo cells. Although inactivated measles vaccines were previously used, they are no longer recommended because of the short-lived immunity produced by these vaccines. In addition, unusual local and systemic reactions have been observed when recipients of these inactivated vaccines later received a live vaccine or encountered natural measles. Children who have received only inactivated vaccines should be given live attenuated vaccine as soon as possible, and their parents should be cautioned about possible local and systemic reactions.

The two attenuated vaccines most commonly used today are the Schwartz and Attenuvax vaccines, which are further attenuated vaccines of the original Edmonston B strain of vaccine, the first widely used live virus vaccine in the U.S.A. The Edmonston strain is associated with febrile reactions in approximately 40% of the recipients, as well as a mild rash resembling the measles rash in 10 to 20% of vaccinated susceptibles within 10 days following immunization. The symptoms may be modified by the use of measles immune globulin (MIG), given at the time of vaccination with the Edmonston B strain. However, since the Schwartz and Attenuvax strains are associated with a much lower percentage of febrile illness, and since they did not require the use of MIG at the time of their administration, they are currently recommended for primary immunization.

<u>Administration</u>: Measles vaccine is given subcutaneously in one dose. It is recommended that this vaccine be administered at 15 months of age. However, during the course of measles epidemics, the vaccine should be given any time after 6 months of age, followed by a second inoculation after 15 months of age (AAP Committee on Infectious Diseases, October 17, 1976). Infants immunized before 12 months have experienced more variable rates of sero-conversion due to the presence of passive antibody from the mother. This passively acquired antibody might interfere with optimal antibody production. Thus, infants who are immunized before 12 months should have a second dose of live attenuated vaccine at 12 to 16 months of age in order to assure optimal immunity. Finally, measles may be administered simultaneously with other live virus vaccines. At present, a measles-rubella vaccine (MR vaccine) and a measles-mumps-rubella vaccine (MMR vaccine) have recently been licensed in the U.S.A.

Contraindications to immunization with the measles vaccine are essentially those previously cited for live virus vaccines. Although reactions to the vaccine in egg-sensitive children is a theoretical risk since the vaccine virus is grown in chick embryo fibroblasts, no adverse effects have been reported. An additional contraindication is the administration of live measles vaccine to infants or children with untreated tuberculosis, because of the theoretical risk of exacerbating the disease. For this reason, and because it was known that natural measles as well as live virus vaccines can produce a transient depression in cell-mediated immunity, it was recommended in the past that a tuberculin test be administered before giving the measles vaccine. However, since depression of cell-mediated immunity does not occur within the first 48 to 72 hours following administration of live virus vaccines, and as such will not affect the tuberculin test, it is no longer necessary to carry out tuberculin testing prior to administration of the measles vaccines. It is now recommended that in most parts of the United States, wherever the prevalence of tuberculosis and risk of exposure are low, that tuberculin testing and measles vaccination be accomplished simultaneously.

Complications and Management: The incidence of febrile reactions following the use of the Schwartz and Attenuvax strain vaccines is less than 15%. This reaction occurs within 10 to 12 days of vaccination, and rarely a brief rash may appear as the fever subsides. These symptoms may be controlled with antipyretics, and the mother should be alerted to the possibility of this reaction in order to prevent anxiety and to avoid unnecessary phone calls.

1.4: RUBELLA VACCINE:

Preparation: Rubella vaccines are prepared in cell cultures of avian and mammalian tissues. The Cendehill vaccine is prepared in rabbit kidney cells, whereas there are two HPV-77 vaccines - one prepared in duck embryo cells and another in dog kidney cells. All three vaccines are highly immunogenic, producing antibody responses in 95% of susceptible recipients. Antibody titers following immunization with these attenuated rubella vaccines are lower than those occurring after natural rubella infection. Nonetheless, these vaccines do protect against illness following either natural exposure or artificial challenge with the rubella virus. Although the vaccines have only been available since 1969, antibody levels have declined little among those who were first immunized and the prospects for lifelong immunity following a single injection of rubella vaccine are likely. However, exact duration of immunity will be established only by continued observation.

Administration: Rubella vaccine may be administered subcutaneously to two populations: 1) routine immunization of all susceptible boys and girls between the ages of 15 months and 12 years; and 2) selective immunization of adolescents and women of child-bearing age. Currently it is common practice to administer this live virus vaccine simultaneously with either measles and/or mumps vaccines at 15 months of age. Immunization of adolescent and adult females should be undertaken with caution because of the risk of administering the vaccine to pregnant women. Under these circumstances, the vaccine should be administered only to susceptible individuals as determined by a rubella hemaglutination-inhibition (HI) antibody test. If the individual has antibodies, then immunization is not necessary. If, on the other hand, the individual has no rubella HI antibodies, then immunization should be carried out only if she agrees to prevent pregnancy for two months following the use of the vaccine. Contraindications for the use of live, attenuated rubella vaccine are those previously given for live virus vaccines in general. Because preparations of rubella vaccines differ with respect to the type of animal or avian tissue culture used, a person known to be hypersensitive to one species, e.g., dog dander, should not receive the vaccine produced in dog kidney tissue culture, but rather the vaccine grown either in rabbit kidney or duck embryo tissue cultues.

Complications and Management: Reactions that follow the use of rubella vaccine are generally mild. Rash and lymphadenopathy occur infrequently, and in children self-limited arthralgias and arthritis occur in fewer than 5% of those vaccinated. The HPV-77 vaccine prepared in dog kidney cells commonly results in a higher antibody level than the other vaccines, but it is also associated with a higher rate of joint manifestations (7 to 15%). The joint symptoms are of greater severity and longer duration than symptoms caused by other vaccines. Also, data suggest that the incidence of arthritis and arthralgia is more frequent and severe in young adult women than in children, but in no instance have these complications been associated with residual disease.

1.5: MUMPS VACCINE:

Preparation: Mumps virus vaccine is prepared in chick embryo cell culture and was first introduced in the U.S.A. in 1967. The vaccine induces immunity in 95% of susceptibles, following an apparent noncommunicable infection induced by vaccination. Like the rubella vaccine, antibody titers are consistently lower after mumps vaccine than those after natural infection, although antibody persistence parallels that of overt mumps. Also like rubella, the duration of the vaccine-induced immunity is unknown, and only by continued observation will the exact duration of immunity be established.

Administration: The mumps vaccine is administered subcutaneously at any age after 12 months; like measles and rubella vaccines, it should not be administered prior to one year of age because of possible interference resulting from passively acquired maternal antibodies. The vaccine may be administered simultaneously with other live virus vaccines, such as measles-mumps-rubella (MMR). These combination live virus vaccines have been shown to be just as effective and safe when administered simultaneously as when they are administered individually.

Contraindications for use of mumps vaccine are similar to those previously cited as general contraindications for all live virus vaccines.

In addition, the mumps vaccine does contain small amounts of neomycin, and thus should not be given to individuals known to be sensitive to this antibiotic.

<u>Complications and Management</u>: To date there have been no side reactions or complications, including fever, attributable to use of the live mumps virus vaccine.

2. SPECIAL IMMUNIZATIONS

2.1: RABIES VACCINE:

Although human rabies is rare in the United States, rabies prophylaxis is a perplexing problem for physicians. Current anti-rabies regimens are complicated by: 1) the adverse reactions related to rabies vaccine, 2) serum sickness induced by equine anti-rabies serum, and 3) the efficacy of active and passive immunization after rabies exposure.

<u>Preparation</u>: Two vaccines, duck embryo vaccine (DEV) and nervous tissue vaccine (NTV), have been used. The effectiveness of the two vaccines is not significantly different, however, neuroparalytic reactions occur more frequently with NTV than with DEV. Therefore, DEV is preferable to NTV.

A new rabies vaccine, produced in human diploid cells (HDCV), has been recently developed. This vaccine appears to be highly immunogenic and has no side effects; it may become useful in protecting high-risk persons in the near future. (Bahmanyar et al., 1976).

<u>Rationale of Treatment</u>: In the United States, the following factors should be considered in the decision of whether or not to immunize patients exposed to animals suspected of being rabid. 1) Species of biting animal: Incidence of rabies is high in skunks, bats, foxes, coyotes, raccoons, dogs, and cats. In the United States, bites of mice, rats, squirrels, gerbils, chipmunks, hamsters, guinea pigs, and rabbits seldom, if ever, require specific anti-rabies prophylaxis. Recently there has been a reduction of rabies in dogs and cats and a relative increase in prevalence of rabies among wild animals in the United States. 2) Circumstances of biting incident: An unprovoked attack is more likely to suggest the animal is rabid. 3) Type of wound: The chance of infection varies with nature of exposure, namely bite wounds (any penetration of skin by teeth) and non-bite wounds (scratches, abrasion or open wounds). 4) Vaccination status of biting animal: Chance of an animal being rabid and transmitting virus is very small in an animal properly immunized against rabies. 5) Presence of rabies in the region and in the species of biting animal involved.

<u>Local Treatment of Wounds</u>: All bite wounds and scratches should be washed immediately with water and soap. This is perhaps the

most effective means of preventing rabies. In addition, tetanus prophylaxis and control of bacterial infections should be given if indicated.

<u>Management of Biting Animal</u>: 1) If a dog or cat is involved, the animal should be captured, confined, and observed by a veterinarian for at least 5, and preferably 10 days. The local health department should be informed if any illness develops during the observation period. If signs of rabies appear, the animal should be sacrificed and the head removed and shipped under refrigeration to a qualified laboratory for examination. 2) If a wild animal is involved, the animal should be killed at once and the brain examined by fluorescent antibody method for evidence of rabies. If the examination is negative for rabies, the exposed individual need not be treated.

<u>Postexposure Prophylaxis</u>: Every exposure to animal bites or scratches must be individually evaluated. A guide for postexposure anti-rabies prophylaxis is shown in Table 25-3. Combined use of a vaccine (active immunization) and an immune globulin (passive immunization) is the best postexposure prophylaxis and is recommended for all bites by animals suspected of having rabies, and for non-bite exposures inflicted by animals suspected of being rabid. A combination of active and passive immunization should be used regardless of the interval between exposure and treatment.

A) <u>Active immunization</u>: When the decision is made to initiate DEV immunization, 23 doses (1 ml. each) of vaccine should be given. Vaccine may be administered either by giving 21 daily subcutaneous injections, or 14 doses in the first 7 days (2 injections per day) followed by 7 single daily injections. To ensure lasting protection, two booster doses should be given on the 10th and 20th days after the completion of the 21 injections. Reactions to vaccine are common. Local reactions include erythema, pruritus, pain, and tenderness. Low-grade fever and, rarely, shock may occur late in the course of therapy. Serious reactions have rarely occurred after the first dose of infection. Antihistamines may be given to patients with a history of hypersensitivity. When the new vaccine (HDCV) becomes available, the number of injections and side effects will be markedly reduced.

B) <u>Passive immunization</u>: Two preparations, <u>rabies immune globulin-human (RIG)</u> and <u>anti-rabies serum-equine (ARS)</u>, are available in the United States. ARS should be used only if RIG is not available. RIG is administered only once at the beginning of anti-rabies therapy. The recommended dose of RIG is 20 IU/kg (or ARS 40 IU/kg). Half of the dose is thoroughly infiltrated around the wound and the rest administered intramuscularly in the buttocks. Since horse serum (ARS) induces an allergic reaction in more than 20% of recipients, a careful history and appropriate tests for hypersensitivity must be performed before administration.

TABLE 25-3: POSTEXPOSURE ANTIRABIES TREATMENT GUIDE*

ANIMAL	ITS CONDITION AT TIME OF ATTACK	TREATMENT
Wild:		
Skunk Fox Coyote Raccoon Bat	Regard as rabid	RIG + V[1]
Domestic:		
Dog Cat	Healthy Escaped (unknown) Rabid or suspected rabid	None[2] RIG + V RIG + V
Other:	Consider individually - see Rationale of treatment	

V = rabies vaccine; RIG = Rabies Immune Globulin, Human.

1. Discontinue vaccine if fluorescent antibody tests of animal killed at the time of attack are negative.

2. Begin RIG + V at first sign of rabies in biting dog or cat during holding period (10 days).

(The above recommendations are only a guide. They should be applied in conjunction with knowledge of the animal species involved, circumstances of the bite or other exposure, vaccination status of the animal, and presence of rabies in the region.)

*Modified from Recommendation of the Public Health Service Advisory Committee on Immunization Practices, MMWR, December 31, 1976.

Pre-exposure Prophylaxis: Because of the relatively low frequency
of reactions to DEV, preexposure prophylaxis should be offered to
individuals in high risk groups: veterinarians, animal handlers,
certain laboratory workers, and persons who have frequent contacts
with dogs, cats and wild animals. Two injections of 1.0 ml of DEV
are given subcutaneously at 4 weeks apart; this should be followed
by a third injection 6 months later. Booster doses should probably
be given every 1 to 3 years to individuals with continuing exposure.

2.2: INFLUENZA VACCINE:

The difficulty associated with the control of influenza is related to
the antigenic variations of influenza virus A and B. Antigenic changes
have occurred in all major epidemics during the past 4 decades. Each
time there is a change in dominant antigenic composition, the majority of the population is again susceptible to infection. Besides the
major epidemics, influenza occurs every year. In recent years,
influenza A epidemics have occurred more frequently and have been
more severe than those of influenza B.

The formulation of influenza vaccines is revised regularly. Bivalent vaccine, containing greater amounts of two recent strains, are
prepared for use on a yearly basis. Because of the rapid changes in
the status of influenza vaccines, it is suggested that physicians con-
sult bulletins published by the Advisory Committee on Immunization
Practice of the Public Health Service before using influenza vaccines.

Currently, routine influenza immunization in normal infants and children is not recommended. Because of the high mortality rate during
epidemics, annual vaccination is recommended only for those high-
risk patients with the following diseases: (1) cardiovascular disease,
such as rheumatic, congenital, arteriosclerotic, and hypertensive
heart disease, especially those with cardiac insufficiency; (2) chronic
bronchopulmonary disease, such as cystic fibrosis, asthma, bronchiectasis, emphysema, and advanced tuberculosis, as well as patients with impaired function of respiratory muscles; (3) diabetes
mellitus and other chronic metabolic diseases; (4) chronic glomerulonephritis or nephrosis; and (5) chronic neurologic disorders. Immunization of persons who provide essential community services
such as those in health services and in occupations involving public
safety may be considered for vaccination if justified by local priorities.

Persons who have not previously received influenza vaccine should
be given 2 doses of inactivated influenza vaccine ("Influenza Virus
Vaccine, Bivalent") subcutaneously, preferably 6 to 8 weeks apart
(dosage and detailed schedule are specified in the package insert).
Persons who were previously vaccinated need only one booster dose
of the vaccine. All immunization should be completed by mid-
November.

Adverse reactions of the vaccine include local redness and induration, fever, malaise, headaches, and muscle aches. Side effects
have been significantly reduced with the use of more highly purified
vaccine preparations. Influenza vaccine is prepared in chick embryos, and therefore should not be given to persons who are allergic
to egg proteins.

2.3: SMALLPOX VACCINE:

The World Health Organization initiated an intensified global smallpox eradication program in 1966. There were 28 countries in which
smallpox was considered to be endemic. By 1976 only a few prov-
inces in Ethiopia continued to report cases of smallpox. In view of
a declining risk of smallpox importation, a reduced likelihood of
spread if it were to be imported, and the occasional risk of adverse
effects of vaccination, most workers agree that it is justified to discontinue routine smallpox vaccination in the United States. However, it is important to realize that until the day smallpox is entirely eradicated from the earth, one must be prepared to recognize
and respond appropriately to any accidentally imported case. Currently, vaccination is necessary only for travel to countries which
require an International Certificate of Vaccination against Smallpox
as a condition for entry, for travel to or from Ethiopia, and for
persons at special risk in laboratories where variola virus or monkeypox virus is handled (Cho et al., 1973). In order to ensure protection, vaccination should be repeated every 3 years.

Smallpox vaccine is a live vaccinia virus, preserved in a glycerin-
ated or in the more stable lyophilized form.

A. Primary vaccination: A small drop of vaccine is placed on the
    dry cleansed skin, and a series of pressures (approximately 10)
    is applied in an area about one-eighth inch in diameter with the
    side of a sharp, sterile needle held tangentially to the skin. The
    remaining vaccine is wiped off with a dry, sterile gauze; no dres-
    sing to the area is needed. A successful vaccination shows a
    typical Jennerian vesicle in 6 to 8 days, followed by pustule and
    crust formation. If a typical Jennerian vesicle is not observed,
    the vaccination technique should be checked and the individual
    revaccinated with a different lot of vaccine until a successful
    result is obtained.

B. Revaccination: A similar technique of vaccination is used, ex-
    cept that 25 to 30 pressures should be made. Two types of re-
    vaccination reaction may be seen: (1) Major reaction - a vesicle
    or pustular lesion or an area of definite palpable induration or
    congestion surrounding a central lesion which may be a crust or
    ulcer. This reaction indicates a successful revaccination and
    virus multiplication. (2) Equivocal reaction - all reactions other
    than a major reaction. This may represent that the immunity is

adequate to suppress virus multiplication, or it may be an allergic reaction to an inactive vaccine. When an equivocal reaction occurs, revaccination procedures should be checked and another lot of vaccine should be used to repeat the revaccination.

Precautions to Vaccination: Smallpox vaccination is contraindicated in the following conditions: (1) skin disorders - persons with eczema and other forms of chronic dermatitis, and in household contacts of persons with skin disorders; eczematous individuals requiring vaccination should be given Vaccinia Immune Globulin (VIG), (2) pregnancy, and (3) altered immune states - dysgammaglobulinemia, leukemia, lymphoma, and other reticuloendothelial malignancies, as well as patients undergoing immunosuppressive therapy.

2.4: YELLOW FEVER VACCINE:

Yellow fever still occurs in Africa and South America. There are two forms of yellow fever: urban and jungle. Urban yellow fever of man is transmitted from person to person by the mosquito Aedes aegypti; the disease can be controlled by eradicating the A. aegypti. Jungle yellow fever occurs among nonhuman hosts, and it is transmitted to animals and man by a variety of mosquitoes. Because infection is from the nonhuman reservoir, the disease in man can be prevented only by immunization of all persons at risk.

Yellow fever vaccine (17D strain) is an attenuated live virus, grown in chick embryos and distributed in a freeze-dried state. Yellow fever vaccines required for international travel must be approved by the World Health Organization and administered at a Yellow Fever Vaccination Center designated by WHO (contact state or local health departments for information).

Those for whom vaccination is indicated include: (1) adults or children over 6 months of age traveling to or living in areas where yellow fever is prevalent, and (2) laboratory personnel who are exposed to virulent yellow fever virus. Over 90% of vaccinated persons develop antibody after one dose of 0.5 ml. vaccine administered subcutaneously. Immunity persists for more than 10 years; therefore, revaccination is not required more frequently than every 10 years.

Reactions to 17D strain of yellow fever vaccine are few and generally mild. Low grade fever, malaise, headache, or myalgia may occur 5 to 10 days after vaccination. The vaccine is prepared in chick embryos; persons hypersensitive to egg proteins should avoid vaccination. Viremia may occur after primary vaccination; therefore the vaccine should not be given to pregnant women or to patients with altered immune states. For persons in whom vaccination is contraindicated, attempts should be made to obtain a waiver. A physician's letter validated by the immunization center indicates that the contraindication to vaccination has been acceptable to some government's quarantine regulations, although this may not be uniformly true. It is important to obtain authoratative advice from the countries one plans to visit regarding quarantine regulations.

2.5: CHOLERA VACCINE:

Cholera vaccines, whether prepared from phenol inactivated classic Inaba and Ogawa strains or E1 Tor strain, are of limited prophylactic value. They provide only about 60% to 80% protection for a period of approximately 6 months. Indications for use of cholera vaccine are limited to travel to or residence in areas where cholera is endemic or epidemic.

A validated cholera immunization within 6 months is usually required by some countries in Asia, the Middle East, and Africa. Some other countries may require evidence of recent vaccination if a person has traveled in areas reporting cholera. Cholera immunization is no longer required for travelers entering the United States.

Travelers to the cholera affected countries should be vaccinated within one to two months before their departure. A full primary immunization consists of 2 doses given subcutaneously or intramuscularly at 1 week to 1 month apart. Booster injections should be given every 6 months when exposure continues. Dosage of vaccine for various age groups is shown in Table 25-4. Vaccination in infants under 6 months of age is not required by most countries.

TABLE 25-4: CHOLERA VACCINE DOSAGE			
	AGE (YEAR)		
DOSE NUMBER	5	5-10	10
1	0.1 ml	0.3 ml	0.5 ml
2	0.3 ml	0.5 ml	1.0 ml
Booster	0.1 ml	0.3 ml	0.5 ml

Most individuals will react to the vaccine with local tenderness and mild swelling for 1 to 2 days. Occasionally, it may be accompanied by mild to moderate fever, malaise, and headache. Serious sensitivity reaction after cholera vaccination is extremely rare. Revaccination in such cases is not recommended.

Cholera is acquired primarily from contaminated water or food. The best protection for travelers is to avoid eating uncooked and potentially contaminated food and water. Cholera vaccine does not prevent transmission of the disease.

2.6: TYPHOID VACCINE:

In recent years, about 400 cases of typhoid fever have been reported annually in the United States. It is doubtful that typhoid vaccine has played a significant role in the continuing decline of incidence of typhoid fever in many parts of the world. More likely, better sanitation and careful follow-up of typhoid cases and carriers are responsible for the downward trend of typhoid fever.

Typhoid vaccine is a killed vaccine, either heat-killed, phenol-preserved, or acetone-killed. These vaccines have been proven in field trials to confer protection in approximately 70% to 90% of susceptibles, particularly in children. Routine vaccination is no longer required in the United States; however, selective immunization is recommended in the following conditions: (1) household exposure to a carrier, (2) outbreaks of typhoid fever in a community, and (3) travel to typhoid endemic areas. Vaccination is no longer recommended for persons going to summer camps or areas with flood conditions.

Adults and children over 10 years old should be given two doses of 0.5 ml. of vaccine subcutaneously at 4-week intervals. Booster injections (0.5 ml. for those over 10 years and 0.25 ml. for those under 10 years) are recommended every 1 to 3 years for persons constantly exposed to typhoid fever.

Local and systemic reactions are commonly seen in vaccine recipients. Local redness, induration, mild lymphadenopathy, malaise, slight fever, headache, and myalgia may occur within 24 hours and usually last 1 or 2 days.

Because of its increased rate of vaccine reactions and its unproved protective effect against paratyphoid A and B, TAB typhoid vaccine (which also contains paratyphoid A and B antigens) is not recommended.

2.7: PLAGUE VACCINE:

Plague is an enzootic infection of wild rodents in Asia, Africa, parts of South America, and the western United States. Disease in man is due to accidental infection from infected rodents.

The plague vaccine is prepared from Yersinia pestis inactivated with formaldehyde. Immunization is recommended only for the following selective groups of persons: (1) those traveling to Vietnam, Cambodia, and Laos; (2) those whose vocation or field work brings them into frequent and regular contact with wild rodents in plague enzootic areas; and (3) laboratory personnel working with Y. pestis or with plague-infected rodents.

Primary immunization series consists of 3 intramuscular injections. The first two doses are given at an interval of 4 or more weeks; the third dose is given 4 to 12 weeks after the second dose. Recommended doses for plague immunization are shown in Table 25-5.

TABLE 25-5: RECOMMENDED DOSES FOR PLAGUE IMMUNIZATION				
	AGE (YEAR)			
DOSE NUMBER	UNDER 1	1-4	5-10	OVER 10
1 and 2	0.1 ml	0.2 ml	0.3 ml	0.5 ml
3 and boosters	0.04 ml	0.08 ml	0.12 ml	0.2 ml

Mild reactions of local pain, erythema, and swelling are commonly seen. With repeated injections, systemic reactions of fever, headache, and malaise occur more frequently and are more pronounced. Sterile abscesses are rarely reported to occur.

2.8: TUBERCULOSIS VACCINE (BCG):

Bacillus Calmette Guerin (BCG), a live attenuated bovine tubercle bacilli vaccine, has been used extensively in countries where tuberculosis is still prevalent. In view of the low incidence of tuberculosis and the high value of the tuberculin skin test for detection of primary tuberculosis, most experts agree that BCG should not be used routinely in the United States. It is recommended for: (1) babies born to mothers with active tuberculosis, and (2) tuberculin-negative persons who live in or plan extensive travel to areas with a high prevalence of tuberculosis. BCG should be given at least 2 months prior to exposure. The tuberculin skin test usually becomes positive when tested 2 or 3 months after vaccination. BCG vaccination may be repeated if the test is negative. BCG and isoniazid should not be given simultaneously, because isoniazid inhibits multiplication of BCG.

BCG vaccination produces a varying degree of immunity (30 to 80%). Natural infection with M. tuberculosis may occur in immunized persons, but the disease is rarely progressive. BCG is given subcutaneously or by the multiple-puncture method. Dosage is 0.05 ml. for newborns and 0.1 ml for older children and adolescents. Complications of vaccination are uncommon; reactions include local induration and, rarely, ulceration. BCG is contraindicated in persons with cellular or combined immunodeficiency states, skin infections, or burns, or in those receiving corticosteroid therapy. Chemoprophylaxis may be used as a substitute for BCG in tuberculin-negative individuals for temporary protection against tuberculosis.

2.9: TYPHUS VACCINE:

There has not been an outbreak of louse-borne (epidemic) typhus since 1922 in the United States, therefore routine vaccination is not warranted. Immunization against typhus is also not required for international travel. Vaccination is recommended only for the following special-risk groups: (1) persons who live in or visit endemic areas or who have regular contact with indigenous populations in such areas, and (2) workers in rickettsial laboratories. Areas affected with epidemic typhus include some rural and remote highland areas of a few countries in Africa, Asia, and South America.

Typhus vaccine (Coxtype) is prepared from inactivated Rickettsia prowazekii grown in chick embryos. Immunity is limited only to louse-borne typhus; it does not protect against murine or scrub typhys. The mortality and severity of typhus fever are diminished among persons who have received 2 or more doses of vaccine. Vaccination during the incubation period may also lessen the severity of illness.

For primary immunization two doses of vaccine can be given subcutaneously 4 weeks apart, using the dosage indicated by the manufacturer. Single booster injections should be given every 6 to 12 months for as long as exposure exists.

Adverse reactions to the vaccine are generally mild. Local pain and tenderness and occasionally low-grade fever may be encountered. The vaccine should not be given to anyone who is hypersensitive to egg proteins.

REFERENCES

GENERAL

Balduzzi, P. and Glasgow, L.A.: Paralytic poliomyelitis in a contact of a vaccinated child. NEJM 276:796, 1967.

Cabasso, V.J., Nozell, H., Ruegsegger, J.M. and Cox, H.R.: Persistence of antibody after oral trivalent poliovirus vaccine (Sabin Strains). NEJM 270:443, 1964.

Foege, W.H. and Eddins, D.L.: Mass vaccination programs in developing countries. Progr. Med. Virol. 15:205, 1973.

Gold, E., Fevrier, A., Hatch, M.H., Herrmann, V.H., Jones, W.L., Krugman, R.D., and Parkman, P.D.: Immune status of children one to four years of age as determined by history and antibody measurement. NEJM 289:231, 1973.

Health information for international travel, 1976. U.S. Public Health Service Center for Disease Control (#76-8280), 1976.

Horstmann, D.M.: Need for monitoring vaccinated populations for immunity levels. Progr. Med. Virol. 16:215, 1973.

Katz, S.L.: Efficàcy, potential and hazards of vaccines. NEJM 270:884, 1964.

Klock, L.E. and Rachelefsky, G.S.: Failure of rubella herd immunity during an epidemic. NEJM 288:69, 1973.

Lamp, G.A. and Feldman, H.A.: Rubella vaccine responses and other viral antibodies in Syracuse children. Am. J. Dis. Child. 122:117, 1971.

Lepow, M.L. and Spence, D.A.: Effect of trivalent oral poliovirus vaccine in an institutionalized population with varying natural and acquired immunity to poliomyelitis. Pediatrics 35:236, 1965.

Levine, M.M., Edsall, G. and Bruce-Chwatt, L.J.: Live-virus vaccines in pregnancy. Risks and recommendations. Lancet 2:34, 1974.

Melnick, J.L., Burkhardt, M., Taber, L.H., and Erckman, P.M.: Developing gap in immunity to poliomyelitis in an urban area. JAMA 209:1181-1185, 1969.

Meyer, H.M., Jr., Parkman, P.D., and Hopps, H.E.: The control of rubella. Pediatrics 44:5, 1969.

Pagano, J.S., Plotkin, S.A., Janowsky, C.C., Richardson, S.M. and Koprowski, H.: Routine immunization with orally administered attenuated poliovirus. A study of 850 children in an American city, JAMA 1973:1883, 1960.

Phillips, C.F.: Children out of step with immunization. Pediatrics 55:877, 1975.

Report of the Committee on Infectious Diseases. Am. Acad. Pediatr., Evanston, 1974.

Rousseau, W.E., Noble, G.R., Tegtmeyer, G.E., Jordan, M.C., and Chin, T.D.Y.: Persistence of poliovirus neutralizing antibodies eight years after immunization with live, attenuated-virus vaccine. NEJM 289:1357, 1973.

Wilson, G.S.: The hazards of immunization. Univ. of London, Athlone Press, 1967.

DIPHTHERIA, PERTUSSIS AND TETANUS

Berg, J.M.: Neurological complications of pertussis immunization. Br. Med. J. 2:24, 1958.

Edsall, G.: Specific prophylaxis of tetanus. JAMA 171:417, 1959.

Fanning, J.: An outbreak of diphtheria in a highly immunized community. Br. Med. J. 1:371, 1947.

Graham, B.S., Blum, H.L., and Green, T.W.: Immunization against tetanus and diphtheria with special combined toxoid. JAMA 166:1586, 1958.

Ipsen, J.: Circulating antitoxin at the onset of diphtheria in 425 patients. J. Immunol. 54:325, 1946.

Levine, L., McComb, J.A., Dwyer, R.C., and Latham, W.C.: Active-passive tetanus immunization. Choice of toxoid, dose of tetanus immune globulin and timing of injections. NEJM 274:186, 1966.

McCarroll, J.R., Abrahams, I. and Skudder, P.A.: Antibody response to tetanus toxoid 15 years after initial immunization. Am. J. Pub. Health 52:1669, 1962.

Miller, L.W., Older, J.J., Drake, J., and Zimmerman, S.: Diphtheria immunization. Am. J. Dis. Child. 123:197, 1972.

Peebles, T.C., Levine, L., Eldred, M.C., and Esdall, G.: Tetanus-toxoid emergency boosters. A reappraisal. NEJM 280:575, 1969.

Preston, N.W.: Effectiveness of pertussis vaccines. Br. Med. J. 2:11, 1965.

Provenzano, R., Wetterlow, L.H. and Sullivan, C.L.: Immunization and antibody response in the newborn infant. I. Pertussis inoculation within twenty-four hours of birth. NEJM 273:959, 1965.

Rubbo, S.D.: New approaches to tetanus prophylaxis. Lancet 2:449, 1966.

Wilkins, J., Williams, F.F., Wehrle, P.F. and Portnoy, B.: Agglutinin response to pertussis vaccine. I. Effect of dosage and interval. J. Pediatr. 79:197, 1971.

MEASLES, MUMPS AND RUBELLA

Bart, K.J., Nankervis, G.A., and Gold, E.: Indicators of mumps immunity and the effect of intradermal antigen and mumps vaccine on antibody level. Am. J. Epidem. 98:39, 1973.

Brickman, H.F., Beaudry, P.H., and Marks, M.I.: The timing of tuberculin tests in relation to immunization with live viral vaccines. Pediatrics 55:392, 1975.

Brunell, P.A., Brickman, A., O'Hare, D., and Steinberg, S.: Ineffectiveness of isolation of patients as a method of preventing the spread of mumps. Failure of the mumps skin test antigen to predict immune status. NEJM 279:1357, 1968.

Cherry, J.D., Feigin, R.D., Lobes, L.A., Jr. and Shakelford, P.G.: Atypical measles in children previously immunized with attenuated measles virus vaccines. Pediatrics 50:712, 1972.

Davis, W.J., Larson, H.E., Simsarian, J.P., Parkman, P.D. and Meyer, H.M., Jr.: A study of rubella immunity and resistance to infection. JAMA 215:600, 1971.

Enders, J.F., Kane, L.W., Maris, E.P. and Stoles, J., Jr.: Immunity in mumps. V. The correlation of the presence of dermal hypersensitivity and resistance to mumps. J. Exper. Med. 84:341, 1946.

Fleet, W.F., Jr., Schaffner, W., Lefkowitz, L.B., Jr., Murphy, G.D., and Karzon, D.T.: Exposure of susceptible teachers to rubella vaccines. Am. J. Dis. Child. 123:28, 1972.

Hardy, J.B., McCracken, G.H., Jr., Gilkeson, M.R. and Sever, J.L.: Adverse fetal outcome following maternal rubella after the first trimester of pregnancy. JAMA 207:2414, 1969.

Horstmann, D.M.: Rubella: The challenge of its control. J. Infect. Dis. 123:640, 1971.

Jabbour, J.T., Duenas, D.A., Sever, J.L., Krebs, H.M., and Horta-Barbosa, L : Epidemiology of subacute sclerosing panencephalitis (SSPE). A report of the SSPE registry. JAMA 220:959, 1972.

Kilroy, A.W., Schaffner, W., Fleet, W.F., Jr., Lefkowitz, L.B., Jr., Karzon, D.T., and Fenichel, G.M.: Two syndromes following rubella immunization. Clinical observations and epidemiological studies. JAMA 215:2287, 1970.

Klock, L.E. and Rachelefsky, G.S.: Failure of rubella herd immunity during an epidemic. NEJM 228:69, 1973.

Krugman, S.: Present status of measles and rubella immunization in the United States: A medical progress report. J. Pediatr. 90:1, 1977.

Krugman, S., Giles, J.P., Jacobs, A.M., and Friedman, M.S.: Studies with live attenuated measles-virus vaccine. Comparative clinical, antigenic and prophylactic effects after inoculation with and without gamma globulin. Am. J. Dis. Child 103:353, 1962.

Meyer, H.M., Jr., Parkman, P.D., and Hopps, H.E.: The control of rubella. Pediatrics 44:5-20, 1969.

Sever, J.L., Hardy, J.B., Nelson, K.B., and Gilkeson, M.R.: Rubella in the collaborative perinatal research study. Am. J. Dis. Child. 118:123, 1969.

Starr, S. and Berkovich, S.: The effect of measles, gamma globulin modified measles, and attenuated measles vaccine on the course of treated tuberculosis in children. Pediatrics 35:97, 1965.

Stokes, J., Jr., Weibel, R.E., Buynak, E.G., and Hilleman, M.R.: Live attenuated mumps virus vaccine. II. Early clinical studies. J. Pediatr. 39:363, 1967.

Stokes, J., Jr., Weibel, R.E., Buynak, E.B. and Hilleman, M.R.: Protective efficacy of duck embryo rubella vaccines. Pediatrics 44: 217, 1969.

Sugg, W.C., Finger, J.A., Levine, R.H., and Pagano, J.S.: Field evaluation of live mumps vaccine. J. Pediatr. 72:461, 1968.

Vaheri, A., Vesikari, T., Oker-Blom, N., Seppala, M., Parkman, P D., Veronelli, J. and Robbins, F.C.: Isolation of attenuated rubella-vaccine virus from human products of conception and uterine cervix. NEJM 286:1071, 1972.

Weibel, R.E., Buynak, E.B., McLean, A.A., and Hilleman, M.R.: Long-term follow-up for immunity after monovalent or combined live measles, mumps and rubella virus vaccines. Pediatrics 56: 380, 1975.

Wyll, S.A. and Herrmann, K.L.: Inadvertent rubella vaccination of pregnant women. Fetal risk in 215 cases. JAMA 225:1472, 1973.

Yeager, A.S., Davis, J.H., Ross, L.A., and Harvey, B.: Measles immunization, successes and failures. JAMA 237:347, 1977.

RABIES, SMALLPOX AND INFLUENZA

Bahmanyar, M., Fayaz, A., Nour-Salehi, S., Mohammadi, M., and Koprowski, H.: Successful protection of humans exposed to rabies infection. JAMA 236:2751, 1976.

Cereghino, J.J., Osterus, H.T., Pinnas, J.L., and Holmes, M.A.: Rabies: a rare disease but a serious pediatric problem. Pediatrics 45:839, 1970.

Cho, C.T. and Wenner, H.A.: Monkeypox virus. Bacteriol. Rev. 37:1, 1973.

Cough, R.B,, Kasel, J.A., Gerin, J.L., Schulman, J.L., and Kilbourne, E.D.: Induction of partial immunity to influenza by a neuraminidase-specific vaccine. J. Infect. Dis. 129:411, 1974.

Francis, T., Jr.: Epidemic influenza: immunization and control. Med. Clin. N.A. 51:781, 1967.

Goldstein, J.A., Neff, J.M., Lane, J.M. and Koplan, J.P.: Smallpox vaccination reactions, prophylaxis, and therapy of complications. Pediatrics 55:342, 1975.

Habel, K.: Rabies: incidence and immunization in the United States. Med. Clin. N.A. 51:693:700, 1967.

Karliner, J.S., Belaval, G.S.: Incidence of reactions following administration of antirabies serum. Study of 526 cases. JAMA 193:359, 1965.

Kempe, C.H.: Studies on smallpox and complications of smallpox vaccination. Pediatrics 26:176, 1960.

Kilbourne, E.D.: Influenza: the vaccines: Hosp. Prac. 6:103, 1971.

Lane, J.M. and Millar, J.D.: Routine childhood vaccination against smallpox reconsidered. NEJM 281:1220, 1969.

Loofbourow, J.C., Cabasso, V.J., Roby, R.E., and Anuskiewixz, W.: Rabies immune globulin (human). Clinical trials and dose determination. JAMA 217:1825, 1971.

Perez-Gallardo, F., Zarzuelo, E., and Kaplan, M.M.: Local treatment of wounds to prevent rabies. Bull. WHO 17:963, 1957.

U.S. Public Health Service Advisory Committee on Immunization Practices: Rabies. Morbidity Mortality Weekly Rep. 25:403, 1976.

APPENDIX I

ANTIMICROBIAL AGENTS COMMONLY USED IN INFANTS AND CHILDREN

Dosage/Kg/day

Drug	Route	Mild-Moderate Infection	Severe Infection
Penicillin G. Crystalline (with K or Na)	IV, IM	25,000-50,000 U. in 4 doses	100,000-400,000 U. in 4-6 doses *(Premature 50,000-150,000 U. full-term 50,000-200,000 U. in 2-3 doses)
Penicillin G. Procaine	IM	25,000-50,000 U. in 1-2 doses	Inappropriate
Penicillin G. Benzathine	IM	300,000-1,200,000 (total) q.15-30 days or 40,000 U/kg	Inappropriate
Penicillin G. Potassium	PO	25-50 mg in 4 doses	Inappropriate
Phenoxymethyl Penicillin	PO	25-50 mg in 4 doses	Inappropriate
Methicillin	IV, IM	100-200 mg in 4 doses	200-300 mg. in 4-6 doses. *(Premature 75 mg. Full-term 100-200 mg. in 2-3 doses)
Oxacillin	IV, IM	50-100 mg. in 4 doses	100-200 mg. in 4-6 doses *(Premature 50-75 mg Full-term 50-100 mg. in 2-3 doses)
	PO	50-100 mg. in 4 doses	Inappropriate

Dosage/Kg/day

Drug	Route	Mild-Moderate Infection	Severe Infection
Cloxacillin	PO	50-100 mg. in 4 doses	Inappropriate
Nafcillin	IV, IM	50-100 mg. in 4 doses	100-200 mg. in 4-6 doses
	PO	50-100 mg. in 4 doses	Inappropriate
Dicloxacillin	PO	12.5-25 mg. in 4 doses	Inappropriate
Ampicillin	IV, IM	50-100 mg. in 4 doses	200-400 mg. in 4-6 doses. *(Premature 100-150 mg. Full-term 100-200 mg. in 2-3 doses)
	PO	50-100 mg. in 4 doses	Inappropriate
Amoxicillin	PO	20-40 mg. in 3 doses	Inappropriate
Carbenicillin	IV, IM	100-200 mg. in 4 doses	400-600 mg. in 4-6 doses. *(Premature 150-200 mg. Full-term 200-300 mg. in 2-3 doses)
Cephalothin	IV, IM	40-80 mg. in 4 doses	100-150 mg. in 4-6 doses
Cephaloridine	IV, IM	30-50 mg. in 2-3 doses	100 mg. in 3-4 doses
Cephaloglycin	PO	25-50 mg. in 4 doses	Inappropriate
Cephalexin	PO	25-50 mg. in 4 doses	Inappropriate

Dosage/Kg/day

Drug	Route	Mild-Moderate Infection	Severe Infection
Cefazolin	IV, IM	50 mg. in 3-4 doses	100 mg. in 4 doses
Erythromycin	PO	25-50 mg. in 4 doses	Inappropriate
Lincomycin	IV, IM	10-20 mg. in 3-4 doses	20 mg. in 3-4 doses
	PO	30-60 mg. in 4 doses	Inappropriate
Clindamycin	IV, IM	10-25 mg. in 4 doses	25-40 mg. in 4 doses
	PO	8-20 mg. in 4 doses	Inappropriate
Kanamycin	IM, (IV only if IM not possible)	15 mg. in 2-3 doses	15 mg. in 2-3 doses *(Premature, full-term 15-20 mg. in 2 doses)
Gentamicin	IM, IV	3-5 mg. in 3 doses	5-6 mg. in 3 doses. *(Premature 3-5 mg. in 2 doses. Full-term 5-7.5 mg. in 3 doses)
Amikacin	IM	7.5-10 mg. in 2 doses	10-15 mg. in 2 doses
Polymyxin B.	IM, IV	Inappropriate	25,000-40,000 U. in 4 doses
	PO	100,000-200,000 U. in 4 doses	Inappropriate
Streptomycin	IM	Inappropriate	20-40 mg. in 3 doses *(Premature 15-20 mg. Full-term 25 mg. in 2 doses)

Dosage/Kg/day

Drug	Route	Mild-Moderate Infection	Severe Infection
Colistin	IM	Inappropriate	5-7 mg. in 4 doses. *(Premature 5 mg., Full-term 5-7 mg)
	PO	10-15 mg. in 4 doses	10-15 mg. in 4 doses. (Premature & Full-term the same)
Neomycin	PO	50-100 mg. in 4 doses	100 mg. in 4 doses. (Premature & Full-term the same)
Sulfadiazine	IV, SC	120 mg. in 4 doses	120 mg. in 4 doses
	PO	120 mg. in 4 doses	Inappropriate
Sulfisoxazole	IV, SC	120 mg. in 4 doses	120 mg. in 4 doses
	PO	120 mg. in 4 doses	Inappropriate
Triple Sulfonamides	IV, SC	120 mg. in 4 doses	120 mg. in 4 doses
	PO	120 mg. in 4 doses	Inappropriate
Trimethoprim Sulfamethoxazole		6-12 mg (TMP) 30-60 mg (Sulf) in 2 doses	20 mg. (TMP) 100 mg. (Sulf) in 4 doses
Chloramphenicol	IV	Inappropriate	50-100 mg. in 4 doses
	PO	Inappropriate	50-100 mg. in 4 doses

Dosage/Kg/day

Drug	Route	Mild-Moderate Infection	Severe Infection
Vancomycin	IV	-	40-50 mg. in 2-4 doses
	PO	40-50 mg. in 2-4 doses	-
Methenamine	PO	50-75 mg. in 3-4 doses	Inappropriate
Nitrofurantoin	PO	5-7 mg. in 4 doses	Inappropriate
Nalidixic acid	PO	50 mg. in 4 doses	Inappropriate
Isoniazid	PO, IM, IV	10-15 mg. (up to 300 mg. total) in 1 dose)	20 mg. (up to 300-500 mg. total) in 1 dose
Ethambutol	PO	15 mg. in 1 dose	15 mg. in 1 dose
Aminosalicylic acid (PAS)	PO	200 mg. in 3 doses	200 mg. in 3 doses
Rifampin	PO	10-15 mg. in 1-2 doses	20 mg. (up to 600 mg. total) in 1-2 doses
Amphotericin B	IV	Begin 0.2-0.25 mg/kg/day, increase by 0.1-0.2 mg/kg/day to a maximum of 1 mg/kg/day or 1.5 mg/kg every other day	
Flucytosine	PO	50-100 mg. in 4 doses	
Nystatin (mycostatin)	PO	600,000-2,000,000 U. total daily dose	
Griseofulvin	PO	10 mg. in 1-2 doses	

APPENDIX II

DISEASES ACQUIRED FROM ANIMALS AND PETS

TABLE A1: INFECTIONS COMMONLY TRANSMITTED BETWEEN DOGS AND MAN	
BACTERIAL AND VIRAL	**MYCOTIC AND PARASITIC**
Colibacillosis	Ringworm
Salmonellosis	Strongyloidiasis
Pasteurellosis	Dog Tapeworm
Tularemia	American trypanosomiasis
Tuberculosis	Pneumocystis infection
Leptospirosis	Flea bite dermatitis
Rocky Mt. Spotted Fever	
Rabies	
Lymphocytic choriomeningitis	

TABLE A2: INFECTIONS CLINICALLY MANIFESTED IN DOGS	
MYCOTIC	**OTHER MICROBIAL ETIOLOGY**
Sporotrichosis	Bacteroides sp.
Blastomycosis	Brucellosis
Histoplasmosis	Anthrax
Coccidioidomycosis	Gas gangrene
Aspergillosis	Nocardiosis
Phycomycosis	Trichinosis
Candidiasis	Toxoplasmosis
Cryptococcosis	Canine distemper

TABLE A3: INFECTIONS COMMONLY TRANSMITTED BETWEEN CATS AND MAN	
BACTERIAL AND VIRAL	**MYCOTIC AND PARASITIC**
Salmonellosis	Ringworm
Pasteurellosis	Strongyloidiasis
Yersiniosis	Schistosomiasis
Tularemia	Dog tapeworm
Tuberculosis	American trypanosomiasis
Rabies	Toxoplasmosis
Cat Scratch Fever	Flea bite dermatitis

TABLE A4: INFECTIONS CLINICALLY MANIFESTED IN CATS	
BACTERIAL AND VIRAL	**MYCOTIC**
Anthrax	Nocardiosis
Leptospirosis	Histoplasmosis
Feline distemper	Aspergillosis
Influenza-like	Cryptococcosis
Feline enteritis	

TABLE A5: INFECTIONS COMMONLY TRANSMITTED BETWEEN RODENTS AND MAN	
BACTERIAL AND VIRAL	**RICKETTSIAL AND PARASITIC**
Salmonellosis	Rocky Mt. Spotted Fever
Pasteurellosis	Murine typhus
Plague	Scrub typhus
Yersiniosis	Schistosomiasis
Tularemia	Mouse or rat tapeworm
Erysipelothrix infection	Dwarf tapeworm
Leptospirosis	American trypanosomiasis
Endemic Relapsing Fever	Leishmaniasis
Lymphocytic choriomeningitis	
Encephalomyocarditis	

TABLE A6: INFECTIONS CLINICALLY MANIFESTED IN RODENTS	
Chlamydiosis	Aspergillosis
Sporotrichosis	Phycomycosis
Histoplasmosis	Cryptococcosis
Coccidioidomycosis	Toxoplasmosis

TABLE A7: INFECTIONS COMMONLY TRANSMITTED BETWEEN DOMESTIC FOWL AND MAN	
BACTERIAL	VIRAL
Colibacillosis	Chlamydiosis
Salmonellosis	Newcastle's disease
Pasteurellosis	Eastern equine encephalomyelitis
Erysipelothrix infection	Western equine encephalomyelitis
Staphylococcal infection	St. Louis encephalitis
Streptococcal infection	
Tuberculosis	

REFERENCES

Bisseru, B.: Diseases of Man Acquired From His Pets. J.B.
Lippincott Co., Philadelphia, 1967.

Hubbert, W T., McCulloch, W.F., Schnarrenberger, P.R.:
Diseases Transmitted From Animals to Man. 6th edition.
Charles C Thomas, Springfield, 1975.